D1587740

Pediatric Thoracic Surgery

Dakshesh H. Parikh • David C.G. Crabbe
Alexander W. Auldist • Steven S. Rothenberg
Editors

Pediatric Thoracic Surgery

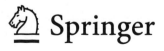

Editors

Dakshesh H. Parikh, MD, FRCS
Department of Paediatric Surgery
Birmingham Children's Hospital
Birmingham
United Kingdom

David C.G. Crabbe, MD, FRCS
Leeds General Infirmary
Leeds
United Kingdom

Alexander W. Auldist, BSc, BM, FRACS
General Surgery Department
The Royal Children's Hospital
Melbourne, Victoria
Australia

Steven S. Rothenberg, MD
The Mother and Child Hospital at
Presbyterian/St. Luke's Medical Center
Denver, Colorado
USA

ISBN 978-1-84800-902-8   e-ISBN 978-1-84800-903-5
DOI 10.1007/b136543

British Library Cataloguing in Publication Data

A catalogue record for this book is available from the British Library

Library of Congress Control Number: 2008944284

Printed on acid-free paper

Springer Science + Business Media
springer.com

Foreword

In most parts of the world the treatment of adults with surgically correctable abnormalities of the thorax and its contents is provided by specially trained thoracic surgeons. On the other hand, in children pediatric general surgeons usually take on this role because of their training in the surgical care of sick infants and children, and their experience with the management of congenital malformations. In an ideal world the treatment of surgical disorders of the thorax in children would be provided by a super specialist, but this is neither practical nor possible. This text provides information that will help bridge the gap for a group of conditions often only encountered rarely by otherwise experienced surgeons.

This book is not designed to be a textbook of operative surgery. Instead the broad scope is to provide important up to date information and reference material relating to most of the thoracic surgical conditions seen in childhood. The editors and contributors have ably met their goal to give the reader the proper medical and surgical principles needed to treat these childhood conditions.

One can't help to note the impressive array of authors from around the world. When I first started out in pediatric surgery only a few pediatric surgeons in a few centers would dare tackle some of the abnormalities noted in these chapters. Others who dared, because they had no other choice, often failed. Now it is clear that globalization has truly come to our discipline. The benefits to children in every corner of the earth cannot be overestimated.

Robert M Filler, MD FRCS(C), OOnt
Professor of Surgery and Pediatrics, Emeritus
University of Toronto
Ontario
Canada

Surgeon-in Chief Emeritus
The Hospital for Sick Children
Toronto, Ontario
Canada

Preface

Most pediatric surgeons operate on the chest. Some operate with confidence, some with trepidation. The concept behind this project was to publish a comprehensive textbook of pediatric thoracic surgery that would assist surgeons in both groups.

The book includes forty seven chapters which provide a broad coverage of thoracic surgical problems in children including diseases of the lung and pleural space, the esophagus, mediastinum, diaphragm and chest wall. Chapters on basic science and respiratory medicine are interspersed with more exclusively surgical chapters partly to gain perspective and partly because successful management of the more complex thoracic problems in children requires close collaboration between physicians and surgeons.

Although we wanted to allow the contributing authors a lot of freedom to express their ideas and experience every effort has been made to achieve a uniform style for each chapter. The general organisation of text includes historical perspective, incidence, investigations, diagnosis, differential diagnosis, management and future perspectives. The chapters are well referenced and, we believe, present a balanced view of contemporary practice.

The editors are experienced paediatric thoracic surgeons from the UK, North America and Australia. The authors have all been chosen carefully for their recognised expertise and we are proud to include experts from all corners of the globe. The effort involved in making this textbook a reality has been exhausting. We hope the final result achieves the original aim.

We would like to acknowledge the thoughtful contributions to the book from all the authors with much gratitude. We also express our thanks to Melissa Morton, Senior Editor at Springer, and her editorial assistants, in particular Lauren Stoney, who provided professional support and encouragement throughout the writing of this book. Finally, we must record our sincere thanks to Sunil Padman, at SPi Technologies, without whom this book would never have reached print.

DHP
DCGC
SSR
AWA

Contents

Contributors

Rosemary J. Arthur, BSc, MBCHB, FRCR
Department of Paediatric Radiology, Leeds Teaching Hospitals NHS Trust, Leeds, West Yorkshire, United Kingdom

Gularaj S. Arul, MD, FRCS
Birmingham Children's Hospital, Birmingham, West Midlands, United Kingdom

Oliver Bagshaw, MB ChB, FRCA
Department of Anaesthesia, Birmingham Children's Hospital, Birmingham, West Midlands, United Kingdom

Ian M. Balfour-Lynn, BSc, MD, MBBS, FRCP, FRCPCH, FRCS(Ed), DHMSA
Department of Paediatric Respiratory Medicine, Royal Brompton Hospital, London, United Kingdom

David J. Barron, MB BS, MD, MRCP(UK), FRCS(CT)
Department of Cardiac Surgery, Birmingham Children's Hospital, Birmingham, West Midlands, United Kingdom

Caroline S. Beardsmore, BSc, PhD
Department of Infection Immunity and Inflammation, University of Leicester, Leicester, East Midlands, United Kingdom

Spencer W. Beasley, MB ChB, MS, FRACS
Department of Paediatric Surgery, Christchurch Hospital, Christchurch, Canterbury, New Zealand

Russell Blakelock BHB, MBchB, FRACS
Department of Paediatric Surgery, Christchurch Hospital, Christchurch, Canterbury, New Zealand

T. J. Bradnock, MRCS(Ed)
Royal Hospital for Sick Children, Glasgow, Scotland, United Kingdom

William J. Brawn, MB BS, FRACS, FRCS
Department of Cardiac Surgery, Birmingham Children's Hospital, Birmingham, West Midlands, United Kingdom

Sarah Brown BSc, MBBS, MRCPCH
Department of Paediatrics, Royal Brompton Hospital, London, United Kingdom

Keith G. Brownlee, MB ChB, FRCPCH
Leeds Regional Paediatric Cystic Fibrosis Centre, Leeds, West Yorkshire, United Kingdom

Philip A. J. Chetcuti, DM, FRCPCH
Department of Paediatrics, Leeds General Infirmary, Leeds, West Yorkshire, United Kingdom

Thomas Clarnette MBBS, MD, SRACS
Department of General Surgery, Royal Children's Hospital, Melbourne, Victoria, Australia

Harriet J. Corbett, MB ChB (Hons), BSc (Hons), MRCS
Department of Paediatric Surgery, The Royal Liverpool Children's Hospital, Liverpool,
North West England, United Kingdom

Joe Crameri MBBS, FRACS
Royal Children's Hospital, Parkville, Victoria, Australia.

Steven Cray, MBBS, FRCA
Department of Anaesthesia, Birmingham Children's Hospital, Birmingham, West Midlands
United Kingdom

Carl F. Davis, FRCS
Royal Hospital for Sick Children, Glasgow, Scotland
United Kingdom

Michael G. Davis, MD, FRCPC
Montreal Children's Hospital, McGill University Health Center, Montreal, Quebec, Canada

Maya Desai, MD, MRCP, MRCPCH
Birmingham Children's Hospital, Birmingham, West Midlands, United Kingdom

Kate Ferguson BSc, MB BS
Austin Hospital, Heidelberg, Victoria, Australia

Hélène Flageole, MD, MSC, FRCPSC, FACS
Montreal Children's Hospital, McGill University Health Center, Montreal, Quebec, Canada

Devendra K. Gupta MS, M.Ch, FAMS, Hony. FAMS, FRCSG (Hony), D.Sc.
All India Institute of Medical Sciences, Ansari Nagar, New Delhi, India

Sundeep Harigopal, MB BS, DCH, MRCPCH
Neonatal Intensive Care Unit, Royal Victoria Infirmary, Newcastle upon Tyne, North East,
United Kingdom

John P. Hewitson, MB, ChB, FCS (SA)
Department of Cardiothoracic Surgery, University of Cape Town and Red Cross Children's
Hospital, Rondebosch, Cape Town, South Africa

Robert E. Kelly, Jr., MD, FACS, FAAP
Department of Surgery, Eastern Virginia Medical School, Norfolk, Virginia, USA

Jennette Kraft, FRCR
Department of Paediatric Radiology, Leeds Teaching Hospitals NHS Trust, Leeds, West
Yorkshire, United Kingdom

Anthony D. Lander, PhD, FRCS(Paed) DCH
Birmingham Children's Hospital, Birmingham, West Midlands, United Kingdom

Jacob C. Langer, MD
Division of Pediatric General Surgery, Hospital for Sick Children, Toronto, Ontario, Canada

David Lasko, MD
Hospital for Sick Children, Toronto, Ontario, Canada

Tim W. R. Lee, MB ChB, BSc, MMedSc, PhD, MRCP(UK), MRCPCH
Leeds Regional Paediatric Cystic Fibrosis Centre, St James's University Hospital, Leeds, West Yorkshire, United Kingdom

Paul D. Losty, MD, FRCSI, FRCS(Eng), FRCS(Ed), FRCS(Paed)
Division of Child Health,
University of Liverpool, Liverpool, North West England, United Kingdom

Ashvini Menon, MRCS
West Midlands Deanery, Birmingham, United Kingdom

Alastair J. W. Millar MB, ChB, FRCS, FRACS, DCh
Paediatric Surgery, University of Cape Town, Rondebosch, Cape town, South Africa

Philip Morreau, MBChB, Dip Obst, FRACS, FRACS (Paeds)
Department of Paediatric Surgery, The Starship Children's Hospital, Auckland, New Zealand

Bommaya Narayanaswamy
Royal Hospital for Sick Children, Edinburgh, United Kingdom

Donald Nuss, MB ChB, FRCS(C), FACS
Eastern Virginia Medical School, Children's Hospital of The King's Daughters, Norfolk, Virginia, USA

Pankaj R. Parekh, MD DCH
Department of Paediatrics, Sir H.N. Hospital and Medical Research Center, Child Health Clinic, Mumbai, India

Juan Carlos Pattillo, MD
Seccion Cirugía Pediatrica, Division de Cirugía, Pontificia Universidad Católica de Chile, Santiago, Chile

Todd A. Ponsky, MD
Department of Surgery, School of Medicine, Case Western Reserve University, Cleveland, Ohio, USA

Heinz Rode
Department of Paediatric Surgery
University of Cape Town, Rondebosch, Cape Town, South Africa

Naeem Samnakay
Department of Paediatric Surgery, Princess Margaret Hospital, Perth, Western Australia, Australia

Khalid Sharif, MBBS, FRCS (Paeds), FCPS Paed Surg (PAK)
The Liver Unit, Birmingham Children's Hospital, Birmingham, West Midlands, United Kingdom

Shilpa Sharma
Department of Pediatric Surgery, All India Institute of Medical Sciences, Ansari Nagar, New Delhi, India

Nigel John Shaw, MB ChB, MD, MRCP, FRCPCH, MA (Clin Ed)
Neonatal intensive Care Unit, Liverpool Women's Hospital, Liverpool, North West England,
United Kingdom

Malcolm Simms, FRCS,
University Hospital Birmingham NHS Foundation Trust, Birmingham, West Midlands,
United Kingdom

David A. Spencer, MBBS (Hons), MD, MRCP, FRCP CH
Department of Respiratory Paediatrics, Newcastle Upon Tyne Hospitals Foundation Trust,
Newcastle Upon Tyne, North East, United Kingdom

Jenny Thomas
Department of Paediatric Surgery, University of Cape Town, Rondebosch, Cape Town,
South Africa

Juan A. Tovar, MD, PhD
Department of Pediatric Surgery, Hospital Universitario "La Paz", Madrid, Spain

Gregor M. Walker, MD, FRCS
Royal Hospital for Sick Children, Glasgow, Scotland, United Kingdom

Section 1
Fundamental Considerations

1
Applied Anatomy

Dakshesh H. Parikh

Introduction

The thorax is a functional anatomical organ that is airtight, compliant and continuously active in response to the bodily demands for oxygen. It provides protection to the thoracic viscera and support for the upper extremities. Successful thoracic surgery requires a good understanding of the normal anatomy and the common variations.

Recent advances in imaging techniques, including computerized tomography and magnetic resonance imaging, with three-dimensional reconstruction, can help accurately define anatomical relationships with pathology. Video-assisted techniques for thoracic surgery, in particular, require a good understanding of the three-dimensional anatomical relationships of the thoracic viscera.

Historical perspective

Modern anatomical knowledge of thorax has developed over generations by transfer of knowledge from the Islamic, Greek and Roman physicians.[1,2] The ancient Islamic contribution to thoracic anatomy and physiology only became known in Europe in the late sixteenth century. The original description in the Süleymaniye library of the contemporary texts and drawings of the trachea, lung, and vascular system in Semseddin-i Itaki's and Ahmed bin Mansur's anatomy texts indicates that knowledge of the thoracic anatomy existed in great depth.[3] In 1924 the text "Christianismi Restitutio" by Michael Servetus (1511–1553) was rediscovered and translated, describing the pulmonary circulation. However, Ibn al-Nafis (1210–1288) of Damascus made the same observations three centuries earlier.[4] Ali bin Abbas wrote that the pulmonary artery wall had two layers and postulated that these layers might have a role in constriction and relaxation of this vessel. He also stated that pulmonary veins branched together with the bronchial tree.[3] The Dutch surgeon and anatomist van Mauden translated the works of Vesalius, Fallopius and Arantius as well as adding his own observations on anatomical variations in a book that,

in his own words, he considered would be helpful to surgeons and trainees.[5]

Thoracic skeleton

Sternum

The sternum is a flat subcutaneous bone in the anterior midline of the chest. It has been likened to an ancient sword - the manubrium representing the handle, the gladiolus representing the blade and the xiphoid process the point of the sword. The sternum forms from a series of segmental ossification centers, the sternebrae, which coalesce between puberty and twenty-five years of age. The manubrium and the first sternebrum contain a single or occasionally two ossification centers situated one above the other. The third, fourth and fifth sternebrae contain two lateral ossification centers and the irregular union between these explains the rare occurrence of a cleft sternum. The xiphisternum joins the sternum around forty years of age. The manubrium articulates with sternum through a synchondrosis although this joint occasionally ossifies in later life.

Ribs

Twelve pairs of ribs form the greater part of the thoracic cage. Occasionally, a cervical or lumbar rib may be encountered and rarely there may be only eleven pairs of ribs. The first six ribs articulate with the spine posteriorly and join the sternum anteriorly through individual costal cartilages. The costal cartilages of the seventh, eighth, ninth and tenth ribs coalesce to form the costal margin. The eleventh and twelfth ribs are floating and lack any connection with the sternum.

Surgical anatomy

- The marrow space in the sternum remains active throughout life and can be sampled for hematological diagnosis.
- Sternal fractures are very uncommon in children because of the elasticity of the ribs.

D.H. Parikh et al. (eds.), *Pediatric Thoracic Surgery*,
DOI: 10.1007/b136543_1, © Springer-Verlag London Limited 2009

- Rib fractures in children are the results of significant force and are often associated with injury to the thoracic or upper abdominal viscera. A rib is most likely to fracture just in front of the angle of the rib, usually as a result of forcible compression of the chest wall. The rib attachments prevent significant displacement but excessive callus formation at the site of a fracture is common because of respiratory movement.
- The shape of the chest wall may change in disease. Classical changes seen in rickets include enlargement of the costochondral junctions, giving rise to a "rickety rosary", pectus deformities and exaggerated Harrison's sulci caused by flaring of the lower ribs from the enlarged abdominal organs often found in malnourished children. In chronic respiratory disease the chest assumes a barrel shape due to a constant pressure exerted by the expanded lungs. Thoracotomy in early life may result in rib crowding which, in turn, may lead to scoliosis in adolescence.
- Drainage of the pleural cavity is best carried out between fifth and sixth intercostal spaces just in front of mid-axillary line. The ribs are easily palpable in this region, the intercostal spaces are wider here than in any other part of the chest and this is the last part of the pleural cavity closed by expansion of the lung.

Cervical ribs

Rudimentary cervical ribs develop during fetal life but usually involute before birth. Cervical ribs persist in approximately 1% of the population, the majority producing no symptoms. The transverse process of a typical cervical vertebra has two tubercles of which the anterior tubercle is the homologue of a rib. Cervical ribs persist in various forms ranging from a complete rib that articulates with the first rib to a fibrous cord.

Cervical ribs cause symptoms by tenting the brachial plexus and the subclavian vessels. The lowest trunks of brachial plexus (C8 and T1) are affected and symptoms generally appear in the second decade of life or later when the muscles of the shoulder girdle loose their tone. Presentation in the teenage years is seen occasionally. Symptoms include neuralgia, sensory deficits, muscular weakness and wasting. Disturbance related to the sympathetic fibers causes circulatory changes such as coldness, cyanosis, edema and paresthesia.

Clavicle

The clavicle is the most frequently broken bone in the human body as it is slender, superficial and connected to the upper limb. The clavicle usually fractures obliquely at the junction between the outer one-third and inner two-thirds which is the weakest point of the bone. The outer fragment is displaced inwards due the nature of the force and hence compound fractures are rare. The subclavius muscle plays an important role protecting the brachial plexus and subclavian vessels from injury when the clavicle fractures.

Thoracic vertebrae

The vertebral column of the thorax comprises twelve vertebrae aligned in a gentle forward concavity (kyphosis). The ribs articulate with the vertebrae by two synovial joints – between the head of the rib and the body of the vertebra and between the tubercle of the rib and the transverse process of the vertebra.

Thoracic wall

The chest wall surrounds and protects the intra-thoracic viscera and its regular movement constitutes the physiology of respiration. Anatomically, the roof of the thoracic cavity above the lung apex is formed by the suprapleural membrane (Sibson's Fascia) at the thoracic inlet and the floor is formed by the diaphragm that separates the thorax from the abdomen. The thorax is circular in shape in infancy and young children and subsequently assumes an oval shape in adulthood. The skeleton of the thoracic wall consists of twelve thoracic vertebrae, twelve pairs of ribs with their costal cartilages and the sternum. The lower ribs, along with the convexity of the diaphragm, cover and protect the solid organs of the upper abdomen.

Three layers of morphologically similar muscles cover the thoracic and abdominal wall. The outer layer comprises a specialized group of muscles including the pectorals, rhomboids, levator scapulae, latissimus dorsi and serratus anterior that are attached to the upper limb. The second, or intermediate, layer is confined to the ribs and comprises the external and internal intercostal muscles with fibers running at right angles to each other. The innermost muscle layer is incomplete, comprising the transversus thoracis and the intercostales intimi, subcostales and sterno-costalis. The neurovascular bundles, containing the intercostal vessels and nerves and their collateral branches, run between the middle and the innermost muscle layers, similar to the abdominal wall.

Intercostal space

The intercostal space between ribs, separated by the intercostal muscles, extends from the vertebral column posteriorly to the sternocostal joint anteriorly and to the costal margin of the lower ribs (Fig. 1.1).

The external intercostal muscle passes obliquely downward and forwards from the rib above to the upper border of the rib below. This muscle extends from costo-transverse ligament posteriorly to the costochondral junction anteriorly where it becomes membranous. The internal intercostal muscle runs downwards and backwards from the subcostal grove to the upper border of the rib below. The internal intercostal muscle runs from the sternum anteriorly to the angle of the rib posteriorly where the posterior intercostal membrane replaces it up to the superior costo-transverse ligament. The transversus, or innermost intercostal muscle layer, comprises three incomplete sheets of thin muscular fibers: (a) subcostales that lie in the paravertebral gutter, each crossing more than one rib

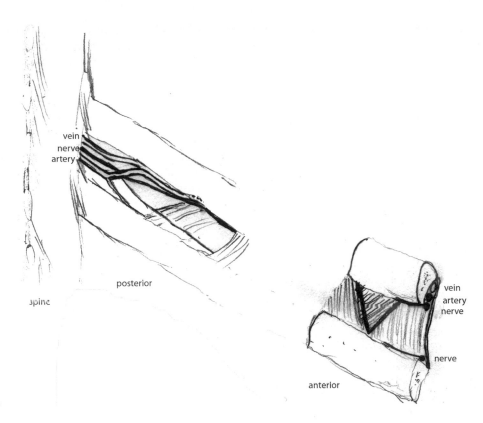

vein
nerve
artery

posterior

spine

vein
artery
nerve

nerve

anterior

FIG. 1.1. Intercostal space

space, (b) intercostales intimi: similar to subcostales these fibers cross more than one rib space and line the lateral thoracic wall (c) sterno-costalis: this muscle arises from the lower end of the sternum where digitations diverge on each side, one to each costal cartilage from second to sixth inclusive. Caudally, the transversus thoracis group of muscles recedes to form the diaphragm.

The intercostal nerves are mixed spinal nerves that emerge from the intervertebral foramina. After giving off a posterior ramus the nerve runs forwards between the internal intercostal and transversus thoracis muscle layers. A collateral branch innervates the intercostal muscles and is sensory to the parietal pleura and the periosteum of the rib. A lateral cutaneous branch pierces the intercostal muscles in the midaxillary line, and divides into anterior and posterior branches to supply skin over the intercostal space. The anterior terminal branch in the upper six spaces pierce the intercostal muscles anterior to the internal mammary artery and supply the skin of the anterior chest wall. The intercostal nerve lies below the intercostal vein and artery during its course through the intercostal space and all three are protected by the downward projection of the rib. The lower five intercostal nerves innervate the abdominal wall. The subcostal nerve passes behind the lateral arcuate ligament into the abdomen, accompanied by the subcostal artery and vein.

The supreme intercostal artery is a descending branch of the costocervical trunk, which arises from the second part of the subclavian artery, and supplies the upper two intercostal spaces. This vessel enters the thorax by passing behind the

scalenus anterior and across the neck of the first rib, with the sympathetic chain on its medial side. The supreme intercostal vein lies between the artery and the sympathetic chain where the first thoracic and inferior cervical ganglia fuse to form the stellate ganglion (Fig 1.3). This knowledge is important to a surgeon dissecting in this region, especially during tumor resection (neuroblastoma). The descending thoracic aorta gives off the next nine posterior intercostal arteries that travel in the neurovascular plane.

The internal mammary artery runs down the lateral border of sternum to supply the anterior body wall from clavicle to umbilicus. The internal mammary artery sends branches to the upper six intercostal spaces anteriorly. In females the branches to the second and third intercostal spaces are large to supply the breast. At the costal margin the internal mammary artery divides into superior epigastric and musculo-phrenic arteries. The superior epigastric passes lateral to xiphisternal fibers of the diaphragm to enter the posterior rectus sheath. The musculophrenic artery passes along the costodiaphragmatic gutter and gives off two anterior intercostal arteries before piercing the diaphragm and ramifying on its abdominal surface. The internal mammary artery is accompanied by two vena commitantes that drain into the innominate vein. The artery also gives off a pericardiophrenic branch, which follows the phrenic nerve and supplies branches to the fibrous and parietal pericardium.

Intercostal veins accompany the intercostal arteries. Paired anterior intercostal veins drain into internal mammary and musculophrenic veins. In the lower eight spaces the posterior intercostal veins drain into the azygos vein on the right and the accessory hemiazygos and hemiazygos veins on the left. The first space is drained by the supreme intercostal vein, which drains into either the vertebral vein or the brachiocephalic vein. The superior intercostal vein collects blood from the second and third intercostal spaces on each side. The superior intercostal vein on right side drains into the azygos vein. The same trunk on the left runs forward over the arch of the aorta, lateral to vagus nerve and medial to the phrenic nerve, to join the brachiocephalic vein.

Muscles and fasciae of the chest wall

The chest wall is covered by the pectoralis major and minor muscles anteriorly, laterally by the serratus anterior, superiorly by the trapezius, inferiorly and laterally by the latissimus dorsi and, on each side of the vertebral column, by the erector spinae muscles. Although these muscles are primarily responsible for shoulder girdle movement and axial stability they are also accessory muscles of respiration.

Pectoralis major arises from the medial half of the clavicle, sternum, the costal cartilages of the first to seventh ribs, and the aponeurosis of the external oblique and rectus sheath. From this extensive origin fibers converge on a flat tendon which inserts into bicipital grove of the humerus. The muscle is covered by the pectoral fascia which is continuous with the axillary fascia. The dominant thoracoacromial neurovascular bundle enters the superior part of the muscle posteriorly in the mid-clavicular line. This allows elevation of a reliable muscle flap that may be used to cover sternal defects after tumor excision or osteomyelitis complicating sternotomy. The pectoralis minor arises from the third, fourth and fifth ribs and inserts onto the coracoid process of the scapula. Both pectoral muscles are absent in Poland's syndrome which sometimes presents late in adolescence with a thoracic wall deformity.

Serratus anterior surrounds the side of the chest wall beneath the scapula. The muscle arises as a series of digitations from the upper eight or nine ribs. The fibers pass backwards to insert into the medial border of the scapula. Serratus anterior is supplied by the long thoracic nerve of Bell which arises from the fourth to seventh cervical nerves. The blood supply and venous drainage of the muscle come from the thoracodorsal vessels and perforators from the chest wall. This muscle is particularly useful as an intrathoracic muscle flap either using a number of digitations[6] or the whole muscle to fill the space left by a post-lobectomy empyema[7]. The serratus anterior rotates the scapula during the elevation of the arm and keeps the scapula applied to the chest wall. Paralysis of the serratus anterior causes the lower angle of the scapula project outwards when the arm is lifted, resulting in a winged scapula. This deformity may be seen as a long-term sequel of a posterior-lateral thoracotomy.

Trapezius is a large triangular muscle that arises from the occiput, occipital protuberance, ligamentum nuchae and the spines of the entire cervical and thoracic vertebral column. The muscle inserts in the outer third of the clavicle, the acromion and the spinous process of the scapula. It aids in rotation of scapula and elevates the shoulder. It is supplied by the spinal accessory nerve that may be injured inadvertently during operations in the posterior triangle of the neck.

Latissimus dorsi is the largest flat muscle of the chest wall. It arises from the spinous processes of the lower six thoracic vertebrae, the lumber fascia, the posterior third of the iliac crest and by digitations from the lower third or fourth ribs. The muscle fibers converge on a long tendon that forms the posterior axillary fold and inserts in the bicipital groove of the humerus. The thoracodorsal neurovascular bundle enters the muscle along the line of the tendon. This provides a robust vascular pedicle that that allows elevation of the muscle as a flap for reconstruction of the chest wall.[8] The latissimus dorsi muscle may also be used to repair a recurrent diaphragmatic hernia when synthetic materials have been unsuccessful.

Erector spinae is a great mass of muscle which runs the full length of the vertebral column, filling the hollows on each side of the spinous processes. Various muscular bundles are inserted into the vertebra by innumerable tendinous slips which have to be divided to expose the spine during a laminectomy.

Suprapleural membrane (Sibson's fascia)

This is a tough fascial layer which forms the roof of the thoracic inlet. The suprapleural membrane is attached circumferentially to the inner border of the first rib and costal cartilage except over the neck of the rib where the first thoracic nerve crosses to join the brachial plexus. The subclavian vessels lie on the suprapleural membrane as they pass laterally into the axilla.

Endothoracic fascia

Outside the pleura, lining the thoracic wall, is a layer of loose areolar tissue similar to the transversalis fascia of the abdomen. The endothoracic fascia is of little anatomical significance although it is the plane of dissection between the parietal pleura and the chest wall which is entered performing a decortication or pleurectomy. Provided dissection is done with care in this plane injury to intercostal vessels and nerves can be avoided.

The diaphragm

The diaphragm is a muscular septum between the thoracic and abdominal cavities derived from the innermost (transversus) layer of the body wall musculature. The muscle fibers of the diaphragm radiate circumferentially from the central tendon to form right and left hemidiaphragms. Diaphragmatic excursion plays a major role in respiration, especially in young infants. The crura arise from the sides of the bodies of the upper lumber vertebrae and insert into the central tendon.

The fibers encircle the esophageal hiatus in the diaphragm with a sling-like loop. The right and left crural fibers together form an arch over the aortic hiatus. The origins of the crura are continuous with the median arcuate ligaments, which are thickenings of the psoas fascia extending from the body of the second lumber vertebra to the transverse process of the first lumber vertebra. From this point the lateral arcuate ligament extends as a thickening of the lumber fascia over the quadratus lumborum muscle to the lower border of the twelfth rib near its tip. Laterally the diaphragm consists of a series of muscular slips arising sequentially from the twelfth through seventh costal cartilages that interdigitate with the transversus abdominis muscle. Anteriorly the muscle sheet of the diaphragm is completed by fibers that pass backwards from the xiphisternum to the central tendon. The central tendon of the diaphragm is a thin aponeurosis in the form of a three-leaf clover. The central tendon of the diaphragm is inseparable from the fibrous pericardium.

The diaphragm derives its blood supply from the right and left phrenic arteries, which run alongside each crus, and peripherally from the lower intercostal vessels.

The phrenic vessels are found on the under surface of the diaphragm and divide into anterior and posterior divisions around the central tendon. The smaller posterior branch anastomoses with the lower five intercostal arteries, while the larger anterior division anastomoses with the pericardiophrenic artery.

The diaphragm is innervated by the phrenic nerves. Injury to the phrenic nerve from obstetric trauma to the brachial plexus during delivery may result in paralysis of the diaphragm. Iatrogenic injury to the phrenic nerve during cardiac surgery and in operations involving the root of the neck is well recognised.[9] Radiologically the paralyzed diaphragm shows eventration and paradoxical movement. Diaphragmatic eventration may require plication if respiration is compromised.

The openings of the diaphragm

There are three main foramina in the diaphragm which admit structures from the abdomen. Their anatomical location and contents are described in Table 1.1.

Surgical incisions in the diaphragm

Incisions through diaphragm are necessary to access the thoracic and abdominal cavities simultaneously (Fig. 1.2).[10,11,12] Incisions in the diaphragm should be made with care to minimize injury to the phrenic nerves with resultant paralysis. In

TABLE 1.1. Openings of the diaphragm.

Foramen	Location	Contents
Esophageal hiatus	A muscular opening left of the midline near the 10th thoracic vertebra	Eesophagus, anterior & posteror vagus nerves, esophageal branches of the left gastric artery and vein
Caval hiatus	Situated in the central tendon to the right of the midline near the 8th thoracic vertebra	Inferior vena cava, right phrenic nerve
Aortic hiatus	A hiatus in the posterior aspect of the diaphragm on the 12th vertebra	Aorta, azygos vein and thoracic duct

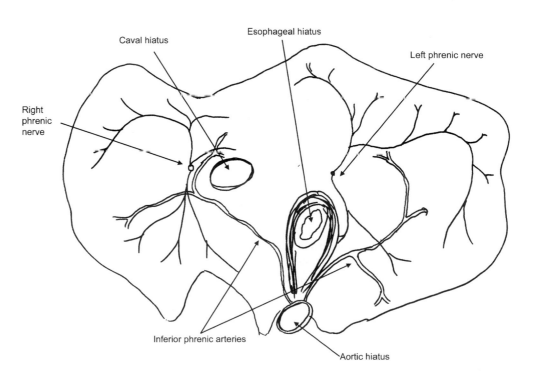

FIG. 1.2. The inferior surface of the diaphragma

general incisions in the diaphragm should be very medial or circumferential. Incisions through the central tendon of the diaphragm are rarely useful. A circumferential incision around the periphery of the diaphragm avoids all the major branches of the phrenic nerve and allows excellent exposure of both the upper abdomen from the chest and the thoracic cavity from the abdomen. On the left side a radial incision can be made from the costal margin down to the esophageal hiatus provided this is taken medial to the point where the phrenic nerve enters the diaphragm. This requires mobilization of the phrenic nerve from the surface of the pericardium which then becomes at risk from retraction injury in the chest.

The mediastinum

The mediastinum is conveniently divided into superior and inferior compartments by a line from the manubriosternal junction (the angle of Louis) backwards to the lower border of the fourth thoracic vertebra. Several important anatomical landmarks lie in the region of this line including the bifurcation of the trachea, the junction of the azygos vein and the superior vena cava and the ligamentum arteriosum. The thoracic duct crosses the mediastinum from right to left at this point. The inferior mediastinum can be subdivided into anterior, middle and posterior compartments.

Superior mediastinum

The trachea and esophagus enter the mediastinum in the midline with vagus and phrenic nerves on each side and the thymus anteriorly. At the level of the thoracic inlet the trachea touches the suprasternal notch and the esophagus lies posteriorly on the body of the first thoracic vertebra. The apices of the lungs lie laterally, separated by vessels and nerves passing between the superior mediastinum and neck. The brachiocephalic artery runs to the right of the midline while the left brachiocephalic vein crosses from left to right to join the superior vena cava.

The arch of the aorta lies in the plane of angle of Louis behind the manubrium as it turns backwards towards the body of the fourth thoracic vertebra, arching over the origin of the left main bronchus and the pulmonary arterial trunk. The brachiocephalic artery, left common carotid and left subclavian artery arise from the aortic arch and run upwards to the neck. The pretracheal fascia blends with the aorta in this region forming the lower limit of the pretracheal space. This fascia fixes the distal trachea to the back of the aortic arch and forms the anatomical basis for aortopexy as a procedure for tracheomalacia. The right recurrent laryngeal nerve loops around the right subclavian artery as it arises from the brachiocephalic artery. The left recurrent laryngeal nerve arises more distally in the mediastinum and hooks around ligamentum arteriosum before returning to the neck in the grove between trachea and esophagus. This nerve is particularly prone to injury during aortic arch surgery.

The right and left brachiocephalic veins, each formed by the confluence of internal jugular and subclavian veins, travel through the superior mediastinum in front of the arteries. The two brachiocephalic veins join to form the superior vena cava which passes vertically downward behind the right edge of the sternum, anterior to the right main bronchus. The left brachiocephalic vein projects slightly above the suprasternal notch when the neck is fully extended and is potentially at risk during tracheotomy. The thoracic duct enters the left internal jugular vein at the point where it joins the subclavian vein to form the brachiocephalic vein. Not infrequently the thoracic duct divides into four or five branches that join the vein separately. The thymus lies in front of the brachiocephalic vein. One or two short wide veins from thymus enter the left brachiocephalic vein directly. These are prone to inadvertent damage during mobilization of the left lobe of thymus.

Trachea

The trachea is a cartilaginous and membranous tube that begins in the neck at the cricoid cartilage and continues until it divides into two main bronchi at the level of the fourth thoracic vertebra. The brachiocephalic artery crosses the trachea obliquely as it courses upward to the right. At one time respiratory symptoms were attributed to tracheal compression from this vessel but this is no longer considered to be a real entity. The left common carotid and subclavian arteries run up along the left side of the trachea. The trachea is crossed obliquely by the brachiocephalic vein just below the sternal notch. Thymus lies anteriorly and extends a variable distance from the anterior mediastinum into the neck. The trachea is in direct contact with the esophagus posteriorly and the recurrent laryngeal nerves travels upward in the grove between the two. The arch of the aorta crosses the front of the trachea just above the carina. The tracheobronchial group of lymph nodes lies around the bifurcation of the trachea.

The blood supply to the trachea in the neck arises from tracheoesophageal branches of the inferior thyroid arteries. In the superior mediastinum the trachea receives a variable blood supply from branches of the supreme intercostal artery and the internal mammary artery. The distal trachea and carina receives a consistent blood supply from the left bronchial arteries. A tracheal branch from the right supreme intercostal artery supplies the proximal right main bronchus in 90% of cases.[13] The tracheal and bronchial vasculature has been studied in detail recently in relation to lung transplantation.[14,15]

Surgical anatomy

- Knowledge of the arterial anastomoses and microcirculation within the trachea is useful for successful tracheal resection and lung transplantation.
- Tracheal cartilage receives its blood supply through a submucosal arterial plexus. Overinflated endotracheal tube cuffs will result in ischaemic injury to the tracheal rings. A detailed description of the microcirculation of the trachea is provided by Salassa et al.[16]

- A variety of structural and congenital anomalies can produce tracheomalacia. Tracheomalacia may only become apparent after surgery for mechanically compressing lesions such as vascular ring or following repair of esophageal atresia. Rarely developmental defects of cartilages cause tracheomalacia.
- Congenital tracheal stenosis is usually associated with absence of the membranous portion of the affected trachea resulting in complete rings of tracheal cartilage.

Phrenic nerve

The phrenic nerves arise in the neck chiefly from the fourth cervical nerve roots, with variable contributions from the third and fifth roots. The nerves run into the thorax on the scalenus anterior muscles and enter the thorax between the subclavian vein and artery. The phrenic nerves run through the mediastinum in front of the lung hila (Figs. 1.3 and 1.4). The right phrenic nerve runs in contact with the right brachiocephalic vein, superior vena cava, right atrium and inferior vena cava before entering the diaphragm. The left phrenic nerve crosses the aortic arch and pericardium over the left ventricle before entering the diaphragm. Both phrenic nerves pierce through the diaphragm and supply it from the abdominal surface. The phrenic nerves contain sensory fibers from the mediastinal pleura, pericardium, diaphragmatic pleura and peritoneum. A pericardiophrenic artery arising from the internal mammary artery accompanies each phrenic nerve.

The long course of the phrenic nerves renders them prone to injury. Iatrogenic damage during cardiac surgery is now more common than birth injury to the brachial plexus. Both may result in eventration of the diaphragm with paradoxical movement of the paralyzed side during respiration.

Vagus nerve

The left vagus nerve enters the thorax alongside the left common carotid artery (Fig. 1.3) before crossing the arch of the aorta, where it gives off the recurrent laryngeal nerve. The vagus then passes behind the hilum of the left lung and continues down into the abdomen along the esophagus. The right vagus nerve runs down the trachea in the superior mediastinum (Fig. 1.4) passing deep to the azygos vein and behind the hilum of the right lung. The vagus then continues into the abdomen along the esophagus. The vagus nerves give branches to the superficial and deep cardiac plexuses. Behind the lung hila branches are given to the pulmonary plexuses. In the posterior mediastinum the two vagus nerves coalesce to form the esophageal plexus from which arise anterior and posterior vagal trunks which accompany the esophagus through the diaphragm into the abdomen.

Thymus gland

The thymus gland arises from ventral diverticula of the third pharyngeal pouch. The diverticula coalesce to form a bilobed structure that descends into the anterior mediastinum. The thymus is large in infants but atrophies during adolescence. The arterial supply to the thymus arises from multiple small branches of the internal mammary arteries that generally give

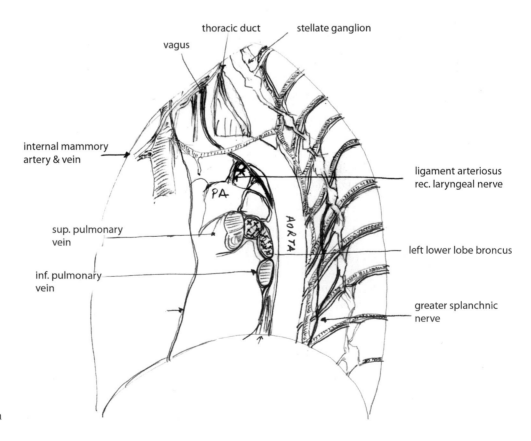

FIG. 1.3. Left mediastinum

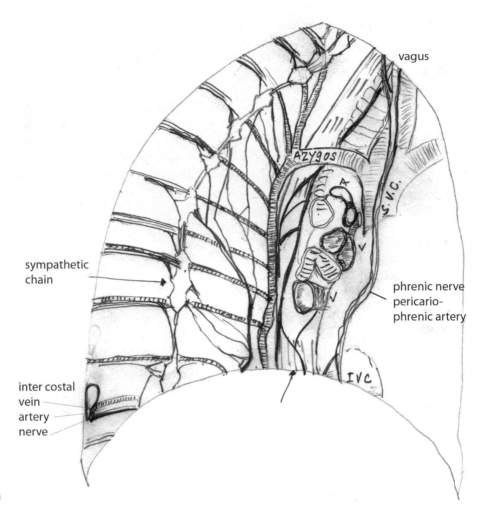

FIG. 1.4. Right mediastinum

no trouble during resection of the gland. The main venous drainage of thymus is a short wide vein on the posterior surface of the gland opening directly into the left brachiocephalic vein. Unless care is taken to ligate this vessel during thymectomy substantial bleeding may ensue.

Middle mediastinum

This division of the mediastinum strictly includes the pericardium, heart and lung roots. The anatomy of the lung hila differ on each side.

Left pulmonary hilum (Figs. 1.3, 1.5, 1.6)

The superior part of the left hilum is occupied by the left pulmonary artery which lies within the concavity of the aortic arch. The left main bronchus slopes from the carina to pass under the aortic arch and lie posteriorly in the hilum. The left main bronchus is sandwiched between the superior pulmonary vein anteriorly pulmonary artery superiorly. The hilum contains two pulmonary veins – the superior pulmonary vein lies in front of the main bronchus and the inferior pulmonary vein lies below the bronchus on the pulmonary ligament. The inferior pulmonary ligament is the dependent part of the sleeve of the mediastinal pleura as it reflects from the lung

root. The inferior pulmonary ligament extends down 1–2 cm and contains no important structures except a small vessel at the lowest point. The pulmonary artery is the most anterior and superior structure in the left hilum. The artery winds around the upper lobe bronchus into an anterior and lateral position. The first branches of the artery supply the apical and posterior segments of the upper lobe. These branches may arise from a common trunk. The left superior pulmonary vein lies anteriorly and inferior to left pulmonary artery and drains three principle tributaries from the apical posterior, anterior and lingular segments. The inferior pulmonary vein lies inferiorly and posterior to the superior pulmonary vein and is found in the apex of the inferior pulmonary ligament.

Right pulmonary hilum (Figs. 1.4 – 1.6)

The structural arrangement of the right hilum is similar to the left except that the upper lobe bronchus leaves the right main bronchus outside the lung. The hilum of the right lung lies within the concavity of the azygos vein as it arches forwards to join the superior vena cava. The right upper lobe bronchus is the most superior and posterior structure in the hilum. The right pulmonary artery enters the hilum anteriorly and inferior to the main bronchus, dividing immediately into superior and

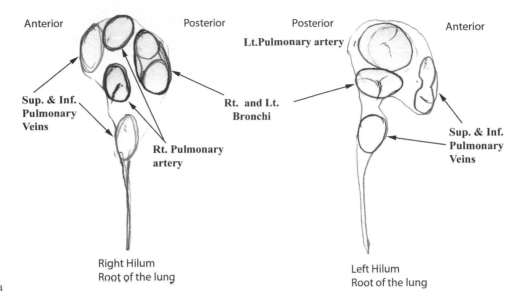

Anterior Posterior Posterior **Lt.Pulmonary artery** Anterior

Sup. & Inf. Pulmonary Veins

Rt. and Lt. Bronchi

Rt. Pulmonary artery

Sup. & Inf. Pulmonary Veins

Right Hilum
Root of the lung

Left Hilum
Root of the lung

FIG. 1.5. Pulmonary hila

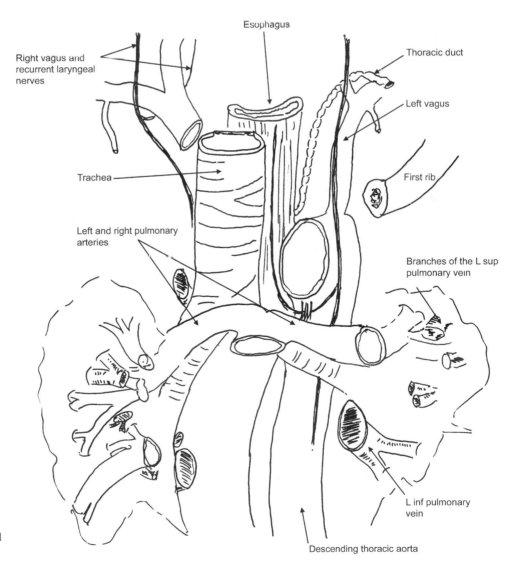

Esophagus

Right vagus and recurrent laryngeal nerves

Thoracic duct

Left vagus

Trachea

First rib

Left and right pulmonary arteries

Branches of the L sup pulmonary vein

L inf pulmonary vein

Descending thoracic aorta

FIG. 1.6. The mediastinum and pulmonary hila

inferior trunks. The superior trunk divides on the upper lobe bronchus into three segmental vessels and the inferior arterial trunk descends on the anterior surface of the bronchus intermedius. The superior pulmonary vein lies in front of the pulmonary artery and receives tributaries from the upper and middle lobes. The inferior pulmonary vein has two principle tributaries – one branch draining the superior segment of the lower lobe and a second comprising the basal segmental branches. The inferior pulmonary ligament is similar to the left side.

Pericardium

The fibrous pericardium is a conical shaped sac which encases the heart. The apex of the pericardium is fused with the roots of the great vessels and the broad base is inseparable from the central tendon of the diaphragm as both are derived embryologically from the septum transversum. Weak sterno-pericardial ligaments unite the pericardium with the posterior surface of the sternum.

The fibrous pericardium is lined by the parietal pericardium which is a serous membrane. This is reflected onto the heart around the great vessels to form the visceral pericardium. Paracentesis of the pericardial cavity can be performed through the diaphragm using a sib-xiphisternal approach or through the fifth intercostal space at the left edge of the sternum to avoid entering the pleural cavity.

Posterior mediastinum

This space extends down to the diaphragm behind the heart and is continuous with the posterior part of the superior mediastinum. The posterior boundary is formed by the vertebral column. The posterior mediastinum includes the paravertebral gutters containing the sympathetic chain.

Descending aorta (Figs. 1.3 and 1.6)

This great arterial trunk commences at the lower border of the fourth thoracic vertebra, where the aortic arch ends. The descending aorta leaves the posterior mediastinum at the level of the twelfth thoracic vertebra, passing behind the diaphragm between the crura. The descending thoracic aorta gives off nine intercostal arteries on each side that enter the posterior ends of the lower nine intercostal spaces. The descending aorta gives off bronchial and esophageal arteries. There are normally two bronchial arteries on the left and one on the right. The second right bronchial artery occasionally arises from the artery to the third intercostal space. The esophageal branches comprise four or five small vessels which provide a segmental supply to the lower esophagus.

Esophagus (Fig. 1. 6)

This muscular tube extends from the cricopharyngeus to the cardiac orifice of the stomach at the level of the tenth thoracic vertebra and left seventh costal cartilage. The cervical portion of the esophagus lies in front of the prevertebral fascia, slightly to the left of the midline, but enters the chest in the midline on the body of the first thoracic vertebra. As a consequence it is preferable to open the left side of the neck to perform a cervical esophagostomy although care must be taken to avoid the left recurrent laryngeal nerve and the thoracic duct. The intrathoracic esophagus traverses the superior mediastinum slightly to the left of the midline. The esophagus remains in contact with the vertebral bodies during its course through the thorax except distally where it inclines forward slightly to pierce the diaphragm to the left of the midline through the esophageal hiatus at the level of the tenth thoracic vertebra.

In the superior mediastinum the arch of the aorta crosses the esophagus on the left and azygous vein on the right. The aortic arch commonly leaves an impression on the left side of the esophagus which is visible on a Barium swallow radiograph.

In the lower mediastinum the thoracic duct runs along the right side of the esophagus, crossing the prevertebral fascia at the level of the fourth thoracic vertebra to continue into the superior mediastinum along the left side of the esophagus.

The muscular wall of the esophagus comprises an outer longitudinal layer and an inner circular layer. In the upper one third of the esophagus this muscle is striated and in the lower two thirds this is replaced by smooth muscle, in common with the remainder of the gastrointestinal tract. The esophagus lacks a serosal covering. The strength of the esophagus lies in the submucosa and consequently it is essential that sutures placed for an esophageal anastomosis include a generous bite of mucosa.

The arterial blood supply to the esophagus in the neck and superior mediastinum arises from esophageal branches of the inferior thyroid arteries. As the esophagus enters the posterior mediastinum it acquires a segmental blood supply from the esophageal branches of the descending aorta. The distal esophagus receives a blood supply from an ascending branch of the left gastric artery. This blood supply has important consequences for the repair of esophageal atresia. The axial nature of the blood supply to the upper esophagus means that the upper esophageal pouch can be mobilized extensively without jeopardizing perfusion. In contrast, excessive mobilization of the distal esophagus must be avoided to preserve the segmental vessels.

The venous return from the upper esophagus enters the brachiocephalic veins. From the middle part the venous drainage enters the azygos system. The lower esophagus drains into tributaries of the left gastric vein, which enters the portal system. Consequently a porto-systemic anastomosis exists in the submucosal venous plexus of the lower esophagus and varices may develop here in children with portal hypertension.

The lymphatic drainage of the esophagus follows the arterial supply. The upper esophagus drains into a posterior-inferior group of deep cervical lymph nodes near the origin of the inferior thyroid artery. The middle portion of the esophagus drains into the preaortic group of lymph nodes and the lower esophagus drains along the left gastric artery to preaortic lymph nodes around the celiac axis.

The esophagus receives an autonomic nerve supply from the vagus and the sympathetic chain. In the neck and superior mediastinum this is conveyed by the recurrent laryngeal nerves and sympathetic fibers running along the inferior thyroid arteries. In the posterior mediastinum the vagus nerves ramify over the lower esophagus in a plexus which receives branches from the upper four thoracic ganglia of the sympathetic trunk. As the esophagus passes through the crural sling on the diaphragm anterior and posterior vagal trunks reform.

The commonest sites for impaction of foreign bodies in the esophagus are at three anatomical narrow points. These are the cricopharyngeus, the level of the aortic arch and at the level of the diaphragm. Foreign bodies must be removed from the esophagus expeditiously to prevent ulceration with resultant mediastinitis or fistulation into the airway or aorta.

Lymphatics of the thorax

The lymphatics of the posterior mediastinum follow a similar pattern to the abdomen. Preaortic nodes on the front of the aorta are visceral and drain the middle reaches of the esophagus. Paraaortic nodes along each side of the aorta are somatic and drain the intercostal spaces. Lymphatic drainage from the anterior region of the intercostal spaces drains into nodes alongside the internal mammary artery. These nodes also receive lymphatic drainage from the medial margins of the breast. Lymphatic drainage from the heart and lungs enters the tracheobronchial chain of lymph nodes which surrounds the trachea and carina. Lymphatics from this group of nodes form right and left mediastinal lymph trunks which may join the thoracic duct but more usually open separately into the ipsilateral brachiocephalic vein.

Thoracic duct (Figs. 1.6 and 1.7)

The thoracic duct is the major lymphatic drainage channel in the body. The anatomy of the thoracic duct is so highly variable that only a general description can be given. The thoracic duct originates from the cisterna chyli which is found in the

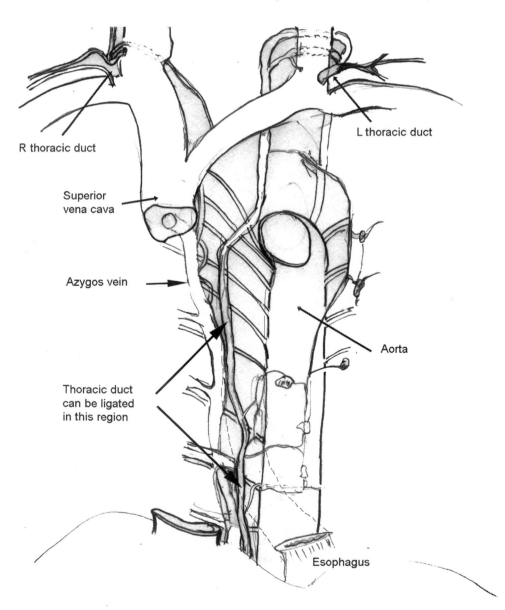

FIG. 1.7. Thoracic duct

midline adjacent to the aorta in the region of the second lumbar vertebra. The thoracic duct enters the thorax through the aortic hiatus of the diaphragm between the vena azygos and the aorta. The thoracic duct can be found reliably in the lower right thorax where it lies on the bodies of the thoracic vertebrae between the azygos vein and the aorta, behind the esophagus.

The thoracic duct typically crosses the midline at the level of the fourth thoracic vertebra. The duct is prone to injury at this point during aortic arch surgery or creation of a Blalock-Taussig shunt. The thoracic duct then ascends into the left side of the neck where it enters the confluence of the internal jugular and subclavian veins from behind. Often the thoracic duct divides in to three or four branches at this point, each entering the venous system separately. There are numerous valves in the thoracic duct along its course although there are no valves at the junction with the venous system.

The thoracic duct conveys the lymph from the lower half of the body, including the gut, and the left side of the thorax. Jugular and subclavian lymphatic trunks from the left arm and left side of head and neck join the thoracic duct at the thoracic inlet. Lymphatics from the right arm, right side of the head and neck and the right side of the thorax drain into lymphatic trunks which either combine or enter the right brachiocephalic vein separately.

This description of "typical" lymphatic anatomy is seen in about 65% of the population.[17, 18, 19] Davies reported nine major anatomical variations[17] while Anson described twelve variations in 1950.[20] The cisterna chyli is absent in approximately 2% of the population. Common variations in the anatomy of the thoracic duct include duplication, found in 5–39% of the population, right-sided termination in 1.6%, bilateral termination 1.8% and, rarely, termination in the azygos vein.[21, 22]

Azygos veins (Figs. 1.3 and 1.4)

The venous drainage from the chest wall and upper lumber region enters the azygos venous system. The azygos veins are derivatives of the cardinal veins which are longitudinal trunks that drain blood from the fetal body wall. The anatomy of the azygos venous system is asymmetrical and somewhat variable, particularly on the left.[23, 24]

On the right side of the body the ascending lumbar vein and the subcostal vein join to form the azygos vein which ascends through the aortic hiatus of the diaphragm, running to the right of the midline behind and lateral to the esophagus. At the level of the fourth vertebra the azygos vein crosses the esophagus and arches forward over the right main bronchus to join the superior vena cava (SVC). The azygos vein receives the lower eight right intercostal veins and, as it turns to join the superior vena cava, it is joined by the right superior intercostal vein which drains the upper intercostal spaces.

The azygos system on the left side of the body is discontinuous. The venous drainage of the upper intercostal spaces enters the accessory hemiazygos vein. The venous drainage of the lower left intercostal spaces, along with the left subcostal

vein and the left ascending lumbar vein, enters the hemiazygos vein. The accessory hemiazygos and the hemiazygos veins may communicate but more usually cross the midline separately behind the esophagus to enter the azygos vein separately.

The paired fetal anterior cardinal veins convey venous drainage from the head and neck to the developing heart. The jugular veins, brachiocephalic veins and superior vena cava are all derivatives of the anterior cardinal veins. The central connection of the left anterior cardinal vein regresses in most cases, as a median anastomosis with the right anterior cardinal vein develops which is destined to become the left brachiocephalic vein. Developmental anomalies are relatively frequent, particularly in association with congenital cardiac malformations. Persistence of a left SVC, which drains into the coronary sinus, is seen in approximately 0.3% of the general population and around 10% of children with cardiac malformations. Abnormalities in the course and union of the inferior vena cava (IVC) are found in 1–4% of population, most without clinical significance. Absence of suprarenal IVC is associated with the biliary atresia-polysplenia syndrome and with congenital heart disease, although it may be an isolated finding.[25] If the IVC is interrupted the venous drainage of the abdomen and lower extremities returns via the azygos vein. If an excessively large azygos vein is encountered at thoracotomy the possibility of an interrupted IVC should be considered because ligation of the azygos vein may prove fatal.

Thoracic sympathetic chain

The thoracic sympathetic chain lies on the necks of the ribs overlying the intercostal vessels and nerves. The first thoracic ganglion is commonly fused with the inferior cervical ganglion to form the stellate ganglion. Sympathetic fibers from the stellate ganglion innervate the head and neck, including the pupil of the eye, and injury to this ganglion results in a Horner's Syndrome. The sympathetic innervation to the hand originates mainly from the second and third thoracic ganglia, while fourth ganglion supplies the axilla. Each ganglion receives a white preganglionic ramus from the corresponding spinal nerve and returns a postganglionic grey ramus to the same thoracic nerve. The heart receives a sympathetic supply from the cervical ganglia through the superficial and deep cardiac plexuses. The lungs and esophagus receive a sympathetic supply from the upper four thoracic ganglia. The pulmonary and esophageal plexuses also receive parasympathetic fibers from the vagus nerves.

The greater and lesser splanchnic nerves arise from the lower eight ganglia of the thoracic sympathetic chain. They pierce the crus of the diaphragm and join the celiac plexus. The lowest (or least) splanchnic nerve leaves the twelfth ganglion to ramify over the renal arteries after piercing the crus of the diaphragm. The sympathetic trunk continues into the abdomen passing behind the median arcuate ligament of the diaphragm to lie on the psoas fascia.

Division of the greater and lesser splanchnic nerves has been performed to relieve debilitating visceral pain.[26] Neurogenic tumors associated with the sympathetic chain are encountered in children. These tumors may extend into the extradural space through the lateral foramina of the vertebral bodies.

Pleura

The parietal pleura lines the chest wall. The diaphragmatic pleura is densely adherent compared to the parietal pleura over the ribs and mediastinum. The pleural membrane is reflected around the hila of the lungs and continues as the visceral pleura which invests all surfaces of the lungs, including the fissures. The pleural cavity provides a frictionless space for lung movement during respiration. The parietal pleura has an abundant sensory nerve supply from the intercostal and phrenic nerves. Consequently the parietal pleura must be anesthetized before pleural aspiration or insertion of a chest drain. Afferents from the visceral pleura are conveyed in the autonomic nerves which enter the lung.

The pleural membrane projects above the medial third of the clavicle and can be penetrated during percutaneous cannulation of the central veins, especially the subclavian veins. The costodiaphragmatic recess is a deep gutter around the lower border of the thoracic cavity where the diaphragm joins the chest wall. Posteriorly this extends below the twelfth rib and is regularly encountered during surgical exposure of the upper pole of the kidney.

The lungs[27]

The right lung is larger than the left and comprises three lobes. The major, or oblique, fissure separates the upper and middle lobes from the lower lobe. The minor, or horizontal, fissure separates the upper and middle lobes. This fissure is commonly incomplete and in approximately 10% of the population it is absent completely. This complicates upper or middle lobectomy and is usually divided once the major vascular and bronchial structures have been dealt with.

The left lung has a concave medial border - the cardiac notch – and comprises two lobes. As with the right lung a major, or oblique, fissure separates the upper and lower lobes.

Bronchopulmonary segments (Figs. 1.8 a, b)

Each lobe of the lung is made up of bronchopulmonary segments which are discrete anatomical units with a bronchus, an arterial supply and a venous drainage. At segmental level the bronchial anatomy is relatively uniform and the arterial supply normally follows the bronchus, albeit with a more variable pattern. The segmental veins do not accompany the bronchus but run in intersegmental planes, a matter of crucial importance for successful anatomical lung resection.[28] Although it is possible to resect individual bronchopulmonary segments this is now of limited importance with the advent of minimally invasive techniques and surgical staplers.

The segmental anatomy of the right and left lungs differs. Both upper lobes comprise three bronchopulmonary segments although the apical and posterior segments of the left upper lobe are commonly fused. The position of the middle lobe segments differs, with these segments comprising the lingula of the left upper lobe and a middle lobe proper on the right. The lower lobe of the left lung lacks a medial basal segment.

Right upper lobe

The right upper lobe bronchus at right angles to the right main bronchus a short distance below the carina. Anomalies involving the origin of the right upper lobe bronchus have

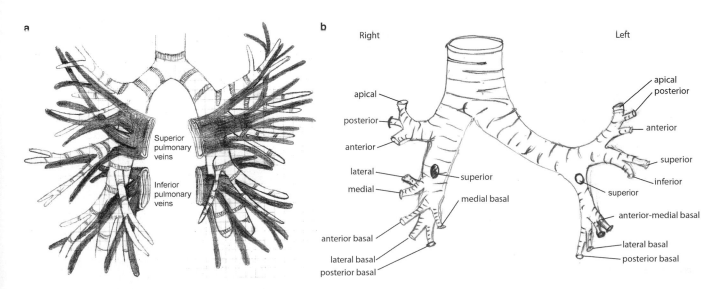

FIG. 1.8. (a) The pulmonary vein, (b) Bronchopulmonary segments

TABLE 1.2. The bronchopulmonary segments.

Bronchopulmonary segments				
Right side ($n = 10$)		Left side ($n = 8$)		
Upper lobe	Apical Anterior Posterior	Upper lobe	Superior	Apical posterior Anterior –
Middle lobe	Lateral Medical	Lingular	Inferior	Sup. lingular Inf. lingular
Lower lobe	Superior Medial basal	Lower lobe		Superior Anteriomedial basal
	Anterior basal Lateral basal Posterior basal			Lateral basal Posterior basal

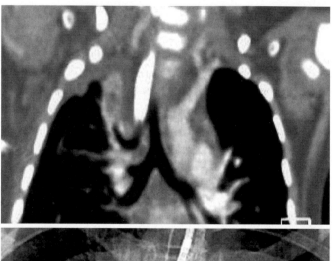

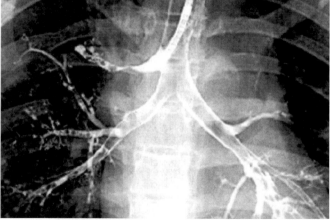

FIG. 1.9. Right upper lobe bronchus from trachea

been described in 3% of population.[29] The upper lobe bronchus arises directly from trachea in 0.5% (Fig. 1.9). The apical segmental bronchus arises directly from the trachea in 1.4%. In 1.1% the right upper lobe bronchus is absent, with the segmental bronchi arising independently from the main bronchus. The right pulmonary artery divides into superior and inferior trunks in the hilum of the lung. The superior trunk lies on the anterior surface of the upper lobe bronchus and supplies the apical and anterior segments. The arterial supply to the posterior segment arises from the inferior trunk of the right pulmonary artery.

Variations of the arterial supply to the right upper lobe are described by Milloy et al.[30] A superior pulmonary artery is found in all cases and in 10% of cases this represents the only supply to the upper lobe. In 3.6% of cases the apical and anterior vessels arise separately from the right pulmonary artery. Ascending branches from the inferior pulmonary trunk supplying the posterior segment of the upper lobe are present in 90% of the population although they vary in number – a single branch in 60%, two branches in 29% and three branches in 1%.

The superior pulmonary vein drains the upper and middle lobes. It is crucial to identify and preserve the right middle lobe vein when resecting the right upper lobe. The venous drainage of the right upper lobe is remarkably constant.

Right middle lobe

After giving off the upper lobe bronchus the right main bronchus continues as the bronchus intermedius. The middle lobe bronchus usually arises as a common stem before bifurcating into medial and lateral segmental bronchi. The inferior trunk of the right pulmonary artery runs down the anterior surface of the bronchus intermedius and is conveniently identified in the major fissure, where the branch or, more commonly, two branches to the middle lobe can be identified.[31] The artery supplying the superior segment of the lower lobe arises directly opposite the origin of the middle lobe vessels. Two segmental veins from the middle lobe join the superior pulmonary vein.

Right lower lobe

The segmental bronchi to the right lower lobe comprise a superior segmental bronchus, which arises directly opposite the middle lobe bronchus, and then four basal segmental branches. The middle lobe bronchus must be identified and protected during a right lower lobectomy as it is easily damaged if the lower lobe bronchus is mass ligated or divided using a stapler. Wragg et al undertook a detailed study of the anatomical variations in this region.[31] A single artery supplies the superior segment of the right lower lobe in the majority of cases. Less frequently there are two arteries. Occasionally the arterial supply to the superior segment arises from the ascending upper lobe posterior segmental artery. The inferior pulmonary vein has two main tributaries - a superior segmental vein and a common basal vein.

Left upper lobe

The left main bronchus enters the hilum passing under the arch of the aorta. The main bronchus then divides into upper and lower lobe bronchi. The upper lobe bronchus immediately bifurcates into a lingular lobe bronchus and a common bronchus to the anterior and apical posterior segments. The arterial supply to the upper lobe is highly variable and described in detail by Milloy et al.[32] The number of branches to the upper lobe vary from one to eight, although the most common arrangement is three branches. The venous drainage to the left upper lobe is also variable comprising two to three major branches which form the superior pulmonary vein.

Left Lower Lobe

The arterial branches to the lower lobe arise from the left pulmonary artery deep in the major fissure. The superior segmental artery arises from the posterior surface of the pulmonary artery opposite, and often slightly proximal, to the lingular segmental vessel. In 26% cases two arteries supply the superior segment and, as with the right lower lobe, rarely there is a common origin with the upper lobe posterior segmental artery. Division of the lower lobe arteries during a a lower lobectomy exposes the lower lobe bronchus. The first branch is the superior segmental bronchus, which originates from the posterior and lateral aspect of the bronchial trunk. This can be divided first to allow division of the main bronchus flush with the upper lobe. The venous drainage of the lower lobe enters the inferior pulmonary vein usually in the form of two tributarics – a superior segmental vein and a common basal vein.

Further Reading

1. Gray H, Pick TP, Howden R. Anatomy, Descriptive and Surgical, Gray's Anatomy. Bounty Books, New York, 1988.
2. Ellis H. Clinical Anatomy, 11th Edition. Blackwell Scientific, Oxford, 2006.
3. Last RJ. Anatomy: Regional and Applied, 7th Edition. Churchill Livingstone, London, 1984.
4. Davis GG. Applied Anatomy. The Construction of the Human Body, 8th Edition. J B Lippincott, Philadelphia, 1929.

References

1. French RK. The thorax in history 4. Human dissection and anatomical progress. Thorax 1978; 33:439–456.
2. French RK. The thorax in history 2. Hellenistic experiment and human dissection. Thorax 1978; 33:153–166.
3. Batirel HF. Early Islamic physicians and thorax. Ann Thorac Surg 1999; 67:578–580.
4. Persaud TV. Historical development of a pulmonary circulation. Can J Cardiol 1989; 5: 12–16.
5. Van Hee R, Lowis S. David van Mauden (± 1538–± 1597), "Sworn medical doctor and surgical prelector of Antwerp", and his book on anatomy. Acta Chir Belg 2006; 106: 130–135.
6. Hallows R, Parikh DH. Surgical management of children with pyo-pneumothorax: serratus anterior digitations myoplastic flap. J Pediatr Surg 2004; 39: 1122–1124.
7. Pairolero PC. Chest wall reconstruction. In: General Thoracic Surgery, 4th Edition, Shields TW (ed). Williams & Wilkins, Malvern, PA, 1994; 589–597.
8. Cormack GC, Lamberty BG. The arterial anatomy of skin flaps, 2nd Edition. Churchill Livingstone, London, 1994.
9. Fell SC. Surgical anatomy of the diaphragm and the phrenic nerve. Chest Surg Clin N Am 1998; 8: 281–94.
10. Merendino KA, Johnson RJ, Skinner HH, Maguire RX. The intradiaphragmatic distribution of the phrenic nerve with particular reference to the placement of diaphragmatic incisions and controlled segmental paralysis. Surgery 1956; 39: 189–98.
11. Perera H, Edward FR. Intradiaphragmatic course of the left phrenic nerve in relation to diaphragmatic incisions. Lancet 1957; 273: 75–77.
12. Sheilds TW. Embryology and anatomy of the diaphragm. In: General Thoracic Surgery, 4th Edition, Shields TW (ed). Williams & Wilkins, Malvern, PA, 1994; 36–40.
13. Cauldwell EW, Siekert RG, Linninger RE, Anson BJ. The bronchial arteries; an anatomic study of 150 human cadavers. Surg Gynecol Obst 1948; 86:395–412.
14. Schreinemakers HHJ, Weder W, Miyoshi S, et al. Direct revascularization of the bronchial arteries for lung transplantation: an anatomical study. Ann Thorac Surg 1990; 49: 44–53; discussion 53–54.
15. Couraud L, Baudet E, Martigne C, et al. Bronchial revascularization in double-lung transplantation: a series of 8 patients. Bordeaux Lung and Heart-Lung Transplant Group. Ann Thorac Surg 1992; 53: 88–94.
16. Salassa JR, Pearson BW, Payne WS. Gross and microscopical blood supply of the trachea. Ann Thorac Surg 1977; 24: 100–107.
17. Davies MK. A statistical study of the thoracic duct in man. Am J Anat 1915; 171: 212.
18. Kausel WH, Reeve TS, Stein AA, et al. Anatomic and pathologic studies of thoracic duct. J Thorac Cardiovasc 1957; 34: 631–641.
19. Kinnaert P. Anatomical variations of the cervical portion of the thoracic duct in man. J Anat 1973; 115: 45–52.
20. Anson BJ. An Atlas of Anatomy. Philadelphia. WB Saunders 1950; 336–337.
21. Miller JI. Anatomy of the thoracic duct. In: General Thoracic Surgery, 4th Edition, Sheilds TW (ed). Williams & Wilkins, Malvern, PA, 1994; 104–107.
22. Meade RH., Head JR, Moen CW. The management of chylothorax. J Thorac Cardiovasc Surg 1950; 19: 709–23.
23. Demos TC, Posniak HV, Pierce KL, et al. Venous anomalies of the thorax. Am J Roentgenol 2004; 182: 1139–1150.
24. Ozbeck A, Dalcik C, Colak T, Dalcik H. Multiple variations of the azygos venous system. Surg Radiol Anat 1999; 21: 83–85.
25. Articol M, Lorenzini D, Mancini P, et al. Anatomic VariationsMultiple variations of the azygos venous systemRadiological evidence of anatomical variation of the inferior vena cava: Report of two cases. J Surg Radiol Anat 2004, 26: 153 156.
26. Stone HH, Chauvin EJ. Pancreatic denervation for pain relief in chronic alcohol associated pancreatitis. Br J Surg 1990; 77: 303–5.
27. Rice TW. Anatomy of the lungs. In: Thoracic Surgery, Pearson FG, Deslauriers J, Ginsberg RJ, Hiebert CA, McKneally MF, Urschel HC (eds). Churchill Livingstone, New York, 1995; 355–369.
28. Ramsey BH. The anatomical guide to the intersegmental plane. Surgery 1949; 25: 533.
29. Le Roux BT. Anatomical abnormalities of the right upper bronchus. J Thorac Cardiovasc Surg 1962; 44: 225–227.
30. Milloy FJ, Wragg LE, Anson BJ. The pulmonary arterial supply to the right upper lobe of the lung based upon a study of 300 laboratory and surgical specimens. Surg Gynecol Obstet 1963; 116: 34–41.
31. Wragg LE, Milloy FJ, Anson BJ. Surgical aspects of the pulmonary artery supply to the middle lobe and lower lobes of the lungs. Surg Gynecol Obstet 1968; 127: 531–537.
32. Milloy FJ, Wragg LE, Anson BJ. The pulmonary arterial supply to the upper lobe of the left lung. Surg Gynecol Obstet 1968; 126: 811–824.

2
Developmental Biology and Embryology of the Thorax

Anthony D. Lander

Introduction

- To understand the mechanisms involved in development of the lung parenchyma, airways, vasculature, diaphragm, vertebrae, and chest wall
- To understand the developmental aberrations that may underlie congenital malformations of the thorax

Ideally this chapter should detail the mechanisms controlling normal development of the thorax and explain the cause of the congenital anomalies we manage. It cannot yet, because the knowledge is not available. However, some important concepts and recent findings are discussed. Were this chapter to fulfill its ideal we would then ask if a complete understanding of the basic science would influence our management of thoracic problems in children. It might, but there is no guarantee that understanding the developmental biology will lead to better surgical treatment.

Is an understanding of the basic science important? Understanding surfactant deficiency has made a big difference to the management of hyaline membrane disease (HMD) in premature babies. One family of genetic defects in surfactant physiology has been described. Understanding neonatal lung physiology has improved the survival of premature infants. Understanding the defect in cystic fibrosis has lead to improvements in genetic diagnosis but gene therapy has yet to show clinical benefit.

Developmental Biology

Insights into the embryology and teratology of the thorax have come from descriptive studies and the application of molecular techniques to study murine, *Xenopus*, chick, and particularly *Drosophila* (fruit fly) development. The head–tail axis (which developmental biologists term the anterior–posterior axis) is segmented. Some positional information along that axis, and how it is interpreted in both normal and abnormal development, is now understood.[1]

Much happens in an embryo before morphogenetic changes in tissues take place. Cells are told what type of cell they are to be and where to go – their fate is "specified." Development is thus the gradual allocation of specific cells to more narrowly defined fates. Developmental biology asks, "How are the cells chosen by position?" and "What are the molecular and cellular events that constitute changes in cell fate?"

Expression of cascades of transcription factors and interacting cofactors regulates normal development. Disruption of normal gene expression can produce congenital anomalies. These are the focus of much current research. Importantly, many different insults can result in the same phenotypic abnormality. Moreover, one gene defect can result in several different phenotypes. Inbred strains of mice with either a genetic defect or a specific teratogen exposure may have a litter of genetically identical offspring demonstrating a wide spectrum of anomalies. These observations often cause surprise to those who presume development to be rigidly prescribed by genes acting as a blueprint for development. The genetic code should rather be thought of as a highly influential script, or program, played out in the chaotic physicochemical environment of individual cells and sheets of cells that interact with one another. It is important to consider the influence of nongenetic effects during development. In susceptible individuals chance variations in levels of morphogens, the timing of the switching on or off of regulatory genes, or minor alterations in the timing of periods of apoptosis or growth may all result in diverse anomalies.

The paradigm of molecular biology is that a gene is transcribed into messenger RNA (mRNA). The mRNA is translated into a protein, which may be modified by posttranslational mechanisms. A cell type is defined to some extent by the genes it expresses because these dictate to a large extent the proteins produced. However, control of protein production is exercised at a number of levels.

Control of gene transcription is a fundamental process in development. This is controlled in part by transcription factors,

D.H. Parikh et al. (eds.), *Pediatric Thoracic Surgery*,
DOI: 10.1007/b136543_2, © Springer-Verlag London Limited 2009

which are proteins and are thus gene products themselves. A good example is the *Hox* gene products. These are an important group of transcription factors containing the homeobox. The homeobox is 180 base pairs in length and codes for 60 amino acids with a specific conformation that allows the protein to bind to DNA itself and thereby influence the expression of other genes. Protein expression is also controlled after transcription into mRNA and at the stage of posttranslational modification, which affects both function and transport.

Embryos can be studied at different times during development, and computer reconstruction of histological sections allows speedier and better descriptive embryology. Immunohistochemistry allows protein expression to be studied, and molecular techniques such as in-situ hybridization allow gene expression to be mapped and followed. Candidate genes can be studied in various ways, and transgenic mice can be created to answer specific developmental questions.

Evolution

Simple extant creatures have a head tail axis and some degree of segmental patterning. We, too, have segmental patterning beautifully evident in the thorax (ribs, vertebral bodies, musculature, dermatomes, cardiac segments), and the thorax is itself a major body segment. Since we share common ancestors, evolutionary biologists can ask how the components of the human thorax relate to structures in drosophila and other extant creatures.

The human thorax may have developed from segments 6, 7, and 9 of an annelid-like common ancestor. However, of importance to mammalian development is knowledge gained from the study of *Drosophila*, which has provided much insight intothe molecular biology of normal development.

Overlapping *Hox* Genes Specify the Different Thoracic Vertebrae and Ribs

In 1971 Lewis Wolpert first hypothesized that animals might share a universal embryonic positional information system and that developing embryos might then read this positional information and interpret it differently depending upon the species.[1] This seems to be the case for much of the head–tail axis, which is specified by the Hox code. In *Drosophila* the cranial limits of expression of a family of homeotic genes specify important embryonic segments. They are organized in two clusters known as the homeotic complex or *HOM-C* genes. During evolution this complex was duplicated twice, and mammals have four complexes of homeotic genes with similar sequence homology to the insect *HOM-C* genes. In the fly the thoracic and abdominal segments are specified by the expression patterns of these genes; in mammals rhombomeres and vertebrae were early examples of specified segments. The expression pattern provides positional information that informs how far along the embryonic antero–posterior axis cells are. For example: in flies the transcription

factor coded for by the Ultrabithorax (*Ubx*) gene is expressed in the third thoracic segment and influences butterflies to develop wings whereas drosophila develops halteres, which are modified balancing organs. The influence of other transcription factors results in the different developmental outputs in different species and in some congenital anomalies. This is entirely consistent with Wolpert's universal positional information model. In the mouse, the cranial expression boundaries of the overlapping Hox code specify the development of individual somites or groups of somites and are involved in the detailed patterning of the different vertebrae. The specification of the different thoracic vertebrae and their different ribs is thus specified by the overlapping hox code. This family of genes is expressed from the posterior of the embryo forward with different anterior limits of expression. Cells know their position along the head–tail axis depending upon which genes are switched on at their location.

Abnormal expression of certain *Hox* genes in mice can cause cranialization of caudal vertebral bodies or caudalization of cranial vertebral bodies. Some of these anomalies are remarkably similar to the abnormalities seen in human esophageal atresia (EA). This suggests that abnormal head–tail patterning at a fundamental level may be responsible for some cases of EA with or without tracheoesophageal fistula (TEF).

In mice, disruption of the type IIB activin receptor (ActRIIB) results in altered *Hox* gene expression and vertebral cranialization. Genetically engineered mice carrying a homozygous knockout of the IIB activin receptor gene (*ActRIIB*–/–) die after birth with complicated cardiac defects including defects of cardiac situs, transposition of the great arteries, and ventricular and atrial septal defects. These findings provide genetic evidence that the ActRIIB-mediated signaling pathway plays a critical role in patterning both anteroposterior and left–right axes in vertebrate animals.[2]

The Foregut

The Origins of the Foregut Endoderm

The primitive foregut forms from definitive endoderm at the cranial end of the trilaminar germ disk (Fig. 2.1). This definitive endoderm arises from primitive ectoderm that has passed through the cranial primitive streak and migrated forward and laterally. It does not arise from the primitive endoderm of the bilaminar germ disk since all of this primitive endoderm migrates out into the extraembryonic tissues. The primitive ectoderm fated to become foregut endoderm may receive some information by pattern-forming phenomena before passing through the primitive streak. Cells that then pass through the streak may be further programmed depending upon their head–tail position along the streak and the time when they pass. Cells passing more caudally through the streak may have different genes switched on to those passing through more cranially. Also those passing through early may have different genes switched on compared with those passing through later. The details of the major genes involved and their products are gradually being discovered.

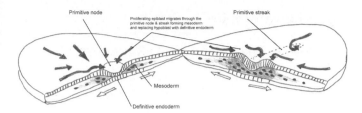

FIG. 2.1. Trilaminar germ disk during gastrulation with a fate map: The fate map shows the primitive ectoderm of the bilaminar germ disk and regional fates at the start of gastrulation. The primitive streak can be seen at the caudal end of the head–tail axis on the fate map. Cells fated to become the notochord migrate forward from the node on the endodermal surface of the disk. Cells fated to become definitive endoderm pass through the cranial end of the primitive streak and migrate laterally, forward and backward. Primitive endoderm is pushed out into extraembryonic tissues. Those definitive endodermal cells at the very cranial end of the streak become foregut endoderm, some of which will become trachea and respiratory tract lining. Cells fated to become extra embryonic mesoderm are shown hashed. These cells pass through the tail end of the streak. After the cells fated to become the notochord and definitive endoderm have migrated the primitive ectoderm cells fated to become mesoderm pass through the streak and come to lie between the layers of endoderm and ectoderm. After all the cells have migrated the definitive ectoderm is left on the dorsal surface fated to become skin and neural tissue. The fate map changes with time.

The embryonic disk pictured above has been cut horizontally at the level of the node that lies at the anterior end of the primitive streak. The posterior part of the streak can be seen on the right hand side of the diagram. Primitive ectodermal cells migrate in the direction of the black lines toward the node and the primitive streak. Those that pass through at the node form the notochord. The notochord later migrates into the mesoderm leaving a continuous sheet of endoderm ventrally. The notochord later helps specify the mesoderm of the future vertebral bodies and the ventro-dorsal patterning of the esophagus and trachea

Products of the Foregut Endoderm

The thyroid, thymus, esophagus, trachea, lung buds, stomach, liver, and pancreas develop at defined positions along the head–tail axis of the foregut. *Hox* genes provide head–tail signaling pathways that govern skeletal and central nervous system patterning. Detail is emerging about the genetic programs that specify foregut organ position, cell fate, morphogenesis, and cellular differentiation. Sonic hedgehog (Shh) is a secreted signaling protein whose endodermal expression specifies boundaries and may influence the differentiation of the stomach, spleen, pancreas, intestines, and respiratory tract. Abnormal Shh expression, or inactivation in mice, leads to defects including TEF, heterotopic pancreas, annular pancreas, and hyposplenism.[3–5] Adriamycin interferes with Shh expression in the rodent model of EA/TEF consistent with this picture.

The Airways and Blood Vessels

The lining of the respiratory tract arises from the ventral foregut endoderm. Extensive branching of the primitive airway involves many bifurcations generating the tree-like structure ending in the alveoli and capillaries needed for postnatal gas exchange. These bifurcations are reduced in congenital diaphragmatic hernia (CDH) accounting for the lung hypoplasia. There is extensive molecular communication between epithelium and mesenchyme, and there may be signal communication between vascular branching and airway branching. The pulmonary mesenchyme arises from lateral plate mesoderm and forms the cartilage of the trachea and main bronchi, the lymphatics and vasculature, smooth muscle, and the pleura. The pulmonary vasculature develops from two sources. Large blood vessels arise from the aortic arches and the left atrium and migrate into the lung parenchyma. The alveolar capillaries arise in the lung mesenchyme near developing epithelial buds and later connect to the larger vessels.[6,7]

Foregut Septation

The Laryngotracheal Groove

When the human embryo is about 3 mm in length and has about ten somites at around 22–23 days after fertilization the foregut has formed and a laryngo-tracheal groove develops in the ventral wall. This groove is close to the fourth and sixth pharyngeal pouches, and it deepens with elongation. It is

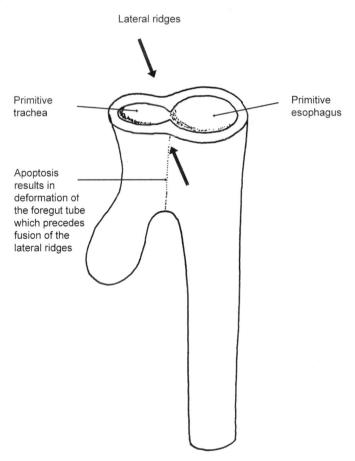

FIG. 2.2. Tracheal separation from the esophagus

initially open to the esophagus throughout its length but two tracheoesophageal folds develop on either side of the groove and fuse gradually from below to separate the trachea from the esophagus (Fig. 2.2).[8–10] Fusion of the tracheoesophageal folds follows coordinated apoptosis of the opposing midsections of the circumference of the foregut tube. An orifice remains at the cranial end of the trachea with mesenchymal swellings developing into the epiglottis, glottis, laryngeal cartilages, and musculature.

After Normal Separation

Tracheoesophageal separation is complete by 36 days and the stomach is then below the future diaphragm. Circular muscle is evident in the esophagus by week 6, and this becomes innervated by the vagus before the longitudinal muscle becomes well defined at 12 weeks. Interestingly innervation of the esophagus is abnormal in the Adriamycin model. This is relevant when we consider the innervation and motility problems frequently seen in children with repaired EA-TEF. On cross section the esophagus is round at first and then by week 5 it flattens dorsoventrally, cranially, and from side-to-side caudally. Longitudinal ridges rotate 90° clockwise as one looks down the esophagus. This rotation is consistent with the rotation of the stomach, which brings the dorsal wall of the stomach to the left. In the 7th and 8th week after fertilization there is marked epithelial proliferation almost occluding the esophagus. This phenomenon may be responsible for the rare esophageal webs. It was once thought that occlusion and failure of recanalization was a possible cause of EA but this now seems most unlikely. The esophageal epithelium is initially ciliated but becomes replaced by a stratified squamous epithelium after 16 weeks. Islands of ciliated mucosa are occasionally still found in the neonatal esophagus.

Septation Failure as a Cause of EA/TEF

If tracheoesophageal separation fails, a cleft of life-threatening importance remains. Some surgeons recommend a bronchoscopy before repairing an EA/TEF combination in all neonates to rule out a larnyngeal cleft as well as to identify the site of the fistula, exclude a possible upper pouch fistula, and assess the degree of tracheomalacia. Failure of septation leaving a TEF is seen in sonic hedgehog null mutant mice, in Gli2/Gli3 compound null mutants, and in null mutations of Nl alpha 2.1.[4,11] This defect has been also associated with deficiencies in Foxf1,[12] Tbx4,[13] and retinoic acid (RA).[14] Failure of septation is also seen in the Adriamycin rat model of EA/TEF. In this animal model a pregnant dam is given intraperitoneal Adriamycin on days 6–9 of gestation. Levels of Shh are abnormally expressed especially dorsoventrally and the notochord is deformed. Furthermore, the Shh level normally declines as the embryo approaches birth but in the Adriamycin-treated rats the level of Shh protein is lower than in normal rats and fails to show temporal changes.

Lung Development

Histological Phases of Lung Development

The lungs have four distinct phases of development recognizable under the microscope: 5–17 weeks pseudoglandular, 16–25 weeks canalicular, 24–40 weeks terminal sac, late fetal-8 years alveolar.

Vertebrate lungs develop from an asymmetric bud arising from the ventral wall of the foregut, which divides into two. The lung bud appears at about 28 days in the human. In amphibians and many reptiles the lungs retain a short connection with the esophagus, but in others the connection elongates into a substantial trachea. Mammalian lungs occupy separate thoracic cavities and are divided into lobes. The number of lobes varies in different mammals. By the fifth week there are three branches on the right and two on the left. The asymmetry in mice is in the same direction but with a single lobe on the left and four on the right. Branching continues for 10 weeks with around 24 bifurcations leading to the terminal bronchioles, which likewise divide to form two respiratory bronchioles and then three to six ducts, ending in an alveolar complex. The pulmonary arteries and veins bifurcate similarly to join extensive angiogenesis around the alveolar complexes.

Terminal epithelial cells differentiate into the important surfactant producing type II pneumocytes. These are cuboidal cells and occupy only 1–5% of the alveolar surface area. Type I pneumocytes are as numerous but they are flat squamous cells that thin out such that by 36 weeks the capillaries are intimate with the future airspaces. Evidence suggests that for up to 3 years after birth new alveoli can be generated by subdivision of existing immature alveoli. Fetal "breathing" of amniotic fluid is thought to have an important role in lung development.

Genes Involved in Foregut and Lung Development

A large number of genes and gene products have been identified that are either involved directly in the initial stages of foregut and lung development or can affect them when mutations are present.[15]

- Fibroblast growth factor-10 is involved in primary tracheal branching. In mice with an FGF-10 null mutation the trachea does not separate from the foregut, and nothing develops distal to the trachea.
- Hox a5 null mutants have tracheal occlusion and surfactant deficiency.
- The forkhead transcription factors Foxp2 and Foxp1 are expressed in the lung. Loss of Foxp2 in the mouse leads to defective postnatal lung alveolarization.[16]
- Fibroblast growth factor receptor-2 and -4 compound null phenotypes have poor neonatal alveolar development and persistent neonatal elastin deposition.

- The epidermal growth factor receptor Egfr is important since impaired branching and deficient alveolization are seen in Egfr$^{-/-}$ mice.[17]

- The sonic hedgehog (*Shh*) gene is involved in left–right axis specification and differentiation of the notochord, floor plate, and limbs. Sonic hedgehog also has a role in foregut and lung development. Sonic hedgehog Shh mutants show impaired branching and TEFs.[4,5,18] Abnormal sonic hedgehog expression is also seen in the Adriamycin rat model of EA/TEF with the spectrum of anomalies seen in the VATER association.[19] We are aware that bronchial branching is reduced in CDH but there is no evidence of reduced branching in human EA/TEF although this might be worth investigating.

- Other proteins thought to be important in lung development include bone morphogenetic protein, retinoic acid, and the Wnt signaling pathways. These agents also have important roles in the development of other systems and are often implicated in tumors. Many genes, especially tumor suppressor genes and growth factors, are important in both embryogenesis and tumors. Interestingly, Shh is yet another example of this.[20]

The Diaphragm

The diaphragm was traditionally described as arising from the septum transversum, pleuroperitoneal folds (PPFs), the dorsal esophageal mesentery, and the body wall (Fig. 2.3).[21,22] The contribution from the body wall is now known not to occur. The septum transversum originates in mesoderm rostral to the primitive cardiogenic mesoderm. Differential growth and ventral folding of the embryo bring this primordium into a position to divide the embryo into a pleuro-pericardial cavity rostrally and a peritoneal cavity caudally. The pleuro-peritoneal canals that lie laterally are then occluded by triangular-shaped PPFs.

The muscular component of the diaphragm was previously thought to arise from the lateral body wall. It is now clear

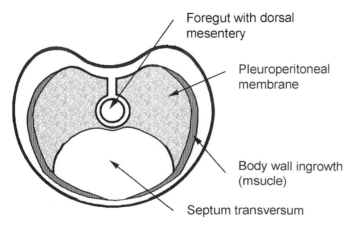

FIG. 2.3. The traditional view of the embryonic contributions to the diaphragm

that this arises from a distinct population of migratory muscle precursor cells (MPCs) from the lateral dermo-myotomal lip. This was concluded from the observation that in c-met null-mutant mice the muscles of the body wall are normal but the diaphragm has no muscle in it. The *c-met* gene encodes a tyrosine kinase receptor, which is involved in the delamination and migration of MPCs.[23] In support of this, Babiuk et al. found no immunological evidence for contributions from the lateral body wall, septum transversum, or esophageal mesenchyme.[24] They found that myogenic cells and axons destined to form the neuromuscular component of the diaphragm coalesce within the pleuro-peritoneal folds. Expansion of these components from the PPFs forms the diaphragm.

CDH has been attributed to abnormal lung development, abnormal phrenic nerve innervation, abnormal myotube formation, and failure of closure of the embryonic pleuroperitoneal canal. The association of lung hypoplasia with a diaphragmatic defect has encouraged this speculation. Some think that given a hernia, pressure from the herniated abdominal viscera damages the lung. Others think that failure of the lung to develop allows the herniation, although both children and animals with absent lungs usually have intact diaphragms, which makes this view unlikely. It is most likely that the abnormal lung development is fundamentally associated with diaphragmatic hernia rather than there being a cause and effect phenomenon. Indeed Guilbert et al. have shown that in the rat nitrofen model lung hypoplasia occurs early.[25]

Animal Models of CDH

There are some interesting observations that support the argument that retinoids and the PPFs are important. Vitamin A-deficient rats have CDH in 25–40% of pups. Defects in the PPFs are described in these animals. The rate of herniation decreases when vitamin A is introduced into the diet mid-gestation. In retinoid receptor double null-mutant mice, lacking both α and β subtypes of retinoic acid receptors (RAR), offsprings have CDH.

Greer's group has examined the developing diaphragm in the nitrofen rat model of CDH. Nitrofen and other teratogens are thought to perturb the retinoid signaling pathway by inhibiting a retinoic acid synthesizing enzyme. Greer's group found that malformation of the postero-lateral PPF mesenchyme in the nitrofen model led to the defects.[24,26] In addition, a mouse with an inactivated gene called *COUP-TFII* has CDH and a PPF defect.[27]

Genetic Associations

CDH usually occurs as an isolated defect although there are some recognized syndromal associations, including Cornelia de Lange syndrome, Fryns syndrome, and Pallister–Killian syndrome (tetrasomy 12p mosaicism). Other chromosomal abnormalities associated with CDH include trisomy 13, trisomy

18, and Turner syndrome (monosomy X). Chromosome deletions are reported on 1q, 8p, and 15q in association with CDH. Fewer than 2% of CDH are familial although pedigrees are described with autosomal recessive, autosomal dominant, and X-linked patterns of inheritance. Anterior diaphragmatic hernias are more common in children with Down's syndrome. Unfortunately none of these genetic defects point toward an etiological mechanism.

Left–Right Asymmetry in the Chest

Left–right asymmetry of the pulmonary anatomy is evident from the time the lung buds first appear. The right pulmonary artery is more bulbous and deflected away from the mid line more than the left. There are normally three lobes to the left lung and two on the right in the human. The main bronchi are of different lengths, inclined at different angles and have different relationships to the pulmonary vasculature. When there are defects in left–right development these arrangements may be reversed; alternatively, there may be isomeric arrangements when the lungs are grossly symmetrical. Bronchial and pulmonary isomerisms have little direct clinical relevance. However, these isomerisms are associated with important cardiac, vascular, splenic anomalies, and sometimes abnormalities of intestinal rotation.

Left bronchial isomerism is associated with left atrial isomerism, bilateral superior caval veins, hemiazygous continuation of the inferior caval vein, a common atrioventricular valve, ambiguous and biventricular atrioventricular connections but a relatively normal ventriculoarterial junction. The majority of infants with left-sided isomerism have multiple spleens and abnormal lateralization of the abdominal viscera, including a short pancreas. About one-third have a confluent suprahepatic venous channel connecting the hepatic veins to the atrium. The pulmonary venous connections are normal with two pulmonary veins on each side.

Right bronchial isomerism is associated with right atrial isomerism and bilateral superior caval drainage. Total anomalous pulmonary venous drainage, including anomalous drainage via a narrow sinus in the roof of atrium, is seen. There is absence of the coronary sinus, a common atrioventricular valve, double inlet or ambiguous atrioventricular connections, and abnormal ventriculoarterial connections such as transposition of the great vessels and pulmonary obstruction. The majority of infants have asplenia and many have abnormal lateralization of the abdominal viscera.

Left is specified from the right when bilateral symmetry is broken by monociliated cells at the primitive node. These cilia beat in an asymmetric way imparting a force on morphogens, so breaking the symmetry. The node lies at the anterior end of the primitive streak and from it cells migrate toward the foregut pocket. As they reabsorb their monocilia they start dividing again. These cells form the notochord.[28] Genes involved in left–right development include the transforming growth factor-beta superfamily members Lefty-1, Lefty-2, nodal transcription factor, and hepatocyte nuclear factor-4 and Shh.

Dynein is an important motor protein in cilia. Dynein abnormalities are associated with primary ciliary dyskinesia (PCD). Patients with PCD may have defects of left–right development.

Surfactant Deficiency

The clinical term respiratory distress syndrome (RDS) and the histological term hyaline membrane disease (HMD) have been used to describe the consequences of surfactant deficiency in immature lungs. Surfactant is produced by type II alveolar cells and stored intracellularly in lamellar bodies. Surfactant is secreted by exocytosis to form a lipid-rich monolayer that coats the lining of the alveoli. Surfactant deficiency leads to alveolar collapse from surface tension, a decreased functional residual capacity, uneven lung expansion, increased capillary permeability, and alveolar edema with hypoxia. Around half of babies born between 26 and 28 weeks and 20–30% of neonates born at 30–31 weeks of gestation develop RDS. Understanding the basic science allows delivery of exogenous surfactant with excellent clinical outcomes.

Respiratory distress syndrome can result from many different causes of surfactant deficiency and is occasionally seen in term babies. The gene for an ATP-binding cassette transporter A3 (ABCA3) is expressed in alveolar type II cells. The protein localizes to lamellar bodies and probably has an important role in transporting phospholipids. Mutations of the ABCA3 gene have been found in newborns with unexplained severe RDS, who also showed abnormal lamellar bodies. In one study of consanguineous families with ABCA3 gene mutations five pairs of siblings were homozygous for the same mutation but unique mutations were found in different families.[29]

Cystic Fibrosis

Cystic fibrosis (CF) is inherited in an autosomal recessive manner and affects 1 in 2,500 newborns. The condition is seen mainly in white babies. The defective gene is carried by 1 in 25 Caucasians. Thus, for 1 couple in 625 (25×25) both parents will have a defective gene and 1 in 4 of their children will be homozygous for a mutation in the CF gene. Thus, 1 child in 2,500 is affected ($2,500 = 4 \times 625$). Cystic fibrosis is caused by mutations in the gene for the cystic fibrosis transmembrane conductance regulator (CFTR). Cloning of the CF gene with subsequent characterization of the CFTR protein by Riordan et al. in 1989 gave hope for gene therapy. The CFTR protein is found in sweat and pancreatic ducts, gut, seminiferous tubules, and the lungs. When CFTR mutations are present abnormal thick secretions are produced limiting bacterial clearance and leading to chronic lung damage. Life expectancy has increased from less than 10 years in the 1960s to 30–40 years with better respiratory, nutritional, and transplant management. Advanced therapies aim to deliver the normal CF gene or protein to the lungs hoping to restore normal cellular function. In vitro transfer of the *CFTR* gene was achieved in 1990 by Rich et al. and in vivo to the airway epithelial cells of transgenic CF mice in 1993.[30-32] There have been over 20 phase I studies in humans using liposome–plasmid complexes or adenoviruses as gene transfer vectors. The amount of gene transferred is similar for both viruses and liposomes. Unfortunately, gene expression lasts only a few days and no trial has yet measured a therapeutic benefit.

References

1. Wolpert L. One hundred years of positional information. Trends Genet 1996; 12: 359–364.
2. Oh SP, Li E. The signaling pathway mediated by the type IIB activin receptor controls axial patterning and lateral asymmetry in the mouse. Genes Dev 1997; 11: 1812–1826.
3. Apelqvist A, Ahlgren U, Edlund H. Sonic hedgehog directs specialised mesoderm differentiation in the intestine and pancreas. Curr Biol 1997; 7: 801–804.
4. Litingtung Y, Lei L, Westphal H, Chiang C. Sonic hedgehog is essential to foregut development. Nat Genet 1998; 20: 58–61.
5. Pepicelli CV, Lewis PM, McMahon AP. Sonic hedgehog regulates branching morphogenesis in the mammalian lung. Curr Biol 1998; 8: 1083 1086
6. deMello DE, Sawyer D, Galvin N, Reid LM. Early fetal development of lung vasculature. Am J Respir Cell Mol Biol 1997; 16(5): 568–581.
7. Gebb SA, Shannon JM. Tissue interactions mediate early events in pulmonary vasculogenesis. Dev Dyn 2000; 217: 159–169.
8. Zaw-Tun HA. The tracheo-esophageal septum-fact or fantasy? Origin and development of the respiratory primordium and esophagus. Acta Anat 1982; 114: 1–21.
9. Sutliff KS, Hutchins GM. Septation of the respiratory and digestive tracts in human embryos: crucial role of the tracheoesophageal sulcus. Anat Rec 1994; 238: 237–247.
10. Ioannides AS, Chaudhry B, Henderson DJ, et al. Dorsoventral patterning in oesophageal atresia with tracheooesophageal fistula: evidence from a new mouse model. J Pediatr Surg 2002; 37: 185–191.
11. Minoo P, Su G, Drum H, et al. Defects in tracheoesophageal and lung morphogenesis in Nkx2.1(–/–) mouse embryos. Dev Biol 1999; 209: 60–71.
12. Lim L, Kalinichenko VV, Whitsett JA, Costa RH. Fusion of lung lobes and vessels in mouse embryos heterozygous for the forkhead box f1 targeted allele. Am J Physiol Lung Cell Mol Physiol 2002; 282: L1012–L1022.
13. Sakiyama J, Yamagishi A, Kuroiwa A. Tbx4-Fgf10 system controls lung bud formation during chicken embryonic development. Development 2003; 130: 1225–1234.
14. Dickman ED, Thaller C, Smith SM. Temporally-regulated retinoic acid depletion produces specific neural crest, ocular and nervous system defects. Development 1997; 124: 3111–3121.
15. Cardoso WV, Lü J. Regulation of early lung morphogenesis: questions, facts and controversies. Development 2006; 133: 1611–1624.
16. Shu W, Lu MM, Zhang Y, et al. Foxp2 and Foxp1 cooperatively regulate lung and esophagus development. Development 2007; 134: 1991–2000.
17. Kheradmand F, Rishi K, Werb Z. Signaling through the EGF receptor controls lung morphogenesis in part by regulating MT1-MMP-mediated activation of gelatinase A/MMP2. J Cell Sci 2002; 115: 839–848.
18. Roberts DJ. Molecular mechanisms of development of the gastrointestinal tract. Dev Dyn 2000; 219: 109–120.
19. Arsic´ D, Cameron V, Ellmers L, et al. Adriamycin disruption of the Shh-Gli pathway is associated with abnormalities of foregut development. J Pediatr Surg 2004; 39: 1747–1753.
20. Arsic´ D, Beasley SW, Sullivan MJ. Switched-on sonic hedgehog: a gene whose activity extends beyond fetal development to oncogenesis. J Pediatr Child Health 2007; 43: 421–423.
21. Bremer JL. The diaphragm and diaphragmatic hernia. Arch Pathol 1943; 36: 539–549.
22. Wells LJ. Development of the human diaphragm and pleural sacs. Carnegie Contrib Embryol #236. 1954; 35: 107–134.
23. Birchmeire C, Brohman H. Genes that control the development of migrating muscle precursor cells. Curr Opin Cell Biol 2000; 12: 725–730.
24. Babiuk RP, Zhang W, Clugston R, et al. Embryological origins and development of the rat diaphragm. J Comp Neurol 2003; 455: 477–487.
25. Guilbert TW, Gebb SA, Shannon JM. Lung hypoplasia in the nitrofen model of congenital diaphragmatic hernia occurs early in development. Am J Physiol Lung Cell Mol Physiol 2000; 279: L1159–L1171.
26. Allan DW, Greer JJ. Pathogenesis of nitrofen-induced congenital diaphragmatic hernia in fetal rats. J Appl Physiol 1997; 83: 338–347.
27. You LR, Takamoto N, Yu CT, et al. Mouse lacking COUP-TFII as an animal model of Bochdalek-type congenital diaphragmatic hernia. Proc Natl Acad Sci USA 2005; 102: 16351–16356.
28. Bellomo D, Lander A, Harrigan I, Brown NA. Cell proliferation in mammalian gastrulation: the ventral node and notochord are relatively quiescent. Dev Dyn 1996; 205: 471–485.
29. Shulenin S, Nogee LM, Annilo T, et al. *ABCA3* gene mutations in newborns with fatal surfactant deficiency. N Engl J Med 2004; 350: 1296–1330.
30. Rich DP, Anderson MP, Gregory RJ, et al. Expression of CFTR corrects defective chloride channel regulation in cystic fibrosis airway epithelial cells. Nature 1990; 347: 358–363.
31. Hyde SC, Gill DR, Higgins CF, et al. Correction of the ion transport defect in cystic fibrosis transgenic mice by gene therapy. Nature 1993; 362: 250–255.
32. Alton EW, Middleton PG, Caplen NJ, et al. Non-invasive liposome-mediated gene delivery can correct the ion transport defect in cystic fibrosis mice. Nat Genet 1993; 5: 135–142.

Further Reading

Bourbon J, Boucherat O, Chailley-Heu B, Delacourt C. Control mechanisms of lung alveolar development and their disorders in bronchopulmonary dysplasia. Pediatr Res 2005; 57: 38R–46R.

Cardoso WV, Lü J. Regulation of early lung morphogenesis: questions, facts and controversies. Development 2006; 133: 1611–1624.

Pauling MH, Vu TH. Mechanisms and regulation of lung vascular development. Curr Top Dev Biol 2004; 64: 73–99.

Williams MC. Alveolar type I cells: molecular phenotype and development. Annu Rev Physiol 2003; 65: 669–695.

3
Applied Physiology and Pulmonary Function Testing

Caroline Beardsmore

Introduction

The main purpose of pulmonary function tests is to identify and quantify abnormalities of respiratory function. Respiratory function tests are rarely diagnostic by themselves although they do contribute to diagnosis. In a surgical setting, tests of respiratory function are important to document preoperative status and whether respiratory function is changing over time. As such, they may help with timing of thoracic surgery. Preoperative respiratory function has long been used in adults to predict postoperative function and likelihood of complications[1] although the range of investigations has increased in recent years.[2] Assessment of postoperative function will document the impact of surgery on the respiratory system. Serial measurements will show how respiratory function changes with time in individual patients. Since growth of the thorax may continue beyond the age of 20 in males it may be necessary to examine respiratory function over an extended time period following surgery in childhood to be sure of the final effect. A further value of respiratory function may be to inform the surgeon and anesthetist of any limitation of function.

There is an extensive range of tests of respiratory function which may provide information pertinent to gas exchange, the mechanical properties of the lungs and chest wall, the functioning of the airways, or a combination of these. Some of the tests are well established and can be performed with children of different ages, whereas others require a level of cooperation that may not be possible in a young child. Tests of respiratory function in infants are possible but usually only available in specialist laboratories. Whatever the setting for testing children (inpatient wards, outpatient clinic, laboratory), it is important that any measurements are performed, evaluated, and reported by a person experienced with children and using appropriate predicted values. Furthermore, they should be used in conjunction with clinical and radiographic findings and not viewed in isolation.

Measurements of Respiratory Function

The measurement of blood gases and monitoring of pulse oximetry can be considered a basic form of respiratory function test, since they may provide evidence that the basic function of the lungs (oxygenation) is adequate. The ability of the cardiorespiratory system to compensate is such that these indicators may be entirely normal in the presence of extensive disease, and a more detailed testing is required. The most common measurements are those of the mechanics of the respiratory system, providing information about the divisions of lung volume and airway function. These can be complimented by assessment of gas mixing, pulmonary blood flow, and diffusion across the alveolar wall. Measurements of respiratory pressures can be used to assess respiratory muscle strength.

Measurements of Spirometry

Equipment

Spirometry remains the most widely used test of lung mechanics, and forced vital capacity (FVC), forced expiratory volume in one second(s) (FEV_1), and FEV_1/FVC are still the most widely quoted measurements. The old-fashioned, mechanical spirometers (e.g., bellows, wedge, or water-sealed spirometers) have been replaced by electronic models that are readily portable. Many devices permit the recording of an inspiratory maneuver as well as expiratory maneuver, which is invaluable in evaluating upper airway function. Criteria have been developed for the minimum technical requirements for these devices,[3] and they may come with a wealth of features. A high-quality graphical display is essential for the operator to assess the technical adequacy of the maneuvers and as an aid in interpretation of the results. An integral printer allows a recording to be inserted into the patient records. Some software packages allow for trends to be recorded, and all will provide predicted values,

D.H. Parikh et al. (eds.), *Pediatric Thoracic Surgery*,
DOI: 10.1007/b136543_3, © Springer-Verlag London Limited 2009

usually based on the age, height, and gender of the subject. Some of the more expensive models will alert the operator if the respiratory maneuver does not accord with preset criteria for technical acceptability,[3] but such criteria relate to adults and may not be appropriate for pediatric use. For example, the duration of a full, forced expiratory maneuver should be 6s or longer in an adult. Most young children find this impossible to achieve.[4] The inclusion of text that provides interpretation of the data is to be eschewed at all costs, since the machine may be unable to distinguish between a poor effort on the part of the subject and adequate effort but deranged lung function. More importantly, the operator should be using his/her critical faculties at all stages of testing, including evaluation of data.

Procedure

Almost all children aged six and above can perform spirometry. Many younger children can perform the necessary maneuvers with appropriate training.[5,6] The use of incentive spirometry, in which the force and the duration of the exhalation influences a computer animation, may improve the success rate and the quality of the maneuvers.[7] Spirometric maneuvers are usually performed with the subject seated. The use of a nose clip is usual for consistency but not essential because the palate will close when mouth pressure is positive, if pharyngeal function is normal. Whatever the age of the child, she/he will require a clear explanation of the maneuver from the operator, which is often best accompanied by a demonstration. The subject is generally asked to breathe quietly through the mouthpiece until tidal respiration is stable, at which point they are asked to take a maximum inspiration, followed immediately by full, forced expiration, which is maintained until residual volume (RV) is reached. At this point they may be asked for another maximal inspiration to complete a flow volume loop. The maneuver should be repeated after short breaks until three reproducible recordings are obtained, unless a maximum of eight attempts have been made without satisfactory readings, in which case testing should be abandoned. Reproducible measurements are defined as the two best measurements of FVC and FEV_1 being within 5% or 200 mL, whichever is the greater,[3] although this may not be achievable in very young or sick children. Recommendations for quality control for spirometry in preschool children have been published.[8]

Infants lack the necessary cooperation to participate actively in lung function testing but measurements of maximal flows can be obtained in infants under mild sedation. Flow and volume are measured from a pneumotachograph attached to a facemask that is positioned around the nose and mouth, and the chest and abdomen are wrapped in an inflatable jacket connected to a pressure source. When the infant is breathing steadily, the jacket can be rapidly inflated at the end of inspiration, causing a forced expiration. A series of measurements is made, with gradual increases in applied pressure, until forced expiratory flow (FEF) ceases to increase in line with applied pressure. The forced maneuver will continue below the resting

end-expiratory level, permitting recording of the maximal flow at functional residual capacity ($V_{max}FRC$), which is the usual index recorded.

The forced maneuver described above yields only a partial flow-volume curve but careful application of pressure at the airway opening during inspiration results in an increase of lung volume toward total lung capacity (TLC). When the forced expiratory maneuver commences at this elevated lung volume, it is possible to record timed expiratory volumes (such as FEV_1), which more closely approximate the measurements in older children. The pressures used to elevate the lung volume and to produce the forced expiration need to be stringently controlled with proper monitoring of the infant at all times. Guidelines are available for the technique.[9]

Indices Derived from Spirometry

The key measurements derived from a flow-volume maneuver are the FVC and FEV_1. Volumes expired in other timed intervals (e.g., forced expired volume in 0.5 s ($FEV_{0.5}$) may also be reported. The peak expiratory flow (PEF) is also generally reported since it has been shown that any discrepancies between PEF derived from a full, forced expiration and from a short, sharp peak flow maneuver are minimal.[10] The ratio FEV_1/FVC is often reported, but may be normal even if both FEV_1 and FVC are abnormal. Additional measurements derived from the expiratory portion of the maneuver relate to flows at defined fractions of the FVC. The nomenclature of these flows has recently been standardized to FEF, and the fraction of FVC to that which has been expired (rather than the portion remaining in the lung). Older reports and textbooks (particularly those of European origin) may use old nomenclature referring to maximum expiratory flows (MEF). Similarly, the average flow across the middle half of the FVC is reported as FEF_{25-75}, rather than maximum mid-expiratory flow (MMEF). The commonly reported indices derived from spirometry are shown (Fig. 3.1).

Inspiratory flows are less commonly reported than their expiratory counterparts. The commonest reported indices are the peak inspiratory flow (PIF) and flow at mid-vital capacity (FIF_{50}). In infant testing, the reported measurements may include $V_{max}FRC$, FEV_1, $FEV_{0.75}$, and $FEV_{0.5}$.

Interpretation

Before interpretation of measurements the operator should inspect the recordings for technical acceptability. The expiratory flow-volume curve should rise rapidly to reach peak flow early in the maneuver and then descend smoothly to RV without being truncated by either closure of the glottis or early onset of inspiration. A maximum inspiratory maneuver should have a smooth outline. The shape of a flow-volume loop provides valuable information about the underlying condition (Fig. 3.2). Both phases of the flow-volume loop should be reproducible on a single occasion in a healthy individual

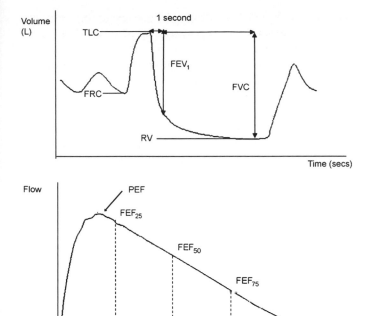

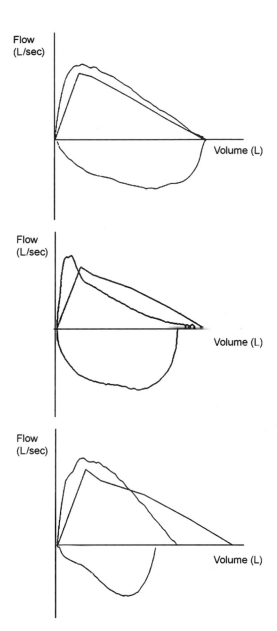

FIG. 3.1. Spirogram (*upper panel*) and expiratory flow volume loop (*lower panel*), annotated to show derivation of indices of spirometry. *TLC* Total lung capacity; *FRC* Functional residual capacity; *RV* Residual volume; *FEV$_1$* Forced expired volume in 1 s; *FVC* Forced vital capacity; *PEF* Peak expiratory flow; *FEF$_{25}$*, *FEF$_{50}$*, *FEF$_{75}$* Forced expiratory flow at 25%, 50%, and 75% vital capacity, respectively

or one with stable disease. An exception to this generalization is a child with respiratory muscle weakness, in whom the flow-volume loop may be variable from one maneuver to the next. A concave shape to the expiratory limb is indicative of intrathoracic airway obstruction, most frequently seen in children with asthma and which is usually improved following administration of a bronchodilator. A reduction in FVC with expiratory flows that are preserved or elevated is found when there is a restrictive disorder, such as scoliosis (Fig. 3.2).

While the shape of the flow-volume loop is informative, the numerical values of PEF, FVC, and FEV$_1$ are important for quantifying the extent of any abnormality. The practice of expressing measurements as percentage of predicted is widespread but does not truly indicate the extent of deviation from prediction as reliably as a standard deviation score (z-score). The ratio FEV$_1$/FVC is constant through most of the childhood (predicted value 84%, range 79–92%) but will tend to be elevated in younger, shorter children (below approximately 115 cm). This is because a healthy child whose height is below 100 cm may well empty their lungs within less than 1 s, so that FEV$_1$/FVC would be 100%, and the proportion of children in whom forced expiration takes longer than 1 s increases with age/height. In children with restrictive disease the ratio tends to increase. The ratio will be artifactually increased

FIG. 3.2. Flow-volume curves in health and disease. *Upper panel* shows recording from a healthy child in whom the vital capacity is normal and the expiratory flow-volume curve is very close to the predicted curve (shown schematically). *Middle panel* shows a recording from a child with an obstructive disorder (severe asthma), with characteristic scooped appearance to the expiratory loop and flows below predicted values for most of the expiration. *Bottom panel* illustrates a restrictive disorder in which the vital capacity is reduced but there is no suggestion of concavity of the expiratory loop. Note that in every case the flow-volume loops are aligned to begin with total lung capacity at the intersection of the axes. This is the usual default display of many spirometers and can mislead the unwary. In the case of restrictive disorders, the deficit in vital capacity is likely to be at total lung capacity, with a normal or near-normal residual volume, in contrast to the display

in children who do not complete full expiration, so that the unwary operator may suspect a restrictive disease where none exists. Differentiating between a child with a restrictive pattern of lung function and one who has not completed a full forced expiration may not be easy, even for a person experienced in pediatric lung function. Highly consistent measurements in which the flow-volume loops can be superimposed would point toward a reliable test. When a child is not blowing out completely the FVC may vary and the flow-volume loop shows evidence of a sudden cessation of flow or early onset of inspiration.

The longstanding and widespread use of spirometry means that there are many reports involving different populations studied with varying protocols.[11] Any laboratory wanting to select prediction equations from the literature could select a study in which the methodology and the population were closely matched to their own, but should be cautious about extrapolating predictions beyond the data. This is especially important when testing adolescents, because the limits of prediction generally become wider during puberty. Prediction equations that are adjusted on the basis of height to take account of puberty are available for white Caucasians, covering the range of spirometric indices.[12] Because FEV_1 may not always be obtainable in small children, either because they cannot sustain expiration until reaching RV or because the maneuver is completed in less than 1 s, alternative timed volumes such as forced expired volumes in 0.75 or 0.5 s ($FEV_{0.75}$ or $FEV_{0.5}$) are becoming more widely used. These allow for growth charts of lung function to be developed from early childhood onward.[13] The amount of published data pertaining to these indices is much less than for FEV_1 but would be expected to increase as interest in lung function in preschool children is expanding.

Application

The main application of spirometry is that of assessment, not diagnosis. The patterns of flow volume loops may be an important clue to site of possible obstruction – and therefore to diagnosis – but monitoring function is much more common. Single measurements may not be particularly helpful, since the limits of prediction are wide, but changes in measurements in response to treatment can be extremely informative. These can be short term (for example the effect of a beta-2 agonist in asthma) or over several days or weeks. Serial measurements over longer periods of time may monitor progression of disease or recovery. Spirometric measurements are often used in respiratory-related clinical trials, epidemiological studies, and research into lung growth and development in both health and disease.

Measurements of Lung Volumes

The volume of air within the lungs at rest is the functional residual capacity (FRC), and is determined by the balance of elastic recoil of the lungs (tending to reduce lung volume) and that of the chest wall. The extent of possible changes from FRC is limited by the mechanical properties of the lungs and the chest wall and the strength of the respiratory muscles. Absolute values of lung volume can be obtained from whole body plethysmography, gas dilution tests, or by gas washout tests, in which case the primary purpose of the test is usually to investigate gas mixing. The methods of measurement are not equivalent, since plethysmography measures the volume of gas in the thorax and will include any trapped gas, whereas other techniques measure the ventilated lung volume only. In healthy individuals the differences will be small, but in the presence of early airway closure resulting from extensive airway disease there may be considerable hyperinflation, which will be better detected by plethysmographic measurements. Because of this difference, lung volume measurements performed by plethysmography are reported as FRC_{pleth}.[14] Having measured FRC, a full vital capacity maneuver will enable TLC and RV to be calculated. Measurements of lung volume are helpful in assessment of restrictive conditions resulting from neuromuscular disease or skeletal abnormalities, and in quantifying the extent of hyperinflation.

Equipment and Procedure for Plethysmographic Measurement of Lung Volume

A whole-body plethysmograph is a cabin in which the subject can be seated that is almost airtight when closed. He breathes through a mouthpiece and pneumotachograph so that flow and volume can be measured. A pressure transducer is situated to measure pressure close to the lips. A nose clip is essential. After a period of acclimatization, a valve or shutter located distal to the pneumotachograph is activated to occlude the external airway for a short time, during which the subject makes one or two respiratory efforts. After the shutter opens he has a very short period of tidal breathing before making a vital capacity maneuver, which enables the divisions of lung volume to be measured.

The basis of the measurement of lung volume is the application of Boyle's law, which states that for a fixed mass of gas at constant temperature, the product of pressure and volume is constant. During the period of airway occlusion the mass of air behind the closed shutter remains constant (oxygen uptake and carbon dioxide production can be disregarded in such a brief measurement) but is subjected to changes in pressure and volume. Shutter closure is timed for the end of a tidal breath, when there is no flow occurring and the pressure at the start of the maneuver is therefore atmospheric. During the respiratory efforts against the occlusion, pressure changes within the lung are transmitted to the airway opening where they are measured directly. The accompanying changes in lung volume (brought about by compression and rarefaction of the fixed mass of gas within the lung) are measured indirectly from the plethysmograph. Since any change in thoracic gas volume is mirrored by an equivalent inverse change in plethysmograph volume, appropriate calibration allows the volume change to be calculated. Thoracic gas volume can then be computed from the following equation

$$V = \frac{\Delta VP}{\Delta P}$$

where V represents thoracic gas volume, P represents atmospheric pressure (measured from the barometer and corrected for water vapor pressure), ΔP represents the pressure change in the thoracic gas volume (measured directly), and ΔV represents the volume change (measured indirectly).

The calculated volume is adjusted for the dead space of the apparatus between the lips and the shutter. In small children being studied by equipment designed for adults, this can represent a considerable adjustment and it is recommended to keep this volume to a minimum, e.g., by selecting pediatric mouthpieces.

The technique assumes that pressure changes are isothermal, i.e., they are not accompanied by temperature change, which would produce artifactual changes in volume. Establishing a respiratory rate that is somewhat faster than that observed naturally at rest prior to occlusion helps to achieve this condition. A second assumption is that pressure change measured at the airway opening is a true reflection of mean alveolar pressure change. A plot of airway opening pressure against plethysmograph pressure during the period of airway occlusion should show a straight line relationship if this condition is met. Any episodes of glottis closure are simple to detect as there will be a sharp deviation from this plot. In cases of advanced airway disease, there may be uneven distribution of pressure change within the lung that give more subtle disturbance to the plot and in these cases the measurement becomes less reliable.[15,16]

Measurements are repeated after short rests, and an average value of FRC_{pleth} is reported. For adults, the reported value should be the mean of at least three values that agree within 5%, and measurements should be repeated until this level of repeatability is obtained.[14] When working with children it may not be possible to achieve such stringent repeatability because of the lack of sustained cooperation and reports based on fewer measurements may be acceptable.[17]

From a practical standpoint, children require careful instruction in the technique before beginning the test, and reinforcement and encouragement at intervals between measurements. After closing the door of the plethysmograph, it is customary to wait for 1 or 2 min before beginning the measurements in order for cabin temperature to stabilize. A game or video can provide a welcome distraction at this point. Good posture is essential to achieve repeatability. The child should be seated upright without flexion or extension of the neck. The height of the seat and the footrest should be adjusted for comfort, or the child may distort the plethysmographic pressure by wriggling. During measurements he should place the palms of his hands on his cheeks to avoid any dissipation of pressure due to undue movement of the cheeks.

It is very rare for children to refuse to enter the plethysmograph because they feel claustrophobic, but young children may not be willing to be separated from parent or caregiver. In such cases, they may be successfully studied while seated on the knee of an adult, provided that the adult holds their breath at the time when measurements are being made. A small adjustment to the plethysmograph calibration then needs to be made to take account of the volume occupied by the accompanying adult.

Infant whole-body plethysmography is possible but requires miniaturized equipment and specially trained staff skilled in the measurement.[18] Infants are studied supine and the nose clip and mouthpiece are replaced by a facemask that is positioned around the nose and mouth with putty to provide an airtight seal. Except in the case of very young infants (up to 1 month of age), they are sedated with chloral hydrate so that they will sleep soundly and tolerate the necessary handling. Contraindications to sedation include past history of apneic events, and known or suspected upper airway abnormality. Infants should be examined by a pediatrician prior to sedation and testing and oxygen saturation monitored throughout the procedure.

Equipment and Procedure for Lung Volume Measurement by Gas Dilution

The equipment for measuring lung volume by gas dilution is a closed circuit including a mechanical spirometer (such as a water or rolling seal spirometer), a gas analyzer, a means of absorbing carbon dioxide and adding oxygen, and a pump to circulate the gases within the circuit (Fig. 3.3).

The subject breathes in and out of the circuit and the displacement of the spirometer needs to be recorded and displayed to the operator. Before beginning the measurement, the circuit is filled with a mixture of gases comprising approximately 69% nitrogen, 21% oxygen, and 10% tracer gas. The commonest tracer gas is helium since it is inert and virtually insoluble. The starting volume of the circuit is determined by calibration and the initial concentration of helium is noted. The subject wears a nose clip and initially breathes room air through a mouthpiece. When respiration is regular the subject is switched at end-expiration to breathe from the circuit. Over the subsequent 1–4 min, the air within the lungs becomes completely mixed with that in the circuit and a new, lower concentration of helium is recorded. As the measurement proceeds, carbon dioxide is absorbed and the operator bleeds in oxygen, to maintain a stable end-expiratory system volume and avoid the risk of hypoxia developing. The volume V_2 (circuit plus lung volume) is calculated from the following equation

$$V_2 = (V_1 C_1) / C_2$$

where C_1 and C_2 are the initial and final concentrations of helium and V_1 is the starting volume of the circuit. Having calculated V_2, FRC is obtained by subtracting initial circuit volume from V_2 and making any adjustment if the subject was switched into the circuit at a volume above FRC. The measurements are made with the circuit at room temperature. By convention, lung volumes are reported under body temperature and pressure, saturated (BTPS) conditions so a final small

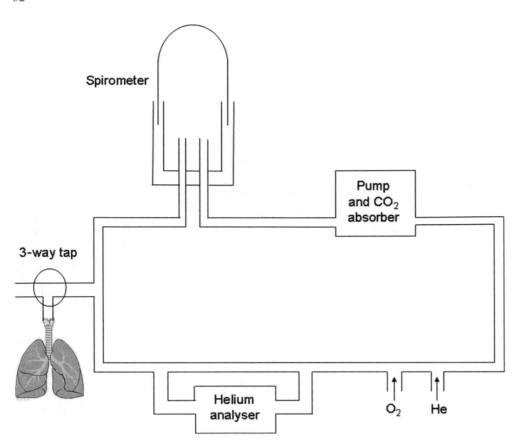

FIG. 3.3. Circuit for measurement of lung volume by closed circuit helium dilution (see text for explanation)

correction is made for this. The duration of each measurement will depend on the efficiency of gas mixing. The test is usually stopped when the helium concentration remains stable for a 15-s period, at which point the subject may be asked for a full vital capacity maneuver to measure the divisions of lung volume. The measurement is critically dependent on maintaining an airtight seal around the mouthpiece, so may not be easy in very young children or those who have difficulty with mouthpieces. Small leaks may be difficult to detect until a washout has progressed for some considerable time and it becomes clear that the concentration of helium is not stabilizing. Before measurements are repeated, time must be allowed for the helium within the lungs to be completely breathed out, i.e., the rest period between tests takes longer than the tests themselves. The reported value for FRC is generally taken as the mean of at least two measurements which vary by less than 10%.

The measurement can be readily applied to sleeping infants by replacing the mouthpiece and nose clip with a facemask positioned around the nose and mouth. However, a miniaturized circuit is essential to reduce dead space and so that the addition of the air from the lungs is sufficient to bring about a measurable change in the helium concentration. The resolution of the system can be improved if the helium analyzer can be modified to add an extra decimal place. With careful modification to the circuit, lung volumes as low as 50 ml can be accurately measured.[19]

Indices

Both plethysmography and gas dilution will provide a measurement that usually equates to end-expiratory lung volume which is quoted in liters for children of school age and in milliliters for infants. In infants, it is frequently reported in mL per kg body weight to facilitate comparison between infants or groups of differing age or size, but this presupposes a linear relationship between weight and lung volume. In practice, height is the best predictor of lung volume for boys and girls at all ages with arm span being a good surrogate in children in whom height cannot be accurately measured. There are many published prediction equations for lung volume in children of school age[20-22] and in infancy.[23-27]

Interpretation

An increased FRC will be found in children who are hyperinflated and is most commonly seen in advanced cystic fibrosis and exacerbations of asthma. It will be accompanied by poor airway function and arise because the small airways, narrowed by a combination of edema of the airway wall, excessive secretions, bronchoconstriction of the airway smooth muscle, and loss of radial traction, will close prematurely during tidal exhalation with consequent gas trapping. The RV is likely to be the most affected division of lung volume in these children. This may be reversible in whole or in part with appropriate treatment, depending on the primary reason for airway narrowing. A reduced FRC may arise as a result of congenital abnormality such as diaphragmatic hernia, in which case the lung on the affected side will be small, or may be acquired through disease such as muscular dystrophy that affect the chest wall. Abnormal stiffness of the lung, such as in hyaline membrane disease in preterm infants or acquired following certain forms of chemotherapy, will make the lung less distensible and result in a reduced lung volume. In such cases the TLC will be most severely affected.

Application

Knowledge of the underlying clinical condition will guide the clinician in the most valuable tests to perform and in the interpretation of results. Single measurements that indicate normal lung volumes may be reassuring but should not be over-interpreted since a hypoplastic lung may be hyperinflated. A normal FRC in this case would not indicate normal alveolar structure. Isolated measurements are less valuable than serial tests, which allow for progression to be monitored. Comparison with reference values is necessary for full interpretation, both for clinical studies[28] and research reports.[29]

Measurements of Ventilatory Efficiency

The efficiency of ventilation can be assessed by multiple breath inert gas washout. The gas of choice may be nitrogen, in which case the subject breathes oxygen during the measurement. If an inert gas such as helium or argon is to be used, the patient must first breathe a gas mix containing the gas of choice until the lungs have reached equilibrium after which she/he breathes room air during the washout procedure. The basis of the measurement is that the rate of clearance of the chosen gas is a measure of ventilatory efficiency. The clearance of the gas is expressed in relation to ventilation. By knowing the starting concentration of the gas and quantifying the volume washed out, a measurement of lung volume can also be obtained.[30-32]

Equipment

The test requires a gas analyzer appropriate for the chosen gas and a means of measuring ventilation. Since the overall gas composition being breathed varies over the course of the measurement, and some types of flow-measuring devices are sensitive to physical properties of the gas, it may be necessary to correct the measurement of ventilation. Equipment for multiple breath wash out is commercially available, but some laboratories combine other standard pieces of equipment for the purpose of the test. The test requires minimal cooperation other than tidal breathing so it can be applied to infants or older children. If infants or preschool children are to be tested, it is particularly important to minimize dead space.

Procedure

The subject breathes through a mouthpiece or a facemask (according to age) until she/he is settled and tidal volume is regular. The sample port for the gas analyzer is positioned close to the mouth or nose. If a nonresident gas is to be used, the subject is switched to breathe a gas mix containing the chosen gas until there is minimal change between the inspired and the expired concentrations, i.e., wash-in is complete. At the beginning of the washout, the subject is switched to breathe oxygen (if nitrogen is the test gas) or air if a nonresident gas is being used. A one-way valve is used to separate the inspired and the expired gases. The recording of gas concentration and ventilation usually continues until the concentration of the test gas in the expirate is below 2%.

Indices

Analysis of the multibreath washout is complex. The mean concentration of test gas in each expired breath is logarithmically transformed and expressed in terms of "lung volumes expired," or turnovers. This has the advantage that patients of different sizes (and therefore lung volumes) can be compared directly. An early index of ventilatory efficiency was the lung clearance index (LCI), which is the number of turnovers required to reduce the concentration of the test gas to 1/40th of the starting concentration. More complex indices (moment ratios) require the plotting of gas concentration against turnover and quantifying the change in the relationship of the two as washout progresses.[33] In more recent years, advances have been made in the analysis of multiple breath washouts, in which each sequential expired breath is treated separately. The change in concentration of the test gas during the plateau phase of each expiration is used to give two measures of ventilation inhomogeneity, one relating to that of the acinus and the other to inhomogeneity within the conducting airways.[34]

Interpretation and Application

Although washout tests have been used in pediatric settings for several years, variations in test procedures and analysis mean that comparison of data from different laboratories is difficult. The technique has demonstrated impaired gas mixing in the lungs of preterm infants, with and without mild lung disease,[35,36] and in children with cystic fibrosis.[31,32]

Maximum Respiratory Pressures

Patients with respiratory muscle weakness may be assessed in different ways. At a certain point the weakness will result in a reduction in vital capacity but the maximal respiratory pressures a patient can generate will be reduced before any effect on vital capacity can be demonstrated. The relationship between lung volume and maximal pressures is not straightforward because the maximal pressures do not depend solely on the force generated by the respiratory muscles but also reflect the recoil pressure of the respiratory system, specifically the lung and the chest wall. At FRC the elastic recoil of the lung and the chest wall are equal and opposite so there should be no net contribution to maximal pressures. At the extremes of vital capacity, the recoil of the respiratory system can make a substantial contribution to the pressures that the individual can generate but the component parts are not usually measured separately. The maximal pressures are taken as a surrogate for respiratory muscle strength.

When there is a substantial degree of diaphragmatic weakness vital capacity is reduced when the patient assumes a supine posture. In normal adults, the fall in vital capacity when the subject moves from seated to supine posture is less than 10%.[37] In severe isolated diaphragmatic weakness it may exceed 50%.[38] Changes in vital capacity with posture can also be observed in children but making measurements in a supine child can be challenging, especially if muscle weakness makes it difficult to maintain a leak-free seal around the mouthpiece. In contrast, maximal inspiratory and expiratory pressures ($P_I$max and $P_E$max) are usually easier to obtain and provide an indication of global respiratory muscle weakness.

The most common measures of maximal respiratory pressures are noninvasive and are measured at the mouth as the subject makes maximal inspiratory and expiratory maneuvers against a blocked external airway. Inspiratory nasal pressure can also be made with a "sniff" maneuver (sniff nasal inspiratory pressure, SNIP) which may be easier for patients to perform.[39] This means that measurements can be obtained in a larger population that includes younger patients. Transdiaphragmatic pressure reflects diaphragmatic function specifically but requires the introduction through the nose of sensors to measure gastric and esophageal pressure. These may be small balloons mounted on catheters such as feeding tubes or miniature transducers built into catheters. These measurements are invasive and require the subject to perform respiratory gymnastics. As a result, they are rarely applicable to children. They may be combined with phrenic nerve stimulation to provide a nonvolitional measure of diaphragmatic strength requiring magnetic stimulation of the phrenic nerve at the neck and recording of the transdiaphragmatic pressure. Maximal respiratory pressures, though less invasive than phrenic nerve stimulation, require cooperation, coordination, and motivation. They have been shown to correlate with nonvolitional measurements in different patient groups.[40]

Equipment and Procedure for Measuring Maximal Respiratory Pressures at the Mouth

The facility to measure maximal respiratory pressures at the mouth is incorporated into many proprietary pieces of lung function equipment since the main requirement is a pressure transducer connected to a mouthpiece. Portable equipment is also available.[41] The type of mouthpiece has been shown to influence the measurement and a cylindrical mouthpiece has been shown to result in greater expiratory pressures than a flanged type in children and adolescents.[42] A flanged mouthpiece, however, provides results that are more reproducible than a simple tube and is generally recommended.[43] Clearly the predicted values that are employed should be derived from studies employing the same equipment and mouthpiece if interpretation is to be meaningful. The mouthpiece should be connected to (1) a rigid tube that has a side arm connected to a pressure transducer and (2) a valve that permits regular respiration prior to the measurement and is then closed as the subject makes respiratory efforts. The dead space of the equipment should be minimized. The apparatus should contain a small leak so that the muscles of the mouth cannot be used to increase $P_E$max artifactually and to prevent glottis closure.[44] The leak may be provided by a tube of internal diameter 1–2 mm and length 20–30 mm. A nose clip is not necessary.

The lung volume at which measurements are made influences the pressures that are generated. The $P_I$max is greatest when measured at or close to RV. The largest values of $P_E$max are obtained close to TLC. By convention, measurements are made close to these extremes of vital capacity as well as at FRC and the lung volume at which measurements are made should be recorded. It has been shown that the posture of the child (seated or standing) does not affect the maximal pressures recorded but subjects are usually studied seated.[45] This provides consistency of approach for those children whose conditions will lead to them becoming wheelchair users. An experienced operator should instruct and coach them and provide verbal encouragement to obtain maximum effort. Ideally, each respiratory effort should be maintained for at least 1.5 s so that the maximum pressure sustained for 1 s can be calculated.[46] There are no firm recommendations relating to the number of attempts to be made. The amount of coaching and number of "practice" attempts needed for the child to produce satisfactory measurements is variable. A minimum of three measurements in which the two best results do not differ by more than 5% has been suggested.[45]

In infants, maximal pressures can be measured during crying. A rubber facemask with cushion rim should be firmly applied round the nose and the mouth, which will usually be sufficient to stimulate crying. The mask should be connected to a pressure transducer and recording system. The operator should occlude the mask at the beginning and end of crying efforts to measure peak inspiratory and expiratory pressures, respectively.[47] The facemask should have a small leak to prevent glottis closure during measurement. The maximal expiratory pressure can be measured as a plateau pressure (as for older children) but maximal inspiratory pressure will be measured as a peak. It is not possible to record the lung volume at which the pressures are measured.

Equipment and Procedure for Measuring Sniff Pressure

SNIP is an easier technique for children to perform than measurement of pressures at the mouth because it avoids the need for a mouthpiece and does not require maintenance of effort for over 1 s. Pressure is measured via a catheter inserted into one nostril which is occluded with any suitable moldable material such as eartips designed for auditory evoked potentials. The pressure change recorded during a sniff is very rapid so the pressure transducer and the recording system need to have a high frequency response. The catheter should be as short as is practicable.[44]

When the catheter has been positioned and the nostril plugged, the child should be seated comfortably and the system checked for leaks. This is done by transiently closing the unobstructed nostril with a finger and asking the child to sniff. Having ascertained that the equipment is properly positioned and leak-free in one nostril, the child is instructed to sniff through the unobstructed nostril while ensuring that the mouth remains closed. Maximal efforts are obtained as the subject makes short, sharp sniffs, and visual feedback (e.g. computer screen) and verbal encouragement from the operator are helpful.[48] Sniffs should be separated by 30 s and commence at the end of a tidal exhalation. A learning effect has been documented in several patient groups[48] such that a series of 20 sniffs is recommended. Not all children were able to perform this number of sniffs but in those who could not the best SNIP was obtained in measurements after the tenth sniff.

Indices

For both SNIP and maximal pressures recorded at the mouth the highest values should be recorded. It is usual to ensure that the two highest recorded values differ by less than 5%. In infants the maximum pressures recorded during crying should be recorded, but these should be interpreted cautiously since predicted values are less well established than those for children.[47] In patients with a severe restrictive ventilatory defect, it is advisable to use both tests.[49]

Interpretation

Predicted values of maximal pressures from children have been reported.[50–52] In all studies, there is considerable variability in the measurements. Pressures are greater in boys than girls, even before puberty. In both sexes, the absolute values are primarily related to age rather than height. The inclusion of height in prediction equations for maximal pressures has a greater impact on variability for boys than girls.

The variability of the indices means that isolated measurements in individuals may be difficult to interpret unless the measurement is well within the range of prediction, which may rule out significant muscle weakness. Sequential measurements are useful in charting progression of condition.

Knowledge of lung volumes aids interpretation. A child with a skeletal abnormality, for example, may have reduced maximal expiratory pressures as a consequence of having a reduced TLC. The pattern of reduction in pressures may also be helpful since normal maximal expiratory pressures in conjunction with reduced maximal inspiratory pressures can be indicative of isolated diaphragmatic weakness, something that could be further investigated by phrenic nerve stimulation.

Application

The primary application of measurements of maximum respiratory pressures is in assessment and monitoring of patients with respiratory muscle weakness. This may be particularly relevant in presurgical assessment since diaphragm contractility has been shown to be reduced during administration of nitrous oxide.[53] Patients with already compromised diaphragmatic function may therefore be potentially placed at risk of diaphragmatic fatigue if nitrous oxide is administered.

Contribution of Respiratory Function Tests

The indications for respiratory function testing are widespread and results are important for medical management, especially for asthma and cystic fibrosis. The contribution of lung function testing to surgical management of children is of equal importance although the number of children involved will be considerably smaller. Respiratory function testing may be important in the evaluation of anesthetic risk, or because of possible respiratory complications after surgery. Whatever the indication, it is important that children are evaluated in a specialist pediatric laboratory if possible, or at least by staff experienced in assessment of children. This is vital for young children, not only because the testing requires that the operator be skilled at working with children but also because the tests require more time, and equipment for testing may need modification such as use of smaller mouthpieces and incorporation of visual incentives for spirometry. Of equal importance is the interpretation of tests since most commercially available pieces of equipment generate predicted values based on sex and height of the patient. These predicted values are rarely derived from populations including children below 115 cm height. When testing a smaller child predicted values will be obtained by extrapolation and therefore should be viewed with extreme caution. Furthermore, the sensitivity and the specificity of any index of lung function may well be different in young children than in adults, so that the classification into "normal" and "abnormal" may have different boundaries. The use of arbitrary cutoffs (e.g., 80% predicted) is to be discouraged in the evaluation of individual patients since it has no basis other than familiarity,[54] although expression of data as percentage of predicted is frequently employed in research studies or reports of patient series.

Respiratory function testing is important to provide data on outcomes of surgical procedures in different conditions. This may have prognostic importance for individuals but is also relevant for healthcare planning. A large follow-up study of respiratory function following repair of diaphragmatic hernia showed a range of outcomes, from individuals with normal function who were able to participate in competitive sports to others with markedly reduced performance.[55] There are two major drawbacks to large follow-up studies. The first is the time period over which data were collected (26 years in this case). Management at the time of intervention and postoperative care may well alter over this time course, which will impact on survival and morbidity. The other drawback may be the relatively small size of the follow-up cohort. Only 45 of the 83 survivors in this example were studied and the outcomes may be subject to bias. Despite these caveats, vital capacity was normal in the 29 patients in whom it was measured. FEV_1 was also within normal limits for these individuals, but none of the group had an FEV_1 greater than the predicted value, i.e., this index of lung function was reduced for the group as a whole. A proportion of those studied had evidence of hyperinflation and others had reduced mid-expiratory flows. Scintigraphic ventilation studies showed normal distribution of ventilation in 77% of those tested, and the abnormal findings were seen in patients with skeletal defects or diaphragmatic adhesions. Although the overall outcome of diaphragmatic hernia repair may be encouraging, emerging tests of function such as hyperpolarized helium-3 MRI scanning[56] will be needed to show whether alveolar size differs between the two lungs. This in turn will show whether the (relatively) normal lung volume results from an increase in number of alveoli of expected size or an overexpansion of a smaller number of alveoli on the affected side.

The relationships between severity of the original condition, clinical findings, and respiratory function are complex and may change with growth and time between studies. In a study of 16 infants with tracheoesophageal fistula repair, abnormalities of lung function measured within 3 months of repair broadly reflected the severity of the clinical problems encountered, and at 1 year of age those who had good function and few symptoms initially remained well.[57] Those shown to have marked abnormalities were more likely to have troublesome symptoms and three went on to have tracheopexy, which resulted in immediate improvement in two of them. The third child also had aortopexy but still failed to improve and subsequently died. Although this study concluded that infant respiratory function testing could provide a general guide to likely clinical progress, this was not entirely borne out by a subsequent study of all survivors at school age.[58] Clinical findings and respiratory function showed limited relationship to status in infancy. Previous studies of respiratory function in adult survivors of tracheoesophageal fistula repair had reported a mildly restrictive pattern of lung function.[59,60] Confirmation of this finding in the study of Agrawal et al. indicated that the restrictive pattern was more likely to result from reduced lung

growth rather than being a concomitant feature of the primary congenital abnormality.

Adolescent idiopathic scoliosis is common, affecting 2% of the population.[61] Impairment of pulmonary function is the most serious consequence of this condition and in severe, untreated cases can lead to cardiopulmonary failure. The relationship between spinal deformity and lung function is complex; the angle of scoliosis alone is not sufficient for pulmonary impairment to be inferred.[62] Extensive studies of radiologic measurements in patients with scoliosis showed that the factors predicting a restrictive pattern of lung function were the angle of scoliosis, number of vertebrae involved, cephalad location of the curve, and loss of normal thoracic kyphosis. Measurements of maximal pressures, FEFs, and gas transfer were also reduced, although the range of function was wide. The assessment of patients with scoliosis should not focus exclusively on the radiological measurements but should include functional measurements in addition.[62] In those patients having surgery for adolescent idiopathic scoliosis, preoperative respiratory function is the most important predictor of function measured 2 years postoperatively, but surgical approach also influenced final outcome.[63] An open anterior thoracic approach and a thoracoplasty were both associated with a small decrease in vital capacity and TLC, although the impact was small.[63]

The options available for treatment of some children with thoracic hypoplasia and scoliosis have widened with the development of the vertical expandable prosthetic titanium rib (VEPTR).[64] In a series of ten children (median age 4.3 years at onset) serial measurements of lung function have been made under anesthesia using a forced deflation device. The lungs can be inflated to a preset pressure ($+40\,cmH_2O$) at the endotracheal tube which can then be connected to a negative pressure reservoir (set to $-40\,cmH_2O$) resulting in a MEF-volume curve, albeit one constrained by the endotracheal tube and with the "TLC" and "RV" determined by the applied pressures.[65] Nevertheless, the unique and valuable data so obtained from serial measurements has demonstrated the absolute increase in FVC in these children, many of whom would be too young for conventional spirometric measurements. In most cases, FVC was reduced at the time of the first surgery but was maintained in line with growth in height.

The commonest chest wall deformity seen by pediatricians and in general practice is that of pectus excavatum, which occurs in approximately 8 per 1,000 live births.[66,67] Although psychological problems may predominate in younger patients,[68] severe defects result in functional abnormalities of variable severity.[69,70] Evaluation of the condition may involve chest radiographs and CT scanning to determine the pectus index and fast MRI scanning to examine the degree of cardiac displacement and unusual diaphragmatic excursions.[71] Spirometry and plethysmography confirm a restrictive pattern of lung function although the reductions in vital capacity and TLC are modest.[72–74] Following surgical correction there may be an initial worsening of lung function which then returns to preoperative levels.[72] Patients usually report subjective improvement in breathlessness and exercise tolerance. Despite the generally good outcome, extensive surgery performed at a young age (below 4 years) can result in marked restriction of chest wall growth so that vital capacity in teenage years is less than half the expected value requiring chest cavity expansion surgery.[75]

Conclusions

Lung function testing in children and infants, once the preserve of a few laboratories with dedicated staff, has become much more important in the past 20 years. The applications have grown in line with improved technology and increased attention to standardization of protocols. Development of robust prediction equations has aided the interpretation of data, both in a clinical setting and in a research. Ongoing development of new measurements and refinement of procedures will continue to provide challenges to the respiratory physiologist and, hopefully, benefits to children with respiratory disorders and those who care for them.

References

1. Auchincloss JH. Preoperative evaluation of pulmonary function. Surg Clin N Am 1974; 54: 1015–1026
2. Cetindag IB, Olson W, Hazelrigg SR. Acute and chronic reduction of pulmonary function after lung surgery. Thorac Surg Clin 2004; 14: 317–323
3. American Thoracic Society. Standardization of spirometry: 1994 update. Am J Respir Crit Care Med 1995; 152: 1107–1136
4. Arets HG, Brackel HJ, van der Ent CK. Forced expiratory manoeuvres in children: do they meet ATS and ERS criteria for spirometry? Eur Respir J 2001; 18: 655–660
5. Zapletal A, Chalupova J. Forced expiratory parameters in healthy preschool children (3–6 years of age). Pediatr Pulmonol 2003; 35: 200–207
6. Eigen H, Bieler H, Grant D, et al. Spirometric pulmonary function in healthy preschool children. Am J Respir Crit Care Med 2001; 163: 619–623
7. Vilozni D, Barker M, Jellouschek H, et al. An interactive computer-animated system (Spirogame) facilitates spirometry in preschool children. Am J Respir Crit Care Med 2001; 164: 2200–2205
8. Aurora P, Stocks J, Oliver C, et al. Quality control for spirometry in preschool children with and without lung disease. Am J Respir Crit Care Med 2004; 169: 1152–1159
9. Lum S, Stocks J, Castile R, Davis S, et al. ATS-ERS Consensus Statement. Raised volume forced expirations in infants: guidelines for current practice. Am J Respir Crit Care Med 2005; 172: 1463–1471
10. Wensley DC, Pickering D, Silverman M. Can peak expiratory flow be measured accurately during a forced vital capacity manoeuvre? Eur Respir J 2000; 16: 673–676
11. Merkus PJFM, de Jongste JC, Stocks J. Respiratory function measurements in infants and children. Eur Respir Mon 2005; 31: 166–194
12. Rosenthal M, Bain SH, Cramer D, et al. Lung function in white children aged 4 to 19 years: I – Spirometry. Thorax 1993; 48: 794–802.
13. Hoo A-F, Dezateux C, Hanrahan J, et al. Sex-specific prediction equations for V'max FRC in infancy: a multicentre collaborative study. Am J Respir Crit Care Med 2002; 165: 1084–1092.
14. Wanger J, Clausen JL, Coates A, et al. Standardisation of the measurement of lung volumes. Eur Respir J 2005; 26: 511–522
15. Beardsmore CS, Stocks J, Silverman M. Problems in the measurement of thoracic gas volume in infancy. J Appl Physiol 1982; 53: 698–702
16. Rodenstein DO, Stanescu DC, Francis C. Demonstration of failure of body plethysmography in airway obstruction. J Appl Physiol 1982; 52: 949–954
17. Beardsmore CS, Paton JY, Thompson JR, et al. Standardising lung function laboratories for multicentre trials. Pediatr Pulmonol 2007; 42: 51–59
18. Stocks J, Godfrey S, Beardsmore CS, et al. Standards for infant respiratory function testing: plethysmographic measurements of lung volume and airway resistance. Eur Respir J 2001; 17: 302–312
19. Beardsmore CS, MacFadyen UM, Moosavi SSH, et al. Measurement of lung volumes during active and quiet sleep in infants. Pediatr Pulmonol 1989; 7: 71–77.
20. Rosenthal M, Cramer D, Bain SH, et al. Lung function in white children aged 9 to 14 years: II – single breath analysis and plethysmography. Thorax 1993; 48: 803–808
21. Manzke H, Stadlober E, Schellauf H-P. Combined body plethysmographic, spirometric and flow-volume reference values for male and female children aged 6 to 16 years obtained from 'hospital normals'. Eur J Pediatr 2001; 160: 300–306
22. Hibbert ME, Lannigan A, Landau LI, Phelan PD. Lung function values from a longitudinal study of healthy children and adolescents. Pediatr Pulmonol 1989; 7: 101–109
23. Moriette G, Chaussain M, Radvanyi Buovet MF, et al. Functional residual capacity and sleep states in the premature newborn. Biol Neonate 1983; 43: 125–133
24. Taussig LM, Harris TR, Lebowitz MD. Lung function in infants and young children. Am Rev Respir Dis 1977; 116: 233–239
25. Tepper RS, Morgan WJ, Cota K, et al. Physiologic growth and development of the lung during the first year of life. Am Rev Respir Dis 1986; 134: 513–519
26. Gappa M, Fletcher ME, Dezateux CA, Stocks J. Comparison of nitrogen washout and plethysmographic measurements of lung volume in healthy infants. Am Rev Respir Dis 1993; 148: 1496–1501
27. Greenough A, Stocks J, Nothen U, Helms P. Total respiratory compliance and functional respiratory capacity in young children. Pediatr Pulmonol 1986; 2: 321–326
28. Dimitriou G, Greenough A, Kavvadia V, et al. Diaphragmatic function in infants with surgically corrected anomalies. Pediatr Res 2003; 54: 502–508
29. Beardsmore CS, Dundas I, Poole K, et al. Respiratory function in survivors of the UK ECMO trial. Am J Respir Crit Care Med 2000; 161: 1129–1135
30. Wall MA, Misley MC, Brown AC, et al. Relationship between maldistribution of ventilation and airways obstruction in children with asthma. Respir Physiol 1987; 69: 287–297
31. Aurora P, Gustaffson PM, Bush A, et al. Multiple breath inert gas washout as a measure of ventilation distribution in children with cystic fibrosis. Thorax 2004; 59: 1068–1073
32. Gustaffson PM, Aurora P, Lindblad A. Evaluation of ventilation maldistribution as an early indicator of lung disease in children with cystic fibrosis. Eur Respir J 2003; 22: 972–979

4
Radiology of the Chest

Rosemary J. Arthur and Jennette Kraft

Introduction

Diagnostic imaging plays a crucial role in the safe practice of pediatric thoracic surgery. The pediatric thoracic surgeon must not only understand current imaging modalities but also appreciate the merits and limitations of each technique. Underlying any request for radiological imaging is the need to obtain information to guide management. This may be to confirm or refute a particular diagnosis, to guide the surgical approach, or to enable the clinician to advise parents and children about prognosis. Increasingly imaging is used to guide interventional radiological procedures including biopsy, abscess and fluid drainage, dilatation of strictures, and vascular embolization.

Requesting Imaging

"Making the Best Use of a Department of Clinical Radiology" published by The Royal College of Radiologists, provides evidence-based guidelines for most imaging investigations.[1] These guidelines draw attention to the common causes of unnecessary investigation. These include performing the wrong examination because of inadequate clinical information on the request card and repeat examinations as a substitute for obtaining imaging and reports from another hospital. Without exception it is better to discuss complex clinical problems directly with the radiologist to ensure that the most appropriate examination is undertaken.

Care of the Patient

Patient safety is of paramount importance. Informed consent for radiological investigation involves discussion with parents and children. Verbal consent is usually sufficient although written consent should be obtained for interventional procedures where there is significant risk of complications. Following the study the results and implications should be communicated to the parents and the child.

Risks and benefits must be considered when requesting a radiological investigation. These include the risks of transportation of a sick child to the radiology department, the risks of the procedure including administration of contrast media, exposure to ionizing radiation, specific procedural risks, and the risks of sedation or anesthesia, if required.

Risks Associated with Ionizing Radiation

Radiography, fluoroscopy, CT scanning, angiography, and nuclear medicine examinations all expose the patient to the potentially harmful effects of ionizing radiation. Although the risk is small, the relative risks of the various investigations should be appreciated (Table 4.1). There is much debate about the precise level of risk but it is generally accepted that radiation risk is cumulative over the lifetime of a patient. Children are at a greater risk of long-term effects because of their longer life expectancy and the greater sensitivity of growing tissues to ionizing radiation. The excess life-time risk of developing fatal cancer following exposure to ionizing radiation in childhood is approximately two to fourfold greater than following identical exposure in adult life. Exposure as a neonate is thought to carry a substantially higher risk of up to 10–15 times. These estimated additional risks must be balanced against the background incidence for the life-time development of fatal cancer of one in three of the population as a whole. Although CT scanning accounts for approximately 5% of all imaging, it is responsible for approximately half of the radiation dose to the population from medical exposure. While CT scanning is undoubtedly an important diagnostic tool, consideration should be given to ultrasound or MRI scanning whenever possible.[1–3]

Use of Contrast Media

Radiographic contrast media are associated with a number of risks depending on the route of administration and the specific properties of the contrast agent. Oral contrast media for outlining the esophagus and stomach include Barium sulphate solution and water-soluble agents. Although Barium sulphate solution

D.H. Parikh et al. (eds.), *Pediatric Thoracic Surgery*,
DOI: 10.1007/b136543_4, © Springer-Verlag London Limited 2009

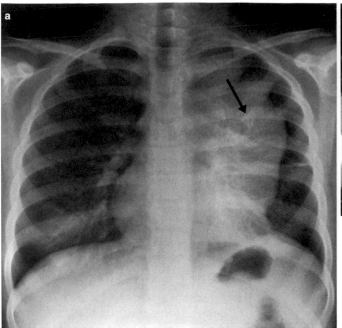

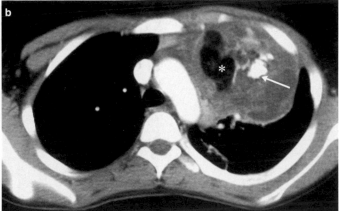

FIG. 4.6. (**a**) Chest X-ray shows widening of the mediastinum with obliteration of the aortic knuckle indicating an anterior or middle mediastinal mass. A faint opacity due to calcification is seen within the mass (*arrow*). (**b**) A contrast-enhanced CT scan demonstrates a complex mass of mixed attenuation containing low density fatty tissue (*asterisk*), calcification (*arrow*). Excision biopsy confirmed the diagnosis of a mature mediastinal teratoma

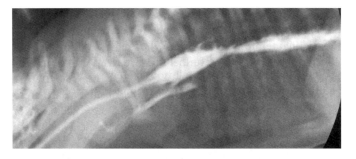

FIG. 4.7. Prone tube injection oesophagram demonstrating an H-type tracheo-esophageal fistula, with contrast medium seen extending obliquely from the junction of the cervicothoracic esophagus to the trachea

The Heart and Great Vessels

The transverse diameter of a normal heart may approach 60% of the transverse diameter of the thorax in an infant. An expiratory phase radiograph may exaggerate the heart size further. Dextroposition of the heart and the position of the gastric air bubble should be noted as complex congenital heart disease is often present where cardiac and visceral situs are incongruent, e.g., dextrocardia with left-sided stomach. A right-sided aortic arch is frequently seen in association with Tetralogy of Fallot and in association with vascular rings.[27]

An increase in cardiac size should prompt a close inspection of the lungs to assess pulmonary vascularity. A reduction in pulmonary blood flow, e.g., in pulmonary atresia is demonstrated by the presence of oligaemic lungs where there is poor visualization of pulmonary vessels in the central half of the lungs. Branches of the pulmonary arteries should not be visible in the peripheral third of the lung and if seen indicate increased pulmonary blood flow often due to a left to right shunt, e.g., a ventricular septal defect. Where there is any suspicion of an underlying cardiac disorder, an echocardiogram is necessary to determine whether the abnormality is structural, i.e., due to congenital heart disease acquired, e.g., a viral myocarditis or due to a pericardial effusion.

Lungs/Pleural Cavities

Both hemithoraces should be of equal size and of symmetrical lung density. The basic patterns of abnormality identified in the lungs and pleural cavities can be divided broadly into general or focal areas of:

- Increased opacification
- Increased translucency
- Ring shadows
- Pulmonary nodule(s)
- Increased pulmonary opacification

Increased opacification of a hemithorax may caused by decreased aeration of the lung, e.g., pulmonary collapse, pulmonary infiltrates (consolidation and interstitial fibrosis, agenesis) or mass (tumor, congenital malformation, pleural fluid/tumor), and abnormalities of the chest wall.

Pulmonary collapse is often focal giving rise to linear densities in the lung, although it can involve the whole of one lobe or whole lung. The hallmark of significant pulmonary collapse is an area of increased opacity associated with loss of volume. The latter will alter the position of the major fissures and/or the hilar shadows. If the whole lung collapses, the mediastinum will shift toward the collapse and the ipsilateral diaphragm will rise.

There are two basic patterns of pulmonary infiltration on a chest X-ray: air space shadowing and interstitial infiltration (Fig. 4.8a, b). Air space shadowing, often referred to as consolidation, is caused by fluid or pus within the alveoli. Infection, aspiration, pulmonary hemorrhage, and pulmonary edema are the commonest causes of air space shadowing, which generally appears as a homogeneous opacity with visible air bronchograms. Consolidation due to infection is frequently segmental or lobar in distribution whereas a more generalized "white out" of both lungs has a wide differential diagnosis including pulmonary edema, cardiac or noncardiac, drowning, aspiration, and opportunistic Infection. Radiological interpretation relies on correlation with the clinical setting. In neonates, surfactant deficiency disease, acute pulmonary edema, and congestive cardiac failure are the most frequent causes.

Interstitial infiltration results from thickening of the pulmonary interstitium or alveolar walls. Likely causes are inflammation, fibrosis, infiltration, and increased interstitial fluid. Interstitial shadowing tends to be more heterogeneous than air space shadowing with a linear or nodular pattern which may be associated with septal lines and bronchial wall thickening due to peribronchial inflammation and edema. In the acute situation, interstitial shadowing is often caused by acute pulmonary edema. In the neonate, this is particularly associated with total anomalous pulmonary venous return with obstructed venous drainage. In an older child, this is seen typically following acute fluid retention and in Mycoplasma pneumonia where there may be a combination of both interstitial and air space shadowing. When associated with a more chronic history, pulmonary interstitial disease is more likely and HRCT may be necessary to clarify the diagnosis.[15,28]

Pleural Fluid

In the supine position, a pleural effusion appears as a generalized increased opacity of the hemithorax, whereas in the erect position the classical crescentic opacity in the pleural space is generally present. Preservation of normal lung markings "through" the opacity is an Indication that the opacification is not arising from within the lung but due to pleural fluid, particularly if loculated. The hallmark of a large pleural effusion is the presence of mass effect with shift of the mediastinum to the contralateral side, as opposed to collapse where there is shift to the ipsilateral side (Fig. 4.9). No mediastinal shift is usually present with lobar consolidation. Pleural effusions may occur in conjunction with collapse of the underlying lung in which case there will be less or no mediastinal shift.

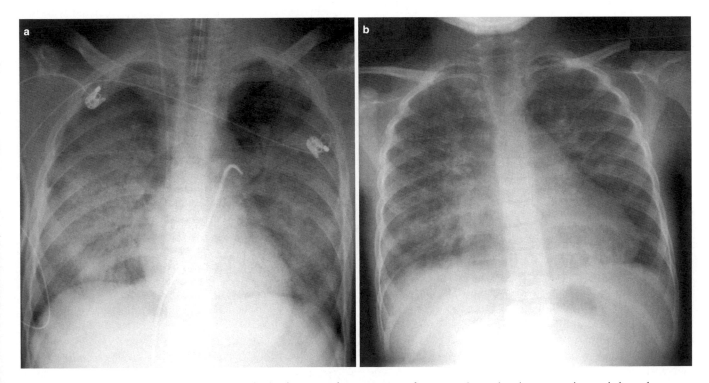

FIG. 4.8. Pulmonary infiltrates. (a) Air space shadowing secondary to acute pulmonary edema showing a prominent air bronchograms. (b) Interstitial shadowing due to acute interstitial pulmonary edema with a predominantly linear pattern

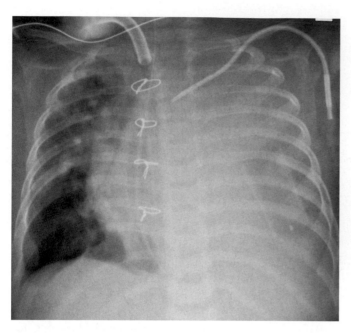

FIG. 4.9. Large left pleural effusion displacing the mediastinum to the right. Note the proximal position of the tip of the central line, which slipped back after placement, causing iatrogenic leakage of the infusate into the pleural cavity

Tumor

A tumor arising in the lung, mediastinum, or chest wall is often manifest by a large opacity or even a completely opaque hemithorax with contralateral shift of the mediastinum due to the mass effect. It may be difficult to differentiate a large tumor from a large pleural effusion on a plain film. The presence of rib destruction or erosion and calcification within a mass all points to an underlying tumor.

Further imaging of pulmonary opacification depends on the clinical situation. Children who present with signs of infection, show typical radiological appearances of lobar pneumonia, and who respond to antibiotics rapidly need no further imaging. There is no good evidence to support the need to follow radiograph in this group.[29] If recovery is incomplete a further chest radiograph may be helpful after an interval of 4–6 weeks. Follow-up radiography should be performed earlier if the clinical condition dictates in case complications such as an empyema, pulmonary abscess, or pneumatocoele are developing. Further investigations are required for children with recurrent pulmonary infections. A contrast swallow and meal possibly supplemented with a prone tube esophagram will be required to investigate suspected aspiration from gastroesophageal reflux or an H-type tracheoesophageal fistula. Swallowing video fluoroscopy will be more appropriate for the child thought to have a swallowing disorder. The possibility of cystic fibrosis and immunodeficiency should also be considered. HRCT is superior to chest radiography to demonstrate bronchiectasis. Repeated infection involving the same lobe or segment, particularly at the left base, should raise the possibility of an extralobar pulmonary sequestration (see below).

An ultrasound examination is the next most appropriate investigation in children with signs of pleural fluid on a plain film. Ultrasound will confirm the size of the effusion and indicate the presence of loculations and the degree of organization and the presence of pleural thickening (Fig. 4.10a, b). The results may help to determine whether aspiration or drainage is feasible in children with an empyema. Ultrasound may demonstrate collapse or consolidation of the underlying lung and sometimes areas of lung necrosis are visible. In complicated pneumonias, CT scanning with intravenous contrast provides better imaging of the lung parenchyma and pleural cavities but this examination should not be considered routine. Although US may demonstrate the presence of tumor or tumor deposits within the pleural space, CT scanning is necessary for staging.

Opacification due to pulmonary collapse associated with an acute asthmatic attack or following surgery does not require follow-up imaging. Bronchoscopy is advised if there is a history of foreign body inhalation or where the cause is uncertain. CT scanning may then be indicated if the pulmonary collapse remains unexplained or if an extrinsic bronchial compression has been demonstrated on bronchoscopy.

Increased Translucency

Generalized increased translucency may be seen if the child makes an exuberant inspiratory effort. This is frequently noted in children with congenital heart disease and metabolic acidosis where compensatory hyperinflation often occurs in the absence of pulmonary disease. Generalized increased translucency due to over inflation is usually associated with low flattened diaphragms and there may be intercostal herniation of lung. Bilateral overinflation is a feature of peripheral air trapping, e.g., in bronchiolitis and cystic fibrosis. Central air trapping is seen secondary to tracheal obstructions from tumor, impacted foreign bodies, and vascular rings. A long-standing esophageal foreign body impacted above the thoracic inlet may result in localized inflammation with subsequent extrinsic compression and narrowing of the trachea.

Asymmetrical translucency of the two hemithoraces is an important sign requiring further investigation. This may be an artifact due to patient rotation but the possibility of air trapping, e.g., from an inhaled foreign body must be considered and a repeat straight radiograph obtained. It may be difficult to determine which side is abnormal when the two lungs are of different densities, but consideration of the following points, as described by Swischuk should help[30]:

- *Pulmonary vascularity:* The side with decreased vascularity is abnormal, whereas the side with increased or normal vascularity is usually normal.
- *Variation in appearance* between inspiratory and expiratory films is particularly valuable. The side which changes least is usually abnormal.
- *The size of the hemithorax* is a useful pointer in which a small completely opaque hemithorax is always abnormal.

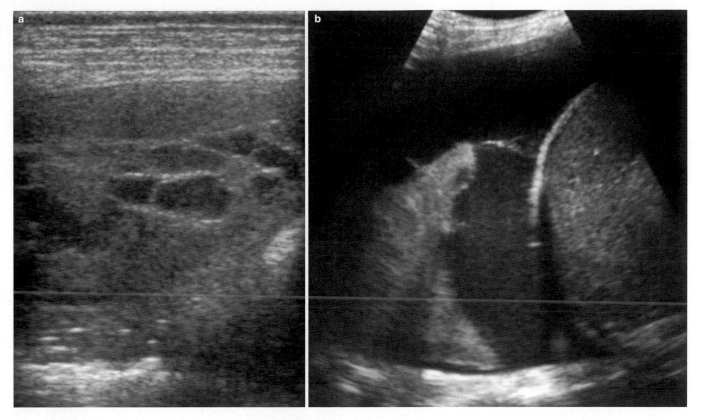

FIG. 4.10. Ultrasound scans of the pleural cavity showing (**a**) organized pleural exudate typical of an empyema and (**b**) free fluid in the pleural cavity. The increased echogenicity of the fluid indicates high protein content, consistent with an exudate or hemorrhage

It may be difficult to perform plain X-rays in both inspiration and expiration in a young child. Fluoroscopic examination is an option. An alternative approach is to obtain two lateral decubitus frontal views of the chest, one with the left side down and one with the left side raised. The dependent lung will effectively be in expiration because of the weight of the mediastinum. The degree of change of each lung can be assessed and air trapping confirmed of excluded.

If unilateral overinflation is present, it is necessary to determine whether this is due to compensatory or obstructive emphysema. Compensatory emphysema occurs following pneumonectomy or in the presence of contralateral collapse or agenesis. In this circumstance, the normal emphysematous lung inflates and deflates appropriately and pulmonary vascularity is normal or increased. In obstructive emphysema, characteristically from an inhaled foreign body, there will be limited or no deflation of the affected lung on expiration and pulmonary vascularity will be decreased. Further investigation depends on the mode of presentation. If the child presents with acute onset respiratory distress, bronchoscopy will be indicated as an inhaled foreign body is likely even when no specific history is given. In younger children an underling lung/bronchial abnormality is more likely, e.g., a pulmonary artery sling or a bronchogenic cyst, obstructing the bronchus resulting in unilateral or bilateral obstructive emphysema.

In congenital lobar emphysema, over inflation is most often confined to a single lobe generally with compression, and subsequent collapse of the other ipsilateral lobes and the contralateral lung. In these cases, contrast-enhanced CT or MRI should identify the underlying cause. Radionuclide scintigraphy can give good functional assessment of both ventilation and perfusion and confirm the presence of air trapping which may be helpful in evaluating asymmetrical hypertranslucency. However, following improvement in CT techniques and difficulties in performing radionuclide scans in young children, this modality is used infrequently.

Air Leaks

Free air is more difficult to detect on a supine chest X-ray than an erect film. Features suggestive of free air include translucency adjacent to the heart border associated with increased sharpness of the mediastinal structures and increased depth and translucency of the lateral costophrenic angle – the deep sulcus sign. If the air leak is large the lung edge may be visible. If the pneumothorax is under tension, the mediastinum will shift to the contralateral side and the diaphragm will flatten or evert. Air–fluid levels within a hydropneumothorax will require a horizontal beam projection for demonstration.

Mediastinal air results in increased clarity of the mediastinal outline. This may extend into the superior mediastinum as linear translucencies and into the neck as surgical emphysema.

It may be difficult to distinguish mediastinal air from a pneumothorax but a lateral decubitus view with the suspicious side raised may demonstrate a free lung edge below the costal margin whereas air in the mediastinum will stay central in position. Air around the thymus, in a lateral shoot through projection, confirms the presence of mediastinal air. CT is very sensitive for detection of small amounts of free air. This is particularly valuable following trauma or where ventilation is increasingly difficult without explanation.[31]

Pulmonary Masses and Nodules

The commonest cause of a round opacity on a chest X-ray is a "round pneumonia" which is often associated with pneumococcal infection. Correlation with clinical features will usually confirm the diagnosis in which case further imaging is not required. Other causes of round opacities include loculated pleural fluid, posttraumatic contusion, fluid-filled peripheral bronchogenic cyst, vascular malformation, and malignancy although primary pulmonary malignancy is rare in children. Although the presence of multiple nodules of varying sizes is suspicious of pulmonary metastatic disease, multifocal nodules may also be caused by infection, including fungal infection, granulomas, papillomatosis, and multiple emboli including septic emboli. Contrast-enhanced CT scanning is particularly helpful in defining the number, nature, and distribution of nodules, and is more sensitive than chest radiography for the development of cavitation suggesting infection as the underlying cause (Fig. 4.11a–c). CT scanning can be used to guide percutaneous abscess drainage and biopsy of larger nodules.

Ring Shadows

The term "ring shadow" is used to describe a well-defined cystic areas of increased translucency. These may be large or small, multiple or solitary. Pneumatocoeles are the commonest case of a solitary ring shadow although the differential diagnosis includes a congenital lung cyst, a solitary bullus, and a loculated pneumothorax. The presence of a thick or irregular wall is suggestive of an abscess or necrotic tumor. Infected pneumatocoeles may contain fluid and appear opaque on a supine X-ray. A number of congenital lesions of the thorax may also present as a solitary lung cyst, but multiple ring shadows in association with mass effect are more frequent and seen in congenital diaphragmatic hernia and congenital cystic adenomatoid malformation (CCAM). Extralobar sequestrations may also present as predominantly cystic lesion. Many congenital thoracic lesions are nowadays diagnosed prenatally. Postnatal ultrasound can readily distinguish a congenital diaphragmatic hernia and a CCAM. Color flow imaging may demonstrate a juxta-diaphragmatic echogenic mass with an aberrant blood supply from the aorta, indicating an extralobar sequestration. CT or MRI is wise prior to surgical resection of a congenital lung lesion to demonstrate the extent of pulmonary involvement, exclude abnormality in other lobes and

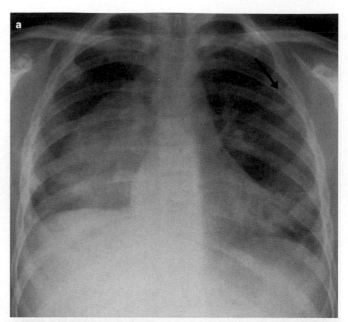

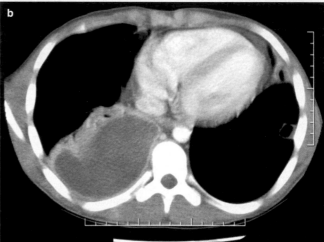

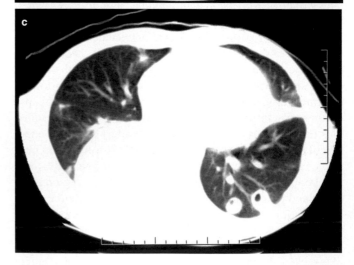

FIG. 4.11. Teenage intravenous drug addict with an empyema and multiple septic emboli. (a) Chest X-ray demonstrates well-demarcated opacity at the right lung base with lung markings clearly visible "through" the opacity due to loculated pleural fluid. Several nodules

identify arterial blood supply and venous drainage. The latter is particularly important with right-sided pulmonary sequestrations which may be associated with anomalous venous drainage of the right lung in the Scimitar syndrome.[32,33]

Diaphragms

Loss of clarity of one or both diaphragms indicates loss of aeration at the lung base either due to pulmonary collapse or due to the presence of a mass/fluid between the lung base and the diaphragm. Loss of clarity of the right hemidiaphragm in association with a small hemithorax secondary to pulmonary hypoplasia should raise a suspicion of Scimitar syndrome. CT or MRI will clarify the pulmonary venous drainage, which may be anomalous.

There are a number of possible explanations for apparent elevation of the diaphragm. These include a congenital diaphragmatic hernia (either the Bochdalek or Morgagni type), traumatic diaphragmatic rupture, diaphragmatic eventration, loss of lung volume, e.g., lung hypoplasia, a subpulmonary effusion and a subphrenic collection. Most congenital diaphragmatic hernias, particularly the Bochdalek type, are readily diagnosed on a plain film which includes the thorax and the abdomen. The differential diagnosis usually lies between a congenital diaphragmatic hernia and a CCAM. In the former, there is a paucity of gas in the abdomen because the midgut has herniated into the thorax and in the latter the intestinal gas pattern is normal. In some cases, particularly right-sided hernias, or if the X-ray has been taken very early before the bowel has filled with air, the appearances may be confusing. Ultrasound may clarify the diagnosis. CT should be performed if diaphragmatic rupture is suspected following trauma, partly to exclude coexisting abdominal visceral injury (Fig. 4.12a, b). The multiplanar capabilities of MRI can be particularly useful as a "problem-solving" tool if there is difficulty distinguishing an eventration from a Bochdalek hernia.

Ultrasound assessment of diaphragmatic movement is an alternative to fluoroscopy for the assessment of diaphragmatic paralysis seen most frequently following cardiac surgery or in children with neuromuscular disorders. The examination must be performed with spontaneous ventilation and no positive end expiratory pressure applied.

Thoracic Skeleton and Soft Tissues

Assessment of the chest X-ray is incomplete until the thoracic skeleton and soft tissues have been assessed. Air in the soft tissues of the neck may be a sign of a retropharyngeal abscess

FIG. 4.11. (continued) are seen in the lungs some of which show central cavitation (*arrow*). CT was performed to assess the extent of the pulmonary involvement. (**b, c**) Contrast-enhanced CT scan defined the number and distribution of the cavitating nodules and confirmed the presence of a loculated pleural effusion but showed no evidence of a necrotizing pneumonia at the right lung base

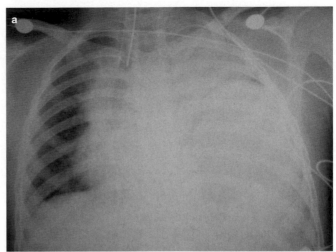

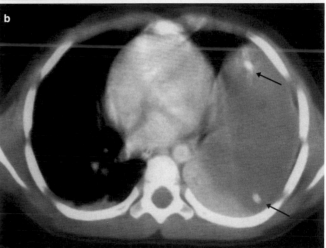

FIG. 4.12. (**a**) Supine chest X-ray following trauma shows opacification of the left hemithorax and displacement of the mediastinum (note endotracheal tube position). (**b**) Contrast-enhanced CT scan shows a nasogastric tube (*arrow*) within the stomach which has herniated through the diaphragm into the left chest to lie at the same level as the heart

or penetrating injury to the neck or pharynx (Fig. 4.13a, b). Surgical emphysema may be seen in association with mediastinal air following esophageal rupture.

Generalized abnormality of the thoracic skeleton is a useful marker of underlying metabolic bone disease, e.g., a rickety rosary or skeletal dysplasia. Detection of an unexplained old or new rib fracture in an infant raises the possibility of non-accidental injury and appropriate pediatric medical advice should be sought. Rib destruction, particularly in association with a soft tissue mass, indicates chest wall infection or malignancy. Displacement and scalloping of a rib and widening of the intervertebral canal are typical of benign neurogenic tumors, e.g., a neurofibroma. Generalized abnormalities of the chest wall may alter the translucency of the lungs. Chest wall thickening from burns or edema will decrease translucency. A decrease in chest wall thickness may be seen in Poland's

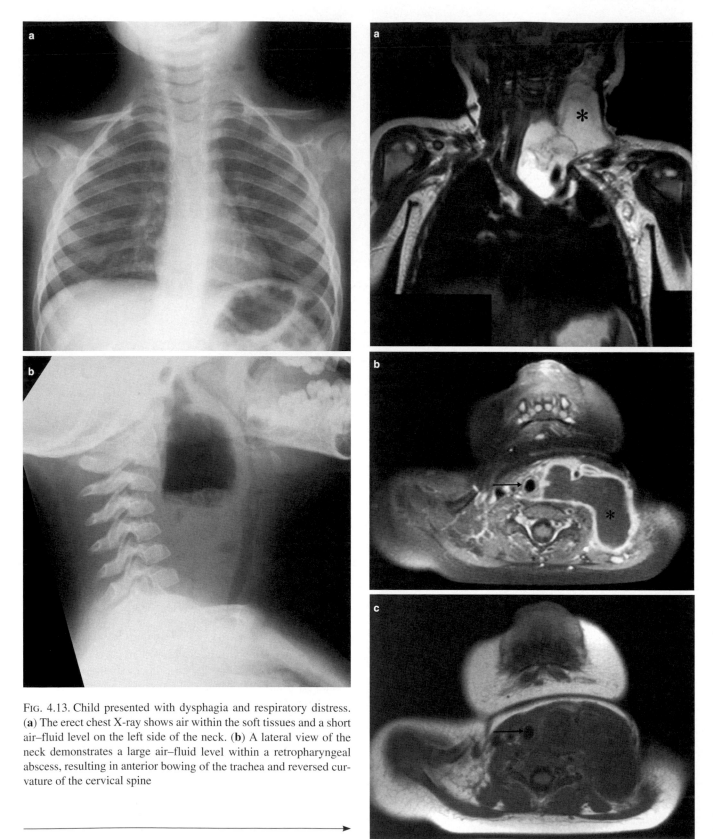

FIG. 4.13. Child presented with dysphagia and respiratory distress. (a) The erect chest X-ray shows air within the soft tissues and a short air–fluid level on the left side of the neck. (b) A lateral view of the neck demonstrates a large air–fluid level within a retropharyngeal abscess, resulting in anterior bowing of the trachea and reversed curvature of the cervical spine

FIG. 4.14. Thoracic MR scan to demonstrate the mediastinal extension of a supraclavicular lymphangioma. (a) T_2 weighted coronal image showing the cystic mass (*asterisk*) extending deeply into the mediastinum displacing the trachea to the right. (b) Unenhanced scan transverse T_1 weighted images. (c) Contrast-enhanced transverse T_1

FIG. 4.14. (continued) weighted images. The wall of the lesion enhances, clearly identifying the extent of the lesion. *Arrow* indicates the displaced trachea. Note that fluid-filled cyst is of high signal on T_2 weighting and low signal on T_1 weighting (*asterisk*)

syndrome. Soft tissue masses seen in neurofibromatosis may project as multiple opacities in the lungs. These should be obvious on clinical examination but occasionally a noncontrast CT examination of the lungs is necessary to exclude coexisting lung disease.

The chest X-ray with additional lateral view may be the only imaging necessary in the assessment of chest wall abnormalities although US is being increasingly used to examine "swelling" of the chest wall due to prominence of the costochondral junctions and exclude the presence of an underlying tumor. CT provides a more objective assessment of the severity of significant deformities. A limited noncontrast CT examination provides useful three-dimensional imaging of pectus deformities. The Haller index, also referred to as the pectus index, provides an objective measure of the severity of the deformity in pectus excavatum. Diameters of the chest are measured on the CT scan at the deepest level of the sternal depression. The ratio of transverse to anteroposterior diameter of the normal chest is approximately 2.5. A ratio greater than 3.25 represents a significant deformity. Asymmetry in the size of the right and the left hemithorax should also be noted because this prejudices the final cosmetic result.

Ultrasound examination, particularly with additional color flow imaging, is invaluable for the initial assessment of a soft tissue mass. Hemangiomas and lymphangiomas can be identified with confidence and distinguished from solid lesions, e.g., malignant tumor of the chest wall. Cross-sectional imaging is necessary prior to surgery in most cases to determine the full extent of the lesion, and to document mediastinal or intrathoracic extension (Fig. 4.14a–c). The choice between MRI and CT must be made on a case by case basis. MRI is generally more appropriate for evaluation of soft tissue lesions, whereas contrast-enhanced CT has the advantage in the assessment and the staging of potentially malignant tumors because it is more sensitive for the detection of pulmonary metastatic disease and the identification of rib involvement.[34]

Although interpretation of the pediatric chest X-ray may seem daunting at first, the structured approach described above should direct the clinician toward the correct diagnosis. However, it remains good practice to discuss the films with an experienced pediatric radiologist prior to surgery.

References

1. Royal College of Radiologists. Making the Best Use of Clinical Radiology Services (6th edition). Royal College of Radiologists, London, 2007.
2. Slovis TL, Berdon WE, Hall EJ. Effects of radiation in children. In: Caffey's Pediatric Diagnostic Imaging. Kuhn PJ, Slovis TL, Haller JO (Editors). Mosby, Philadelphia 2004.
3. Martin CJ and Shand J. Risks from radiological examination. In: Medical Imaging and Radiation Protection for Medical Students and Clinical Staff. Martin CJ, Denby PP, Corbett RH (Editors). British Institute of Radiology, London, 2003.
4. Royal College of Radiologists. Standards for Iodinated Intravascular Contrast Agent Administration to Adult Patients. Royal College of Radiologists, London, 2005.
5. Morcos SK. Adverse reactions to iodinated contrast media. Eur Radiol 2001; 11: 1267–1275.
6. Thomsen HS and Morcos SK. Contrast-medium-induced nephropathy: Is there a new consensus? A review of published guidelines. Eur Radiol 2006; 16: 1835–1840.
7. Ionising Radiation (Medical Exposure) Regulations 2000 (Statutory Instrument 2000 No. 1059). UK HMSO, London, 2000.
8. Coley BD. Pediatric chest ultrasound. Radiol Clin North Am 2005; 43: 405–418.
9. Frush DP, Donnelly LF, Chotas HG. Contemporary pediatric thoracic imaging. Am J Roentgenol 2000; 175: 841–851.
10. Frush DP. Pediatric CT: Practical approach to diminish the radiation dose. Pediatr Radiol 2002; 32: 714–117.
11. Siegel MJ. Multiplanar and three-dimensional multi-detector row CT of thoracic vessel and airways in the pediatric population. Radiology 2003; 229: 641–650.
12. Pappas JN, Donnelly LF, Frush DP. Reduced frequency of sedation of young children with multisection helical CT. Radiology 2000; 215: 897–899.
13. Kosucu P, Ahmetoglu A, Koramaz I, et al. Low-dose MDCT and virtual bronchoscopy in pediatric patients with foreign body aspiration. Am J Roentgenol 2004; 183: 1771–1777.
14. Haliloglu M, Ciftci AO, Oto A, et al. CT virtual bronchoscopy in the evaluation of children with suspected foreign body aspiration. Eur J Radiol 2003; 48: 188–192.
15. Brody AS. Imaging considerations: Interstitial lung disease in children. Radiol Clin North Am 2005; 43: 391–403.
16. Brown MA and Semelka RC. MR imaging abbreviations, definitions, and descriptions: A Review. Radiology 1999; 213: 647–662.
17. Malik TH, Bruce IA, Kaushik V, et al. The role of magnetic resonance imaging in the assessment of suspected extrinsic tracheobronchial compression due to vascular anomalies. Arch Dis Child 2006; 91: 52–55.
18. Golding S. Magnetic resonance imaging. In: Medical Imaging and Radiation Protection for Medical Students and Clinical Staff. Martin CJ, Denby PP, Corbett RH (Editors). British Institute of Radiology, London, 2003.
19. Johnson K. Ventilation and perfusion scanning in children. Paediatr Respir Rev 2000; 1: 347–357.
20. Hogan MJ. Neonatal Vascular catheters and their complications. Radiol Clin North Am 1999; 37: 1109–1125.
21. Frush DP and Herlong JR. Pediatric thoracic CT angiography. Pediatr Radiol 2005; 35: 11–25.
22. Beekman RP, Hazekamp MG, Sobotka MA, et al. A new diagnostic approach to vascular rings and pulmonary slings: the role of MRI. Magn Reson Imaging 1998; 16: 137–145.
23. Roebuck DJ. Pediatric interventional radiology. Imaging 2001; 13: 302–320.
24. Franco A, Mody NS, Meza MP. Imaging evaluation of paediatric mediastinal masses. Radiol Clin North Am 2005; 43: 325–353.
25. Laffan EL, Danemann A, Ein SH, et al. Tracheoesophageal fistula without oesophageal atresia: Are pull-back tube oesophagrams needed for diagnosis? Pediatr Radiol 2006; 36: 1141–1147.
26. Fordham LA. Imaging of the esophagus in children. Radiol Clin North Am 2005; 43: 283–302.

27. Burton EM and Brody AS. Cardiovascular system. Essentials of Pediatric Radiology. Thieme Medical Books, New York, NY, 1999.

28. Langton-Hewer SC. Is limited computed tomography the future for imaging the lungs of children with cystic fibrosis? Arch Dis Child. 2006; 91: 377–378.

29. Heaton P and Arthur K. The utility of chest radiography in the follow-up of pneumonia. N Z Med J 1998; 111: 315–317.

30. Swischuk LE and John SD. Chest. In: Differential Diagnosis in Pediatric Radiology. Swiscuk LE (Editor). Williams and Wilkins, Baltimore, 1995.

31. Westra SJ and Wallace EC. Imaging evaluation of pediatric chest trauma. Radiol Clin North Am 2005; 43: 267–281.

32. Kang MP, Khandelwal N, Ojili V, et al. Multidetector CT angiography in pulmonary sequestration. J Comput Assist Tomogr 2006; 30:926–32.

33. Fefferman NR and Pinkey LP. Imaging evaluation of chest wall disorders in children. Radiol Clin North Am 2005; 43: 355–370.

34. Bush CH and Kalen V. Three-dimensional computed tomography in the assessment of congenital scoliosis. Skeletal Radiol 1999; 11: 632–637.

5
Anesthesia for Thoracic Surgery

Oliver Bagshaw and Steven Cray

Introduction

Pediatric thoracic procedures provide an enormous challenge for even the most experienced pediatric anesthesiologist. Patients are often small and may have significant respiratory disease, surgery is technically difficult and may compromise both the cardiovascular and respiratory systems, and the procedures can result in severe postoperative pain.

Thoracic conditions can generally be classified as congenital, infective, neoplastic, and traumatic. Patients may present with their condition at any age, from antenatal diagnosis (congenital lobar emphysema, cystic adenomatoid malformation), through the neonatal period (tracheoesophageal fistula, congenital diaphragmatic hernia), childhood (pulmonary sequestration, empyema), and up to adolescence (mediastinal mass, pectus excavatum). Unlike adult patients, children are often completely asymptomatic and diagnosis of their underlying condition may be coincidental. The quality of the nondiseased parts of the lungs is generally good and therefore there is often better tolerance of single-lung ventilation (SLV), although this can be negated in younger children by adverse physiological consequences.

The major considerations for the anesthesiologist are the age of the patient, associated pathology, the preoperative patient condition, the use of invasive monitoring, lung isolation, and postoperative analgesia.

Historical Perspective

Thoracic anesthesia has developed as a subspecialty since the 1930s, when the introduction of endotracheal intubation and positive pressure ventilation into routine clinical practice greatly improved the operating conditions for the surgeons and the outcomes for the patients.[1,2] Before that anesthesiologists and surgeons had struggled to overcome the adverse physiological effects of an open pneumothorax in a spontaneously breathing, anesthetized patient, undergoing major surgery. The first recorded attempt at a pulmonary resection by the surgeon H.M. Block, in East Prussia, ended in tragedy, with the death of the patient. It was soon understood by the surgeons of the time, that to open the chest was to kill the patient. Dieffenbach qualified this with the maxim "stop at the pleura." Thus thoracic surgery was limited to chest wall procedures and the drainage of pleural fluid collections and the evolution of thoracic surgery as a subspecialty ground to a halt for many years, until the problem of how to overcome the adverse physiological consequences of the open chest was conquered.[3]

Most anesthetics in the early part of the twentieth century consisted of the administration of either ether or chloroform by facemask, to a patient spontaneously breathing room air. In thoracic surgery, access was limited by the size of the thoracotomy wound the patient would tolerate. Often the lung had to be used as a plug to prevent enlargement of the pneumothorax created when the pleura was opened and the surgeons had to work quickly, before there was a significant deterioration in the patient's respiratory status.

Despite experimentation from the mid-nineteenth century onward, it was not until the late 1920s that a practical design for an endotracheal tube (ETT) was introduced, and the early 1930s before the use of positive pressure ventilation during surgery became routine. In both cases, this was due to the work of Arthur Guedel.[1,2] This was further facilitated by the introduction of neuromuscular blockade with curare into clinical practice by Harold Griffith in 1942.[4]

The next challenge was recognition of the need for lung isolation with surgery for conditions such as hemoptysis, lung abscess, and bronchopleural fistula (BPF). Selective one-lung intubation and ventilation was first employed by Gale and Waters in 1931, by advancing a cuffed rubber ETT into a bronchus and inflating the cuff.[5] Soon afterward bronchial blockers were introduced into clinical practice, with a view to isolating the nonoperative lung from contamination by purulent secretions.[6,7] These required considerable skill and experience to place accurately and maintain in position during surgery. The first double-lumen endotracheal tube (DLT) was designed by the Swedish physiologist, Carlens.[8] He initially

D.H. Parikh et al. (eds.), *Pediatric Thoracic Surgery*,
DOI: 10.1007/b136543_5, © Springer-Verlag London Limited 2009

TABLE 5.1. Effect of different physiological states on FRC and V/Q ratio in adults in the LDP.

	Dependent lung FRC	Nondependent lung FRC	V/Q ratio
LDP awake	Normal	High	$\rightarrow$
LDP anesthesia	Low	Normal	$\downarrow$
LDP chest open	Very low	High	$\downarrow\downarrow$

TABLE 5.2. Effect of different physiological states on FRC and V/Q ratio in infants in the LDP.

	Dependent lung FRC	Nondependent lung FRC	V/Q ratio
LDP awake	Low	Normal	$\downarrow$
LDP anesthesia	Low	High	$\downarrow\downarrow$
LDP chest open	Very low	High	$\downarrow\downarrow\downarrow$

Lateral decubitus position: Children

The main difference between children and adults is the position of the lungs on the compliance curve. It has been speculated that the increased compliance of the child's chest wall allows further compression of the dependent lung and a greater reduction in that lung's FRC, such that it approaches residual volume. This allows the closing volume to impinge on tidal ventilation, so that airways in the dependent lung collapse and no longer contribute to gas exchange. More ventilation is therefore distributed to the nondependent lung than would be the case in an adult.[36–38] In both ventilated and spontaneously breathing anesthetized infants, this effect has been shown to cause an overall increase in FRC, due to a shift of the nondependent lung to a more favorable position on the compliance curve. It only decreases again once the pleura is opened and retraction of the upper lung occurs.[39,40] The overall effect of these ventilatory changes, in conjunction with more perfusion to the dependent lung due to the effects of gravity, is to increase V/Q mismatch and physiological deadspace.[41,42] There is also a less-marked effect of the abdominal pressure gradient on the mechanical properties of the dependent diaphragm, such that the mechanical advantage seen in adults does not seem to occur in small children.

Perfusion may also be affected by changes in pulmonary vascular resistance. Pulmonary vascular resistance increases at the extremes of lung volume, due to the mechanical effects of the lung on vessel diameter.[43,44] Theoretically this would cause a similar redistribution of blood flow to the upper lung, although this has not been proven in children. Indeed, the small size of the child's chest means that the hydrostatic pressure gradient in the lungs is less than in adults, so that the beneficial effect of the gradient in terms of matching ventilation and perfusion is less marked.[45]

In both adults and children, opening the chest leads to a further increase in V/Q mismatch, as the nondependent lung becomes more compliant and easier to ventilate, while the dependent lung is further compressed by the unopposed weight of the abdominal and mediastinal contents. This causes an additional reduction in the movement of the dependent diaphragm, exacerbating the hypoventilation. It would be impossible for the patient to effectively breathe spontaneously in this situation and positive pressure ventilation becomes mandatory. In practical terms, this mismatch can be obviated by reducing ventilation to the nondependent lung by employing either SLV or surgical retraction.

To some extent these changes are mitigated by hypoxic pulmonary vasoconstriction (HPV), whereby underventilated areas of lung have their blood supply reduced by a reflex increase in vascular resistance.[46] Under normal circumstances the dependent lung receives about 60% of the pulmonary blood flow, but only 40% of the ventilation. HPV reduces blood flow in the nondependent lung by about half, to around 20% of total pulmonary blood flow. Anesthesia may have a small inhibitory effect on the reflex, but this is dose dependent and not normally clinically significant.[47,48] Coupled with the measures described above to reduce ventilation of the nondependent lung, HPV improves V/Q matching sufficiently to allow SLV to be undertaken. However, in pure physiological terms, infants tolerate SLV less well than older children and adults, and are at significant risk of oxygen desaturation and hypoxia during any procedure (Table 5.2).

In reality, there may be alterations to the normal physiological state and responses, due to the presence of pathology in the nondependent lung. Certainly, lesions such as congenital lobar emphysema, cystic adenomatoid malformation, and intrathoracic tumors may produce significant effects on the V/Q relationships within the lung, such that SLV has less of a detrimental effect on gas exchange.

Investigations

Patients presenting for thoracic surgery often require an extensive workup, including a number of investigations. The anesthesiologist will need to review these as part of the preoperative assessment, and occasionally may be involved in providing anesthesia, so that the investigations can be undertaken.

Chest Roentgenogram

Initial investigation of any respiratory pathology should involve the use of plain radiography. It is the quickest and the simplest radiological investigation to undertake, and many lesions will be apparent and identifiable, having characteristic features. Roentgenograms may also give information on the extent of any disease process, including involvement of vital structures such as the trachea, bronchi, diaphragm, and major blood vessels.

Computed Tomography

Computed tomography (CT) is probably the second commonest investigation used in the assessment of thoracic pathology. It provides diagnostic information, allows the extent of the pathology to be ascertained, along with determination of

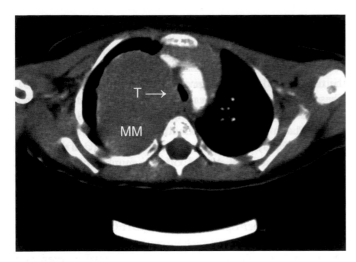

FIG. 5.2. CT of the chest in a child with a large mediastinal mass (MM), demonstrating deviation and compression of the lower trachea (T)

involvement of other organ systems. For the anesthesiologist it is particularly useful for imaging the tracheobronchial tree, which may be essential in conditions such as mediastinal mass, where compression may occur (Fig. 5.2). Three-dimensional and angiographic images can be created. Modern spiral CT scanners are extremely fast and there is rarely a need to provide anesthesia for this imaging modality, except where arrested respiration is essential during imaging and the patient is too young to cooperate with this. The latest multidetector-row scanners may reduce this need even further.[49]

Magnetic Resonance Imaging

Magnetic resonance imaging (MRI) generally provides the most detailed anatomical, pathological, and even physiological information on thoracic lesions. Most children can be imaged with either sedation or nothing at all. However, uncooperative or failed sedation patients may need anesthesia for the scan to be successfully undertaken. The main considerations are the isolated location, the magnetic environment, the need for specialized equipment, the patient's underlying disease state, and the duration of the procedure.

Thoracic Sonography

There are obvious limitations to thoracic sonography, given its poor performance in the presence of air and bone, and it has now been largely superseded by CT in thoracic imaging. However, it is accessible, inexpensive, safe, and provides real-time imaging of the patient.

Bronchoscopy

Bronchoscopy is the definitive investigation for suspected lesions involving the airway. However, the invasive nature of the procedure means that it nearly always requires a general anesthetic, irrespective of whether a rigid or flexible scope is used. Ideally, the patient should be kept breathing spontaneously, which can be a challenge for the anesthesiologist, when the patient has significant airway pathology and the airway is being instrumented. This is covered in more detail below.

Bronchography

Bronchography is useful in the diagnosis of dynamic airway disease and bronchiectasis in children, and can be used as an alternative to bronchoscopy or as part of the bronchoscopic evaluation. The need to inject radiological dye into the airway limits the investigation to patients who already have the airway instrumented, either as part of their general anesthetic or as part of their intensive care management. There are potential problems associated with sharing the airway with the radiologist and spontaneous respiration needs to be maintained if potential dynamic airway disease is being investigated. The presence of an ETT may also mask dynamic airway disease affecting the trachea.

Echocardiography

Echocardiography is undertaken in a number of situations when children present for thoracic surgical procedures. Neonates with conditions such as esophageal atresia and tracheoesophageal fistula, should have this done preoperatively, because of the possibility of the VACTERL association and the implications to the surgeon of a right-sided aortic arch. Upper airway obstruction may be related to vascular anomalies such as double-aortic arch and pulmonary artery sling. Penetrating thoracic trauma may lead to occult cardiac injuries, which may be picked up on echocardiography.[50,51] Chest wall abnormalities, such as pectus excavatum, may be associated with congenital heart disease[52,53] Pericardial involvement in patients with mediastinal tumors is rare, but about 5% will have a pericardial effusion, although most will not need draining.[54]

Angiography

Angiography may be used to diagnose vascular abnormalities such as those described above. However, it is an invasive procedure which usually requires general anesthesia, and has been largely superseded by CT for noncardiac conditions.

Pulmonary Function Tests

Pulmonary function tests (PFTs) may give useful information on a child's underlying lung function in damaging or progressive conditions such as cystic fibrosis and bronchopulmonary dysplasia. It may also be useful in conditions leading to restriction of the chest wall movement, including scoliosis and pectus excavatum. Patient cooperation is a problem under the

TABLE 5.5. Sizes of pediatric univent endotracheal tubes.

Internal diameter	Outside diameter (mm)	Equivalent standard ETT
3.5-mm Univent (uncuffed)	8.0	6.0 mm ID
4.5-mm Univent (cuffed)	9.0	6.5 mm ID

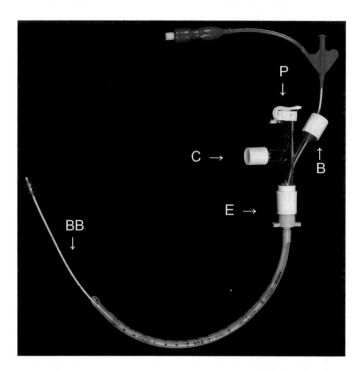

FIG. 5.4. Arndt endobronchial blocker (BB), with multiport adaptor. It connects to the endotracheal tube (E), with an anesthetic circuit attaching at the side (C). The bronchial blocker is passed through the blocker port (B) and fixed in place, while a suction catheter or bronchoscope can be passed through the spare port at the top (P)

TABLE 5.6. Endotracheal tube (ETT) and fiber-optic bronchoscope (FOB) sizing for placement of a 5-FG Arndt endobronchial blocker.

Endotracheal tube size (mm)	Bronchoscope size (mm)	Comments
3.0–4.0	2.2	Blocker must be placed outside endotracheal tube
4.5–5.0	2.2	
5.5	2.8	
6.0	3.4	

of bronchoscope and lubricate the blocker and bronchoscope well to allow both devices to move freely within the lumen of the ETT. A 7-FG Arndt bronchus blocker may be used in older children as an alternative to a double lumen tube. This is particularly useful in cases where intubation is difficult. The 7-FG blocker may be used with an ETT of internal diameter 6.0 mm or greater.

There is a risk that a bronchus blocker will move during patient positioning for surgery. If the balloon is left inflated and the blocker is inadvertently pulled up into the trachea, obstruction to ventilation is likely to occur. The balloon should

therefore be deflated during patient positioning and the correct placement of the blocker rechecked with a FOB once the patient is in the LDP. Bronchus blockers provide reliable lung isolation and if they incorporate a central lumen, CPAP may be applied to the lung on that side or gentle suction may be used to aid lung deflation. At the conclusion of surgery the blocker is deflated or removed to enable reinflation of the operated lung.

Postoperative Analgesia

Thoracic surgery is associated with considerable postoperative pain.[66] The provision of effective analgesia is essential to allow the patient to breathe and cough effectively after surgery. Chronic pain is a frequent problem after thoracic surgery in adults. Although thoracoscopic surgery is less invasive, it may also be accompanied by significant postoperative pain. Effective pain relief after thoracic surgery is best achieved by the use of a combination of drugs and techniques of administration with effective trouble shooting to deal with inadequately controlled pain. If a technique such as epidural analgesia proves inadequate in an individual patient, then alternatives should be substituted urgently.

Epidural analgesia is frequently used after thoracic surgery. In order to produce analgesia using local anesthetic solutions, it is desirable for the tip of the epidural catheter to be positioned at the dermatomal level that corresponds with the surgical incision. There are a number of approaches to the epidural space that may be used to achieve this aim. In infants, an epidural catheter can be reliably advanced to the thoracic region from a caudal approach.[67] This avoids the risk of direct spinal cord trauma from more cephalad insertion. In older children, an epidural may be placed by a direct approach at T4 to T8. This is almost invariably performed after the induction of general anesthesia, in contrast to adult practice.[68] Trauma to the spinal cord during thoracic epidural placement in children has been described;[69] although the incidence of serious complications appears to be low (<1:10,000),[70] there is a paucity of reliable data from the very large series needed to demonstrate safety and limited evidence to show improvements in outcome with different analgesic techniques in children.[71,72] Attempts to position the tip of the epidural catheter in the thoracic region using a lumbar approach are less likely to be successful, although analgesia may be achieved with the use of large volumes of either local anesthetic or opioids.[73]

It is usual to use a combination of dilute local anesthetic and an opioid for epidural analgesia after thoracic surgery (Table 5.7). Commonly used local anesthetics include ropivacaine, levobupivacaine, and bupivacaine, with, or without, epinephrine. Ropivacaine and levobupivacaine are less likely to cause cardiac toxicity than bupivacaine. Neonates are at greater risk of local anesthetic toxicity because of reduced protein binding and immature metabolic pathways.[74–76] The addition of opioids to the epidural local anesthetic solution provides optimal analgesia. Lipophilic drugs such as fentanyl may act predominantly through systemic absorption into

TABLE 5.7. Examples of epidural infusion regimes for management of postoperative pain.

Epidural solution	Infusion rate (mL/kg/h)	Comments
Bupivacaine 0.125% + Fentanyl 2 mg/mL	0.1 to 0.3 mL/kg/h	
Bupivacaine 0.1% + Hydromorphone 0.003 mg/mL	0.3 mL/kg/h	
Ropivacaine 0.2%	0.1 to 0.3 mL/kg/h	In neonates/infants
Ropivacaine 0.25% + Diamorphine 20 micrograms/mL	0.1 to 0.3 mL/kg/h	Diamorphine not licensed by FDA

TABLE 5.8. Examples of regimes for patient controlled analgesia (PCA), nurse controlled analgesia (NCA), and continuous morphine infusion for management of postoperative pain

Regime	Drug concentration	Continuous infusion (mL/h)	Bolus dose (mL)	Lockout period (min)
PCA	Morphine 1 mg/kg body weight in 50 mL	0.2	1	5
NCA	Morphine 1 mg/kg body weight in 50 mL	0.5	1	30
Continuous infusion	Morphine 1 mg/kg body weight in 50 mL	1–2		

epidural veins, or spread very little in the subarachnoid space.[77] Morphine, on the other hand, may reach opioid receptors in the spinal cord far from the site of administration. Unfortunately, epidural morphine may spread as far as the brain stem causing delayed respiratory depression.[78] Other common side effects of epidural opioids include nausea and vomiting, pruritis, and urinary retention.[79] Drugs such as hydromorphone or diamorphine (not licensed by the FDA) may be the most satisfactory options as they provide effective analgesia with less risk of serious side effects than morphine.[80,81] Thoracic epidural local anesthetics block sympathetic outflow from the spinal cord, but hypotension is less likely in children because of their lower resting sympathetic tone compared to adults and alternative causes, such as postoperative hemorrhage, should be considered.

There are situations in which epidural analgesia may be contraindicated, not accepted by the patient or parents, or not possible. Contraindications to epidural analgesia include coagulopathy and local or systemic infection. The mainstay of analgesia in these circumstances is intravenous opioids. Morphine may be administered as a continuous infusion or preferably using a patient-controlled[82] or nurse-controlled analgesia system (Table 5.8). Although opioids are associated with respiratory depression, poorly controlled postoperative

pain will lead to an inadequate depth of breathing and reluctance to cough and must be avoided.

Other local anesthetic techniques have been used in children after thoracic surgery. Intercostal nerve blocks are easy to place either percutaneously or under direct vision and may be a useful adjunct to systemic opioids. The risks of pneumothorax are usually minimized by the routine placement of chest drains after thoracotomy. However, the duration of analgesia will be limited to a few hours and there is rapid absorption of the local anesthetic solution that may lead to toxicity without careful attention to dosing.

Paravertebral administration of local anesthetics can produce similar analgesia to an epidural on the side of the operation. A catheter may be placed in the paravertebral space percutaneously or under direct vision for continued local anesthetic administration.[83] Local anesthetic solutions may also been instilled via a catheter into the pleural cavity, although there are varying reports of the efficacy of this technique.[84]

Even with a well-positioned epidural catheter, patients may have pain that the block does not cover. A common example is shoulder pain from irritation of the diaphragm. Nonsteroidal antiinflammatory drugs such as diclofenac or ibuprofen, or acetaminophen are useful adjuncts.

Specific Procedures

Rigid Bronchoscopy

In children, the indications for rigid bronchoscopy will often require that an anesthetic technique is chosen that preserves spontaneous ventilation. For example, the diagnosis of dynamic airway abnormalities such as bronchomalacia will be impossible if muscle relaxants are used. Spontaneous ventilation is often preferred during foreign body removal,[85] although assisted ventilation may also be used.[86]

Pediatric rigid bronchoscopes, such as the Storz system (Karl Storz, Inc., Culver City, CA, USA), enable an anesthetic breathing circuit to be connected to a side port (Fig. 5.5). It is important that the appropriate size bronchoscope is chosen for the diameter of the trachea as this enables breathing to be assisted with hand ventilation if necessary, otherwise the patient can breathe spontaneously from the anesthetic circuit. Anesthesia is usually induced with a volatile anesthetic agent such as sevoflurane or halothane in oxygen. Atropine, given either as premedication or following induction of anesthesia, will act as an antisialogogue and mitigate against the effects of vagal stimulation. Once a deep plane of anesthesia is achieved, laryngoscopy is performed and the vocal cords and subglottic area are sprayed with lidocaine. It is important to provide effective topical anesthesia of the airway as this reduces the chances of coughing during bronchoscopy. The dose of local anesthetic needs to be carefully controlled because there is the potential for rapid systemic absorption from the tracheal mucosa with a risk of systemic toxicity. The dose of lido-

with a risk of rupture into both the pleural cavity and the lung tissue itself. The latter may lead to soiling of the airway, with infected material contaminating the opposite lung. BPF may occur as a complication of the pneumonic process, following tube thoracostomy or after surgery for decortication. Cavitatory lung disease occurs in about 20% of cases of empyema and of these, a further 20% are likely to go on and develop a BPF.[102] This can lead to difficulties with positive pressure ventilation in the perioperative period and increase the risk of the patient developing a tension pneumothorax.

Perhaps the most controversial aspect of management is the decision as to whether or not to use epidural analgesia in the face of possible systemic infection. Most anesthesiologists will avoid the use of epidural analgesia in this situation because of the risks of seeding infection within the spinal epidural space. However, spinal epidural abscesses are extremely rare in children. All patients will have been commenced on a course of intravenous antibiotics and most will have no evidence of systemic sepsis, although about 10% will yield positive blood cultures.[101] Fluid or pus removed from the thoracic cavity at the time of surgery often proves to be sterile, with only about one-third of samples subsequently culturing microorganisms. Increasingly, there is a move toward early surgical intervention in empyema, either with minithoracotomy or with thoracoscopic procedures. This may increase the likelihood of patients presenting for surgery during the acute phase of their illness, when systemic infection is more likely. However, as thoracoscopic surgery becomes more popular, the role of epidural analgesia in these cases is likely to diminish, as postoperative pain is less.[103] The emphasis is more likely to be on nurse-controlled analgesia, patient-controlled analgesia, or even nonparenteral analgesic regimes.

Bronchiectasis often develops as a complication of severe pulmonary infection. Other causes include congenital, cystic fibrosis and immune deficiency. Patients present for surgery for a number of reasons, including persistent lung infection, hemoptysis, lung parenchymal destruction, and BPF. Pulmonary resection of the affected lung is the most common procedure undertaken and consideration needs to be given to the presence of active infection at the time of surgery, despite regular courses of antibiotics.

Anterior Mediastinal Mass

Anesthesia in a child with an anterior mediastinal mass is associated with significant risks of severe airway and/or cardiovascular compromise and may lead to significant morbidity and even death.[104,105] Careful consideration must be given to the timing of interventions requiring general anesthesia. In many cases, the risks of anesthesia may be substantially reduced by prior treatment with steroids or other chemotherapy to reduce the tumor bulk (Fig. 5.6).

Anesthetic Considerations

Lymphomas are probably the commonest anterior mediastinal tumors in children. They may present with signs of airway obstruction (stridor, dyspnea, orthopnea), pain, or with evidence of superior vena cava (SVC) compression (facial swell-

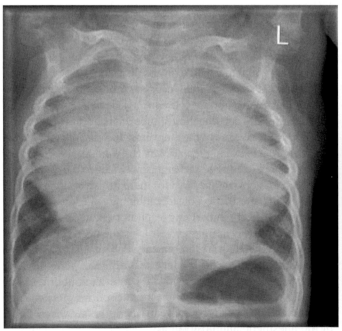 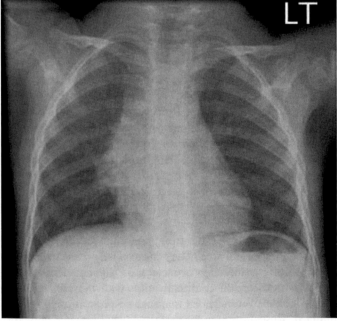

FIG. 5.6. Chest X-rays of a child with an anterior mediastinal tumor (lymphoma) showing the effect of 5 days of treatment with dexamethasone

ing). When general anesthesia is induced, the loss of muscle tone in the chest wall allows the tumor to compress either major airways or the SVC leading to respiratory or cardiovascular collapse. Because the tumor frequently extends beyond the level of the carina, conventional tracheal intubation may fail to reestablish a patent airway.

The anesthesiologist should evaluate the child's history and physical examination carefully. There may be episodes of acute dyspnea that wake the child from sleep or they may not be able to tolerate lying supine – these all suggest airway compromise. Unfortunately, the absence of abnormal findings does not preclude collapse after induction of anesthesia.[106] The most useful preoperative investigation is the CT scan.[107] The anesthesiologist should assess the position of the mass in relation to airways and major blood vessels, and also ascertain the extent of paratracheal and bronchial lymph node involvement. Pericardial effusions may be present in some children, and an echocardiogram should be obtained.[54]

In the patient judged to be at risk for serious complications during general anesthesia, consideration should be given to either shrinking the tumor with steroids, chemotherapy, or radiotherapy beforehand or performing the procedure (e.g., tumor biopsy) under local anesthesia with or without sedation. If general anesthesia cannot be avoided, the recommended approach is to induce anesthesia with a volatile agent maintaining spontaneous breathing. Intravenous access should be placed in the lower extremity to avoid the effects of SVC compression. Endotracheal intubation may be performed under deep volatile anesthesia. The use of intravenous anesthetic agents and/or muscle relaxants is associated with sudden changes in the muscle tone of the chest wall and may precipitate cardiorespiratory collapse. If the airway becomes compromised, application of CPAP may be useful or the patient may be turned lateral or prone. A rigid bronchoscope may be lifesaving in situations where airway compression is beyond the reach of an ETT. The use of cardiopulmonary bypass via the femoral vessels should also be considered in severely compromised patients.

Thoracic Trauma

Children are less likely to be involved in trauma than adults and deaths secondary to trauma have declined in the past 10 years, due to better preventative measures and improvements in clinical management. Thoracic trauma is rare, accounting for less than 4–8% of cases of pediatric major trauma.[108-110] The vast majority is associated with blunt trauma, secondary to falls, motor vehicle accidents, and nonaccidental injury. Penetrating trauma with weapons such as knives and firearms may be responsible. However, despite its low prevalence, it is the second leading cause of death in pediatric trauma, after head injuries.[111]

The high compliance of the chest wall in children means that considerable force can be transmitted to the structures

within the thoracic cavity, with very little evidence of external injury. The most common injuries seen are pulmonary contusion, rib fractures, pneumothorax, and hemothorax.[108,110,112,113] About two-thirds will have associated injuries in other organ systems.[113] Common associated factors include low systolic BP, tachypnoea, abnormal thoracic examination (including auscultation), femoral fracture, and a Glasgow Coma Score of less than 15.[110] Most will not require surgery. The overall mortality rate has been quoted at 7–26% and varies depending on the type of injury, the number of thoracic injuries, and other associated injuries.[108,112,113] Mortality is highest with heart and great vessel involvement and may be as much as 75%.[108] Other indicators of poor outcome include hemothorax, lung laceration, and rib fractures.[108,112,113] The latter is not a good indicator of the severity of injury, because rib fractures are absent in half of patients with significant intrathoracic injuries.[112] Overall, the commonest cause of mortality is from an associated head injury.

Thoracic CT has been found to be superior to plain chest roentgenogram in diagnosing chest complications in the severely injured patient.[114,115] Up to two-thirds of patients will have pathology not picked up from the radiograph.[114-116] However, pneumothoraces diagnosed by scan and not plain radiograph, rarely require intervention.[117]

Overall, only 6–8% of children with thoracic trauma require a thoracic surgical procedure, and the commonest surgical procedure performed is tube thoracostomy.[108,112,113] However, they may need anesthesia for imaging or surgery for other injuries that the child has sustained. Emergency thoracotomy may be required for evacuation of pericardial tamponade, control of intrathoracic hemorrhage or massive air embolism, internal cardiac massage, and cross-clamping of the descending aorta. Unfortunately, in both blunt and penetrating trauma, injuries requiring such procedures are associated with a high mortality, and quoted survival rates are rarely above 10%.[118-120] Esophageal perforation and diaphragmatic rupture may rarely occur, although, the latter would normally necessitate a laparotomy rather than a thoracotomy, unless the diagnosis is delayed and adhesions have formed.

Anesthetic Considerations

The anesthesiologist may be involved in the initial resuscitation and stabilization of the patient. Consideration should be given to the possibility of cervical spine injury in any case of major trauma and care should be taken to ensure the c-spine is immobilized from the outset and remains so throughout the resuscitation and treatment period. Evidence of stridor, abnormal voice, or upper airway obstruction may indicate a laryngeal injury. Breathing difficulties may be the result of pulmonary contusion, pneumothorax, hemothorax, flail chest, and diaphragmatic rupture. Unresolved pneumothorax or pneumomediastinum should raise the possibility of a tracheobronchial tear and air leaks, including BPF. Tracheal injuries can often be managed conservatively, but bronchial injuries require diagnosis by bronchoscopy, followed by thoracotomy and surgical repair.[121,122] Hemodynamic instability results from tension pneumothorax, massive hemothorax, cardiac tamponade, myocardial contusion, and spinal cord injury. These may be further exacerbated by the presence of significant head injury. Evidence from animal and adult studies suggests that outcome may be improved by avoiding overaggressive volume replacement and accepting a degree of controlled hypotension prior to definitive surgery, so as not to "pop the clot."[123–125] What is not clear is whether or not any benefit from this strategy applies in cases of blunt trauma, significant head injury, and the pediatric population in general.[126] IPPV in the presence of a pneumothorax increases the risks of tension developing; therefore consideration should be given to inserting a chest drain, either before or soon after the commencement of IPPV. Difficulties with ventilation may occur if pulmonary contusion is severe and complicated by pulmonary hemorrhage or edema. This often necessitates a high PEEP ventilation strategy from the outset and occasionally high-frequency oscillatory (HFO) ventilation. Flail chest is generally managed by either prolonged IPPV or operative stabilization, with the use of epidural analgesia or patient-controlled analgesia to control pain. Although an adult study has demonstrated benefit from using CPAP rather than intubation and IPPV, by reducing the incidence of pneumonia and overall mortality.[127] Thoracic trauma patients will usually require radiological procedures such as CT scan, ultrasound scan, and angiography, as part of the diagnostic workup. Care must be taken to ensure that patient's condition is stable prior to transfer for such investigations to be undertaken.

Thymectomy

The thymus gland has been shown to be important in the development of myasthenia gravis, through T-cell sensitization to acetylcholine receptors and production of antibodies. Thymectomy is generally reserved for older patients with a diagnosis of juvenile myasthenia gravis, as concerns have been raised about the long-term effects on immune function in younger children and other forms of myasthenia gravis (MG) do not seem to benefit from the procedure.[128–134]

Traditionally, thymectomy has been undertaken via a transsternal approach, although the transcervical route has been described and increasingly thoracoscopic removal is being reported, with good results.[135–139]

Anesthetic Considerations

The main anesthetic considerations are the degree of muscle weakness, the muscle groups involved, sensitivity to neuromuscular blocking drugs (NMBDs) and volatile agents, and the anticipated surgical approach. Anesthesia needs to be tailored accordingly, with the emphasis on avoiding exacerbation of symptoms, preventing complications, and effective postoperative analgesia.

Preoperative preparation involves imaging to exclude thymoma, optimization of medical management and a clinical assessment of the patient's condition. Pulmonary function tests are often performed, but may give unreliable results depending on patient cooperation, disease progression, and recent treatments. The mainstay of treatment remains anticholinergic drugs, such as pyridostigmine and neostigmine. Patients are often receiving corticosteroids and supplementation may be required in the perioperative period. In more severely affected cases, treatments such as plasmapheresis and immunoglobulin therapy have been used to improve the patient's condition prior to surgery. Anesthetic assessment should be aimed at ascertaining the nature and severity of the condition, particularly the presence of bulbar symptoms and episodes of respiratory failure requiring PICU admission and respiratory support.

Anticholinergics are often omitted on the day of surgery, particularly if nondepolarizing muscle relaxants are to be used. However, consideration needs to be given to the patient's preoperative condition and the possible need for postoperative ventilation, as the prolonged nature of the procedure may mean the patient goes several hours without a dose. Anesthesia can be induced with either an intravenous induction agent or an anesthetic vapor. The anesthetic technique depends on surgical requirements and the knowledge and expertise of the anesthesiologist. Most would favor an inhalational anesthetic technique, with or without the use of NMBDs. Many adult practitioners advocate the use of a total intravenous anesthesia (TIVA) technique, using propofol and remifentanil, thus avoiding the use of NMBDs altogether. There seems to be less experience of this technique in pediatric practice, with few reports in the literature.[140,141] Safe administration of NMBDs, such as atracurium and vecuronium, has been used in MG patients, although there is evidence to show that they can increase the requirement for postoperative ventilation.[142] The dose needs to be much reduced and monitoring of neuromuscular function is mandatory, due to the unpredictable nature of their action. Succinylcholine is best avoided, as there is relative resistance to its effects in MG and recent plasmapheresis causes a depletion of plasma cholinesterase, leading to a prolonged duration of action. Remifentanil metabolism remains unaffected following plasmapheresis, probably because metabolism is primarily by tissue esterases.[140] Intraoperative analgesia can be provided using either opioids, such as morphine, fentanyl or remifentanil, or regional techniques such as epidural analgesia. If the surgical approach is via a median sternotomy, high thoracic epidural analgesia is necessary to be effective. This has the potential for cardiorespiratory compromise from a high block, including bradycardia, hypotension, and loss of intercostal muscle function. However, these risks may be offset by the superior analgesia afforded and by avoiding the side-effects of opioids in the postoperative period.

Predictors of the need for postoperative ventilation have been defined in the adult population, but these do not apply to juvenile MG and if the transcervical or thoracoscopic routes are used.[143–145]

Nuss Procedure

The Nuss procedure is a minimally invasive technique for correction of pectus excavatum.[146,147] Under thoracoscopic guidance, a pre-bent metal bar is passed beneath the anterior chest wall and then flipped through 180° to push out the lower sternum and rib cage. Some children with pectus excavatum will have underlying lung disease, Marfan's syndrome, or cardiac abnormalities, and the preoperative work-up should include PFTs and an echocardiogram. However, most patients will have normal findings.

Potential complications of the Nuss procedure include pneumothorax, myocardial injury, and bar displacement. Management of general anesthesia includes the use of a muscle relaxant and endotracheal intubation.[148] SLV is not usually necessary.[149] The patient's arms need to be positioned to enable access to the lateral aspect of the chest wall, but the arms should not be brought up above the head as this has been associated with brachial plexus injury.[150] Postoperative pain is a significant problem and thoracic epidural analgesia with a combination of local anesthetic and opioid is appropriate.[151] In some cases, intravenous patient controlled analgesia with morphine may be required to supplement epidural local anesthetic. Pain may continue for several weeks following the procedure, requiring the use of oral opioid and nonsteroidal antiinflammatory drugs.

References

1. Guedel AE, Waters RM. A new endotracheal catheter. Curr Res Anesth Analg 1928; 7: 238–9
2. Guedel AE, Treweek DN. Ether apnoeas. Anesth Analg 1934; 13: 263–4
3. Grannis FW. "Stop at the pleura": The problem of the open chest and the early history of thoracic surgery (http://www.smokinglungs.com/theop1a.htm accessed 11/1/07)
4. Griffith HR, Johnson GE. Use of curare in general anesthesia. Anesthesiology 1942; 3: 418–20
5. Gale JW, Waters RM. Closed endobronchial anesthesia in thoracic surgery. J Thorac Surg 1931; 1: 432–7
6. Archibald E. A consideration of the dangers of lobectomy. J Thorac Surg 1935; 4: 335–51
7. Magill IW. Anaesthetics in thoracic surgery with special reference to lobectomy. Proc R Soc Med 1936; 29: 643–53
8. Carlens E. A new flexible double-lumen catheter for bronchospirometry. J Thorac Surg 1949; 18: 742–6
9. Bjork VO, Carlens E. The prevention of spread during pulmonary resection by the use of a double-lumen catheter. J Thorac Surg 1950; 20: 151–7
10. Robertshaw FL. Low resistance double lumen endotracheal tubes. Br J Anaesth 1962; 34: 576–9
11. Vale R. Selective bronchial blocking in a small child. Case report. Br J Anaesth 1969; 41: 453–4
12. Tobias JD, Lowe S, O'Dell N, Holcomb GW 3rd. Thoracic epidural anaesthesia in infants and children. Can J Anaesth 1993; 40: 810–2
13. Gunter JB, Eng C. Thoracic epidural anesthesia via the caudal approach in children. Anesthesiology 1992; 76: 935–8
14. Meurat I, Delleur MM, Levy J, Esteve C, Saint-Maurice C. Continuous epidural anaesthesia for major abdominal surgery in young children. Eur J Anaesthesiol 1987; 4: 327–35
15. Eng J, Sabanathan S. Continuous paravertebral block for postthoracotomy analgesia in children. J Pediatr Surg 1992; 27: 556–7
16. Shah R, Sabanathan S, Richardson J, Mearns A, Bembridge J. Continuous paravertebral block for post thoracotomy analgesia in children. J Cardiovasc Surg (Torino) 1997; 38: 543–6
17. Keens TG, Bryan AL, Levison H, et al. Development pattern of muscle fiber types in human ventilatory muscles. J Appl Physiol 1978; 44: 909–13
18. Rudolph AM, Heymann MA. Cardiac output in the fetal lamb: The effects of spontaneous and induced changes of heart rate on right and left ventricular output. Am J Obstet Gynecol 1976; 124: 183–92
19. Kenny J, Plappert T, Doubilet P, et al. Effects of heart rate on ventricular size, stroke volume, and output in the normal human fetus: A prospective Doppler echocardiographic study. Circulation 1987; 76: 52–8
20. Kirkpatrick SE, Pitlick PT, Naliboff J, Friedman WF. Frank–Starling relationship as an important determinant of fetal cardiac output. Am J Physiol 1976; 231: 495–500
21. Agata Y, Hiraishi S, Oguchi K, et al. Changes in left ventricular output from fetal to early neonatal life. J Pediatr 1991; 119: 441–5
22. Gordon JB, Rehorst-Paea LA, Hoffman GM, Nelin LD. Pulmonary vascular responses during acute and sustained respiratory alkalosis or acidosis in intact newborn piglets. Pediatr Res 1999; 46: 735–41
23. Lee KJ, Hernandez G, Gordon JB. Hypercapnic acidosis and compensated hypercapnia in control and pulmonary hypertensive piglets. Pediatr Pulmonol 2003; 36: 94–101
24. Ostrea EM, Villanueva-Uy ET, Natarajan G, Uy HG. Persistent pulmonary hypertension of the newborn: Pathogenesis, etiology, and management. Paediatr Drugs 2006; 8: 179–88
25. Guignard JP, Torrado A, Da Cunha O, Gautier E. Glomerular filtration rate in the first three weeks of life. J Pediatr 1975; 87: 268–72
26. Polacek E, Vocel J, Neugebauerova L, et al. The osmotic concentrating ability in healthy infants and children. Arch Dis Child 1965; 40: 291–5
27. McDonald JW, Johnston MV. Physiological and pathophysiological roles of excitatory amino acids during central nervous system development. Brain Res Brain Res Rev 1990; 15: 41–70
28. Ben-Ari Y. Excitatory actions of gaba during development: The nature of the nurture. Nat Rev Neurosci 2002; 3: 728–39
29. Anand KJS, Hickey PR. Pain and its effects in the human neonate and infant. N Eng J Med 1987; 317: 1321–9
30. Gerhardt T, Reifenberg L, Hehre D, Feller R, Bancalari E. Functional residual capacity in normal neonates and children up to 5 years of age determined by a N2 washout method. Pediatr Res 1986; 20: 668–71
31. Gerhardt T, Hehre D, Feller R, Reifenberg L, Bancalari E. Pulmonary mechanics in normal infants and young children during first 5 years of life. Pediatr Pulmonol 1987; 3: 309–16
32. von Ungen-Sternberg BL, Hammer J, Schibler J, Frei FJ, Erb TO. Decrease of functional residual capacity and ventilation homogeneity after neuromuscular blockade in anesthetized young infants and preschool children. Anesthesiology 2006; 105: 670–5
33. Rothen HU, Sporre B, Engberg G, et al. Re-expansion of atelectasis during general anaesthesia: A computed tomography study. Br J Anaesth 1993; 71: 788–95

34. Tusman G, Bohm SH, Tempra A, et al. Effects of recruitment maneuver on atelectasis in anesthetized children. Anesthesiology 2003; 98: 14–22

35. Froese AB, Bryan AC. Effects of anesthesia and paralysis on diaphragmatic mechanics in man. Anesthesiology 1974; 41: 242–55

36. Heaf DP, Hehns P, Gordon I, et al. Postural effects of gas exchange in infants. N Eng J Med 1983; 308: 1505–8

37. Davies H, Kitchman R, Gordon I, et al. Regional ventilation in infancy. N Eng J Med 1985; 313: 1626–8

38. Davies H, Helms P, Gordon I. Effect of posture on regional ventilation in children. Pediatr Pulmonol 1992; 12: 227–32

39. Larsson A, Jonmarker C, Joqi P, Werner O. Ventilatory consequences of the lateral position and thoracotomy in children. Can J Anaesth 1987; 34: 141–5

40. Larsson A, Jonmarker C, Lindahl SG, Werner O. Lung function in the supine and lateral decubitus positions in anaesthetized infants and children. Br J Anaesth 1989; 62: 378–84

41. Fletcher R. Gas exchange during thoracotomy in children. A study using the single-breath test for CO2. Acta Anaesthesiol Scand 1987; 31: 391–6

42. Puri GD, Hariwir S, Chari P, Gujral JS. Respiratory variables during thoracotomy for PDA ligation. Anaesth Intensive Care 1996; 24: 375–8

43. Burton AC, Patel DJ. Effect on pulmonary vascular resistance of inflation of the rabbit lungs. J Appl Physiol 1958; 12: 239–46

44. Whittenberger JL, McGregor M, Berglund E, Borst HG. Influence of state of inflation of the lung on pulmonary vascular resistance. J Appl Physiol 1960; 15: 878–82

45. Bhuyan U, Peters AM, Gordon I, Davies H, Helms P. Effects of posture on the distribution of pulmonary ventilation and perfusion in children and adults. Thorax 1989; 44: 480–4

46. Benumof JL. Mechanism of decreased blood flow to atelectatic lung. J Appl Physiol 1979; 46: 1047–8

47. Rogers SN, Benumof JL. Halothane and isoflurane do not decrease P_aO_2 during one-lung ventilation in intravenously anaesthetized patients. Anesth Analg 1985; 64: 946–54

48. Benumof JL, Augustine SD, Gibbins J. Halothane and isoflurane only slightly impair arterial oxygenation during one-lung ventilation in patients undergoing thoracotomy. Anesthesiology 1987; 67: 910–5

49. Dawn SK, Gotway MB, Webb WR. Multidetector-row spiral computed tomography in the diagnosis of thoracic diseases. Respir Care 2001; 46: 912–21

50. Nagy KK, Lohmann C, Kim DO, Barrett J. Role of echocardiography in the diagnosis of occult penetrating cardiac injury. J Trauma 1995; 38: 859–62

51. Meyer DM, Jessen ME, Grayburn PA. Use of echocardiography to detect occult cardiac injury after penetrating thoracic trauma: A prospective study. J Trauma 1995; 39: 902–7

52. Willekes CL, Backer CL, Mavroudis C. A 26-year review of pectus deformity repairs, including simultaneous intracardiac repair. Ann Thorac Surg 1999; 67: 511–8

53. Shamberger RC, Welch KJ, Castaneda AR, Keane JF, Fyler DC. Anterior chest wall deformities and congenital heart disease. J Thorac Cardiovasc Surg 1988; 96: 427–32

54. Bashir H, Hudson MM, Kaste SC, Howard SC, Krasin M, Metzger ML. Pericardial involvement at diagnosis in pediatric Hodgkin lymphoma patients. Pediatr Blood Cancer 2007; 49: 666–71

55. Hammer GB. Pediatric thoracic anesthesia. Anesth Analg 2001; 92: 1449–64

56. Cheney FW. The American Society of Anesthesiologists closed claims project: What have we learned, how has it affected practice, and how will it affect practice in the future? Anesthesiology 1999; 91: 552–6

57. Hammer GB. Methods for single lung ventilation in pediatric patients. Anesth Analg 1999; 89: 1426–9

58. Hammer GB, Brodsky JB, Redpath JH, et al. The univent tube for single-lung ventilation in paediatric patients. Paediatr Anaesth. 1998; 8: 55–7

59. Kubota H, Kubota Y, Toshiro T, et al. Selective blind endobronchial intubation in children and adults. Anesthesiology 1987; 67: 687–9

60. Lammers CR, Hammer GB, Brodsky JB, et al. Failure to isolate the lungs with an endotracheal tube positioned in the bronchus. Anesth Analg 1997; 85: 944.

61. Cay DL, Csenderits LE, Lines V, et al. Selective bronchial blocking in children. Anaesth Intensive Care 1975; 3: 127–30

62. Guruswamy V, Roberts S, Arnold P, et al. Anaesthetic management of a neonate with congenital cyst adenoid malformation. Br J Anaesth 2005; 95: 240–2

63. Arndt GA, DeLessio ST, Kranner PW, et al. One-lung ventilation when intubation is difficult – presentation of a new endobronchial blocker. Acta Anaesthesiol Scand 1999; 43: 356–8

64. Wald SH, Mahajan A, Kaplan MB, et al. Experience with the Arndt paediatric bronchial blocker. Br J Anaesth 2005; 94: 92–4

65. Hammer GB, Harrison TK, Vricella LA, et al. Single lung ventilation in children using a new paediatric bronchial blocker. Paediatr Anaesth 2002; 12: 69–72

66. Gottschalk A, Cohen S, Yang S, et al. Preventing and treating pain after thoracic surgery. Anesthesiology 2006; 104: 594–600

67. Bosenberg AT, Bland BA, Schulte-Steinberg O, et al. Thoracic epidural anesthesia via the caudal route in infants. Anesthesiology 1988; 69: 265–9

68. Drasner K. Thoracic epidural anesthesia: Asleep at the wheal? Anesth Analg 2004; 99: 578–9

69. Kasia T, Yaegashi K, Hirose M, et al. Spinal cord injury in a child caused by an accidental dural puncture with a single-shot thoracic epidural needle. Anesth Analg. 2003; 96: 65–7.

70. Goldman LJ. Complications in regional anesthesia. Paediatr Anaesth 1995; 5: 3–9

71. Chalkiadis G The rise and fall of continuous epidural infusions in children Paediatr Anaesth 2003; 13: 91–3

72. Wilson GA, Brown JL, Crabbe DG, et al. Is epidural analgesia associated with an improved outcome following open Nissen fundoplication? Paediatr Anaesth. 2001; 11: 65–70

73. Blanco D, Llamazares J, Rincon R, et al. Thoracic epidural anesthesia via the lumbar approach in infants and children. Anesthesiology 1996; 84: 1312–6

74. Chalkiadis GA, Anderson BJ, Tay M. Pharmacokinetics of levobupivacaine after caudal epidural administration in infants less than 3 months of age. Br J Anaesth 2005; 95: 524–9

75. Hansen TG, Ilett KF, Reid C, et al. Caudal ropivacaine in infants: Population pharmacokinetics and plasma concentrations. Anesthesiology 2001; 94: 579–84

76. Peutrell JM, Holder K, Gregory M. Plasma bupivacaine concentrations associated with continuous extradural infusions in babies. Br J Anaesth 1997; 78: 160–2.

77. Guinard JP, Carpenter RL, Chassot PG. Epidural and intravenous fentanyl produce equivalent effects during major surgery. Anesthesiology 1995; 82: 377–82

78. Henneberg SW, Hole P, Madsen de Haas I, et al. Epidural morphine for postoperative pain relief in children. Acta Anaesthesiol Scand 1993; 37: 664–7

79. Moriarty A. Postoperative extradural infusions in children: Preliminary data from a comparison of bupivacaine/diamorphine with plain ropivacaine. Paediatr Anaesth 1999; 9(5): 423–7

80. Wilson PT, Lloyd-Thomas AR. An audit of extradural infusion analgesia in children using bupivacaine and diamorphine. Anaesthesia 1993; 48: 718–23

81. Goodarzi M.Comparison of epidural morphine, hydromorphone and fentanyl for postoperative pain control in children undergoing orthopaedic surgery. Paediatr Anaesth 1999; 9: 419–22.

82. Berde CB, Lehn BM, Yee JD, et al. Patient-controlled analgesia in children and adolescents: A randomized, prospective comparison with intramuscular administration of morphine for postoperative analgesia. J Pediatr 1991; 118: 460–6

83. Cheung S, Booker PD, Franks R, et al. Serum concentrations of bupivacaine during prolonged continuous paravertebral infusions in young infants. Br J Anaesth 1997; 79: 9–13

84. Giaufre E, Bruguerolle B, Rastello C, et al. New regimen for interpleural block in children. Paediatr Anaesth 1995; 5: 125–8

85. Farrell PT. Rigid bronchoscopy for foreign body removal: Anaesthesia and ventilation. Paediatr Anaesth 2004; 14: 84–9

86. Soodan A, Pawar D, Subramanium R. Anesthesia for removal of inhaled foreign bodies in children. Paediatr Anaesth 2004; 14: 947–52

87. Midulla F, de Blic J, Barbato A, et al. Flexible endoscopy of paediatric airways. Eur Respir J 2003; 22: 698–708

88. Nussbaum E, Zagnoev M. Pediatric fiberoptic bronchoscopy with a laryngeal mask airway. Chest 2001; 120: 614–6

89. Tunkel DE, Fisher QA. Pediatric flexible fiberoptic bronchoscopy through the laryngeal mask airway. Arch Otolaryngol Head Neck Surg 1996; 122: 1364–7

90. Diaz LK, Akpek EA, Dinavahi R, Andropoulos DB.Tracheoesophageal fistula and associated congenital heart disease: Implications for anesthetic management and survival. Paediatr Anaesth 2005; 15: 862–9

91. Myers CR, Love JW. Gastrostomy as a gas vent in repair of tracheoesophageal fistula. Anesth Analg 1968; 47: 119–421

92. Richenbacher WE, Ballantine TV. Esophageal atresia, distal tracheoesophageal fistula, and an air shunt that compromised mechanical ventilation. J Pediatr Surg 1990; 25: 1216–8

93. Ratan SK, Rattan KN, Ratan J, et al. Temporary transgastric fistula occlusion as salvage procedure in neonates with esophageal atresia with wide distal fistula and moderate to severe pneumonia. Pediatr Surg Int 2005; 21: 527–31

94. De Gabriele LC, Cooper MG, Singh S, Pitkin J. Intraoperative fibreoptic bronchoscopy during neonatal tracheo-oesophageal fistula ligation and oesophageal atresia repair. Anaesth Intensive Care 2001; 29: 284–7

95. Andropoulos DB, Rowe RW, Betts JM. Anaesthetic and surgical airway management during tracheo-oesophageal fistula repair. Paediatr Anaesth 1998; 8: 313–9

96. Al-Salem AH, Qaisaruddin S, Srair HA, Dabbous IA, Al-Hayek R. Elective, postoperative ventilation in the management of esophageal atresia and tracheoesophageal fistula. Pediatr Surg Int 1997; 12: 261–3

97. Frankel LR, Anas NG, Perkin RM, Seid AB, Peterson B, Park SM. Use of the anterior cricoid split operation in infants with acquired subglottic stenosis. Crit Care Med 1984; 12(4): 395–8

98. Raghavendran S, Diwan R, Shah T, Vas L. Continuous caudal epidural analgesia for congenital lobar emphysema: A report of three cases. Anesth Analg 2001; 93: 348–50

99. Thomson AH, Hull J, Kumar MR, Wallis C, Balfour Lynn IM. Randomised trial of intrapleural urokinase in the treatment of childhood empyema. Thorax 2002; 57: 343–7

100. Cohen G, Hjortdal V, Ricci M, et al. Primary thoracoscopic treatment of empyema in children. J Thorac Cardiovasc Surg 2003; 125: 79–84

101. Schultz K, Fan L, Pinsky J, et al. The changing face of pleural empyemas in children: Epidemiology and management. Pediatrics 2004; 113: 1735–40

102. Ramphul N, Eastham KM, Freeman R, et al. Cavitatory lung disease complicating empyema in children. Pediatr Pulmonol 2006; 41: 750–3

103. Goldschlager T, Frawley G, Crameri J, Taylor R, Auldist A, Stokes K. Comparison of thoracoscopic drainage with open thoracotomy for treatment of paediatric parapneumonic empyema. Pediatr Surg Int 2005; 21: 599–603

104. Azizkhan RG, Dudgeon DL, Colombani PM, et al. Life-threatening airway obstruction as a complication to the management of mediastinal masses in children. J Pedatr Surg 1985; 20: 816–22

105. Bray RJ, Fernandes FJ. Mediastinal tumour causing airway obstruction in anaesthetised children. Anaesthesia 1982; 37: 571–5

106. Hammer GB. Anaesthetic management for the child with a mediastinal mass. Pediatr Anesth 2004; 14: 95–7

107. Shamberger RC, Holzman RS, Griscom NT, Tarbell NJ, Weinstein HJ. CT quantitation of tracheal cross-sectional area as a guide to the surgical and anesthetic management of children with anterior mediastinal masses. J Pediatr Surg 1991; 26: 138–42

108. Peclet M, Newman KD, Eichelberger MR, Gotschall CS, Garcia VF, Bowman LM. Thoracic trauma in children: An indicator of increased mortality. J Pediatr Surg 1990; 25: 961–6

109. Cooper A, Barlow B, DiScala C, String D. Mortality and truncal injury: The pediatric perspective. J Pediatr Surg 1994; 29: 33–8

110. Holmes JF, Sokolove PE, Brant WE, Kuppermann N. A clinical decision rule for identifying children with thoracic injuries after blunt torso trauma. Ann Emerg Med 2002; 39: 492–9

111. Cooper A. Thoracic injuries. Semin Pediatr Surg 1995; 4: 109–15

112. Nakayama DK, Ramenofsky ML, Rowe MI. Chest injuries in childhood. Ann Surg 1989; 210: 770–5

113. Balci AE, Kazez A, Eren S, Ayan E, Ozalp K, Eren MN. Blunt thoracic trauma in children: A review of 137 cases. Eur J Cardiothorac Surg 2004; 26: 387–92

114. Trupka A, Waydhas C, Hallfeldt KK, Nast-Kolb D, Pfeifer KJ, Scweiberer L. Value of thoracic computed tomography in first assessment of severely injured patients with blunt chest trauma: Results of a prospective study. J Trauma 1997; 43: 405–11

115. Renton J, Kincaid S, Ehrlich PF. Should helical CT scanning of the thoracic cavity replace the conventional chest x-ray as a primary assessment tool in pediatric trauma? An efficacy and cost analysis. J Pediatr Surg 2003; 38: 793–7

116. Civit CJ, Taylor GA, Eichelberger MR. Chest injury in children with blunt abdominal trauma: Evaluation with CT. Radiology 1989; 171: 815–8

117. Holmes JF, Brant WE, Bogren Hg, London KL, Kuppermann N. Prevalence and importance of pneumothoraces visualized on abdominal computed tomography scan in children with blunt trauma. J Trauma 2001; 50: 516–20

118. Nance ML, Sing RF, Reilly PM, et al. Thoracic gunshot wounds in children under 17 years of age. J Pediatr Surg 1996; 31: 931–5

119. Brown SE, Gomez GA, Jacobsen LE, et al. Penetrating chest trauma: Should indications for emergency room thoracotomy be limited? Am Surg 1996; 62: 530–3

120. Hunt PA, Greaves I, Owens WA. Emergency thoracotomy in thoracic trauma – a review. Injury 2006; 37: 1–19

121. Grant WJ, Meyers RL, Jaffe RL, Johnson DG. Tracheobronchial injuries after blunt chest trauma in children – hidden pathology. J Pediatr Surg 1998; 33: 1707–11

122. Cay A, Imamoqlu M, Sarihan H, Kosucu P, Bektas D. Tracheobronchial rupture due to blunt trauma in children: Report of two cases. Eur J Pediatr Surg 2002; 12: 419–22

123. Chudnofsky CR, Dronen SC, Syverud SA, Hedges JR, Zink BJ. Early versus late fluid resuscitation: Lack of effect in porcine hemorrhagic shock. Ann Emerg Med 1989; 18: 122–6

124. Krausz MM, Landau EH, Klin B, Gross D. Hypertonic saline treatment of uncontrolled hemorrhagic shock at different periods from bleeding. Arch Surg 1992; 127: 93–6

125. Bickell WH, Wall MJ Jr, Pepe PE, et al. Immediate versus delayed fluid resuscitation for hypotensive patients with penetrating torso injuries. N Engl J Med 1994; 331: 1105–9

126. Revell M, Porter K, Greaves I. Fluid resuscitation in prehospital trauma care: A consensus view. Emerg Med J 2002; 19: 494–8

127. Gunduz M, Unlugenc H, Ozalevli M, Inanoglu K, Akman H. A comparative study of continuous positive airway pressure (CPAP) and intermittent positive pressure ventilation (IPPV) in patients with flail chest. Emerg Med J 2005; 22: 325–9

128. Masaoka A, Yamakawa Y, Niwa H, et al. Extended thymectomy for myasthenia gravis patients: A 20-year review. Ann Thorac Surg 1996; 62: 853–9

129. Venuta F, Rendina EA, De Giacomo T, et al. Thymectomy for myasthenia gravis: A 27-year experience. Eur J Cardiothorac Surg 1999; 15: 621–4

130. Adams C, Theodorescu D, Murphy EG, et al. Thymectomy in juvenile myasthenia gravis. J Child Neurol 1990; 5: 215–8

131. Lindner A, Schalke B, Toyka KV. Outcome in juvenile-onset myasthenia gravis: A retrospective study with long term follow-up in 79 patients. J Neurol 1997; 244: 515–20

132. Anlar B, Ozidirum E. Thymectomy in children with myasthenia gravis (letter). Neuropediatrics 1999; 30: 49

133. Essa M, El-Medany Y, Hajjar W, et al. Maximal thymectomy in children with myasthenia gravis. Eur J Cardiothorac Surg 2003; 24: 187–9

134. Raksadawan N, Kankirawatana P, Balankura K, et al. Childhood onset myasthenia gravis. J Med Assoc Thai 2002; 85(Suppl 2): S769–77

135. Kogut KA, Bufo AJ, Rothenberg SS, Lobe TE. Thoracoscopic thymectomy for myasthenia gravis in Children. J Pediatr Surg 2000; 35: 1576–7

136. Kolski HK, Kim PC, Vajsar J. Video-assisted thoracoscopic thymectomy in juvenile myasthenia gravis. J Child Neurol 2001; 16: 569–73

137. Kumar A, Kumar S, Ghanta R, et al. Thoracoscopic thymectomy for juvenile myasthenia gravis. Indian Pediatr 2002; 39: 1131–7

138. Skelly CL, Jackson CC, Wu Y, et al. Thoracoscopic thymectomy in children with myasthenia gravis. Am Surg 2003; 69: 1087–9

139. Seguier-Lipszyc E, Bonnard A, Evrard P, et al. Left thoracoscopic thymectomy in children. Surg Endosc 2005; 19: 140–2

140. Hepaguslar H, Oztekin S, Capar E, Elar Z. Recovery from remifentanil after plasmapheresis in a paediatric patient with myasthenia gravis. Paediatr Anaesth 2003; 13: 842–4

141. Bagshaw O. A combination of total intravenous anesthesia and thoracic epidural for thymectomy in juvenile myasthenia gravis. Pediatr Anesth 2007; 17: 370–4

142. Chevalley C, Spiliopoulos A, de Perrot M, et al. Perioperative medical management and outcome following thymectomy for myasthenia gravis. Can J Anaesth 2001; 48: 446–51

143. Leventhal SR, Orkin FK, Hirsch RA. Prediction of the need for postoperative mechanical ventilation in myasthenia gravis. Anesthesiology 1980; 53: 26–30

144. Eisenkraft JB, Papatestas AE, Kahn CH, et al. Predicting the need for postoperative mechanical ventilation in myasthenia gravis. Anesthesiology 1986; 65: 79–82

145. Naguib M, el Dawlatly AA, Ashour M, et al. Multivariate determinants of the need for postoperative ventilation in myasthenia gravis. Can J Anaesth 1996; 43: 1006–13

146. Nuss D, Kelly RE Jr, Croitoru DP, et al. A 10-year review of a minimally invasive technique for the correction of pectus excavatum. J Pediatr Surg 1998; 33: 545–52

147. Croitoru DP, Kelly RE Jr, Goretsky MJ, et al. Experience and modification update for the minimally invasive Nuss technique for pectus excavatum repair in 303 patients. Pediatr Surg 2002; 37: 437–45

148. Futagawa K, Suwa I, Okuda T, et al. Anesthetic management for the minimally invasive Nuss procedure in 21 patients with pectus excavatum. J Anesth 2006; 20: 48–50

149. Maxwell LG. Anesthesic and Pain Management Considerations for the Nuss Procedure, Available from: http://www.pedsanesthesia.org/meetings/2006winter/pdfs/R5_Maxwell.pdf

150. Fox ME, Bensard DD, Roaten JB, et al. Positioning for the Nuss procedure: Avoiding brachial plexus injury. Paediatr Anaesth 2005; 15: 1067–71

151. McBride WJ, Dicker R, Abajian JC, et al. Continuous thoracic epidural infusions for postoperative analgesia after pectus deformity repair. J Pediatr Surg 1996; 31: 105–7

6
Thoracoscopic Surgery

Steven S. Rothenberg

Introduction

Thoracoscopy is a technique that has been in use since the early 1900s but has undergone an exponential increase in popularity over the last decade. The first experience in humans was reported by Jacobeus in 1910 who used a cystoscope inserted into the pleural space through a rigid trocar to lyse adhesions to allow complete collapse of a lung as treatment for tuberculosis. He later reported the first significant experience with a series of over 100 patients.[1] During the next 70 years thoracoscopy gained some favor, primarily in Europe, for the biopsy of pleural-based tumors and limited thoracic explorations in adults; however, widespread acceptance was minimal.[2,3]

In the 1970s and 1980s the first significant experience in children was reported by Rodgers.[4,5] Equipment modified for pediatric patients was used to perform biopsies, evaluate various intrathoracic lesions, and perform limited pleural debridement in cases of empyema.[6] During this period there was an increasing recognition of the morbidity associated with a standard thoracotomy, especially in small infants and children, including scoliosis, muscle girdle weakness, and chest wall deformity.[7] This clear documentation of the effects of thoracotomy on children led to attempts to minimize the morbidity by various muscle-sparing approaches but all of these limited exposure and were still associated with large thoracotomy scars.[8] It was not until the early 1990s with the dramatic revolution in technology associated with laparoscopic surgery in adults that more advanced diagnostic and therapeutic procedures began to be performed in children.[9–11] The development of high-resolution microchip and, more recently, digital cameras, smaller instrumentation, and better optics has enabled pediatric surgeons to perform even the most complicated intrathoracic procedure thoracoscopically.[12,13] Now every thoracic lesion from empyema to esophageal atresia has been approached and successfully managed using a thoracoscopic approach, drastically reducing the pain, recovery, and long-term morbidity of these procedures.

Indications

Today there are wide varieties of indications for thoracoscopic procedures in children (Table 6.1), and the number continues to expand with advances and refinements in technology and technique. Currently, thoracoscopy is being used extensively for lung biopsy and wedge resection in cases of interstitial lung disease (ILD) and metastatic lesions. More extensive pulmonary resections including segmentectomy and lobectomy have also been performed for infectious diseases, cavitary lesions, bullous disease, sequestrations, lobar emphysema, congenital adenomatoid malformations, and neoplasm. Thoracoscopy is also extremely useful in the evaluation and treatment of mediastinal masses. It provides excellent access and visualization for biopsy and resection of mediastinal structures such as lymph nodes, thymic and thyroid lesions, cystic hygromas, foregut duplications, ganglioneuromas, and neuroblastomas.[14,15] Other advanced intrathoracic procedures such as decortication for empyema, patent ductus arteriosus closure, repair of hiatal hernia defects, esophageal myotomy for achalasia, thoracic sympathectomy for hyperhydrosis, anterior spinal fusion for severe scoliosis, congenital diaphragmatic hernia repair, and most recently primary repair of esophageal atresia have also been described in children. The basic premise is that thoracoscopy provides better exposure because of the proximity and magnification that the optical system affords the surgeon. Couple this with the decreased morbidity associated with the minimal access techniques, thoracoscopy should be the preferred approach for nearly all pediatric thoracic procedures.

Preoperative Workup

The preoperative workup varies significantly depending on the procedure to be performed.[16] Most intrathoracic lesions require routine radiographs as well as a CT or MRI scan. A thin-cut high-resolution CT scan is especially helpful in

D.H. Parikh et al. (eds.), *Pediatric Thoracic Surgery*,
DOI: 10.1007/b136543_6, © Springer-Verlag London Limited 2009

TABLE 6.1. Thoracoscopic procedures in children

Lung biopsy	Patent ductus artcriosus ligation
Lobectomy	Thoracic duct ligation
Sequestration resection	Esophageal atresia repair
Cyst excision	TEF repair
Decortication	Aortopcxy
Foregut duplication resection	Mediastinal mass excision
Esophageal myotomy	Thymectomy
Anterior spine fusion	Sympathectomy
Diaphragmatic hemia/placation	Pericardial window

evaluating patients with ILD as it can identify the most affected areas and help determine the site of biopsy as the external appearance of the lung is usually not helpful (Fig. 6.1).[17] CT-guided needle localization can also be used to direct biopsies for focal lesions, which may be deep in the parenchyma and therefore not visible on the surface of the lung during thoracoscopy. This is usually performed just prior to the thoracoscopy with the radiologist marking the pleura overlying the lesion with a small blood patch or dye (Fig. 6.2).[18,19] As intraoperative ultrasound imaging improves

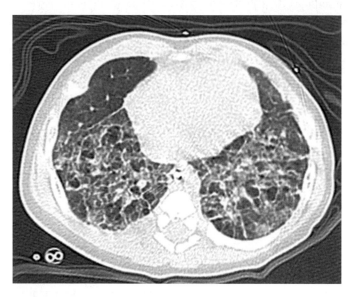

FIG. 6.1. High-resolution CT scan showing interstitial lung disease

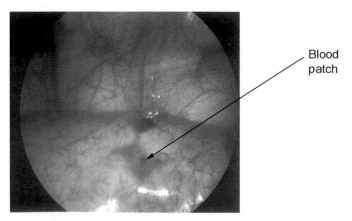

FIG. 6.2. Blood patch marks the pleural surface of an underlying lung lesion

this may provide a more sensitive way for the surgeon to detect lesions deep to the surface of the lung and make up for the lack of tactile sensation. At present, this technology is still unreliable. A MRI scan may be more useful in evaluating vascular lesions or masses, which may arise from or encroach on the spinal canal or in the case of vascular rings. These studies can be extremely important in determining positioning of the patient and initial port placement.

A major consideration for the successful completion of most thoracoscopic procedures is whether or not the patient will tolerate single-lung ventilation, thus allowing for collapse of the ipsilateral lung to ensure adequate visualization and room for manipulation. Unfortunately, there is no specific preoperative test that will yield this answer. However, most patients, even those who are ventilator dependent, can tolerate short periods of single-lung ventilation. This generally allows adequate time to perform most diagnostic procedures such as lung biopsy. In cases where single-lung ventilation cannot be tolerated other techniques may be used, and these will be discussed later.

Anesthetic Considerations

While single-lung ventilation is achieved relatively easily in adult patients using a double-lumen endotracheal tube, the process is more difficult in the infant or small child. The smallest available double-lumen tube is a 28 Fr, which can generally not be used in a patient under 30 kg. Another option is a bronchial blocker. This device contains an occluding balloon attached to a stylet on the side of the endotracheal tube. After intubation the stylet is advanced in the bronchus to be occluded and the balloon is inflated. Unfortunately, size is again a limiting factor as the smallest blocker currently available is a 6.0 tube. For the majority of cases in infants and small children selective intubation of the contralateral mainstem bronchus with a standard uncuffed endotracheal tube is effective. This can usually be done blindly without the aide of a bronchoscope simply by manipulating the head and neck. It is also important to use an endotracheal tube one-half size smaller than for standard intubation, or the tube may not pass into the mainstem bronchus, especially on the left side.

At times, this technique will not lead to total lung collapse as there may be some overflow ventilation because the endotracheal tube is not totally occlusive. This problem can be overcome by the routine use of a low-flow (1 L/min), low-pressure (4 mmHg) CO_2 infusion during the procedure to help keep the lung compressed. If adequate visualization is still not achieved then the pressure and flow can be gradually turned up until adequate lung collapse is obtained. Pressures of 10–12 mmHg can be tolerated for short periods of time without significant respiratory or hemodynamic consequences in most cases. This requires the use of a valved trocar rather then nonvalved port (Thoracoport™, Autosuture, Norwalk, USA). This technique can also be used on patients who cannot tolerate single-lung ventilation. By using small tidal volumes, lower peak pressures, and a higher respiratory rate, enough lung collapse can be achieved to allow for adequate exploration and biopsy. In neonates with TEF or other congenital malformations CO_2 alone can be used to deflate the lung. Once the lung is collapsed it will stay that way until the anesthesiologists makes a conscious effort to reexpand it. The surface tension of the collapsed alveoli in the newborn keeps the lung collapsed without excessive pressures being used.

This technique is also useful if bilateral procedures are being performed such as in the case of sympathectomy.[20] A slight tension pneumothorax gives adequate exposure to visualize the sympathetic chain without the need of changing which lung is isolated. Whatever method is chosen it is imperative that the anesthesiologist and surgeon have a clear plan and good communication to prevent problems with hypoxia and excessive hypercapnia and to ensure the best chance at a successful procedure.[21]

Positioning

Positioning depends on the site of the lesion and the type of procedure. Most open thoracotomies are performed with the patient in a lateral decubitus position. Thoracoscopic procedures should be performed with the patient in a position that allows for the greatest access to the areas of interest and uses gravity to aid in keeping the uninvolved lung or other tissue out of the field of view.

For routine lung biopsies or lung resections, the patient is placed in a standard lateral decubitus position (Fig. 6.3). This position provides for excellent visualization and access to all surfaces of the lung. This position is also the most beneficial set up for decortication, pleurodesis, and other procedures where the surgeon may need access to the entire pleural or lung surface. For anterior mediastinal masses the patient should be placed supine with the affected side elevated 20–30° (Fig. 6.4). This allows for excellent visualization of the entire anterior mediastinum while allowing gravity to retract the lung posteriorly without the need for extra retractors. The surgical ports may then be placed between the anterior and midaxillary lines giving clear access to the anterior mediastinum. This position should be used for thymectomy, aortopexy, or biopsy or resection of anterior tumors or lymph nodes. For posterior mediastinal masses, foregut duplications, esophageal atresia, and work on the esophageal hiatus the patient should be placed in a modi-

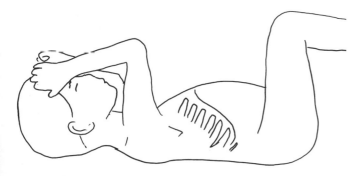

FIG. 6.3. Lateral decubitus position for thoracoscopy

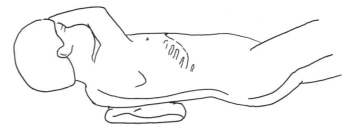

FIG. 6.4. Patient position for access to the anterior mediastinum

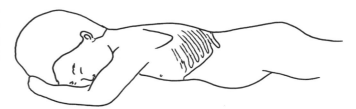

FIG. 6.5. Modified prone position for access to the posterior mediastinum

fied prone position with the effected side elevated slightly (Fig. 6.5). This maneuver again allows for excellent exposure without the need for extra retractors. The patient can then be placed in Trendelenburg or reverse Trendelenburg position as needed to help keep the lung out of the field of view.

Once the patient is appropriately positioned and draped, the monitors can be placed in position. For most thoracoscopic procedures it is advantageous to have two monitors, one on either side of the table. The monitors should be placed between the patient's shoulders and hips depending on the site of the lesion. The goal as always with endoscopic procedures is to keep the surgeon in line with the camera, in line with the pathology, and finally with the monitor. This allows the surgeon to work in the most efficient and ergonomic way. In some cases such as decortication the field of interest may constantly change. In this case the monitors should be placed at shoulder level and moved as necessary.

The majority of operations can be performed with the surgeon and one assistant. The surgeon should stand on the side of the table opposite the area to be addressed so that he can work in line with the camera as he performs the procedure. In most lung cases such as biopsies, it is preferential to have the assistant on the same side of the table as the surgeon so that he is not working in a paradox (against the camera), as he is responsible for operating the camera and providing retraction as necessary. This concept is even more important when the field of dissection is primarily on one side. Cases such as a mediastinal masses, esophageal atresia, or more complicated lung resections require greater surgical skill. It is imperative that both the surgeon and the assistant are working in line with the field of view to prevent clumsy or awkward movements. In cases such as decortication where the field of view and dissection are constantly changing and the majority of movements are relatively gross, having the surgeon and assistant on opposite sides of the table is appropriate and may actually expedite the procedure.

Trocar Placement

Positioning of the trocars varies widely with the procedure being performed and the site of the lesion. Thoughtful positioning of the trocars is more important then with laparoscopic surgery because the chest wall is rigid and therefore the mobility of the instruments will be somewhat restricted as compared to that in the abdomen. The most commonly performed procedures, such as lung biopsy for ILD or decortication for empyema, may require wide access to many areas in the thoracic cavity, and therefore the ports are placed in such a fashion as to facilitate this. However, this may result in some degree of paradox during portions of the procedure. Other operations are directed toward a very restricted area, and therefore the trocars are placed to allow for the best visualization and access to this specific spot. In general, the camera port should be placed slightly above and between the working ports to allow the surgeon to look down on the field of view, much as in open surgery. This will also minimize instrument dueling, which can be a significant problem in smaller infants.

For example with lung biopsies the trocars should usually be placed between the fourth and eighth intercostal space. The camera port is usually in the midaxillary line at the fifth or sixth interspace. If an endoscopic stapler is being used it requires a 12-mm port and therefore should be placed in the lowest interspace possible, especially in smaller children, as these are the widest and better able to accommodate the larger port. If the lesion is anterior it should be positioned closer to the posterior axillary line and visa versa. This is to allow the greatest amount of space between the chest wall insertion and the lesion, as the working head of the stapler requires at least 45–50 mm of space. The third or grasping port is placed closer to the lesion and provides traction on the lesion during biopsy. This arrangement allows the surgeon, camera, and primary working port to be in line with the area to be biopsied. The midaxillary port should be placed first to allow for modification of the other two ports once an initial survey of the chest cavity has been completed. A triangular arrangement of the trocars has also been recommended because it allows for rotation of the telescope and instruments between the three ports giving excellent access to all areas. However, the surgeon can find himself working against the camera, a situation which can make the simplest procedure very difficult. Also, especially in children, the number of large ports should be limited. Therefore, careful planning should go into port placement to limit the number and size of ports needed. Generally, trocar placement can be tentatively planned based on preoperative imaging studies and then modified once the initial trocar is placed.

Instrumentation

The equipment used for thoracoscopy is basically the same as that for laparoscopy. In general 5- and 3-mm instrumentation is of adequate size, and therefore 5-mm and smaller trocars can be used (Fig. 6.6). In most cases valved trocars are used for the reasons previously discussed. Basic equipment

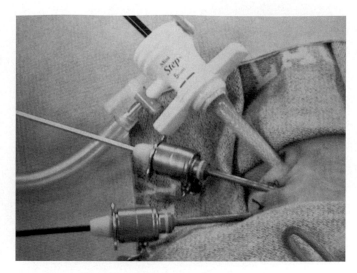

FIG. 6.6. 3- and 5-mm thoracoscopy ports

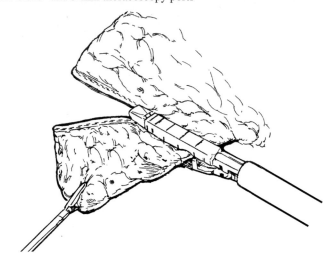

FIG. 6.7. Endo-GIA stapler

should include 5-mm 0° and 30° lenses (most procedures are best performed with a 30° lens). If procedures are being performed in smaller children and infants it is also helpful to have smaller lenses such as a short (16–18-cm long), 3- or 4-mm-diameter, 30° scopes and specifically designed shorter instruments. These tools enable the surgeon to perform much finer movements and dissection allowing advanced procedures to be performed in infants as small as 1 kg. A good quality digital camera and light source are also extremely important to allow for adequate visualization especially when using smaller scopes, which transmit less light. Basic instrumentation should include curved dissecting scissors, curved dissectors, atraumatic clamps (i.e., 3- and 5-mm atraumatic bowel clamps), fan retractors, a suction/irrigator, and needle holders. Disposable instrumentation that should be available includes hemostatic clips, endoloops (pretied ligatures), and an endoscopic linear stapler. The linear stapler is an endoscopic version of the GIA stapler (Autosuture, Norwalk, USA) used in open bowel surgery. It lays down six to eight rows of staples and divides the tissue between them, providing an air- and watertight seal (Fig. 6.7). This is an excellent tool for performing wedge resections of the lung but unfortunately its current size requires placement of a 12-mm trocar precluding its use in patients much under 10 kg because of the limited size of their thoracic cavity. There are also a number of energy sources available, which provide hemostasis and divide tissue. These include monopolar and bipolar cautery, the ultrasonic coagulating shears, and the Ligasure™ (Valleylab, Colorado, USA), all of which can be helpful in difficult dissections. It is also helpful to have one of the various tissue glues available for sealing lung and pleural surfaces.

Postoperative Care

Postoperative care in the majority of patients is straightforward. Most patients following biopsy or limited resection can be admitted directly to the surgical ward with limited monitoring (i.e., pulse oximetry for 6–12 h). These patients are generally suitable for 23-h observation, and a number of patients are actually ready for discharge the same evening. If a chest tube is left it can usually be removed on the first postoperative day. Pain management has not been a significant problem. Local anesthetic is injected at each trocar site prior to insertion of the trocar, and then one or two doses of IV narcotic are given in the immediate postoperative period. By that evening or the following morning most patients are comfortable on oral codeine or acetametaphine. It is very important, especially in patients with compromised lung function, to start early and aggressive pulmonary toilet. The significant decrease in postoperative pain associated with a thoracoscopic approach results in much less splinting and allows for more effective deep breathing. This has resulted in a decrease in postoperative pneumonia and other pulmonary complications.

Conclusions

The recent advances in technology and technique in endoscopic surgery have dramatically altered the approach to intrathoracic lesions in the pediatric patient. Most operations can now be performed using a thoracoscopic approach with a marked decrease in the associated morbidity for the patient. This has allowed for an aggressive approach in obtaining tissue for diagnostic purposes in cases of ILD or questionable focal lesions in immunocompromised patients without the fear of significant pulmonary complications previously associated with a standard thoracotomy. In general, a lung biopsy can now be done with little more morbidity than a transbronchial biopsy, yet the tissue obtained is far superior. The same is true for mediastinal masses or foregut abnormalities. Patients undergoing limited procedures may be discharged home on the day of surgery, and lesions such as esophageal duplications can be excised thoracoscopically with the patient ready for discharge the following day. Even patent ductus arteriosus closures are now performed safely thoracoscopically with a hospitalization of less than 24 h. While a thoracoscopic approach may not always result in a significant decrease in hospital days it may result in a significant decrease in the overall morbidity for the patient, such as in the case of severe scoliosis patients in whom a thoracoscopic anterior spinal fusion results in earlier extubation, a decreased intensive care unit stay, and in general earlier mobilization. Thoracoscopic surgery has clearly shown significant benefits over standard open thoracotomy in many cases, and with continued improvement and miniaturization of the equipment the procedures we can perform and the advantages to the patient should continue to grow.

References

1. Jacobeus HC. The practical importance of thoracoscopy in surgery of the chest. Surg Gynecol Obstet 1921; 4: 289–296
2. Bloomberg HE. Thoracoscopy in perspective. Surg Gynecol Obstet 1978; 147: 433–443
3. Page RD, Jeffrey RR, Donnelly RJ. Thoracoscopy: a review of 121 consecutive surgical procedures. Ann Thorac Surg 1989; 48: 66–68
4. Rodgers BM, Moazam F, Talbert JL. Thoracoscopy in children. Ann Surg 1979; 189: 176–180
5. Rodgers BM. Pediatric thoracoscopy. Where have we come, what have we learned? Ann Thorac Surg 1993; 56: 704–707
6. Kern JA, Rodgers BM. Thoracoscopy in the management of empyema in children. J Pediatr Surg 1993; 28: 1128–1132
7. Vaiquez JJ, Murcia J, Diez Pardo JA. Morbid musculoskeletal sequelae of thoracotomy for tracheo-esophageal fistula. J Pediatric Surg 1985; 20: 511–514
8. Rothenberg SS, Pokorny WJ. Experience with a total muscle sparing approach for thoracotomies in neonates, infants and children. J Pediatr Surg 1992; 27: 1157–1160
9. Rogers DA, Philippe PG, Lobe TE, et al. Thoracoscopy in children: an initial experience with an evolving technique. J Laparoendosc Surg 1992; 2: 7–14
10. Rothenberg SS. Thoracoscopy in infants and children. Semin Pediatr Surg 1994; 3: 277–282
11. Rothenberg SS. Thoracoscopic pulmonary surgery. Semin Pediatr Surg 2007; 16: 231–237
12. Laborde F, Noirhomme P, Karam J, et al. A new video assisted technique for the interruption of patent ductus arteriosus in infants and children. J Thorac Cardiovasc Surg 1993; 105: 278–280
13. Rothenberg SS. Thoracoscopic repair of tracheo-esophageal fistula and esophageal atresia in newborns. J Pediatr Surg 2002; 37: 869–872
14. Partrick DA, Rothenberg SS. Thoracoscopic resection of mediastinal masses in infants and children: an evolution of technique and results. J Pediatr Surg 2001; 36: 1165–1167
15. Kogut KA, Bufo AJ, Rothenberg SS. Thoracoscopic thymectomy for myasthenia gravis in children. J Pediatr Surg 2000; 35: 1576–1577
16. Rothenberg SS, Wagener JS, Chang JH, Fann LL. The safety and efficacy of thoracoscopic lung biopsy for diagnosis and treatment in infants and children. J Pediatr Surg 1996; 31: 100–104
17. Fan LL, Kozinetz CA, Wojtczak HA, et al. Diagnostic value of transbronchial, thoracoscopic, and open lung biopsy in immunocompetent children with chronic interstitial lung disease. J Pediatr 1997; 131: 565–569

18. Smith TJ, Rothenberg SS, Brooks M, et al. Thoracoscopic surgery in childhood cancer. J Pediatr Hematol Oncol 2002; 24: 429–435
19. Holcomb GW, Tomita SS, Hasse GM, et al. Minimally invasive surgery in children with cancer. Cancer 1995; 76: 121–128
20. Cohen Z, Shinar D, Levi I, Mares AJ. Thoracoscopic upper sympathectomy for primary hyperhidrosis in children and adolescents. J Pediatr Surg 1995; 30: 471–473
21. Tobias JD. Anesthesia for minimally invasive surgery in children. Best Pract Res Clin Anesthesiol 2002; 16: 115–118

7
Thoracic Incisions and Operative Approaches

Dakshesh H. Parikh and David C.G. Crabbe

Illustrations drawn by Naseeba Hussain, Birmingham Children's Hospital

Introduction

Most open thoracic operations in children can be performed through a lateral thoracotomy. In the past a posterolateral thoracotomy was used as a matter of routine but now this full-length incision is rarely necessary. The potential for late chest wall deformity following extensive muscle division and rib resection associated with conventional thoracotomy has encouraged most surgeons to use the muscle-sparing lateral thoracotomy in children.

Video-assisted thoracic surgery (VATS) is being used increasingly in children. In skilled hands most procedures performed conventionally by open surgery can be adapted to VATS. Median sternotomy has a limited role in pediatric thoracic surgery for access to mediastinal structures and simultaneous access to both lungs. The purpose of most thoracic approaches is to provide optimal access and adequate exposure of the viscera requiring surgical attention. Unsatisfactory exposure of the operative field results in unnecessary intraoperative and postoperative morbidity.

Historical Perspective

The early history of thoracic surgery is linked inextricably to empyema, bronchiectasis, and tuberculosis. General anesthesia for thoracic operations really only became safe with the development of endotracheal intubation and mechanical ventilation. At the beginning of the last century Sauerbruch attempted to operate on the chest using a negative pressure "hypobaric" operating chamber (Fig. 7.1) but this proved impossibly cumbersome. Vesalius described positive pressure ventilation with endotracheal intubation in experiments on pigs but this remained forgotten until the end of the nineteenth century when the French surgeon Tuffier used this technique for lung resection.[2]

The early lobectomies and pneumonectomies were performed using tourniquets around the lung hilum and mass ligation. Anatomical dissection for lobectomy was introduced in the 1930s. The first successful staged operations for esophageal atresia were performed in 1939 by Leven and then by Ladd. In 1941, Haight performed the first successful single-stage repair through a left thoracotomy. In 1958, Ravitch introduced the western world to surgical staplers, which had been developed in Russia.

General Considerations

Knowledge of the surface anatomy of the chest wall provides a reference for incisions to expose the intrathoracic viscera. These landmarks become increasingly important when minimally invasive techniques are used for chest surgery. The subject is discussed further in the chapter on anatomy.

The surgeon should assume responsibility for positioning the patient correctly on the operating table. The anesthetized child is placed in a lateral decubitus position with a role under the chest to open the rib spaces of the uppermost side (Fig. 7.2). The child should be secured in this position with sandbags or tape. The uppermost arm can be supported by adequate padding and rotated forward. In adolescents the arm can be placed in an arm trough. The legs should be separated by a pillow with the lower leg flexed at the knee and the upper leg straight. Padding should be placed under pressure points. Heat loss from infants and babies can be minimized using Bair Hugger® blankets (Arizant Inc., Eden Prairie, Minnesota, USA).

- The lateral decubitus position affords the best access to the lung hilum. If access to the abdomen or a thoracoabdominal extension to the incision is anticipated the child should be placed in a half-lateral position with a role behind the uppermost scapula.
- The surgeon should note the anatomical landmarks of the nipple, scapula, and vertebral column.
- In a prepubertal girl the skin incision should remain at least two fingerbreadths away from the nipple to avoid scarring of the future breast.

D.H. Parikh et al. (eds.), *Pediatric Thoracic Surgery*,
DOI: 10.1007/b136543_7, © Springer-Verlag London Limited 2009

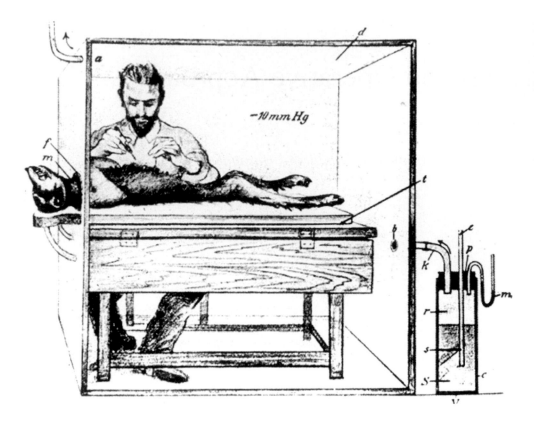

FIG. 7.1. Sauerbruch's "hypobaric" operating chamber[1] (with permission from *Interactive Cardiovascular and Thoracic Surgery*, http://icvts.ctsnetjournals.org/)

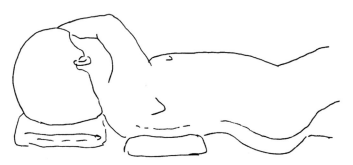

FIG. 7.2. Lateral decubitus position for thoracotomy

- Overenthusiastic rib retraction is a major cause of postoperative pain and should be avoided.
- The method of rib approximation during wound closure remains controversial. The conventional choice is between pericostal sutures and sutures taken through holes drilled in the ribs. Alternatively if the pleural cavity has been entered through the bed of a rib the periosteum can be closed by suture. This closure is secure and avoids the rib crowding often seen with pericostal sutures.
- The divided chest wall muscles are repaired with absorbable sutures. The choice of suture material is individual but the suture size will vary according to the age of the child. There is no benefit from nonabsorbable sutures. For adolescents a 2/0 or 3/0 suture is appropriate, and for small children 3/0, for infants and babies 4/0 sutures are adequate.

- Careful placement of intercostal chest drains at the time of thoracotomy is important. Chest drains exiting behind the posterior axillary line are painful and likely to kink, particularly if the child lies supine. The ideal course for a chest drain inserted at thoracotomy is to exit the costodiaphragmatic recess and then the lateral chest wall between the anterior and mid-axillary lines. This route avoids the major bulk of the latissimus dorsi, pectoralis major, and serratus anterior muscles. Chest tubes should run an oblique course through the body wall, exiting the skin approximately two intercostal spaces below the site where they exit the pleural cavity.

Thoracic Incisions

Posterolateral Thoracotomy

This approach is suitable for a wide variety of thoracic procedures, providing good access to the lung, esophagus, mediastinum, descending aorta, and diaphragm.

Palpate the inferior angle and vertebral border of the scapula, the spine, and note the position of the nipple. The standard incision extends from the anterior axillary line to a point midway between the spine and the vertebral border of the scapula, at the level of the fourth thoracic vertebra. The incision may be extended anteriorly along the course of the rib and posteriorly upward, bisecting a line between the vertebral border of the scapula and the vertebral column. The latissimus dorsi and trapezius muscles are divided. The serratus anterior muscle may be divided in the line of the incision but with minimal difficulty this muscle can be elevated and retracted anteriorly, and this should be a matter of routine. The origins of the serratus anterior muscle are easily divided from the underlying ribs using diathermy. The neurovascular bundle supplying this muscle is preserved and "winging" of the scapula is avoided.

By convention the thorax is opened through the bed of the fifth rib or intercostal space. The surgeon may count the ribs from above placing his hand below the scapula. Entry into the pleural cavity may be obtained either through an intercostal space or through the periosteal bed of a rib. The former is easier if an extrapleural dissection is contemplated for repair of an esophageal atresia. The latter approach is preferable for older children.

Entry into the pleural cavity through an intercostal space is made by using cautery to divide the intercostal muscles close to upper border of the lower rib. Small sections of intercostal muscle can be lifted with a hemostat and then divided. The parietal pleura is then identified. If an extrapleural approach is intended then the pleura is gently separated from the inside of the chest wall using a small damp gauze. If a transpleural approach is necessary the anesthetist should be asked to suspend positive pressure ventilation for a short time as the pleura is opened. Air enters the pleural cavity and the underlying lung collapses facilitating subsequent exposure without injury to the lung.

The pleural space can also be opened through the bed of a rib. The periosteum is cauterized along the length of the chosen rib and then using a periosteal elevator. The posterior periosteum can be opened using diathermy to gain entry to the thoracic cavity. If difficulty is encountered or wide access is necessary this can be achieved by either excising a segment of posterior rib or by removing the whole rib.

Limited (Mini) Thoracotomy: Muscle-Sparing Incisions

With familiarity most thoracic operation in children can be performed safely through a smaller and muscle-sparing incision. The incision must be placed strategically to allow best access and also so that the wound can be extended safely if greater exposure is required. Many muscle-sparing thoracotomy incisions have been described.[3–7] The general principle is retraction rather than division of the chest wall muscles.

The skin incision for a lateral muscle-sparing thoracotomy runs from the anterior axillary line to a point midway between the spine and the vertebral border of the scapula, at the level of the fourth thoracic vertebra. The anterior and anteroinferior edges of the wound should be undermined with diathermy to expose the latissimus dorsi and serratus anterior muscles. The anterior border of the latissimus dorsi muscle is easily defined and freed. This allows posterior retraction of the muscle to expose serratus anterior. The neurovascular bundle can be seen

running vertically down on the surface of this muscle. With further retraction of the latissimus dorsi the posterior border of the serratus anterior can be delineated. This is incised with diathermy allowing the muscle to be retracted anteriorly. As the dissection progresses, the digitation of serratus anterior can be detached sequentially from the rib cage. Perforating vessels from the intercostal arcades run through these muscle slips and require meticulous diathermy to avoid unnecessary bleeding. As the serratus anterior muscle is detached it can be rolled up and "tucked away" under the scapula. The pleural space is then entered in the manner described previously.

The muscle-sparing technique can also be used to enter the chest through the triangle of auscultation. The boundaries of this "space" are trapezius superiorly, the posterior border of latissimus dorsi inferiorly, and laterally by the vertebral border of the scapula (Fig. 7.3). If the scapula is drawn forward parts of the sixth and seventh ribs and the interspace between them become subcutaneous and available for auscultation (hence the name). The skin incision for this approach is best made slightly more posteriorly than for a lateral thoracotomy. The edges of the incision should be undermined above and below. The anterior border of trapezius is defined to allow

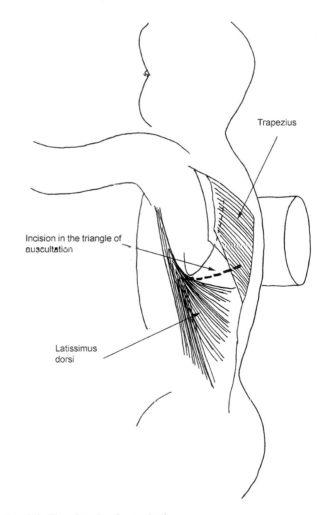

FIG. 7.3. The triangle of auscultation

this muscle to be retracted posteriorly. The posterior border of latissimus dorsi is similarly defined to allow retraction forward. Additional undermining of the inferior skin flap may be required at this stage to allow the latissimus dorsi to be retracted sufficiently to gain decent access. The thorax can then be opened at the desired level.

Closure of muscle-sparing thoracotomy incisions is simple and rapid. The edges of the mobilized muscles are tacked into place with fine interrupted sutures to provide a secure closure.

Subcutaneous emphysema and wound seromas are common. The former is often dramatic and causes concern in the early postoperative period. The tendency for air in the pleural cavity to egress into the tissue planes can be reduced to a considerable degree by the following. The chest drain should be connected to an underwater seal prior to closing the thoracotomy, and the anesthetist should be asked to increase the positive end expiratory pressure. Extubation is inevitably accompanied by a paroxysm of coughing by the patient. Immediately prior to extubation the surgeon should clasp the side of the child's chest firmly with a gloved hand. This encourages pleural air to exit through the chest drain and not into the subcutaneous tissues.

Wound seromas typically appear at around 1 week postoperatively. If small they can be ignored but if large they should be aspirated. Occasionally the aspiration needs to be repeated two or three times.

Axillary Thoracotomy

This incision has been used for most thoracic operations over the years.[3,4,8] The skin incision can be vertical or horizontal although a horizontal incision is cosmetically more pleasing. The subcutaneous tissue and fascia are divided to expose the serratus anterior. Tissue planes are developed between the superficial fascia and the muscle layers. Care should be taken to avoid the intercostobrachial and long thoracic nerves. Latissimus dorsi is retracted posteriorly, and the serratus anterior muscle is elevated to expose the desired rib space for thoracotomy.

The third intercostal space is best suited for operations on the sympathetic chain, apical lung lesions, and patent ductus arteriosus. The fourth space is used for wedge resection, upper lobectomy pleurodesis, and biopsy of mediastinal lesions. Bianchi successfully used this approach for the repair of esophageal atresia in neonates.[9] The fifth intercostal space is employed for lobectomy or pneumonectomy and the sixth or seventh space for diaphragmatic surgery.

Median Sternotomy

Median sternotomy is the incision of choice for most cardiac operations. The incision is also useful if access to both lungs is required, e.g., resection of pulmonary metastases, resection of apical bullae, and pleurectomy. Resection of upper and middle lobes can be accomplished relatively easily through a sternotomy although access to the lower lobes is unsatisfactory

because of cardiac rotation and displacement. Median sternotomy is a useful incision to expose the trachea, particularly if surgery is to involve cardiopulmonary bypass. Anterior mediastinal tumors are best approached through this incision, as is the thymus gland.

The anesthetized child is placed supine on the operating table. A sandbag is placed behind the shoulders, and the arms are allowed to lie by the side of the patient. The neck is extended slightly. A midline skin incision is made from the suprasternal notch to 1 in. below the xiphisternum. The incision is deepened down to the periosteum over the sternum using diathermy. The linea alba immediately below the xiphisternum is opened but the peritoneum should be left intact. In the upper end of the incision the anterior jugular vein is divided, and the lowest portion of the infrahyoid strap muscles is separated in the midline. The cautious surgeon then insinuates one finger from above through the gap in the strap muscles and a second finger though the gap in the linea alba to develop a plane behind the sternum (Fig. 7.4). In small children this is easy and the two fingers will touch. In older children this maneuver is more difficult, and the length of the sternum may preclude digital contact.

The sternum is then divided using a power saw with a reciprocating blade. The anesthetist should temporarily suspend ventilation at this point to avoid laceration of the pleural membranes. Although it is possible to divide the sternum in an infant using heavy scissors this should be resisted because it rarely leaves a straight edge and also risks fragmentation of the cartilaginous regions of the sternum. After the sternum has been divided each edge should be wrapped in a damp swab. Careful attention should be paid to hemostasis at this point using diathermy and Horsley's bone wax. A Finochietto or similar self-retaining

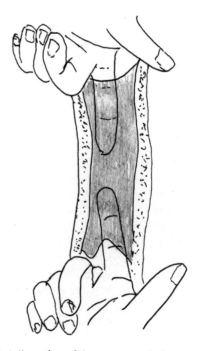

FIG. 7.4. Digital dissection of the retrosternal plane

retractor is then placed in the lower end of the incision. As the retractor is opened tough connective tissue overlying the thymus will need to be divided to allow the chest to open.

Closure of a median sternotomy is quick and reliable. Pleural or mediastinal drains are bought out through stab wounds below the main incision. Stainless steel wire is used to approximate the two halves of the sternum. In infants no. 2 wires are used, in older children no. 4 wires, and in teenagers no. 5 wires. The wires can be driven through the sternum or taken round the edge of the sternum between sternocostal junctions (Fig. 7.5). The ends of the wires are twisted together, cut short, and then buried in the sternal tissues. Between five and seven wires should be sufficient. There is no benefit from trying to close the sternum in a small child with absorbable sutures because it is impossible to tie these sufficiently tightly to prevent movement, which is painful. The linea alba should be closed with one or two interrupted heavy absorbable sutures and the strap muscles approximated with absorbable sutures of a finer grade.

Reopening a median sternotomy can be a challenging procedure. It is essential to determine whether the pericardium is intact and whether there is a space behind the sternum. This may require a CT or MR scan. If the pericardium has been opened previously, particularly if it has been left open, facilities for cardiopulmonary bypass must be available immediately. Consideration should be given to exposure and cannulation of the femoral vessels prior to reopening the sternum in high-risk cases. Unless access to the heart is required the surgeon is advised to consider an alternative approach.

In general it is relatively straightforward to reopen a sternotomy that has been used to resect pulmonary metastases. The pericardium is intact and the thymus gland is more or less intact. The incision is reopened in a similar way to the previous description. The previous wires should be cut and

removed. It may be impossible to redevelop the plane behind the sternum by blunt finger dissection. The sternum should be divided cautiously using an oscillating power saw. Once the bone has been divided the edges can be carefully separated using sharp dissection to release adhesions from the previous surgery. Closure is as described previously.

Thoracoabdominal Incisions

The indications for a thoracoabdominal incision in pediatric practice are few. In almost every occasion adequate exposure can be obtained through either a thoracotomy or a laparotomy. Thoracoabdominal incisions are unduly painful. There is a significant risk of late chest wall deformity associated with division of the costal margin. Rarely, a right-sided retroperitoneal tumor can be mobilized more easily through a thoracoabdominal incision.

The anesthetized child should be placed on the operating table in a half-lateral position. If the position is too lateral access to the abdominal viscera will be difficult. Sandbags should be placed behind the scapula and pelvis. An incision should be made along the line of the ninth rib. The incision is continued through the layers of the abdominal wall, which are divided with cautery. The thorax should be entered through the bed of the rib, as described previously. Rib resection is not required. The costal margin should be transected cleanly with a scalpel. The diaphragm will need to be divided. This is best performed from above. The diaphragm should be detached circumferentially from the chest wall using cautery, leaving a rim of diaphragm approximately 1 cm wide to allow reattachment. Radial incision of the diaphragm will denervate a significant portion of the muscle (see Chap. 40) and, although marginally simpler, adds nothing to the subsequent exposure.

Closure of the incision commences with reattachment of the diaphragm using interrupted heavy absorbable sutures. The costal margin should be approximated next using either a similar heavy absorbable suture or no. 2 stainless steel wire. The advantage of the latter is that two sutures can be inserted a right angles to the long axis of the costal margin and then twisted to bring the edges into apposition. The abdominal wall muscles are closed in a conventional manner.

Intercostal Chest Tube Insertion and Management

Wherever possible, intercostal chest tubes should be inserted under general anesthesia in young children. General anesthesia is invariably safer than intravenous sedation in children for this type of procedure and it is the preferred option for noncooperative children. If a chest drain has to be inserted under local anesthesia equipment for resuscitation and monitoring must be available along with a nurse and an assistant for the surgeon.

In an elective setting informed consent should be obtained. It is incumbent on the operating surgeon to confirm the correct

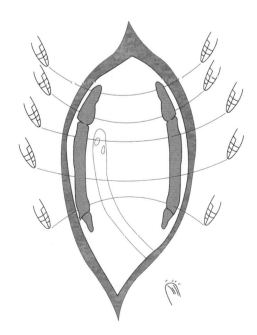

FIG. 7.5. Median sternotomy closure

side for drainage and to ascertain that the necessary equipment are available. Emergency insertion of chest drains will be necessary to treat a tension pneumothorax, parapneumonic effusion, or a traumatic hemothorax where there is respiratory impairment from mediastinal shift. This should be preceded by aspiration of the chest through a 14- or 16 G intravenous cannula, which should result in an immediate improvement in the clinical condition of the patient.

Chest drains should be inserted with an aseptic technique. Whether general anesthesia is used or not local anesthetic should be infiltrated into the chest wall for postoperative analgesia. Plain bupivacaine 0.25% with a maximum dose of 2 mg/kg (0.8 ml/kg)) will provide anesthesia for several hours. Local anesthetic should be infiltrated into the skin, subcutaneous layers, and the intercostal muscles. Intercostal nerve blocks using bupivacaine provide an excellent alternative.

Chest drains should be placed using the open technique described in the ATLS/APLS guidelines. The "safe triangle" for insertion of a chest drain is outlined by the lateral border of pectoralis major, a horizontal line at the level of the nipple, and posteriorly by the anterior border of the latissimus dorsi (Fig. 7.6).[10] Siting a drain in this position avoids damage to the breast and chest wall muscles. The skin should be incised over the fifth rib in the mid-axillary line. The subcutaneous tissues are separated by blunt dissection down to the rib using a hemostat. At this point a track through the intercostal muscles over the upper border of the fifth rib should be created using the hemostat. A distinct pop will be felt as the parietal pleura is breached, and this will be rewarded by drainage of fluid or air through the incision (Fig. 7.7). This use of chest drains with trocars is to be deprecated, and the technique described renders this redundant.

The choice of size of chest tube will depend on the underlying pathology. A pneumothorax can be drained adequately with a 10–16 F catheter; a haemothorax will require a larger catheter of 20–28 F. The choice of catheter for empyema drainage is controversial. Conventional surgical practice dictates the use of a 16–24 F chest tube but recent experience with fibrinolytic agents suggests that small-bore catheters 12–14 F may be sufficient. Small-bore chest drains are now available commercially with Seldinger introduction kits, which are simple to use and avoid the need for dissection through the chest wall.

It is vital that a chest tube is well secured after insertion to prevent inadvertent displacement. A very heavy gauge non-absorbable suture should be used (e.g., no. 1 silk). A generous bite of skin should be taken and the suture knotted at this point. The suture should then be tied repeatedly around the chest tube. The latter knots should be tied sufficiently tightly that a visible waist around the drain is created by the suture. Some centers have found custom dressings/fixation devices to retain chest tubes beneficial, particularly for small-bore tubes (Drain-Fix®, Maersk Medical Ltd, Stonehouse UK). The use of "purse-string" sutures, which are tied to produce an air-tight seal after drain removal, is unnecessary. Purse-string sutures are painful and produce a cosmetically unacceptable scar. The

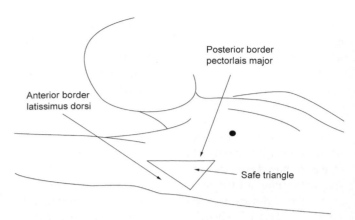

FIG. 7.6. Safe triangle for insertion of a chest drain

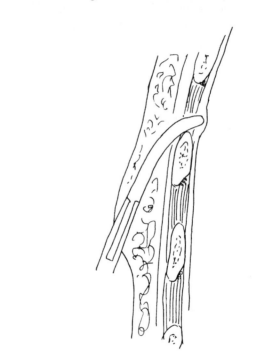

FIG. 7.7. Technique: insertion of chest drain

chest drain should be connected immediately to an underwater seal. The tip of the drainage tube should be 1–2 cm below the water level. A chest radiograph postchest drain insertion is mandatory. The position of the drain can be confirmed, and resolution of the pleural collection can be noted.

The application of suction to chest drains is controversial. The use of low-pressure suction (5–10 cm of water) has been suggested as a method of preventing blockage of small-bore tubes by debris, although this is of doubtful value. In general suction is a poor alternative to an adequate-size chest tube. If suction is to be applied to a chest tube a low-pressure high-volume wall-mounted suction regulator should be used. If this is not available then low-pressure suction can be improvised using three chest drain bottles (Fig. 7.8). Short-term suction is of benefit when there is a large air leak from the lung. Provided air is evacuated from the pleural space more rapidly

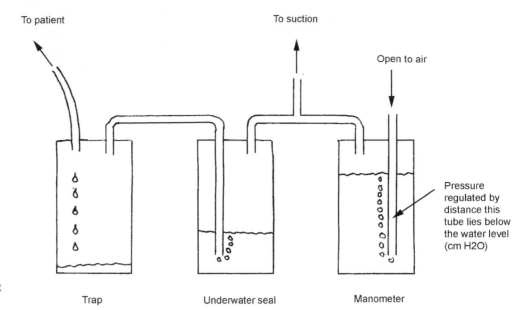

To patient

To suction

Open to air

Pressure regulated by distance this tube lies below the water level (cm H2O)

FIG. 7.8. Chest drain suction using three bottles

Trap

Underwater seal

Manometer

than it can accumulate, the lung will reexpand fully and this provides the best opportunity for an air leak to seal spontaneously. Once the air leak has ceased there is no benefit in continuing suction.

Chest Drain: Ward Management

1. Specially trained nursing staff should manage patients with chest drains.
2. The underwater seal bottle should be kept upright and below the chest at all times. The end of the chest drain tube should be covered by at least 1–2-cm water.
3. A daily record must be kept of the drainage, whether the drain is bubbling, and the presence of respiratory swing. Regular temperature, pulse, and respiration charts should be kept along with a fluid balance chart.
4. If a large pleural effusion is being drained the chest tubes should be clamped for 1 h after 10 ml/kg of fluid is removed to avoid reexpansion pulmonary edema.[11,12]
5. Medical personnel giving instructions for chest drain clamping should record these in writing in case notes.
6. Bubbling chest drains should never be clamped.
7. In presence of chest pain or breathlessness the chest drain should be unclamped immediately.
8. Parents and patients should be encouraged to take joint responsibility for the chest tube and underwater seal bottle. Connections and tapes attaching the drain to the chest wall must be secure at all times.
9. Blockage or a kink of the tubing should be suspected if drainage ceases suddenly. Obstruction may be cleared out by carefully flushing the drain with 10–15 ml of normal saline under aseptic conditions. If the drain cannot be rescued it may need replacing.

10. Chest drains are removed once the lung is fully expanded. In older cooperative children the tube can be removed while the patient performs a Valsalva maneuver. In younger children the drain should be removed as quickly as possible during expiration. The chest drain exit site should be covered immediately with an airtight occlusive dressing that should remain in place for 48 h.
11. A chest radiograph may be taken after drain removal although this is not considered essential.

Complications of chest drain insertion are well reported. Ill-advised placement of chest drains may result in penetration of the liver or spleen. This can be avoided if the "safe triangle" is used. Forcible insertion of a chest tube using a trocar has been associated with puncture of the heart and esophagus, with fatal consequences. The open technique for chest drain insertion will avoid this risk. Inadvertent puncture of the lung is very unlikely in a child breathing spontaneously using the open technique. If the child is attached to a mechanical ventilator this should be disconnected transiently as the pleura is opened and the drain inserted to avoid injury to the underlying lung.

General Techniques for Pulmonary Resection

Technical considerations for pulmonary resection for various pediatric conditions will be discussed in detail in the respective chapters. Surgeons undertaking lung resection in children should be proficient in the basic techniques of dissection and control of large blood vessels, dissection and closure of bronchi, and management of the raw surface of the lung. Specific techniques for endoscopic lung resection will be discussed in detail in the chapter on VATS.

Dissection and Control of Major Arteries and Veins

The pulmonary arteries are thin walled and prone to unintentional injury. Simultaneous traction and countertraction should be avoided. It is also important and essential to avoid traction on branches of the pulmonary artery as they can be avulsed with significant bleeding. Both blunt and sharp dissection is necessary to define the branches of the main pulmonary artery. The fascial envelope around the artery is divided longitudinally, and the vessel underneath is freed by gentle blunt dissection from the underlying fascia. If the vessel is large it should be doubly ligated proximally with a nonabsorbable suture. Reliable surgical knots are essential, and sequential throws must be placed squarely. Tension should be avoided when dividing a vessel between ligatures, as a loosely tied knot may be pulled off accidentally with predictable consequences.

Pulmonary veins can be managed in a similar fashion to the arteries. The walls of the veins are slightly stronger than the arteries. It is a misconception that ligating veins first cause the lung to become congested. Miller showed experimentally that ligating a pulmonary vein causes reflex shunting, which directs arterial flow to other parts of the lung.[13] Additional security can be gained by transfixion ligating the main pulmonary arteries using a nonabsorbable suture. In terms of pediatric pathology it is almost never necessary to divide the pulmonary veins inside the pericardium.

Should inadvertent vascular injury occur during dissection the following well-accepted techniques should be used. Direct pressure should be applied to the site of the bleeding with a gauze sponge. Care should be taken to avoid further injury to the bleeding vessel. The anesthetist should be warned that a vessel has been damaged, and blood can be bought into theatre and checked prior to transfusion.

Vascular clamps should be opened and suction set up. An attempt should then be made to expose the vessel and obtain proximal and distal control. It may be possible to control the injured vessel with a fine vascular clamp. The vessel should then be repaired using a fine vascular suture (4/0 or 5/0 Prolene, preferably on the vascular CC needle).

Dissection and Control of Major Bronchi

The main bronchus is usually the last structure to be divided during a pneumonectomy. On right side the bronchus can be dissected up to the carina without difficulty. On the left side the surgeon has to be more cautious during dissection within the aortic window. It is important to leave behind a short bronchial stump to avoid leaving a diverticulum on the trachea. Particular care should be taken when dissecting a main stem bronchus from the surrounding hilar nodes to avoid damage to the investing fascia and blood

supply because this may jeopardize healing of the bronchial closure. Many surgeons use mechanical staplers for bronchial closure. These devices are simple to use and offer reliable stump closure but they can be difficult to negotiate into the correct position in small children. For this reason the surgeon should be proficient at manual closure of a bronchus. The bronchus should be occluded with a noncrushing clamp distal to the proposed site of resection. The bronchus is then partially divided and the stump closed sequentially with 4/0 or 5/0 Prolene nonabsorbable suture. Interrupted single or mattress sutures are used to approximate the posterior membranous layer of the bronchus to the anterior cartilaginous wall. Once closure is complete the stump is tested for any air leak. Lobar and segmental bronchi can be closed in a similar fashion to the main bronchus. Subsegmental bronchi can be secured by simple ligation.

Occasionally an air leak is identified from the stump of a bronchus. Sometimes the posterior membranous portion of the bronchus has been torn accidentally. This may be closed using additional sutures. Occasionally surrounding tissues may be approximated to buttress the repair. Unnecessary devascularization of the bronchial stump should be avoided.

Raw Surface of the Lung

The raw surface of the lung parenchyma can be the source of a major air leak or bleeding. The raw surface should be inspected carefully for bleeding and air leak after the lung has been reinflated before the closure of the thoracotomy. Small alveolar leaks tend to stop spontaneously after the lung is fully expanded. However, leakage from smaller bronchioles must be recognized and controlled. Various techniques are used to control the raw surface of the lung including closure of the parenchyma by bringing the two surfaces together and applying fibrin glue. These should be unnecessary if meticulous care is taken to control air leaks and bleeding from the raw surface. One advantage of using linear staplers to divide lung parenchyma either during nonanatomical resections or to divide incomplete fissures is that air leaks are very uncommon.

Lobectomy

Lobectomy is the commonest lung resection performed in children. Lung resection may be required for benign conditions including pulmonary infections and bronchiectasis or for congenital anomalies of the lung, including lobar emphysema. Primary lung tumors are very rare in children, and metastases are usually removed by local resection rather than lobectomy.

The techniques for lobectomy are well established. The chest is opened through a posterolateral or a lateral muscle-sparing incision. Opening the thorax at the level of the fifth rib provides good access to the hilum for all lobectomies in children. Once the pleural space is entered any adhesions between the lung and pleura should be divided. Incomplete lobar fissures are common. Hilar dissection is performed in order to identify, ligate, and then divide first artery, then the vein and lastly the lobar bronchus. However, this is not always possible especially if there are dense adhesions and florid lymphadenopathy around the hilum. In this circumstance it may be safer to divide the vein after the bronchus has been sectioned.

Specific Technical Considerations

Right upper lobectomy: The pleura over the main pulmonary artery should be incised to expose the upper lobe branches. The superior trunk of the pulmonary artery is identified, and the branches to the apical and anterior segments of the upper lobe are individually ligated and divided (Fig. 7.9). The tributaries of the superior pulmonary vein are identified and divided next, taking care to avoid the veins draining the middle lobe (Fig. 7.10). The posterior segmental artery to the upper lobe can be divided at this point. The horizontal fissure is then opened or divided using an endo-GIA™ or TA™ stapler (Tyco Healthcare, Mansfield, MA, USA). At this point all that remains is to divide the upper lobe bronchus. This is best performed from behind the hilum. The bronchial stump should

be closed flush with the bronchus intermedius either with a hand-sewn closure, as described previously, or using a stapler. Once the lobectomy is complete the inferior pulmonary ligament may be divided to allow the lower lobe to elevate. If the oblique fissure is complete it is prudent to make sure that the middle lobe cannot volve. If this seems likely then a series of fine sutures should be placed to attach the edge of the middle lobe to the lower lobe.

Right lower lobectomy: During this operation the dissection begins in posterior part of the oblique fissure to identify the artery to the apical segment of the lower lobe. This vessel is divided, taking care to avoid the branch(es) to the middle lobe, which arise at the same level (Fig. 7.10). It may help at this stage to ligate and divide the apical segmental bronchus. The arteries to the basal segments can then be divided. The inferior pulmonary ligament is then divided and the lung reflected forward. This allows the inferior pulmonary vein to be identified and divided. Attention is then turned back to the anterior surface of the lung, and the trunk of the lower lobe bronchus is followed proximally to permit identification of the bronchus or bronchi supplying the middle lobe. These arise at a similar level, but diametrically opposite to the apical segmental bronchus of the lower lobe. The bronchus is divided at this point. This can be achieved conveniently using a stapler or hand sewn.

Right middle lobectomy: Resection of the middle lobe is more difficult than any other lobectomy. The horizontal fissure must be opened to identify the inferior pulmonary artery. Usually there are two vessels supplying medial and lateral segments of the middle lobe although not uncommonly these arise as a single trunk diametrically opposite the origin of the apical segmental artery to the lower lobe, which must be preserved (Fig. 7.11). The middle lobe vein(s) join the superior pulmonary vein, and this can be divided after incising the pleura over the anterior surface of the hilum. The trunk of the middle lobe bronchus is most easily secured from the posterior aspect of the hilum. The relationship of the middle lobe bronchus to the bronchus supplying apical segment of the lower lobe is similar to the arteries. Great care needs to be exercised to ensure that the middle lobe bronchus is divided flush with the bronchus intermedius in a manner that does not narrow the lower lobe apical segmental bronchus.

Left upper lobectomy: The lobe should be retracted anteriorly and downward to allow the pleura over the pulmonary artery to be incised. As the left pulmonary artery spirals down over the main bronchus to enter the fissure a series of branches enter the upper lobe. These have a variable configuration – they may arise as individual branches or as a common trunk. Precision is needed to secure these vessels, which are easily avulsed inadvertently from the pulmonary artery (Fig. 7.12). The lingular segmental vessels will be identified within the fissure, and the lowest branch arises at the same level, or sometimes even distally, to the lower lobe apical segmental artery, which must be preserved. Branches of the superior pulmonary vein are best ligated individually at segmental level. The main trunk of the vein can then be

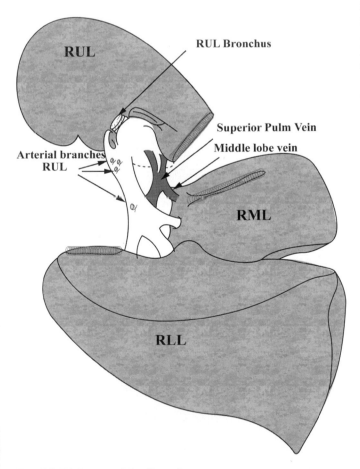

FIG. 7.9. Right upper lobe dissection

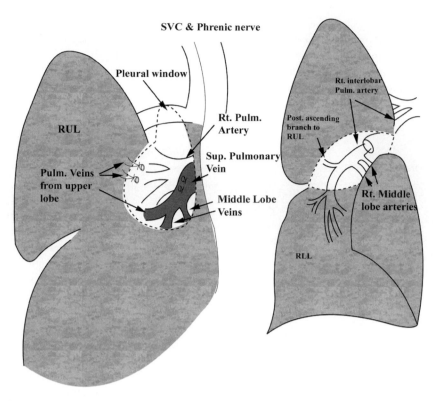

FIG. 7.10. Anatomy of the hilum of the right lung during a right upper lobectomy

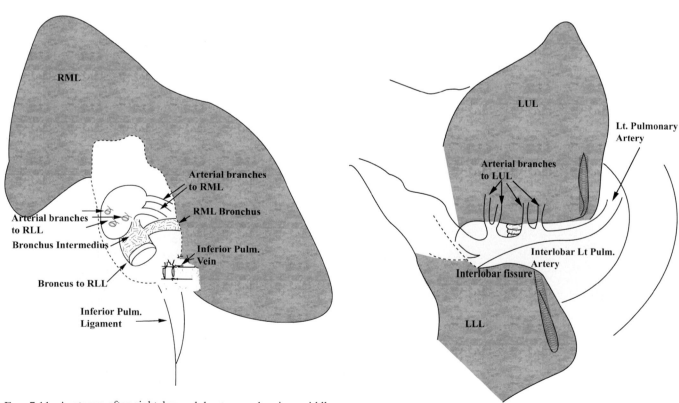

FIG. 7.11. Anatomy after right lower lobectomy, showing middle lobe vessels

FIG. 7.12. Left upper lobectomy

transfixion ligated for additional security. The upper lobe bronchus must be divided flush with the main bronchus and closed by either stapling or hand suture.

Left lower lobectomy: This is probably the simplest lobe to resect. The pulmonary artery is identified in the fissure. The apical segmental artery should be identified and divided first. This vessel often arises above the level of the lingular branches. The apical segmental bronchus may also be divided at this stage. The basal segmental arterial branches can be then divided individually or at the level of the common trunk. The inferior pulmonary ligament is divided next and the pleural reflection over the anterior surface of the hilum incised to expose the inferior pulmonary vein. This vessel should be transfixion ligated and then divided.

The lower lobe bronchus lies immediately below the artery and is easily identified and managed in the way described previously.

Segmental Resection

Individual ligation and division of the corresponding bronchovascular structures allows anatomical resection of a single bronchopulmonary segment of lung. Segmental resection is technically more demanding than lobectomy, requiring a three-dimensional understanding of bronchovascular anatomy. In most situations a nonanatomical or "wedge" resection using a surgical stapler is simpler and more reliable.

The general principles of segmental resection are as follows. The lobe should be mobilized completely to facilitate the exposure required for segmental resection and subsequent reexpansion. The most reliable landmark of a segment is its bronchus, which is rarely anomalous. The segmental bronchi of the right upper and lower lobes and left lower lobe can be identified relatively easily prior to ligation of the segmental artery. This is more difficult in the left upper lobe, where the arteries obscure the segmental bronchi.

The intersegmental plane can be identified by occluding the segmental bronchus and then allowing the surrounding lung to inflate. Occasionally the reverse is necessary to identify a diseased segment. The whole lung is inflated first and the segmental bronchus occluded as the lung is deflated. The diseased segment remains inflated, delineating the margins of the intersegmental plane.

The segmental veins are divided last after completing the intersegmental dissection. It is essential to ensure that the venous drainage of the adjacent segments is intact before completing segmentectomy.

Air leaks should be controlled with fine sutures and bleeding with bipolar diathermy. Air leaks are common after segmental resection, which is one reason why nonanatomical stapled wedge resection is usually preferable. Management of an air leak depends on the severity of the air leak, the general condition of the patient, and the state of the surrounding lung. A continuing significant air leak often requires a second-look thoracotomy. It may be possible to seal the leak

with a muscle flap, but if this is not possible a completion lobectomy will be required.

Pneumonectomy

Pneumonectomy is rarely necessary in children. Occasionally a hilar tumor or a massive congenital lung malformation may necessitate pneumonectomy. Pneumonectomy is usually straightforward in absence of hilar lymphadenopathy and vascular adhesions. Hilar dissection permits identification of the pulmonary artery and then the superior and inferior pulmonary veins. These vessels are large and require double ligation or transfixion ligation with nonabsorbable sutures. The bronchus is closed flush with the edge of the trachea either by hand or using a stapler. The bronchial stump should be leak tested by filling the hemithorax with sterile saline and inflating the contralateral lung to $35\,cm\ H_2O$ pressure. If an air leak is identified this may be closed with an additional suture or by bringing surrounding tissues over the bronchial stump. Chest drainage is probably best avoided following pneumonectomy in children because of the risk of mediastinal displacement.

Complications

Intraoperative Complications and Their Management

Thoracic surgery in children can be associated with life-threatening complications. These include catastrophic bleeding, hypoxia, and contralateral pneumothorax. Lung dissection is invariably associated with some bleeding into the airway. If severe this will compromise ventilation, particularly if compounded by pus released from a bronchiectatic lobe. Ventilation may improve with endobronchial suction but occasionally an emergency change of endotracheal tube is necessary. This is a challenging procedure for even the most experienced anesthetist when the child is fixed to the operating table in a lateral position with the wound open. The surgeon can facilitate this difficult task in several ways. Firstly, the drapes can be lifted or even removed to improve access. Secondly, the surgeon can palpate the trachea and confirm arrival of a new tube. Thirdly, if profound hypoxia develops before the tube can be reinserted the surgeon may need to open the airway from inside the thorax and temporarily insert an endobronchial tube, which can be connected to the anesthetic circuit. This is relatively easy to do through a lobar bronchus or through a direct incision in the main bronchus. After the orotracheal airway has been resecured the transthoracic tube is removed and the bronchotomy closed.

Paraplegia is a rare but disastrous complication, which can occur during dissection of a tumor encroaching on the vertebral column. Monopolar cautery should be avoided in this region as should the temptation to packing Surgicell or similar material into an intercostal space near the intervertebral foramen to stem bleeding.[14–16] The fragile dura is damaged easily and a hematoma may collect in the spinal canal. Some recovery may be possible with early recognition and urgent decompression.

Postoperative Complications

Postoperative bleeding after pulmonary resection usually arises from a bronchial artery, which has been overlooked or from a chest wall vessel. Postoperative bleeding of more than 10 ml/ kg per hour on two consecutive hours is likely to be associated with signs of shock and represents an indication for immediate reexploration. It should be noted that a chest drain may block with clotted blood. In this situation shock will be accompanied by respiratory distress. The diagnosis will be confirmed by an urgent chest X-ray. Reexploration is essential.

Postoperative atelectasis is usually related to retained secretions. This may be compounded by postoperative sedation from analgesia leading to poor respiratory effort. In children this will generally respond to good pain management and physiotherapy. Very rarely bronchoscopy is necessary to aspirate retained secretions.

Subcutaneous emphysema is not uncommon after lobectomy. This has been discussed in detail in the section on muscle-sparing thoracotomy.

Postpneumonectomy syndrome is a rare but serious complication, which may follow right pneumonectomy in infants and young children. Following resection of the right lung the mediastinum will displace and rotate into the right thorax. As the child grows the left main bronchus becomes angulated and stretched between the aortic arch and the pulmonary artery. This gradually occludes the bronchus causing progressively worsening dyspnea from bronchomalacia. The condition has been reported in children with agenesis of the right lung. Treatment is generally unsatisfactory. Prevention is probably the best option by implanting a tissue expander into the thorax at the time of pneumonectomy, which can be progressively inflated as the child grows.

Residual air spaces following lobectomy in children occur occasionally. They are considerably less common than in adults because of the better condition of the pediatric lung. The majority cause no symptoms and resolve over a period of a few months as nitrogen is absorbed slowly from the air space and the adjacent lung expands.

Minor air leaks following lung resection are relatively common. The majority will settle within a few days after the residual lung expands completely. Applying low pressure (10–20 cm H_2O) to the chest drain may help. Provided the child remains well and afebrile patience is usually rewarded by eventual resolution of the air leak.

A persistent air leak after resection of a bronchiectatic lobe is more complicated because the bronchopleural fistula will usually be associated with an empyema. This will prejudice healing and may leave reexploration as the only option. In this situation a muscle flap may need to be taken into the thorax to close a leaking bronchus with healthy vascularized tissue. The simplest muscle flap to raise for intrathoracic use is from serratus anterior.

References

1. Naef AP: The mid-century revolution in thoracic and cardiovascular surgery. Interact Cardiovasc Thorac Surg 2003; 2: 219–226.
2. Naef AP: The Story of Thoracic Surgery: Milestones and Pioneers. Huber, Toronto. 1990.
3. Becker RM, Munro DD. Transaxillary minithoracotomy: the optimal approach for certain pulmonary and mediastinal lesions. Ann Thorac Surg 1976; 22: 254–259.
4. Mitchell R, Angell W, Wuerflein R, Dor R. Simplified lateral chest incision for most thoracotomies other than sternotomy. Ann Thorac Surg 1976; 22: 284–286.
5. Heitmiller RF. The serratus sling: a simplified serratus-sparing technique. Ann Thorac Surg 1989; 48: 867–868.
6. Kittle CF. Which way in? The thoracotomy incision. Ann Thorac Surg 1988; 45: 234.
7. Bethencourt DM, Holmes EC. Muscle sparing posterior-lateral thoracotomy. Ann Thorac Surg 1988; 45: 337–339.
8. Massimiano P, Ponn RB, Toole AL. Transaxillary thoracotomy re-visited. Ann Thorac Surg 1988; 45: 559–560.
9. Bianchi A, Sowande O, Alizai NK, Rampersad B. Aesthetics and lateral thoracotomy in the neonate. J Pediatr Surg 1998; 33: 1798–1800.
10. Laws D, Neville E, Duffy J. BTS guidelines for the insertion of a chest drain. Thorax 2003; 58 (Suppl II): ii53–ii59.
11. Trapnell DH, Thurston JGB. Unilateral pulmonary oedema after pleural aspiration. Lancet 1970; i: 1367–1369.
12. Adegboye VO, Falade A, Osinusi K, Obajimi MO. Reexpansion pulmonary oedema as a complication of pleural drainage. Niger Postgrad Med J 2002; 9: 214–220.
13. Miller GE, Aberg THJ, Gerbode F. Effect of pulmonary vein ligation on pulmonary artery flow in dogs. J Thorac Cardiovasc Surg 1968; 55: 668–671.
14. Short HD. Paraplegia associated with the use of oxidised cellulose in posterolateral thoracotomy incisions. Ann Thorac Surg 1990; 50: 288–290.
15. Walker WE. Paraplegia associated with thoracotomy. Ann Thorac Surg 1990; 50: 178.
16. Benfield JR. Invited commentary of Short HD: paraplegia associated with the use of oxidised cellulose in postero-lateral thoracotomy incisions. Ann Thorac Surg 1990; 50: 290.

Section 2
Infection

8
Pneumonia

Tim W.R. Lee, Keith G. Brownlee, and Philip A.J. Chetcuti

Introduction

Pneumonia can be defined either on clinical grounds alone, or in combination with the radiological appearance. The World Health Organization defines pneumonia as cough or difficulty in breathing combined with tachypnea greater than 50 breaths per minute when less than 1 year of age, and greater than 40 breaths per minute from 1 year of age and older.[1] Radiological features of alveolar consolidation are generally thought to be suggestive of bacterial pneumonia.[2,3]

Historical Perspective

The introduction of antibiotics in the mid-twentieth century dramatically altered the natural history of bacterial pneumonia. From being one of the leading causes of death in childhood, pneumonia is now predominantly a treatable condition with low mortality. In the developing world morbidity and mortality remain significant, principally because of poor nutrition and limited access to healthcare services.[4,5]

Basic Science and Pathogenesis

Etiology

Studies examining the etiology of community-acquired pneumonia are hampered by the frequent difficulty in culturing organisms from either respiratory secretions or blood. In addition, serology or sensitive polymerase chain reaction assays may be coincidentally positive for potential viral pathogens, due to their ubiquitous nature.

In approximately 20–60% of children with pneumonia no pathogen can be identified.[6] In children less than 5 years of age viruses are more likely to be causal, whereas in older children bacterial and atypical infections are common.[7] In the neonatal period group B streptococci, gram-negative enteric bacteria, and *Chlamydia trachomatis* are causes of pneumonia.

The commonest bacterial cause of pneumonia in childhood is *Streptococcus pneumoniae*, followed by *Haemophilus influenzae*, which is particularly prevalent in children under the age of 3. Atypical infections with *Mycoplasma pneumoniae* and *Chlamydia pneumoniae* are common in older children.[7] Table 8.1 illustrates the common pathogens associated with pneumonia in the immunocompetent child.

Epidemiology

Studies in the developed world suggest the incidence of radiologically confirmed community-acquired pneumonia is approximately 36 per 1,000 per year in children less than 5 years of age, and 16 per 1,000 per year in the age range 5–14 years, when all children are included, whether hospitalized or not.[8] If only hospitalized children with radiologically confirmed community-acquired pneumonia are considered the incidence is approximately 3 per 1,000 per year.[9,10] Mortality related to community-acquired pneumonia in the developed world is estimated to be approximately 0.1 per 1,000 per year, although this figure is based on one death in one study.[9]

Clinical Features

The clinical course, severity, and likely pathogens of community-acquired pneumonia are closely linked with the age of the patient. Neonates and infants can deteriorate rapidly, and they can be susceptible to unusual organisms, so the clinical approach is best undertaken in an age-dependent manner. Table 8.2 summarizes the clinical features for each age.

Neonatal Period

Tachypnea greater than 60 breaths per minute is the commonest and most useful sign of pneumonia in the neonate.[6] Indeed, a respiratory rate greater than 70 breaths per minute has 63% sensitivity and 89% specificity for hypoxemia.[11] Signs of respiratory distress such as intercostal and subcostal recession,

D.H. Parikh et al. (eds.), *Pediatric Thoracic Surgery*,
DOI: 10.1007/b136543_8, © Springer-Verlag London Limited 2009

TABLE 8.1. Common pathogens causing pneumonia in the immunocompetent child, grouped by child's age.

Age	Likely pathogens
Neonate (≤4 weeks)	Group B streptococcus
	Gram-negative enteric bacteria
5 weeks – 4 months	Viruses, such as respiratory syncitial virus (RSV), Parainfluenza, Influenza, Adenovirus
	Chlamydia trachomatis
	Bordetella pertussis
4 months – 5 years	Viruses, such as respiratory syncitial virus (RSV), Parainfluenza, Influenza, Adenovirus
	Hemophilus influenzae
	Streptococcus pneumoniae
5 years – 15 years	*Streptococcus pneumoniae*
	Mycoplasma pneumoniae
	Chlamydia pnemoniae
	Viruses, such as respiratory syncitial virus (RSV), Parainfluenza, Influenza, Adenovirus

In each cell pathogens are listed in approximate order of relative importance and prevalence at each age. Table adapted from British Thoracic Society Standards of Care Committee[6] and from Stein and Marostica[7]

TABLE 8.2. Common clinical features of bacterial lower respiratory tract infection, grouped according to age.

Age	Temperature	Respiratory rate	Features
Neonate (≤4 weeks)	38.5°C	>60 per min	Intercostal and subcostal recession, tracheal tug, nasal flaring, head bobbing, expiratory grunting May have features of septicemia
5 weeks – 1 year	38.5°C	>50 per min	Intercostal and subcostal recession, tracheal tug, nasal flaring, head bobbing, expiratory grunting May have cough May have focal crackles or bronchial breathing If wheezy then viral lower respiratory tract infection more likely
>1 year	38.5°C	>40 per min	Intercostal and subcostal recession, tracheal tug, expiratory grunting May have cough May have focal crackles or bronchial breathing If wheezy > 5years of age consider mycoplasma

Table adapted from British Thoracic Society Standards of Care Committee[6] and from Coote and McKenzie[54]

tracheal tug, nasal flaring, and expiratory grunting are often seen.[12] High-grade fever >38.5°C is common although hypothermia can also occur. The more severely affected infant may be septicemic. Auscultation of the chest is usually not helpful. Clinical deterioration can occur extremely rapidly in this age group.

Herpes virus pneumonia presents classically in the newborn period and follows asymptomatic shedding of the virus by the mother.[13] Rapidly progressive respiratory distress occurs at about 6–10 days of age, often in association with pyrexia but without an associated vesicular eruption, particularly in the initial phase. Diagnosis requires viral culture or polymerase chain reaction analysis of airway secretions, and treatment is with acyclovir.[14]

Older Children

Pneumonia in infants beyond the newborn period will usually present with tachypnea greater than 50 breaths per minute and pyrexia >38.5°C. Signs of respiratory distress may be present. Auscultation can be helpful as bilateral wheeze or crepitations in the pyrexial preschool child is much more suggestive of a viral etiology for the lower respiratory tract infection. Focal crackles and/or bronchial breathing suggest a lobar focus for the pneumonia. These features have a sensitivity of 75% and specificity of 57% for predicting radiological consolidation.[11]

One specific classical presentation in early infancy is *Chlamydia trachomatis* pneumonia, which occurs from 4 weeks to 4 months of age (Fig. 8.1). Typically, these infants have conjunctivitis (50% of cases), tachypnea, a "staccato" cough, and are afebrile.[6] From 1 year of age tachypnea greater than 40 breaths a minute becomes significant. In children 5 years and over an acute wheezy episode with insidious onset, cough, malaise, headache, and low-grade fever is typical of *Mycoplasma pneumoniae* infection.

Pneumonia Presenting with Acute Abdominal Pain

The surgeon should remember that pneumonia can present as abdominal pain, particularly right lower lobe pneumonia.[15] Approximately 2.5–5% of pediatric abdominal pain is due to pneumonia.[16,17] Referred pain from diaphragmatic inflammation is the usual explanation. Pneumonia should be considered

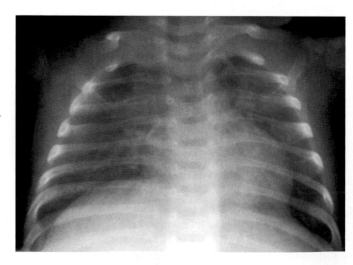

FIG. 8.1. Radiological appearance of Chlamydia trachomatis pneumonia in a 2-month-old child. Hyperinflation is also a common feature

when children with abdominal pain have an unremarkable abdominal examination yet have a significant pyrexia. Respiratory examination may be normal.

Immunocompromised Children

Children with immunocompromise from any cause, including post transplant, undergoing chemotherapy for malignancy, HIV infection, are susceptible to severe and life-threatening pneumonia from both typical and atypical pathogens (see Table 8.3). Infections may be newly acquired pathogens or may be due to reactivation of organisms that had previously been latent or commensal. Immunosuppressed children deteriorate rapidly, and early expert advice from a pediatric respiratory specialist and/or immunologist is recommended. All bacteria normally associated with community-acquired pneumonia should be considered as well as Gram-negative organisms. Atypical organisms must also be considered including *Pneumocystis jiroveci* (previously termed *Pneumocystis carinii*), Aspergillus, and mycobacteria. Common causes of viral pneumonia in the immunocompromised host include respiratory syncytial virus (RSV), influenza, adenovirus, and parainfluenza virus. A recent study suggests that 40% of such pneumonias are hospital-acquired,[18] and mortality rates of up to 67% have been reported.[19] More rarely varicella zoster, measles, cytomegalovirus (CMV), and Epstein Barr virus can cause viral pneumonitis.[19,20] Neutropenic patients are particularly at risk of bacterial and fungal infections, whereas lymphopenic patients are most susceptible to *Pneumocystis jiroveci* and viral infections. In practice considerable overlap occurs.[21,22] Tachypnea and a fever >38.5°C are the usual presenting features, although decreased oxygen saturation may be prominent, particularly in *Pneumocystis jiroveci* pneumonia. Sputum and productive cough is rarely seen in immunocompromised patients due to the relative leucopenia.

TABLE 8.3. Common potential respiratory pathogens in immunocompromised children.

Organism	Examples
Bacteria	*Streptococcus pneumoniae*
	Hemophilus influenzae
	Staphylococcus aureus
	Streptococcus pyogenes
	Klebsiella
	Pseudomonas
Viruses	Respiratory syncitial virus (RSV)
	Parainfluenza
	Influenza
	Adenovirus
	Cytomegalovirus (CMV)
	Measles
	Herpes viruses
Atypicals	*Chlamydia pneumoniae*
	Mycoplasma pneumoniae
	Mycobacteria (tuberculous and nontuberculous)
Fungi	Aspergillus
	Candida
	Pneumocystis jiroveci

Investigations in these children should include full blood count to assess degree of neutropenia and lymphopenia, blood cultures, and a chest X-ray. Serology is rarely helpful due to the immunosuppression.[19] If fungal disease is suspected blood can be sent for candida and aspergillus antigens. Respiratory secretions should be sent for viral detection and culture, requesting parainfluenza, influenza, RSV, adenovirus, and CMV as a minimum. The chest X-ray may show characteristic appearances of a particular pathogen, for example, bilateral perihilar infiltrates with ground-glass shadowing are often seen with *Pneumocystis jiroveci* or CMV pneumonia. (Fig. 8.2). The chest X-ray may be normal and in such cases high-resolution chest CT (HRCT) should be considered.[23] In children unresponsive to treatment or where there is diagnostic uncertainty bronchoalveolar lavage can be used in an attempt to identify the causal pathogen. Ideally, this should be performed early, as once significant respiratory compromise develops bronchoscopy often precipitates the need for mechanical ventilation.[24] It is important to treat these children with broad-spectrum antibiotics to cover both Gram-positive and Gram-negative bacterial pneumonia.

Inhaled Ribavarin should be considered if RSV or parainfluenza virus infection is confirmed, although evidence of benefit is weak.[19] Zanamavir and Oseltamavir have activity against influenza A and influenza B but should be started within 48 h of the onset of symptoms.[25] Aciclovir is given for varicella zoster pneumonitis, and Ganciclovir and Foscarnet are used in CMV pneumonitis, although both have significant toxicity.[19]

Pneumocystis jiroveci pneumonia presents with gradual onset of dyspnea, cyanosis, and a dry cough. Fever is not a major feature. Auscultation of the chest is usually unremarkable. Chest X-ray is often helpful, as described earlier. The diagnosis is

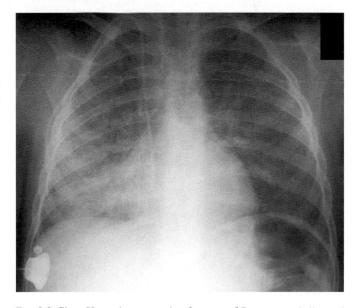

FIG. 8.2. Chest X-ray demonstrating features of *Pneumocystis jiroveci* pneumonia with characteristic "ground-glass" interstitial shadowing. In the early stages perihilar streaky shadowing can give a "bat's wing" appearance

confirmed by specific staining or polymerase chain reaction (PCR) analysis of induced sputum or bronchoalveolar lavage fluid.[26,27] Treatment is with high-dose Septrin, or Pentamidine if Septrin is not tolerated,[27] and the addition of corticosteroids should be considered if there is severe hypoxemia.[28]

Diagnosis of candida pneumonia is complicated by frequent oropharyngeal colonization in immunocompromised subjects. The chest X-ray and clinical findings are generally indistinguishable from *Pneumocystis jiroveci* pneumonia. High-resolution CT is helpful with a characteristic miliary-nodular pattern, although a halo sign and cavitating lesions may also be seen.[29] Treatment options include Amphotericin, Fluconazole, or Caspofungin.[30]

The most common presentation of Aspergillus infection in the immunocompromised host is invasive pulmonary aspergillosis (IPA).[31] The presence of Aspergillus in the respiratory secretions of an immunocompromised individual must be considered pathogenic until proven otherwise because this is associated with a 50–70% risk of invasive aspergillosis.[32] The chest X-ray may show patchy consolidation (Fig. 8.3). High-resolution CT is more informative with characteristic centrilobular nodules, a halo sign, and cavitating lesions.[29,31] Aspergillus antigen is highly specific for invasive aspergillosis but the sensitivity of this test is poor and it often only becomes positive after HRCT features are already apparent.[33] First-line therapy is intravenous Amphotericin B, either standard or liposomal. Amphotericin can also be nebulized as an adjunct to the intravenous route. In patients unresponsive or allergic to Amphotericin second-line agents including Caspofungin and Voriconazole must be used.[31] In neutropenic patients the degree of inflammatory response around the cavitating lesions

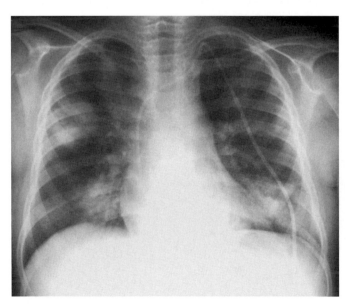

FIG. 8.3. Classical radiological appearance of Aspergillosis in the immunocompromised host, with diffuse patchy consolidation and centrilobular nodules. Later in the infective process cavitation may be seen

increases as the neutrophil count recovers, and this may precipitate life-threatening hemorrhage. Surgical resection of lesions that are central or adjacent to large vessels should be considered. Mortality is high at 30–40%, and prolonged antifungal therapy is required.[34]

Children with Sickle Cell Disease

Children with sickle cell disease are particularly susceptible to pneumococcal, hemophilus, or salmonella infections. This is due to functional asplenia and impaired serum opsonizing activity. The risk of invasive pneumococcal disease is 30–100 times greater than in normal children. This risk can be reduced 3–10 fold by penicillin prophylaxis and pneumococcal vaccination.[35] Parents of children with sickle cell disease are advised to seek medical attention for any chest symptoms or any temperature greater than 38.5°C. In this group there should be a low threshold for admission to hospital for investigation and intravenous broad-spectrum antibiotics.[36] Lower respiratory tract infection can precipitate an acute chest syndrome, with chest pain, pyrexia, tachypnea and cough, or wheeze. Hypoxemia often develops and the chest X-ray reveals segmental consolidation.[37] Acute chest syndrome can also be precipitated by general anesthesia, surgery, fat embolism following infarction within a long bone, and pulmonary infarction. Urgent aggressive treatment with high flow oxygen, broad-spectrum antibiotics, analgesia, and blood transfusion, depending on the hemoglobin and percentage of sickle hemoglobin, are necessary. Early advice from hematology should be sought.[36] Often the oxygen requirement persists for many days, and it is very important to ensure that oxygen saturations above 93% can be maintained before oxygen is discontinued as these patients are at high risk of developing pulmonary hypertension.

Postoperative Children

There is little research on the prevention and treatment of postoperative pneumonia in children. Generally children are at low risk of postoperative pneumonia compared with adults. Obese children are more likely to develop pneumonias postoperatively due to a relative reduction in lung volume.

Children with preexisting lung disease, however, require special consideration. Children with cystic fibrosis require careful preoperative assessment and may benefit from a preoperative course of antibiotics. Postoperatively intensive chest physiotherapy should be performed to mobilize secretions and reduce areas of atelectasis, and prophylactic antibiotics are generally recommended.[38]

In choosing antibiotics for postoperative pneumonia, consideration should be given to the possibility that unusual organisms, for example, Gram-negative bacteria from the gastrointestinal tract, may be implicated.

Unusual Organisms: Actinomycoses, PVL producing MRSA

Actinomyces species are usually found in the oral cavity, particularly in association with poor oral hygiene and dental plaque. With general improvements in oral hygiene actinomyces chest infections have become rare. Children who aspirate are at increased risk. Radiological signs of consolidation and cavitation may be present (Fig. 8.4).[39] Treatment involves a prolonged course of high-dose intravenous penicillin.[40]

Community-acquired methicillin-resistant *Staphylococcus aureus* (MRSA) is an emerging pathogen. Of particular concern are strains positive for the exotoxin Panton-Valentine leukocidin (PVL). PVL is a marker of virulence, which is associated with rapidly progressive disseminated sepsis and necrotizing pneumonia. Mortality rates of 75% have been reported.[41] Teenagers seem at particular risk, and there is an association with influenza infection.[42] Early high-dose intravenous antibiotics active against MRSA are required. Intensive care support is often needed, and intravenous immunoglobulin therapy in unresponsive cases may also have a role.[43,44]

Children with Neurodisability

This group of children is at an increased risk of developing pneumonia, and when pneumonia occurs the associated risks of morbidity and mortality are higher than in neurologically normal children. Up to three-quarters of deaths in severely disabled children may be due to pneumonia.[45] The four main factors predisposing children with neurodisability to the

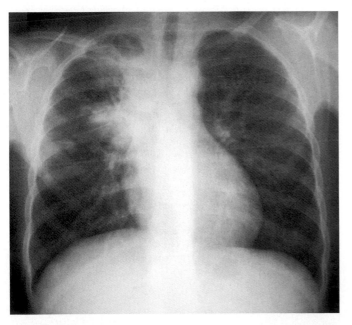

FIG. 8.4. Actinomyces pneumonia in a 10-year-old child. Such infection classically spreads across tissue planes, crossing pulmonary fissures as seen here. Radiological changes are generally slow to resolve

development of pneumonia are recurrent aspiration, ineffective cough, impaired lung function, and immobility.

Bulbar muscle dysfunction can lead to direct aspiration during swallowing.[46] This tends to be worse with liquids compared with solids.[47] In addition, children with neurodisability are prone to gastroesophageal reflux, with rates between 32 and 75%, depending on the diagnostic criteria used.[48] Both direct aspiration and gastroesophageal reflux independently increase the risk of pneumonia but when they are combined there is a particularly high risk of recurrent and severe pneumonia, presumably due to aspiration of stomach contents.[46]

If direct aspiration is suspected clinically this may be documented using a videofluoroscopic contrast swallow, although a negative test does not exclude it.[49] Interventions for direct aspiration include thickened feeds, nasogastric tube feeding, or gastrostomy feeding.[48] Gastroesophageal reflux is usually investigated with 24-h esophageal pH monitoring and/or barium swallow. Initial medical treatment involves feed thickeners, prokinetic agents, and acid suppression, but frequently antireflux surgery is necessary.[48]

In neuromuscular disease coughing is often ineffective due either to poor coordination of forced expiration and glottic closure or to generalized muscle weakness. As a result there is impaired clearance of lower airway secretions, which is a particular problem when viral or bacterial lower respiratory tract infections occur.[48]

The increasing weakness of the respiratory muscles in progressive neuromuscular conditions contributes to a relentless deterioration in lung function. Even in stable neuromuscular conditions lung function may decline due to incremental damage from recurrent pneumonias or aspiration. Lung function measurements can be useful but they are difficult or impossible in small children and children with intellectual impairment. Impaired lung function increases the morbidity and mortality of pneumonia dramatically. In some neuromuscular diseases such as Duchenne muscular dystrophy noninvasive ventilation may reduce respiratory morbidity and improve survival and quality of life, although this needs to be considered very carefully.[50]

Children with Tracheostomies

As these children do not have the physiological benefit of the nasopharynx to warm, humidify, and filter inspired air, they are at increased risk of pneumonia. The trachea may become colonized with *Staphylococcus aureus* or *Pseudomonas aeruginosa*. If isolated on routine culture from an asymptomatic child with a tracheostomy, treatment is not routinely indicated. Presentation of pneumonia in a child with a tracheostomy is similar to child without a tracheostomy. However, the increased secretions require frequent tracheal suction, and this often necessitates admission to hospital for additional humidity.[51]

Diagnosis

Pulse Oximetry

An oxygen saturation of <93% indicates the need for supplemental oxygen.[52] Measurement of oxygen saturation is recommended for every child admitted to hospital with pneumonia.[6]

Acute Phase Reactants

White blood cell count, erythrocyte sedimentation rate, and C-reactive protein are not helpful in differentiating between bacterial and viral pneumonia.[53]

Blood Cultures

Although positive in only 5–10% of children with pneumonia, blood cultures should be routine. They can be useful, for example, in alerting the clinician to organisms demonstrating antimicrobial resistance.[54]

Sputum Culture

Children with pneumonia rarely expectorate, so sputum culture is often not possible. However, in children with neurodisability, children with a tracheostomy, and children with chronic respiratory conditions such as primary ciliary dyskinesia and cystic fibrosis, sputum culture may be extremely helpful in identifying pathogens. There is little data regarding the use of cough swabs or induced sputum samples in normal nonexpectorating children with pneumonia but these techniques are valuable in children with cystic fibrosis.[55]

Nasopharyngeal Aspirates

Detection of RSV, parainfluenza virus, influenza virus, and adenovirus viral antigens in nasopharyngeal aspirates is approximately 80% sensitive for infection.[56] Detection of viral antigen will not usually alter the management of the immunocompetent child but is still useful for cohort isolation and other infection control measures.[6]

Serology

Serology may detect a number of viral, bacterial, and atypical pathogens, but sensitivity and specificity are often poor.[54] In practice, mycoplasma serology is the most relevant. Mycoplasma pneumonia can be difficult to diagnose and can be associated with a number of postinfection extrapulmonary inflammatory syndromes (see section on complications later).

Other

Any ill child with pneumonia should have their urea and electrolytes measured. Inappropriate secretion of antidiuretic hormone is relatively common and results in fluid retention and a fall in the serum sodium. Modest restriction and isotonic intravenous fluids may be indicated. If the initial serum sodium level is below the normal range regular monitoring is indicated to ensure that it corrects slowly (less than 16 mmol/24 h) to avoid damaging rapid swings in intracellular fluid volume.[57]

Radiology

Alveolar shadowing (consolidation) on chest X-ray is a reliable and recognizable indicator of pneumonia in childhood, with 74% specificity for bacterial infection (Fig. 8.5).[2] However, in the outpatient setting a randomized controlled trial has demonstrated that chest radiography does not affect the outcome of children with suspected lower-respiratory tract infection.[58] The indications for a chest X-ray in children thought to have pneumonia require careful consideration.

In a Child <5 Years with Pyrexia of Unknown Origin

Studies suggest that 25% of children less than 5 years of age with significant pyrexia have radiographic signs of pneumonia, even in the absence of any clinical chest signs.[59] A chest X-ray may be clinically useful.

In Children Presenting with Clinical Signs Suggestive of Parapneumonic Pleural Effusion/Empyema

Empyema is considered in a separate chapter. Pleuritic chest pain and/or focally reduced expansion and dullness to percussion

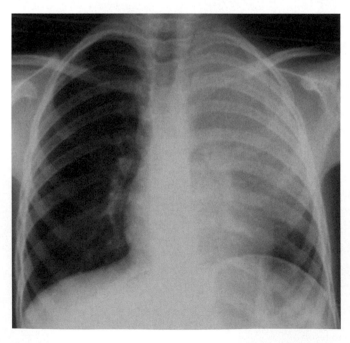

FIG. 8.5. Chest X-ray demonstrating classical left upper lobe pneumonia, without any evidence of lobar collapse

with reduced breath sounds should alert the clinician to the possibility of an empyema, and a chest X-ray is indicated.[60]

In Children Admitted for Treatment of Pneumonia Where There Is No Clinical Improvement After 48h antibiotic Therapy

Children remaining pyrexial or unwell 48h after commencement of antibiotic therapy may have an empyema, atypical infection, or a complicated infection such as staphylococcal pneumonia, and a chest X-ray is indicated.[54,60]

As Follow-Up in Children Who Have Had Lobar Collapse

There is a concern that bronchiectasis may be a sequel of pneumonia when lobar collapse persists (Fig. 8.6). The evidence for this is weak but it remains a common practice to perform a follow-up film at approximately 6 weeks in such cases.[54] Children with consolidation without collapse who are asymptomatic at follow-up 6 weeks later do not require a repeat film.[61]

In Children with Any History Suggestive of an Inhaled Foreign Body

Management of children with an inhaled foreign body is discussed in a separate chapter but the clinician must remember

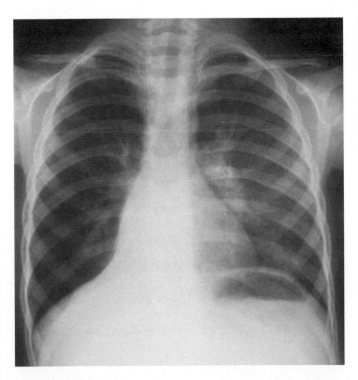

FIG. 8.6. Radiological appearance of right middle lobe collapse, with volume loss of right middle lobe, loss of right heart border, and compensatory hyperinflation of right lower lobe. This child requires radiological follow-up

that these children can present late with symptoms and signs of pneumonia. If a foreign body is suspected a chest X-ray should be performed and bronchoscopy arranged.

Differential Diagnosis

Bronchiolitis

This is predominantly a disease of infancy. A low-grade pyrexia is sometimes present. Auscultation of the chest reveals widespread fine inspiratory crepitations often with widespread expiratory wheeze.

Inhaled Foreign Body

This is considered in a separate chapter, but should always be suspected with focal wheeze or diminished air entry, even in the absence of a suggestive history.

Empyema

Pleuritic chest pain, stony dullness to percussion, diminished air entry, or pneumonia failing to respond to treatment are classical features of an empyema.

Management

Evidence-based guidelines for the management of community-acquired pneumonia in childhood have been published by the British Thoracic Society.[6] As yet no similar guidelines have been produced by the American Thoracic Society.

Infants and children with mild to moderate respiratory distress can be managed safely at home with oral antibiotics. Parents should be advised to seek medical attention if further deterioration occurs, or if there is no improvement after 48h of treatment.[6]

Criteria for Admission

- Oxygen saturation < 93%
- Respiratory rate > 70 breaths per minute in an infant or >50 breaths per minute in older children
- Difficulty in breathing
- Intermittent apneas or grunting
- Inability to feed or signs of dehydration
- Family not able to provide appropriate observation or supervision

These criteria are based principally on a prospective study performed in rural Zambia assessing risk factors for mortality in children under 5 years of age with pneumonia.[11] It should be noted that presence of consolidation on chest X-ray is not a criterion for admission by itself.[6]

Monitoring

Although there is little evidence, it is recommended that children requiring oxygen should be monitored at least four-hourly by oximetry, heart rate, temperature, and respiratory rate. With increasing severity of illness continuous oxygen saturation monitoring is indicated.[6]

Oxygen

As mortality is increased in children with oxygen saturation < 93%, it is recommended that supplemental oxygen is delivered to maintain saturations ≥ 93%. Nasal cannulae are often well tolerated up to flow rates of approximately 2 L per minute, equivalent to an inspired oxygen concentration of around 30–40%.[62] If greater concentrations of oxygen are required a headbox should be used in infants and a rebreathing mask in older children. These devices can deliver an inspired oxygen concentration up to approximately 60%. If the child is still not maintaining satisfactory oxygen saturations an arterial blood gas sample should be taken to measure the PaO_2 and transfer to an intensive care unit arranged.[6,62]

Fluid Management

Children with pneumonia may be unable to drink adequately due to breathlessness and are at risk of dehydration. Babies less than 2 kg with respiratory distress are further compromised by nasal obstruction caused by nasogastric tubes. These babies should receive intravenous fluids.[63] Pneumonia can cause inappropriate secretion of antidiuretic hormone (SIADH). Children requiring intravenous fluid should usually be restricted to 80% of maintenance requirements. Isotonic intravenous fluids should be used, and the serum sodium should be monitored.[6,62]

Antipyretics

Antipyretics are recommended because fever increases insensible fluid losses and also the work of breathing, particularly in infants.[62]

Physiotherapy

Chest physiotherapy is not helpful in previously normal children with pneumonia and should not be performed.[64]

Antibiotic Therapy

Usually when the decision is made to commence antibiotics the causal organism is unknown but empirical treatment can be started based on the age of the child and presenting clinical features.[6,7,62,65] A suggested approach is presented in Table 8.4. Children with preexisting lung disease, neurodisability, or immunocompromise require a more specific approach.

TABLE 8.4. Approach to childhood pneumonia, based on clinical features and age of child.[6,7,62,65]

Age	Clinical features	Chest X-ray features	Inpatient treatment	Outpatient treatment
Neonate (≤4 weeks)	Respiratory distress	Focal consolidation	Intravenous broad spectrum antibiotics (e.g., amoxicillin and gentamicin)	Not recommended
5 weeks – 4 months	Respiratory distress, pyrexia	Focal consolidation	Amoxicillin or penicillin	Amoxicillin
5 weeks – 4 months	Staccato cough, afebrile, tachypnea, conjunctivitis	Interstitial shadowing	Macrolide (e.g., erythromycin)	Macrolide (e.g., erythromycin)
5 months – 15 years	Focal crackles, tachypnea, pyrexia	Focal consolidation	Amoxicillin or penicillin	Amoxicillin
5–15 years	Dry cough, wheeze, pyrexia	Interstitial shadowing	Macrolide (e.g., erythromycin)	Macrolide (e.g., erythromycin)

Antibiotic Resistance

Worldwide surveillance suggests that 10–40% of pneumococcal isolates display resistance to penicillin with particularly high rates in France, Spain, and the USA.[66] This resistance is often not absolute and can be overcome with adequate drug doses. Penicillins remain the antibiotic of choice for pneumococcal infection.[65] Macrolides should only be used against suspected pneumococcal infection in children who are penicillin allergic.[67]

Treatment failure has been described with macrolide-resistant pneumococci.

If *Mycoplasma pneumoniae* or *Chlamydia pneumoniae* are suspected, such as in children older than 5 years with features such as dry cough, fever, wheeze, crackles, and headache, macrolides should be administered.[6,65] Erythromycin is commonly used but this is required four times a day, which reduces compliance. Newer macrolides such as Clarithromycin and Azithromycin can be given twice daily or less but they are more expensive.[68,69]

Route of Administration

There are few studies comparing oral with parenteral antibiotic administration for pneumonia. Two randomized controlled trials suggest that oral amoxicillin is as effective as parenteral penicillin.[70,71] However, in the vomiting or severely unwell child the parental route is more reliable and recommended.[6]

Duration of Antibiotic Treatment

There are no relevant studies regarding either timing of the switch from intravenous to oral antibiotics or the total duration of antibiotic treatment. Generally a total of 7–10 days antibiotic therapy is recommended for pneumonia.[6,65]

Criteria for Transfer to Intensive Care

- Transfer of the child to the pediatric intensive care unit should be considered when:
- The child fails to maintain oxygen saturations of 93% or above in 60% inspired oxygen.
- The child is shocked.
- There is clinical evidence of exhaustion with rise in pulse and respiratory rate. The arterial pCO_2 may be elevated.
- There are recurrent apneas or irregular slow breathing.[6,62]

Complications

The following may occur as complications of childhood pneumonia: empyema, lung abscess, bronchiectasis, pneumatoceles, syndrome of inappropriate antidiuretic hormone (SIADH), and pericarditis (see Table 8.5).[62] Empyema and/or lung abscess should be suspected in any child with pneumonia who remains unwell with a spiking fever 48 h after commencing antibiotic treatment. Management is described in a separate chapter. Mycoplasma pneumonia has a number of specific potential inflammatory sequelae.

Bronchiectasis

Bronchiectasis is defined as abnormal and permanent dilatation of bronchi and is thought to be caused by inflammatory damage to the airway.[72] It is a common feature of cystic fibrosis-related lung disease. Noncystic fibrosis bronchiectasis has a prevalence of approximately 0.2 per 1,000 in children, and a retrospective study suggests that approximately 30% of these cases are associated with previous pneumonia in otherwise normal children.[73] Children with persisting lobar collapse following pneumonia may be at particular risk and require careful follow-up as previously described.[54] Children presenting with bronchiectasis should be screened for cystic fibrosis, primary ciliary dyskinesia, and immunodeficiency.[72]

TABLE 8.5. Complications of childhood pneumonia.

Complications of childhood pneumonia
Empyema
Lung abcess
Bronchiectasis
Pneumatoceles
Syndrome of inappropriate antidiuretic hormone
Pericarditis
Bronchiolitis obliterans
Extrapulmonary inflammatory complications following mycoplasma pneumonia

Pneumatoceles

Pneumatoceles are small multiple thin walled air-filled cysts caused by alveolar and bronchiolar necrosis. They are most commonly associated with *Staphylococcus aureus* pneumonia, when they are seen in approximately 85% of cases, but can also be observed with *Haemophilus influenzae* and Group A Streptococcus pneumonia.[62,74] Progression to pneumothorax or pyopneumothorax has been described but is unusual. In the long term, the prognosis is good with spontaneous resolution and normal lung function, although this may take several months.[75,76]

SIADH

Approximately one-third of children with pneumonia develop hyponatremia due to SIADH.[77] This is thought to be caused by resetting of the thoracic baroreceptors.[62] The excess antidiuretic hormone causes fluid retention by the renal tubules leading to dilutional hyponatremia. Hyponatremia is associated with a 60% longer hospital stay and 3.5-fold increase in mortality.[77] Fluid restriction and regular monitoring of serum electrolytes are the mainstay of treatment. The SIADH resolves as the pneumonia improves.

Pericarditis

This is a rare but life-threatening complication of bacterial pneumonia, with a high mortality.[78] Persistent fever, muffled heart sounds, and signs of right heart failure such as hepatomegaly are the presenting features. Chest X-ray may show a pericardial effusion, and echocardiogram is diagnostic. Treatment includes 4–6 weeks intravenous antibiotics and pericardial drainage.

Bronchiolitis Obliterans

Bronchiolitis obliterans is a poorly understood inflammatory obliteration of small airways resulting in obstructive lung disease with focal areas of air trapping. A characteristic "mosaic" appearance is seen on HRCT (see Fig. 4.3). This complication is particularly seen after adenovirus or mycoplasma pneumonia, especially when contracted in infancy.[79] Bronchiolitis obliterans frequently causes long-term respiratory impairment, and follow-up by a respiratory pediatrician is recommended.

Extrapulmonary Inflammatory Complications Following Mycoplasma Pneumonia

Approximately 25% of those affected by mycoplasma pneumonia will go on to develop extrapulmonary manifestations, most commonly affecting the central nervous system.[80] Such sequelae normally occur within 2 weeks of a *Mycoplasma pneumoniae* infection and may be caused either by direct infectious dissemination, as evidenced by positive culture and PCR analysis of nervous tissue or cerebrospinal fluid, or by an immune-mediated mechanism, as suggested by the development of autoantibodies against components of myelin.[80,81]

Central nervous system manifestations include encephalitis, meningoencephalitis, aseptic meningitis, cerebellar syndrome, cranial nerve palsies, radiculitis, and transverse myelitis. Commonly complete resolution occurs but long-term deficits in motor or cerebral function can occur.

The skin can be involved with erythema multiforme and Stevens–Johnson syndrome, a combination of conjunctivitis, stomatitis, and erythematous rash.[80]

In approximately 14% of cases generalized myalgia, myositis, arthralgia, or polyarthropathy is described. Less common is cardiac involvement including pericarditis, myocarditis, and pericardial effusion. Hemolytic anemia, renal involvement such as glomerulonephritis, hepatitis, and pancreatitis have all been described.[6,80]

For the treatment of the extrapulmonary manifestations of *Mycoplasma pneumoniae* specialist advice should be sought. Generally macrolide antibiotics are recommended. Steroids are used to treat some of the central nervous system manifestations.[80,82]

Rare and Usual Cases

When to Suspect Congenital Abnormality

The respiratory pediatrician must remain alert to the possibility that a child may have developed pneumonia as a result of an underlying congenital abnormality (see Table 8.6). A lobar pneumonia resistant to treatment may be the presenting feature of congenital cystic adenomatoid malformation (CCAM), intralobar sequestration, or bronchogenic cyst.[83] Recurrent pneumonia, particularly if occurring in the same lobe, suggests an underlying congenital abnormality. A study defining recurrent childhood pneumonia as two episodes of pneumonia within a year or three episodes in a lifetime revealed that only 8% of children hospitalized with pneumonia suffer recurrent infection.[84] Of those who did meet the criteria for

TABLE 8.6. Conditions to be considered when pneumonia is either resistant to treatment or recurrent.

Potential underlying causes of recurrent or persistent pneumonia
Congenital abnormality
Congenital cystic adenomatoid malformation
Intralobar sequestration
Bronchogenic cyst
H-type trache-oesophageal fistula
Laryngeal cleft
Immunodeficiency
Cystic Fibrosis
Primary ciliary dyskinesia
Aspiration due to oropharyngeal incoordination
Congenital heart defects

recurrent pneumonia an underlying cause was found in 92%, although the exact diagnostic criteria are unclear. Pneumonia was attributed to aspiration from oropharyngeal incoordination in 48%, congenital cardiac defects in 9%, and congenital pulmonary anomalies in 8%.[84] An H-type tracheesophageal fistula or a laryngeal cleft should be considered in this group of children.[49] Children with recurrent pneumonia affecting the same lobe should, therefore, be investigated to exclude a congenital abnormality.

When to Consider Immunodeficiency, Cystic Fibrosis, or Primary Ciliary Dyskinesia

Immunodeficiency should be considered when a child has had two significant infections requiring intravenous antibiotics. 10% of children identified as having recurrent pneumonia were found to have an immune disorder. These pneumonias did not tend to recur in the same lobe but classically were bilateral and interstitial.[84] Unusual or opportunistic pathogens should also alert the clinician to the possibility of immune deficiency. A careful history of previous infections should be taken including skin infections and episodes of oral thrush. Initial investigations include full blood count for white cell indices, serum immunoglobulins, and functional antibodies. More specialized immunological testing may be necessary in consultation with an immunologist.

Cystic fibrosis classically presents with recurrent chest infections, chronic productive cough, failure to thrive, and loose fatty offensive stools. The diagnosis should be considered in any child who has had two episodes of pneumonia requiring intravenous antibiotics. There may be digital clubbing, unusual pathogens such as *Pseudomonas aeruginosa* detected on sputum culture, and features of bronchiectasis on chest X-ray. Cystic fibrosis is caused by mutations of the gene encoding the cystic fibrosis transmembrane conductance regulator (CFTR) protein. These mutations cause decreased function of this protein resulting in thick viscid pulmonary secretions and reduced clearance of bacteria. Once chronic pulmonary infection develops progressive lung damage occurs and life expectancy is reduced to about 45 years at best.[85] Early diagnosis of cystic fibrosis is extremely important because intensive treatment of early infection, measures to reduce cross-infection, and appropriate pancreatic enzyme and nutritional support are all associated with improved outcome.[86–88] The sweat test remains the gold standard for confirming the diagnosis of cystic fibrosis.[89] A sweat sodium and chloride value of >60 mmol/L is positive, between 40 and 60 mmol/L equivocal, and <40 mmol/L negative. Cystic fibrosis genotyping may be helpful if positive but because of the large number of cystic fibrosis mutations a negative genotype does not exclude cystic fibrosis.[89] 90% of patients with cystic fibrosis are pancreatic insufficient, thus measurement of fecal elastase can also be useful in equivocal cases.[90]

Primary ciliary dyskinesia should also be considered in children who have had two episodes of pneumonia requiring intravenous antibiotics. Primary ciliary dyskinesia is caused by abnormal structure or function of cilia and has a wide spectrum of severity.[91] In approximately 50% of cases there is dextrocardia due to cilial dysfunction during embryogenesis. Ciliary dysfunction in the upper respiratory tract is responsible for chronic rhinosinusitis and secretory otitis media. In the lower respiratory tract chronic productive cough, recurrent pneumonia, and bronchiectasis can occur. Digital clubbing may be present. Diagnosis is by cilial biopsy. Other useful screening investigations include the saccharin test and nasal nitric oxide measurement.[91] Diagnosis allows appropriate treatment including daily chest physiotherapy with early and prolonged courses of oral antibiotics for any increase in respiratory symptoms. The prognosis is usually good, with near normal life expectancy.[91]

Controversies

When Is Treatment Indicated?

There is only one randomized controlled trial in children diagnosed with pneumonia comparing children treated with antibiotics with those not receiving antibiotics.[92] The diagnosis of pneumonia was based on either fine crepitations on auscultation or consolidation on chest X-ray, and children with severe dyspnea, cyanosis, or preexisting lung disease were excluded. Approximately half the children were diagnosed as having viral pneumonia, principally RSV. Although outcome was comparable between the two groups, interpretation of the study is difficult as many of the subjects probably had bronchiolitis rather than pneumonia. Thus, there is little evidence to support the use of antibiotics for community-acquired pneumonia. It is difficult to differentiate reliably between viral and bacterial pneumonias in children either clinically or by using acute phase reactants. The following pragmatic approach is recommended. Preschool children (age less than 4 years) with wheeze as a presenting feature are unlikely to have bacterial pneumonia and should not normally require antibiotics. Children with alveolar shadowing (consolidation) on chest X-ray have 74% specificity for bacterial infection and should receive antibiotics.[2] For other children with respiratory signs, such as focal bronchial breathing or crackles, there is very little direct evidence either for or against treatment, although with these focal signs most clinicians would commence antibiotic therapy.[6]

Aspiration as an Etiological Factor

Aspiration may be due to swallowing dysfunction or gastroesophageal reflux[49] and may be associated with wheeze, stridor,[93] and pneumonia.[94] Children with neurological disease are the most likely to have swallowing dysfunction although it can be seen in otherwise normal children.[49] Proving aspiration as the cause of recurrent pneumonia is often difficult as the literature in the area is limited to describing association rather than

cause, and all the relevant investigations have limitations.[49] For example, normal videofluoroscopic swallow or normal esophageal pH studies do not exclude infrequent aspiration or gastroesophageal reflux, respectively. Gross aspiration or gastroesophageal reflux on such studies, when associated with recurrent respiratory exacerbations, would encourage many to consider treatment such as gastrostomy with fundoplication. Where doubt exists as to the contribution of aspiration to the respiratory symptoms, a trial of nasogastric or, where gastroesophageal reflux is present, nasojejunal feeds may be diagnostically valuable.[49]

If recurrent aspiration is occurring it is important to exclude anatomical causes such as H-type tracheoesophageal fistula, as specific treatment of such abnormalities may be curative.[49]

Duration of Treatment

There are no randomized controlled trials comparing differing total duration of antibiotic treatment or duration of intravenous antibiotic treatment prior to switching to oral antibiotics in the treatment of childhood pneumonia.[6,65] Generally children who have commenced intravenous antibiotics for pneumonia and who are improving can be switched to oral antibiotics at approximately 1–2 days and total treatment duration varies from 5 to 10 days.[65]

Investigations

In children who do not meet the criteria for admission to hospital (see earlier) there is no indication for any investigations. In children admitted to hospital blood cultures may be useful and in sick children serum electrolytes should be performed to assess for any evidence of SIADH.[6] Acute phase reactants are not useful and probably overperformed.[53] Similarly chest X-ray is not routinely indicated in straightforward pneumonia and is probably overrequested.[54] Pulse oximetry should be part of the general assessment of the child at presentation and as part of routine monitoring of children admitted to hospital.[6]

Prognosis and Long-Term Outcome

Bacterial pneumonia, with the exception of that caused by PVL+ve MRSA, has an excellent outcome with complete resolution expected in children with normal nutrition and no underlying disease. Adenoviral pneumonia has a more guarded prognosis, with a mortality in children under 2 years of age of 16.7%,[95] and an increased risk of developing the chronic obstructive lung disease bronchiolitis obliterans.[96]

Conclusions and Future Perspective

The assessment of a child with suspected pneumonia is predominantly clinical. Many children can be treated at home with oral antibiotics. Those who meet the criteria for hospital admission are usually treated initially with intravenous antibiotics. Complications should be suspected if the child is not improving after 48 h of appropriate treatment. The clinician should be aware that underlying conditions should be considered in children suffering two or more episodes of pneumonia requiring hospital admission, or where there are other atypical features.

Several aspects of pneumonia treatment require further study, including the route of administration of antibiotics and the duration of treatment. It will be interesting to see what impact pneumococcal vaccination programs have on the prevalence of pneumonia over the next few years.

References

1. World Health Organization. The management of acute respiratory infections in children. Practical guidelines for outpatient care. Geneva: WHO, 1995
2. Korppi M, Kiekara O, Heiskanen-Kosma T, et al. Comparison of radiological findings and microbial aetiology of childhood pneumonia. Acta Paediatr 1993; 82: 360–363
3. Davies HD, Wang EE, Manson D, et al. Reliability of the chest radiograph in the diagnosis of lower respiratory tract infections in young children. Pediatr Infect Dis J 1996; 15: 600–604
4. Rudan I, Tomaskovic L, Boschi-Pinto C, et al. Global estimate of the incidence of clinical pneumonia among children under five years of age. Bull World Health Organ 2004; 82: 895–903
5. Enwere G, Biney E, Cheung Y, et al. Epidemiologic and clinical characteristics of community-acquired invasive bacterial infections in children aged 2–29 months in The Gambia. Pediatr Infect Dis J 2006; 25: 700–705
6. British Thoracic Society Standards of Care Committee. Guidelines for the management of community acquired pneumonia in childhood. Thorax 2002; 57 (Suppl I): i1–i24
7. Stein RT, Marostica PJC. Community-acquired pneumonia. Paediatr Resp Rev 2006; 7S: S136–S137
8. Jokinen C, Heiskanen L, Juvonen H, et al. Incidence of community-acquired pneumonia in the population of four municipalities in eastern Finland. Am J Epidemiol 1993; 137: 977–988
9. Korppi M, Heiskanen L, Kosma T, et al. Aetiology of community-acquired pneumonia in children treated in hospital. Eur J Pediatr 1993; 152: 24–30
10. Weigl JA, Puppe W, Belke O, et al. Population-based incidence of severe pneumonia in children in Kiel, Germany. Clin Padiatr 2005; 217: 211–219
11. Smyth A, Carty H, Hart CA. Clinical predictors of hypoxaemia in children with pneumonia. Ann Trop Paediatr 1998; 18: 31–40
12. Campbell H, Byass P, Lamont AC, et al. Assessment of clinical criteria for identification of severe acute lower respiratory tract infections in children. Lancet 1989; i: 297–299
13. Rudnick CM, Hoekzema GS. Neonatal herpes simplex virus infections. Am Fam Physician 2002; 65: 1138–1142
14. Andersen RD. Herpes simplex virus infection of the neonatal respiratory tract. Am J Dis Child 1987; 141: 274–276
15. Kanegaye JT, Harley JR. Pneumonia in unexpected locations: An occult cause of paediatric abdominal pain. J Emerg Med 1995; 13: 773–779
16. Winsey HS, Jones PF. Acute abdominal pain in childhood: Analysis of a year's admissions. BMJ 1967; 1: 653–655
17. Jona JZ, Belin RP. Basilar pneumonia simulating acute appendicitis in children. Arch Surg 1976; 111: 552–553
18. Mendoza Sanchez MC, Ruiz-Contreras J, Vivanco JL, et al. Respiratory virus infections in children with cancer or HIV infection. J Pediatr Hematol Oncol 2006; 28: 154–159
19. Soldatou A, Davies EG. Respiratory virus infections in the immunocompromised host. Paediatr Resp Rev 2003; 4: 193–204
20. Heath PT. Epidemiology and bacteriology of bacterial pneumonias. Paediatr Resp Rev 2000; 1: 4–7
21. Pizzo PA, Rubin M, Freifeld A, et al. The child with cancer and infection. II. Non-bacterial infections. J Pediatr 1991; 119: 845–857
22. Pizzo PA. Management of fever in patients with cancer and treatment-induced neutropenia. N Engl J Med 1993; 328: 1323–1332
23. Copley SJ. Application of computed tomography in childhood respiratory infections. Br Med Bull 2002; 61: 263–279
24. Labenne M, Hubert P, Gaillard JL, et al. Diagnosis of pulmonary infections in critically ill immunocompromised children. Pediatr Pulmonol 1997; 16 Suppl: 59–60
25. Johny AA, Clark A, Price N, et al. The use of zanamivir to treat influenza A and B infection after allogeneic stem cell transplantation. Bone Marrow Transplant 2002; 29: 113–115
26. Graham SM. Non-tuberculosis opportunistic infections and other lung diseases in HIV-infected infants and children. Int J Tuberc Lung Dis 2005; 9: 592–602
27. Huang L, Morris A, Limper AH, et al. An official ATS workshop summary: Recent advances and future directions in pneumocystis pneumonia (PCP). Proc Am Thorac Soc 2006; 3: 655–664
28. Briel M, Bucher HC, Boscacci R, et al. Adjunctive corticosteroids for *Pneumocystis jiroveci* pneumonia in patients with HIV-infection. Cochrane Database Syst Rev 2006; 19: 3
29. Althoff Souza C, Muller NL, Marchiori E, et al. Pulmonary invasive aspergillosis and candidiasis in immunocompromised patients: A comparative study of the high-resolution CT findings. J Thorac Imaging 2006; 21: 184–189
30. Pagano L, Caira M, Fianchi L. Pulmonary fungal infection with yeasts and pneumocystis in patients with hematological malignancy. Ann Med 2005; 37: 259–269
31. Pound MW, Drew RH, Perfect JR. Recent advances in the epidemiology, prevention, diagnosis, and treatment of fungal pneumonia. Curr Opin Infect Dis 2002; 15: 183–194
32. Perfect JR, Cox GM, Lee JY, et al. The impact of culture isolation of Aspergillus species: A hospital-based survey of aspergillosis. Clin Infect Dis 2001; 33: 1824–1833
33. Kami M, Tanaka Y, Kanda Y, et al. Computed tomographic scan of the chest, latex agglutination test and plasma (1AE3)-beta-D-glucan assay in early diagnosis of invasive pulmonary aspergillosis: A prospective study of 215 patients. Haematologica 2000; 85: 745–752
34. Herbrecht R, Denning DW, Patterson TF, et al. Voriconazole versus Amphotericin B for primary therapy of invasive aspergillosis. N Engl J Med 2002; 347: 408–415
35. O'Brien KL, Swift AJ, Winkelstein JA, et al. Safety and immunogenicity of heptavalent pneumococcal vaccine conjugated to CRM197 among infants with sickle cell disease. Pediatrics 2000; 106: 965–972
36. American Academy of Pediatrics, Section on Hematology/Oncology and Committee on Genetics. Health supervision for children with sickle cell disease. Pediatrics 2002; 109: 526–535
37. Vichinsky EP, Neumayr LD, Earles AN, et al. Causes and outcomes of the acute chest syndrome in sickle cell disease. National

Acute Chest Syndrome Study Group. New Engl J Med 2000; 342: 1855–1865

38. Weeks AM, Buckland MR. Anaesthesia for adults with cystic fibrosis. Anaesth Intensive Care 1995; 23: 332–338

39. Conant EF, Wechsler RJ. Actinomycosis and nocardiosis of the lung. J Thorac Imaging 1992; 7: 75–84

40. Yildiz O, Doganay M. Actinomycoses and Nocardia pulmonary infections. Curr Opin Pulm Med 2006; 12: 228–234

41. Gillet Y, Issartel B, Vanhems P, et al. Association between Staphylococcus aureus strains carrying gene for Panton-Valentine leukocidin and highly lethal necrotising pneumonia in young immunocompetent patients. Lancet 200; 359: 753–759

42. Hageman JC, Uyeki TM, Francis JS, et al. Severe community-acquired pneumonia due to *Staphylococcus aureus*, 2003–4 influenza season. Emerg Infect Dis 2006; 12: 894–899

43. Gauduchon V, Cozon G, Vandenesch F, et al. Neutralization of *Staphylococcus aureus* Panton-Valentine leukocidin by intravenous immunoglobulin in vitro. J Infect Dis 2004; 189: 346–353

44. Hampson FG, Hancock SW, Primhak R. Disseminated sepsis due to a Panton-Valentine leukocidin producing strain of community acquired methicillin resistant *Staphylococcus aureus* and use of intravenous immunoglobulin therapy. Arch Dis Child 2006; 91: 201

45. Plioplys AV, Kasnicka I, Lewis S, et al. Survival rates among children with severe neurological disabilities. South Med J 1998; 91: 161–172

46. Morton RE, Wheatley R, Minford J. Respiratory tract infections due to direct and reflux aspiration in children with severe neuro-disability. Dev Med Child Neurol 1999; 41: 329–334

47. Mirrett PL, Riski JE, Glascott J. Videofluoroscopic assessment of dysphagia in children with severe spastic cerebral palsy. Dysphagia 1994; 9: 174–179

48. Seddon PC, Khan Y. Respiratory problems in children with neurological impairment. Arch Dis Child 2003; 88: 75–78

49. Boesch RP, Daines C, Willging JP, et al. Advances in the diagnosis and management of chronic pulmonary aspiration in children. Eur Resp J 2006; 28: 847–861

50. Simonds AK. Respiratory complications of the muscular dystrophies. Semin Respir Crit Care Med 2002; 23: 231–238

51. Eber E, Oberwaldner B. Tracheostomy care in the hospital. Paediatr Resp Rev 2006; 7: 175–184

52. Poets CF. When do infants need additional inspired oxygen? A review of the current literature. Pediatr Pulmonol 1998; 26: 424–428

53. Nohynek H, Valkeila E, et al. Erythrocyte sedimentation rate, white blood cell count, and serum C-reactive protein in assessing etiologic diagnosis of acute respiratory infections in children. Pediatr Infect Dis J 1995; 6: 484–490

54. Coote N, McKenzie S. Diagnosis and investigation of bacterial pneumonias. Paediatr Resp Rev 2000; 1: 8–13

55. Ho SA, Ball R, Morrison LJ, et al. Clinical value of obtaining sputum and cough swab samples following inhaled hypertonic saline in children with cystic fibrosis. Pediatr Pulmonol 2004; 38: 82–87

56. Korppi M, Heiskanen-Kosma T, Leinonen M, et al. Antigen and antibody assays in the aetiological diagnosis of respiratory infection in children. Acta Paediatr 1993; 82: 137–141

57. Siragy HM. Hyponatremia, fluid-electrolyte disorders, and the syndrome of inappropriate anti-diuretic hormone secretion: Diagnosis and treatment options. Endocr Pract 2006; 12: 446–457

58. Swingler GH, Hussey GD, Zwarenstein M. Randomised controlled trial of clinical outcome after chest radiograph in ambulatory acute lower-respiratory infections in children. Lancet 1998; 351: 404–408

59. Bachur R, Perry H, Harper MB. Occult pneumonias: Empiric chest radiographs in febrile children with leukocytosis. Ann Emerg Med 1999; 33: 166–173

60. Balfour-Lynn IM, Abrahamson E, Cohen G, et al., on behalf of the Paediatric Pleural Diseases Subcommittee of the BTS Standards of Care Committee. BTS guidelines for the management of pleural infection in children. Thorax 2005; 60 (Suppl 1): i1–i21

61. Gibson NA, Hollman AS, Paton JY. Value of radiological follow-up of childhood pneumonia. BMJ 1993; 307: 1117

62. Russell-Taylor M. Bacterial pneumonias: Management and complications. Paediatr Resp Rev 2000; 1: 14–20

63. Stocks J. Effect of nasogastric tubes on nasal resistance during infancy. Arch Dis Child 1980; 55: 17–21

64. Levine A. Chest physical therapy for children with pneumonia. J Am Osteopath Assoc 1978; 78: 122–125

65. Hale KA, Isaacs D. Antibiotics in childhood pneumonia. Paediatr Resp Rev 2006; 7: 145–151

66. Low D, Pichichero ME, Schaad UB. Optimising antibacterial therapy for community-acquired respiratory tract infections in children in the era of bacterial resistance. Clin Pediatr 2004; 43: 135–151

67. Jacobs MR, Johnson CE. Macrolide resistance: An increasing concern for treatment failure in children. Pediatr Infect Dis J 2003; 22(8 suppl): S131–S138

68. Harris JA, Kolokathis A, Campbell M, et al. Safety and efficacy of azithromycin in the treatment of community acquired pneumonia in children. Pediatr Infect Dis J 1998; 17: 865–871

69. Block S, Hedrick J, Hammerschlag MR, et al. *Mycoplasma pnemoniae* and *Chlamydia pneumoniae* in pediatric community-acquired pneumonia: Comparative efficacy and safety of clarithromycin vs. erythromycin ethylsuccinate. Pediatr Infect Dis J 1995; 14: 471–477

70. Tsarouhas N, Shaw KN, Hodinka RL, et al. Effectiveness of intramuscular penicillin versus oral amoxicillin in the early treatment of outpatient pediatric pneumonia. Pediatr Emerg Care 1998; 14: 338–341

71. Addo-Yobo E, Chisaka N, Hassan M, et al. Oral amoxicillin versus injectable penicillin for severe pneumonia in children aged 3–59 months: A randomised multicentre equivalency study. Lancet 2004; 364: 1141–1148

72. Fall A, Spencer D. Paediatric bronchiectasis in Europe: What now and where next? Paediatr Resp Rev 2006; 7: 268–274

73. Eastham KM, Fall AJ, Mitchell L, et al. The need to redefine non-cystic fibrosis bronchiectasis in childhood. Thorax 2004; 59: 324–327

74. Oviawe O, Ogundipe O. Pneumatoceles associated with pneumonia: Incidence and clinical course in Nigerian children. Trop Geogr Med 1985; 37: 264–269

75. Ceruti E, Contreras J, Neira M. Staphylococcal pneumonia in childhood. Long term follow-up including pulmonary function studies. Am J Dis Child 1971; 122: 386–392

76. Soto M, Demis T, Landau LI. Pulmonary function following staphylococcal pneumonia in children. Aust Paediatr J 1983; 19: 172–174

77. Singhi S, Dhawan A. Frequency and significance of electrolyte abnormalities in pneumonia. Indian Pediatr 1992; 29: 735–740

78. Sinzobahamvya N, Ikeogu MO. Purulent pericarditis. Arch Dis Child 1987; 62: 696–699

79. Castro-Rodriquez JA, Daszenies C, Garcia M, et al. Adenovirus pneumonia in infants and factors for developing bronchiolitis obliterans: A 5-year follow-up. Pediatr Pulmonol 2006; 41: 947–953

80. Waites KB, Talkington DF. Mycoplasma pneumoniae and its role as a human pathogen. Clin Microbiol Rev 2004; 17: 697–728

81. Guleria R, Nisar N, Chawia TC, et al. Mycoplasma pneumoniae and central nervous system complications: A review. J Lab Clin Med 2005; 146: 55–63

82. Carpenter TC. Corticosteroids in the treatment of severe mycoplasma encephalitis in children. Crit Care Med 2002; 30: 925–927

83. Laberge JM, Puligandla P, Flageole H. Asymptomatic congenital lung malformations. Semin Pediatr Surg 2005; 14: 16–33

84. Owayed AF, Campbell DM, Wang EEL. Underlying causes of recurrent pneumonia in children. Arch Pediatr Adolesc Med 2000; 154: 190–194

85. FitzSimmons SC. The changing epidemiology of cystic fibrosis. J Pediatr 1993; 122: 1–9

86. Frederiksen B, Koch C, Hoiby N. Antibiotic treatment at time of initial colonisation with *Pseudomonas aeruginosa* postpones chronic infection and prevents deterioration in pulmonary function in patients with cystic fibrosis. Pediatr Pulmonol 1997; 23: 330–335

87. Farrell PM, Kosorok MR, Rock MJ, et al. Early diagnosis of cystic fibrosis through neonatal screening prevents severe malnutrition and improves long term growth. Wisconsin Cystic Fibrosis Neonatal Screening Study Group. Pediatrics 2001; 107: 1–13

88. Lee TWR, Brownlee KG, Denton M, et al. Reduction in prevalence of chronic *Pseudomonas aeruginosa* infection at a regional paediatric cystic fibrosis centre. Pediatr Pulmonol 2004; 37: 104–110

89. Rosenstein BJ, Cutting GR, for the Cystic Fibrosis Consensus Panel. The diagnosis of cystic fibrosis: A consensus statement. J Pediatr 1998; 132: 589–595

90. Cade A, Walters MP, McGinley N, et al. Evaluation of faecal elastase-1 as a measure of pancreatic exocrine function in children with cystic fibrosis. Pediatr Pulmonol 2000; 29: 172–176

91. Bush A, Cole P, Hariri M, et al. Primary ciliary dyskinesia: Diagnosis and standards of care. Eur Respir J 1998; 12: 982–988

92. Friis B, Andersen P, Brenoe E et al. Antibiotic treatment of pneumonia and bronchiolitis. A prospective randomised study. Arch Dis Child 1984; 59: 1038–1045

93. Sheikh S, Allen E, Shell R, et al. Chronic aspiration without gastro-oesophageal reflux as a cause of chronic respiratory symptoms in neurologically normal infants. Chest 2001; 120: 1190–1195

94. Berquist WE, Rachelefsky GS, Kadden M, et al. Gastro-oesophageal reflux-associated recurrent pneumonia and chronic asthma in children. Pediatrics 1981; 68: 29–35

95. Videla C, Carballal G, Misirlian A, et al. Acute lower respiratory infections due to respiratory syncitial virus and adenovirus amongst hospitalised children from Argentina. Clin Diagn Virol 1998; 10: 17–23

96. Colom AJ, Teper AM, Vollmer WM, et al. Risk factors for the development of bronchiolitis obliterans in children with bronchiolitis. Thorax 2006; 61: 503–506

9
Empyema Thoracis

Dakshesh H. Parikh

Introduction

Empyema thoracis is defined as an accumulation of pus within the pleural cavity. While the morbidity and mortality of this condition have undoubtedly improved over recent years debate continues regarding the nature and timing of surgical intervention. The management planning and the selection of the most appropriate treatment option require good understanding of the empyema disease process. Moreover, the incidence of empyema thoracis in children has increased significantly in recent years in the western world.[1,2] The incidence of parapneumonic effusion and empyema is approximately 3.3 cases per 100,000 children.[3] It has been estimated that 1 in every 150 children hospitalized with pneumonia will develop an empyema.[4]

Historical Perspective

The natural history of empyema thoracis was described by Hippocrates who realized that drainage could result in cure.[5] He observed that death was likely "if pus that flows after opening was mixed with blood, muddy and foul smelling."[5] He also remarked that if the empyema was drained "with knife or cautery" and the pus was "pale and white" the patient would survive.[6,7] The brilliant French surgeon Pare described evacuation of infected blood from the pleural cavity in the sixteenth century. These early physicians understood the importance of early diagnosis and drainage to avoid mortality in this disease. Browditch[8] described thoracocentesis while Wyman performed the first therapeutic pleural aspiration, describing the method in a letter to Sir William Osler.[9] Commenting on pleural space infections, Osler later wrote "It is sad to think of number of lives which are sacrificed annually by the failure to recognise that empyema should be treated as an ordinary abscess by free incision."[10] Sir William Osler himself underwent a rib resection and drainage of parapneumonic empyema in his home in 1819.

Playfair modified the technique of thoracocentesis to closed tube drainage in 1875.[11] Schede introduced thoracoplasty in

1890.[12] Fowler reported the first decortication in 1893 and soon became apparent that release of the trapped lung was a better procedure in chronic nontuberculous empyema than thoracoplasty.[12-15] A survey carried out by the Surgeon General of the United States of America in 1918 concluded that the high mortality (30%) following rib resection in acute empyema was related to the open pneumothorax.[16] This US commission, headed by Graham, recommended closed drainage for the management of acute empyema. This single act reduced the mortality from empyema dramatically to 5–10%.[17] In addition, it was realized that prevention of chronicity by complete obliteration, sterilization of the empyema cavity, and careful attention to the nutrition was responsible for better results.[18]

Pathogenesis and Basic Science

Etiology

The majority of empyemas in children follow acute bacterial lobar pneumonia.[19] During recovery from viral infections such as chicken pox and measles children are more susceptible to lower respiratory tract infections and therefore empyema. Underlying conditions such as chronic pulmonary diseases, diabetes mellitus, long-term steroid therapy, organ transplantation with associated immune suppression, and recurrent aspiration could predispose the child to empyema.

Empyema may follow secondary infection of a traumatic hemothorax or lung contusion.[20,21] Occasionally a secondary empyema follows a penetrating injury of the chest or after infection in the pleural space following thoracotomy. More commonly secondary empyema in children invariably follows intrathoracic rupture of the esophagus either as a result of a leaking anastomosis or rupture following dilatation of an esophageal stricture.[22] Secondary infection of a sympathetic effusion has been reported after acute pancreatitis and a subphrenic abscess. Pneumonia and empyema have been reported in the postoperative period in children with acute appendicitis. In these cases the empyema probably occurs as a result

D.H. Parikh et al. (eds.), *Pediatric Thoracic Surgery*,
DOI: 10.1007/b136543_9, © Springer-Verlag London Limited 2009

a

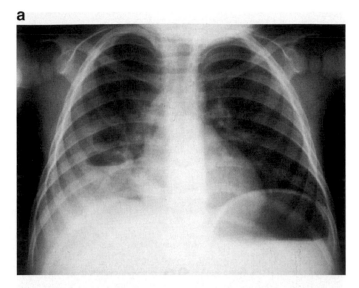

b

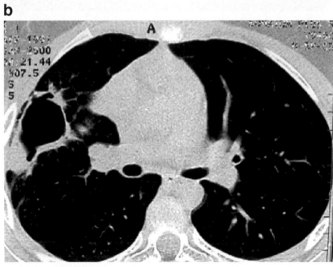

FIG. 9.3. Congenital lung malformation presenting with recurrent pneumonia: (a) Chest X-ray showing consolidation with pneumatoceles in the right lower lobe (b) convalescent CT scan compatible with a cystic adenomatoid malformation, confirmed after a right lower lobectomy

monest causative organism is *Staphylococcus aureus*.[20,21,36] *Haemophilus influenzae, Streptococcus pyogenes* and, less often, *Klebsiella pneumoniae, Bacteroides*, and other anaerobes are isolated from childhood empyemas. There are sporadic reports of empyemas due to *Pseudomonas aeruginosa*, rare species of *Streptococci, Proteus, Salmonella*, and *Yersinia*.[37]

The bacterial profile in developing countries differs with *S. aureus* being the predominant pathogen, especially during the hot and humid months when staphylococcal skin infections are prevalent.[38] There has been a decline in culture-positive *Streptococcus pneumoniae*, probably because of prior antibiotic use.[38] Various Gram-negative organisms (e.g., Enterobacteriaceae such as *Klebsiella* spp. and *Pseudomonas aeruginosa*) are also more common than in the UK. This may be related to protein energy malnutrition.[36,38–40] Tuberculous empyema

may result from progressive pulmonary tuberculosis. It has been reported to account for up to 6% of all empyema cases[41] worldwide although it is seldom seen in the UK.[26]

Fungal empyemas are rare in immunocompetent children.[42,43] *Histoplasma* infection may be related to environmental exposure.[44] *Mycoplasma* is rarely associated with empyema. Mycoplasma serology confirms the association.[45] *Legionella pneumophila*, adenovirus, and influenza[46–48] may be primary agents causing pneumonia associated with a pleural effusion but the contribution of these agents to a subsequent empyema is probably small.

Immunodeficiency predisposes children to infection and overwhelming sepsis. In this context consideration has to be given to opportunistic pathogens as well as organisms recognized to cause empyema. Nocardia and other rare infections have been reported. Conversely if an unusual causative organism is encountered in an empyema, the child should be investigated for an immunodeficiency. These children are usually malnourished and have a history of recurrent infection.

Clinical Features

Clinical History

Symptoms of pneumonia in children such as, cough, breathlessness, fever, malaise, fetor, and loss of appetite precede symptoms related to the pleural collection/empyema. Younger children tend to present early with tachypnea and fever, lethargy, and cough. Some children also complain of pleuritic chest pain. Infection in the lower lobes may present with abdominal pain. In children already on treatment for pneumonia, a spiking fever and lack of improvement after 48 h of antibiotics may signal the presence of an effusion. A comprehensive history should be taken including recent antibiotic therapy, previous medical history, and contact with tuberculosis. The possibility of an inhaled foreign body should not be forgotten in children.

Physical Examination

Almost all children with an empyema will have an intermittent pyrexia, tachycardia, and an increased respiratory rate. Some children will be cyanosed, although this may be difficult to detect in the presence of anemia. Measurement of oxygen saturation (SaO_2) by pulse oximetry is particularly important, with levels below 92% in room air indicating severe disease.[49] Clinical examination must include assessment of the child's state of hydration and a full physical examination.

Clinical signs in the thorax include decreased chest expansion, stony dullness to percussion, reduced or absent breath sounds, and scoliosis. If a large effusion is present mediastinal shift may be detectable by tracheal deviation and displacement of the apex beat to the opposite side although this is relatively uncommon because the effect of the effusion is counterbalanced by collapse of the infected lung. Consolidation of the underlying lung causes bronchial breathing and reduced air entry apparent on auscultation. Regular physical examinations and keeping good clinical records can help a clinician monitor child's condition and pneumonia effectively, and help reduce reliance on blood and radiological parameters.

Diagnosis

Investigations

Acute Phase Reactants

The white blood cell count is invariably raised in a child with an empyema, with a neutrophilia and frequently associated with anemia. C-reactive protein (CRP) and other inflammatory markers such as procalcitonin are also elevated. These have been used as markers to assess response to treatment.

Although it is commonly believed that elevated levels of acute phase reactants such as white cell count, total neutrophil count, CRP, ESR, and procalcitonin will distinguish bacterial infections from viral infections of the respiratory tract several recent prospective studies have shown this to be incorrect.[50-54]

There is no correlation between levels of acute phase reactants in acute bacterial pneumonia and empyema formation. In addition, there is no evidence in the literature supporting the view that trends in acute phase reactants correlate with clinical progress, although clinical practice has shown that serial measurements of CRP and the white cell count can be helpful in monitoring response to treatment.

Biochemistry, Hematology, and Coagulation Studies

Routine measurement of urea and electrolytes forms part of the assessment of the state of hydration. Hyponatremia is relatively common in children with severe sepsis, and this must be corrected preoperatively. Hyponatremia may be due to inappropriate ADH (SIADH) and/or hypotonic intravenous fluid infusions (4% dextrose 0.18% saline). Correction involves modest fluid restriction and, if intravenous fluids are necessary, 5% dextrose with 0.45% saline or 0.9% saline should be used. The serum albumin is invariably low.

Virtually all children with an empyema will be anemic. Usually this is a normochromic normocytic anemia but occasionally hemolysis occurs, particularly in association with pneumococcal infections. The direct Coomb's test will be positive in these children, and specific advice from a hematologist should be sought. Occasionally abnormalities in coagulation are seen in children with empyemas and it is important to recognize this prior to surgery.

Microbiology

Blood, pleural fluid, and sputum should all be sent for culture as a matter of routine in a child with an empyema. In an ideal world these samples should be taken prior to the administration of antibiotics.[49] Microbial culture should always include bacterial and tuberculosis culture. A Mantoux test should be performed if there is suspicion of tuberculosis.

A recent large retrospective study of 540 children with community-acquired pneumonia, 153 of whom subsequently developed an empyema, confirmed the value of these investigations.[55] Blood cultures were positive in 15/153 (10%) of children who developed an empyema and in 25/387 (6.4%) of those with pneumonia alone. In a series of 76 children with complicated parapneumonic effusions blood cultures were positive in 22%, compared with pleural fluid that was positive in 33% cases.[33] Hardie et al. reported a series of 56 children with pneumococcal effusions.[3] Blood cultures were positive in 10/56 cases (18%), and in 7/10 children with positive blood cultures the pleural fluid was sterile.

Diagnostic Pleural Aspiration

Thoracocentesis is not mandatory but is recommended prior to starting antibiotics in a child with a suspected empyema. Pleural fluid should be sent for urgent microscopy, Gram stain, culture, and differential cell count. Cytological examination of the pleural fluid in an empyema classically shows a predominance of polymorphonuclear leukocytes. A lymphocytic preponderance should raise the possibility of either tuberculosis or malignancy[56] although it is important to note that in at least 10% of tuberculous effusions there is a neutrophil preponderance. Most malignant effusions in children are blood stained although cytological examination of the pleural fluid may not show malignant cells.[57]

On many occasions pleural fluid is sterile because of prior antibiotic administration.[58] A diagnostic tap will be unsuccessful if the parietal peel is very thick or the pus particularly viscid. In the event of a failed diagnostic tap, it is mandatory to evaluate all clinical and radiological evidence of empyema thoroughly before undertaking definitive management.

Sophisticated laboratory analysis may reveal causative organisms when conventional culture fails. Latex agglutination tests are available for detection of pneumococcal antigens.[35] Polymerase chain reaction techniques are available for the detection of pneumococcal DNA[34,35] and mycobacterial DNA.[59]

Routine biochemical analysis of the pleural fluid is unnecessary and does not contribute to the management of empyema in childhood. Pleural fluid taken from children with an empyema shows a glucose concentration $< 2.2\,\mathrm{mMol/L}$, pH $<$ 7.2, LDH $> 1,000\,\mathrm{I/dL}$, protein $> 25\,\mathrm{g/L}$, and a specific gravity > 1.018. Pleural fluid from a child with a sterile clear or sympathetic effusion will show a pH > 7.2 and a glucose concentration $> 2.2\,\mathrm{mMol/L}$.

Radiology

First radiological investigation is usually a plain chest X-ray. Pneumonic consolidation will be seen. The appearance of a pleural effusion is signaled by a fluid meniscus. As the effusion enlarges mediastinal shift is rare (Fig. 9.4a). A lung abscess, pneumatoceles, and a pyopneumothorax (Figs. 9.5 and 9.6)

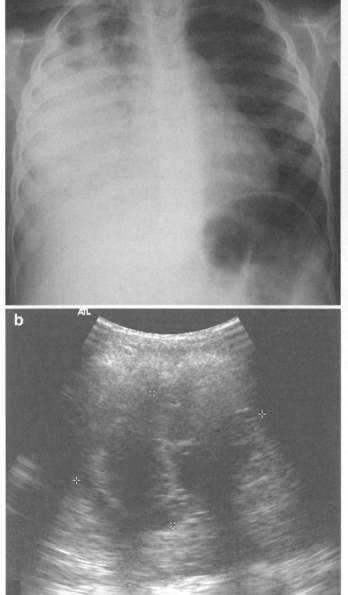

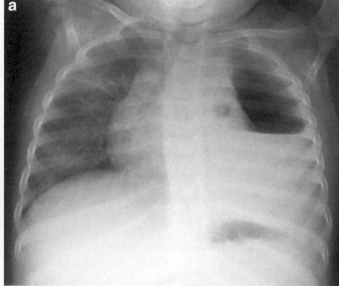

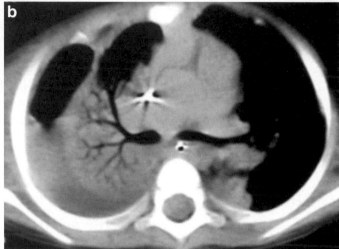

FIG. 9.5. Pyopneumothorax: (**a**) Chest X-ray showing a fluid level in the pleural collection. (**b**) CT scan with IV contrast showing a rupture of a pneumatocele as a cause of a bronchopleural fistula

FIG. 9.4. Empyema: (**a**) Plain chest X-ray showing meniscus sign and consolidation with little or no mediastinal shift, which would suggest consolidation rather than collapse related to pleural effusion. (**b**) Ultrasound showing loculations and septa with the pleural effusion containing debris suggestive of empyema

are all visible on a chest X-ray. The plain X-ray cannot differentiate an empyema from a tumor. A pulmonary blastoma is commonly mistaken for an empyema as the clinical presentation and some of the radiological features are similar.[60,61] Therefore, the plain chest radiograph especially in the fibrinopurulent and organization phases of an empyema is suggestive but not diagnostic of empyema.

Ultrasonography is particularly valuable for imaging the child with a suspected empyema. Ultrasound is portable and thereby available for immediate bedside examination of critically ill children. Fluid in the pleural space is easy to identify. Ultrasound is most useful to determine whether an effusion is loculated (Fig. 9.4b).[62] Although an impression of the density and echogenicity of the pleural fluid can be gained from ultrasound this does not correlate well with the pathological stage of the empyema.[63] Akhan et al. reported a characteristic appearance of tuberculous effusions on ultrasound, noting the presence of diffuse small nodules on the pleural surface.[64]

Ultrasound may be used to guide chest drain insertion or thoracocentesis. The optimum site for drainage or aspiration can be marked on the skin by the radiologist.[65,66] The key limiting factors of sonographic evaluation of the chest are based

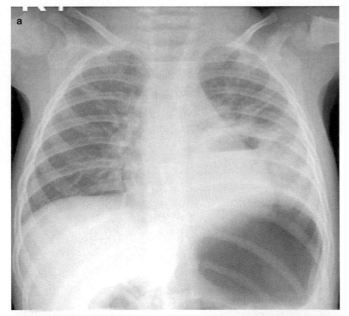

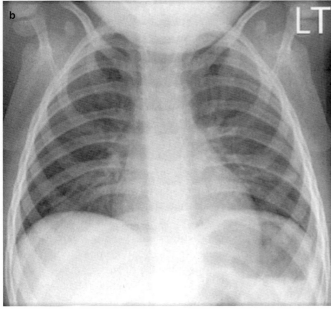

FIG. 9.6. (a) Chest X-ray showing consolidated lung, a cavity containing fluid level (an abscess) and empyema. (b) Follow-up chest X-ray showing complete resolution of the cavity. The management consisted of empyema debridement and drainage without resection of the cavity

on the physical limitations of the ultrasound beam. As the intercostal spaces narrow, the value of ultrasound becomes limited.[67] Occasionally, homogenous solid lesions are mistaken for fluid collections on sonography.

Computed tomography (CT) with intravenous (IV) contrast complements ultrasonography for imaging children with complicated pneumonia.[67,68] Parenchymal lung pathology can be identified clearly. CT with IV contrast distinguishes the rare lung tumors presenting as empyema in childhood as well as identifying mediastinal pathology.[61] Thickened pleural rind, consolidated lung, and associated

lung pathology, such as a lung abscess, are all clearly visible on CT[63,69,70] (Fig. 9.5b). An empyema associated with lung necrosis, pneumatoceles, or a lung abscess invariably takes a more protracted postoperative course than a simple empyema. Furthermore, the presence of underlying lung pathology will require prolonged follow-up and monitoring. While unnecessary for most cases of pediatric empyema, CT undoubtedly has a role in complicated cases (including initial failure to aspirate pleural fluid and failing medical management) and in immunocompromised children.

Bronchoscopy

Routine bronchoscopy is unnecessary unless a foreign body is suspected. Bronchoalveolar lavage may be useful in identifying the infective organism but it is considered unnecessary when pleural fluid is available for culture.

Differential Diagnosis

Intrathoracic Tumors Presenting as Empyema

Thoracic tumors presenting as an empyema appear in literature as case reports.[60,71–75] Initial clinical, biochemical, and radiological findings in all these cases were consistent with a diagnosis of empyema. Although diagnostic pleural aspiration and cytology is not routinely performed in children, if a high lymphocyte count is found underlying malignancy should be suspected and investigated. Most malignant effusions in children are blood stained although it is uncommon for malignant cells to be identified on cytology.

The author reported a series of eight children with intrathoracic tumors mimicking empyema.[62] Ultrasound was performed in four children but failed to identify the presence of intrathoracic tumor in all. Preoperative CT scans without IV contrast were misleading and failed to identify the underlying pathology. Four children underwent thoracotomy for debridement of the empyema, with substantial blood loss in two cases. A third child, with a pleuropulmonary blastoma, developed a tumor implantation nodule at the site of thoracotomy incision necessitating excision of the chest wall with residual tumor in the left lower lobe. In the remaining four cases CT scans with IV contrast correctly identified the intrathoracic tumors preoperatively.

It is possible that in spite of careful preoperative evaluation intrathoracic tumors will occasionally be diagnosed only at the time of emergency thoracotomy. In this situation the surgeon should take a biopsy and then achieve hemostasis before closure. Although incidence of tumors presenting as empyema is thought to be low, the eight children we reported represented 5.3% of all empyemas presenting to us during that period.

In the pediatric population pleuropulmonary blastoma, benign cystic teratoma (Fig. 9.7), primitive neuroectodermal tumors and lymphomas have all been mistaken for empyemas.[61,75]

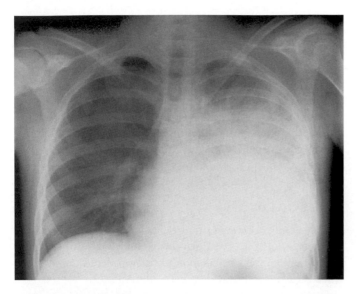

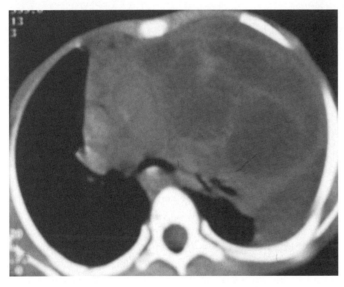

FIG. 9.7. Infected cystic mediastinal teratoma with effusion: (a) Chest X-ray showing signs of pleural collection, ultrasound confirmed pleural collection but failed to identify mediastinal pathology (b) CT scan with IV contrast showing the mediastinal pathology which was resected and the empyema was drained. The CT scan prompted an open thoracotomy approach rather than VATS debridement of the empyema alone.

Clinical vigilance and careful preoperative evaluation are necessary. A nonresolving empyema, blood-stained pleural effusion, and pleural fluid with a raised lymphocyte count and a very large pleural effusion are all potentially suspicious where a preoperative CT scan with IV contrast is recommended.

Management

The cardinal principles of empyema management are administration of appropriate intravenous antibiotics in combination with adequate drainage to achieve full expansion of the lung.

Medical Management

- Optimum perioperative medical management should be an integral component of a successful management strategy of childhood empyema.

Early recognition and treatment of lobar pneumonia in children reduces the incidence of empyema. Lack of clinical improvement after 48 h suggests that either the choice of antibiotic is inappropriate or that there is an associated empyema. The chest radiograph should be repeated, and if there is any suspicion of an effusion an ultrasound examination is requested.

Small sympathetic effusions are commonly associated with acute lobar pneumonia, and these usually resolve with antibiotics alone.

Supportive medical therapy is essential. This includes oxygen, fluids/nutrition, analgesia, and respiratory physiotherapy. Humidified oxygen should be administered to maintain oxygen saturations above 95%. Isotonic intravenous fluids should be given to correct dehydration and electrolyte imbalances. Antipyretics and analgesics should be given regularly. Children who fail to improve clinically and radiologically should be referred to a center with expertise in surgery of empyema drainage procedures.

Antibiotics

Response to antibiotics is dependant upon the pathogen involved, the stage of empyema, and the immune status of the child. In the early exudative stage high concentrations of antibiotics alone may be effective treatment whereas antibiotics are unlikely to be effective in more advanced disease without surgical intervention.[76] Unless a pathogen with known sensitivity to antibiotics has been isolated first-line treatment with high doses of a cephalosporin is recommended. In the authors' institution first-line treatment comprises IV cefuroxime at 50 mg/kg doses three times daily. In the event of impaired renal function reduced doses are recommended. Recommendations for antibiotic therapy for childhood empyema are not evidence based but based on local patterns of bacterial resistance. Other antibiotics such as flucloxacillin, amoxycillin, gentamicin, and meropenem may be necessary depending on the sensitivity of organisms isolated from blood or pleural aspirate culture.

Occasionally despite adequate drainage sepsis continues. This is usually related to necrotizing pneumonia or occasionally to a distant septic focus. In these circumstances, clindamycin or rifampicin may be useful to manage infection with Gram-positive organisms. In these complex empyemas it is usually necessary to give combination therapy with more than one antibiotic. Advice from microbiology is essential.

Pleural Aspiration

Parapneumonic effusions can be drained with either by repeated thoracocentesis or by closed tube thoracostomy. Repeated aspiration is not a satisfactory option in children as it is painful and requires considerable cooperation from the patient. Closed chest drainage is the preferred option.

Traditionally this involves insertion of a 16–20F chest drain through the fifth intercostal space between the anterior and mid-axillary lines under either local or general anesthesia. Practice is changing in many centers in favor of small-bore tubes or pigtail catheters placed under ultrasound guidance.

Surgical Management

- The goal of surgery is to achieve full expansion of the lung and resolution of the empyema.
- Early surgical intervention in childhood empyema reduces morbidity.
- Treatment failure should be recognized early to avoid disease progression.

Surgical practice for the management of childhood empyema varies around the world. The principal problem, however, is establishing the pathological stage of the empyema preoperatively. By the time the child arrives in the hands of a surgeon it is safe to assume that the empyema is in the fibrinopurulent phase even if the pus aspirated is not thick. Effective drainage with lung expansion in this phase is imperative to reduce morbidity and progression of the disease to the organization phase.

A large meta-analysis of literature search from 1984 to 2004 by Avinsino et al. concluded that primary operative therapy is associated with reductions in mortality, reintervention rate, length of hospital stay, time with tube thoracostomy, and duration of antibiotic therapy, compared with nonoperative treatment.[77]

Intercostal Tube Drainage and Fibrinolytics

Closed intercostal tube insertion with administration of IV antibiotics may be successful in early stage empyemas and in some later stage cases if loculation is minitmal. Some authors advocate intrapleural fibrinolytic therapy[58] to improve drainage.

It is important to recognize when conservative therapy is failing to reduce the morbidity associated with delayed referral for surgery. Persistent sepsis with a pleural collection after a maximum of 7 days conservative management is an absolute indication for surgical referral.[56] Seven days is an arbitrary period chosen to acknowledge different rates of disease progression yet provide a clear limit on the duration of medical therapy.

The author recommends pediatricians managing empyemas in peripheral hospitals to seek surgical advice after 3 days of intrapleural fibrinolytics if there is continuing pyrexia and a persisting pleural collection.

There are conflicting studies in the literature concerning the use of intrapleural fibrinolytics. It must be emphasized that the use of fibrinolytics is an adjunct to improve drainage, which should not change the underlying principles of empyema management.

Technique: Intercostal Chest Tube Drainage

Intercostal chest tubes in young children are best inserted under general anesthesia by a pediatric surgeon using an open technique. In some centers pigtail catheters or small-bore catheters are inserted using the Seldinger technique by respiratory physicians or interventional radiologists using intravenous sedation and local anesthesia.

Informed consent must be obtained. The procedure should be explained to the child. The operating surgeon must ensure that the chest radiographs are available to confirm the diagnosis and the side of the empyema.

If conscious IV sedation and local anesthesia is to be used then it is helpful to apply topical anesthetic (EMLA® or Ametop®) to the skin 1–2h prior to the procedure. The safety of the child is paramount and this necessitates that the person administering the sedation should be competent in airway management and resuscitation of children. General anesthesia is safer than intravenous sedation in a child with respiratory compromise and certainly this is the preferred option for noncooperative children.

Chest drains should be inserted using an aseptic technique. Whether conscious sedation or general anesthesia is used, local anesthetic should be instilled to minimize postoperative discomfort. Plain bupivacaine 0.25% to a maximum dose of 2 mg/kg (0.8 ml/kg) can be infiltrated into the skin and deeper layers or, alternatively, used for intercostal nerve blocks.

In some centers ultrasound is used to mark the optimum site (location of the pleural fluid) for chest drain insertion. If this technique is used it is important to document patient position when the spot is being marked.[78–80] Catheter placement using CT guidance has been recommended for difficult cases.[80–85]

The safest site for an open method of intercostal chest drain is the fifth intercostal space between the anterior and mid-axillary lines. This region is termed the "safe triangle."[86] The safe triangle is outlined by the anterior border of the latissimus dorsi muscle, the lateral border of the pectoralis major muscle, and a horizontal line at the level of the nipple. This region minimizes the risk to underlying structures, avoids damage to muscle, breast tissue, and an unsightly scar. A more posterior position is uncomfortable and risks the drain kinking. A more anterior position risks inadvertent laceration of an intercostal artery.

The skin should be incised and a track dissected down to the pleura on the upper border of the rib using an artery forceps. This track should be developed to allow direct insertion of the chest drain without force. Forceful insertion of a chest tube or use of an introducer risks damaging intrathoracic organs with potentially fatal consequences and should be avoided. The drain must be well secured after insertion to prevent inadvertent displacement. This involves a heavy-gauge nonabsorbable suture placed through the skin and tied tightly repeatedly around the drain. An airtight occlusive dressing should be applied. A purse-string suture is unnecessary. Special dressings and fixation devices are available to hold small pigtail catheters in place instead of a conventional suture (e.g., Drain-Fix®, Maersk Medical Ltd, Stonehouse UK).

urokinase therapy.[111] Open thoracotomy results in significant postoperative pain and inevitably leaves behind a scar causing rib crowding and subsequent chest deformity and scoliosis.

Technique of Minithoracotomy and Debridement

The anesthetised child is placed in a lateral decubitus position. An incision is made along the fifth or sixth intercostal space from posterior axillary line to anterior axillary line. A muscle cutting approach involves cutting through both latissimus dorsi and serratus anterior muscles in the line of the incision. A muscle-sparing incision involves mobilization of the latissimus dorsi muscle from its anterior margin, retracting it posteriorly, and then either splitting the serratus anterior between digitations or reflection of the lower digitations after detaching them from the chest wall, which is preferred. Muscle-sparing incisions are believed to be less painful. The thorax can then be opened through an intercostal space or after subperiosteal resection of a segment of rib. Debridement is carried out and all the purulent material is evacuated under direct vision. The collapsed lung is seen to expand before the thoracotomy is closed. One of two chest drains are placed before closure and connected to an underwater seal.

Video-Assisted Thoracic Surgery (VATS) Debridement

With the advent of video-assisted techniques, many surgeons are challenging the traditional approaches to empyema management in children. Kehr and Rodgerson were the first to describe thoracoscopic drainage in children. VATS techniques offer advantages in terms of accurate disease staging and debridement of the fibrinous pleural disease, separating the loculi under vision.[115] The technique is less invasive than thoracotomy yet in experienced hands as effective and safe. There have been no comparative trials in children to suggest that early surgery is superior to drainage and fibrinolytics. A small study included in the Cochrane review, randomized 20 patients with empyema to receive intrapleural streptokinase for 3 days via a chest drain with immediate VATS. The surgical group had a high treatment success rate 10/11. Five of nine patients who failed to respond to streptokinase therapy were salvaged by VATS. The VATS patients required chest drainage for shorter periods and had shorter hospital stays.[116] However, this study can be criticized based on small sample size and an unusually high failure rate following fibrinolysis.

Proponents of early endoscopic surgery claim that if general anesthesia is used for insertion of a chest drain then the procedure should be combined with VATS.[117] Early VATS has been shown to benefit lung reexpansion and improve the drainage of the empyema.[117–119] Loculi can be separated allowing thick pus to drain effectively.[108,115,120–122] Many series have shown reduced postoperative pain, shorter hospital stay, and better cosmetic results when VATS is compared with conventional thoracotomy.[108,120,123,124] Unfortunately VATS is difficult in children when first-line management

with fibrinolytics has failed,[124] and it is not suitable for advanced empyemas.[108,118] Several studies comparing conventional thoracotomy and VATS debridement[115,125,126] have favored VATS approach claiming reduced duration of hospital stay, reduced blood loss, less discomfort, and reduced chest drainage. However, Goldschlager's study showed no difference in length of postoperative chest drainage or hospital stay. Although most studies are retrospective containing small number, VATS has proven effective, with minimal complications, and was well tolerated.

Thoracoscopy requires expertise and a well-trained operating team familiar with the equipment. In the presence of a thick pyogenic membrane covering the visceral and parietal pleura, the likelihood of damaging the inflamed lung while removing the pyogenic membrane is high. Conversion to open thoracotomy is necessary when access to the pleural cavity proves impossible because of a thick pyogenic rind or if there is excessive bleeding. Minithoracotomy and debridement or decortication in these instances is safer and curative.[110,127,128]

Technique of VATS Debridement

VATS is performed under general anesthesia with a single lumen endotracheal tube in majority of cases. Selective endobronchial intubation, or the use of bronchial blocker in young children where double lumen tubes are not available, may be useful in selected cases to avoid contamination of the contralateral lung. The child is placed in a lateral decubitus position with the involved side upward. The best site for trocar placement is determined by needle aspiration of pleural fluid. Firstly a 5-mm port is inserted under direct vision in order to avoid damage to the inflamed lung. This port is usually inserted in the fifth or sixth intercostal space in the posterior axillary line. Creation of a working space is essential. A $0°$ or $30°$ telescope is used for visualization. Liquid pus is aspirated before insufflation with CO_2 at 5–8 mmHg pressure. Carbon dioxide insufflation is not mandatory throughout the length of the procedure because the lung will often collapse sufficiently to allow visualization of the empyema cavity. A second port for instrumentation is placed under thoracoscopic visualization. Two ports are usually sufficient if debridement is performed early.

The empyema cavity is irrigated with warm saline, and pyogenic material is gently removed either with the suction aspirator or with the help of Yohan's or equivalent atraumatic forceps. Pleural debris should be sent for culture. The entire pleural cavity can be debrided effectively under vision. In majority of cases the lung starts to reexpand at this stage of operation. All surfaces of the lung, including the fissures, should be inspected, and a chest drain is left in place through one of the port sites. Local anesthetic is infiltrated around the port sites or used for intercostal nerve blocks.

Most children can be managed safely on a pediatric surgical ward postoperatively with nurse- or patient-controlled analgesia. The chest X-ray is repeated the following day to confirm lung expansion and assess the extent of lung consolidation. Fibrinolytics may be helpful in the postoperative period after thoracoscopic debridement if lung expansion is incomplete. This is especially useful when the surgeon is in the learning phase of thoracoscopic debridement or if debridement is known to be incomplete. The chest drain should remain in place until the losses reduce to less than 30 ml/day and become clear. The child is kept in hospital on intravenous antibiotics until afebrile for at least 24 h. A further chest X-ray should be taken following drain removal.

Thick membrane is seen on occasions encasing the lung not allowing expansion; a peanut sponge is used gently to peel the membrane off the visceral pleura. Conversion to open thoracotomy is indicated in cases of failure of separation of the fibrous rind from the visceral pleura after the thoracoscopic maneuvers, excessive bleeding, inadequate visualization, and failure of lung reexpansion.

Thoracotomy and Decortication

Decortication of an organized empyema carries a significant morbidity from bleeding and air leaks.[27,129–131] Decortication requires removal of the thickened fibrous parietal peel and sharp dissection to remove the visceral peel encasing the lung. This is best performed through a conventional posterolateral thoracotomy. The aim of decortication is to free the encased lung to allow reexpansion and to free the chest wall to allow proper respiratory excursion. Excision of the pleural rind may result in substantial bleeding and an air leak and occasionally nerve damage. Blood must be available. Early recognition of the fibrous stage and prompt intervention minimize these risks. Provided decortication is complete, the prognosis for lung function is excellent in most cases. However, inadequate management places the child at risk of chronic ill health with continuing sepsis, restrictive lung disease, failure to thrive, and anemia. The child becomes a respiratory cripple. The chest X-ray shows persistent lung collapse, loss of volume, and a scoliosis attributable to progressive fibrosis.[130]

Technique of Decortication

Decortication is carried out using a conventional posterolateral thoracotomy.

The chest is usually entered through sixth intercostal space although the rib resection may be necessary to achieve sufficient exposure. The empyema cavity is entered through the organizing parietal peel, which is usually thick and very dense. The cavity is evacuated with samples taken for bacterial culture. The parietal peel is stripped from the inside of the chest wall by digital dissection. This can be difficult but as the chest wall is freed the thoracotomy will open progressively. The peel should not be disturbed over the mediastinal surface because of the risk of damaging vital structures.

Separating the peel from the diaphragm is generally unsatisfactory because it is often impossible to find a plane of cleavage.

The encased lung is then freed. This involves gentle finger dissection around the edge of the lung and between the fissures. The thick visceral rind is carefully incised with knife down to the plane immediately beneath the cicatricial coat and the visceral pleura. The visceral pleura if possible should be left intact if possible. Development of this plane invariably results in significant bleeding and often multiple air leaks. Once the correct plane is entered blunt dissection is generally adequate to liberate the collapsed lung.

After decortication is complete the anesthetist expands the lung gradually to identify any air leaks and to allow excision of any remaining restrictive peel. Injury to the lung parenchyma should be repaired if possible. At least one large-bore chest drain should be placed and sometimes two are necessary. The thoracotomy is then closed using standard techniques. Application of low-pressure suction to the drain helps lung expansion in presence of an air leak.

Major complications from decortication are related to persistent air leak, bleeding, and sepsis. Air leaks up to 10–14 days after surgery are not uncommon in advanced cases. Residual blood in the pleural space may become secondarily infected defeating the purpose of the operation because of ensuing fibrosis. While the mortality following decortication in experienced hands should be low, some series have reported mortalities between 1.3 and 10%.[27,129,131,132] Death is fortunately rare but invariably due to hemorrhage or septic complications.

A chronic empyema causes significant derangement of lung function. Both ventilation and perfusion of the collapsed lung are markedly reduced, particularly perfusion. Physiological improvement following successful decortication depends largely on the nature and extent of any residual parenchymal lung disease, which, in turn, depends on the infecting organism and the duration of the chronic empyema. Functional improvement continues for many months after decortication.

Thoracoplasty

This is rarely necessary in childhood empyema and is to be avoided if at all possible. There are two indications for thoracoplasty: First, if the underlying lung is so badly damaged that it is incapable of reexpansion despite decortication (this leaves a large residual intrapleural space, which will become reinfected unless the chest wall is collapsed), and second, if there is a bronchopleural fistula that fails to close after decortication. In this situation vascularized tissue must be brought into the thorax to cover the damaged lung surface. A pedicled muscle flap thoracoplasty is usually the best solution.

Management of Complex Empyemas

Empyema with Lung Abscess and Necrotizing Pneumonia

The outcome of this type of empyema depends on adequate postoperative lung expansion and appropriate antibiotic therapy. Pneumatoceles will generally resolve after debridement or decortication of the empyema.[109,133] Similarly most lung

10
Pulmonary Tuberculosis

Pankaj R. Parekh

Introduction

Mycobacterium tuberculosis is one of the most successful infective organisms affecting one third of global population and responsible for over two million deaths each year[1]. Tuberculosis (TB) is causing worldwide concern because strains resistant to standard anti-tuberculosis chemotherapy are being isolated with increased frequency[2]. The rising incidence of TB in developed countries is largely attributable to immigration.

Following primary infection in childhood the initial host immune response is usually capable of localizing the infection but unfortunately falls short of completely eradicating the pathogen. The ability of the TB to persist after initial infection within a healed tubercle is referred to as latent TB and this is central to the biology of tuberculous disease. Latent TB poses a significant risk to the host from reactivation in adult life and it also represents a major obstacle to the eradication of the disease.

Over the last century attempts to control tuberculosis have centered on mass immunization with bacille Calmette-Guérin (BCG), early identification of infection, treatment with anti-tuberculous therapy and improvements in hygiene, sanitation and nutrition.

Epidemiology

The Director General of World Health Organization (WHO) declared TB a global public health emergency in 1993 with an estimated global incidence of 1.3 million and a mortality rate of 450,000 children per year. The recently released WHO global TB control report shows that the incidence of TB peaked in 2004 and has remained constant since 2005[3]. The majority of new cases are reported in densely populated countries like India and China but the highest prevalence is seen in sub-Saharan Africa, the Indonesian archipelagos, Afghanistan and Bolivia[4]. The substantial increase in the prevalence of TB in Africa in recent years (almost 80% of the global TB burden) is largely attributable to HIV/AIDS[5]. The incidence of TB in children is much more difficult to estimate accurately because of the lack of systematically collected data. In the past childhood TB has been given a low priority. However, it is estimated that 20–40% of all notifications represent TB infection in childhood. In India alone more than ten million children a year are at risk from contracting TB from a smear-positive adult.[6,7]

Most countries in Western Europe have TB notification rates below 10 per 100,000, while some countries in Eastern Europe, including the former Soviet Union, report case detection rates of more than 100 per 100,000. The percentage of TB cases occurring in children is estimated to vary from 15 % in developing countries to below 5 % in the United States and Europe[4]. In 2002 the US Center for Disease Control and Prevention (CDC) estimated the incidence of TB to be 5.6 new cases per million[8]. Between 1984 and 1992 the incidence of TB increased in the USA as a result of a deteriorating public health infrastructure and the rising incidence of HIV. Pediatric TB, however, fell from 3.1 new cases per 100,000 in 1992 to 1.5 per 100,000 in 2001. The incidence of TB in the UK is increasing. In 2000 there were 12.9 new cases per 100,000 population in England and Wales[9].

Historical Perspective

Hippocrates described a dangerous disease causing death to many by consumption - *"many of those who had been long gradually declining, took to bed with symptoms of phthisis..... many, and, in fact, the most of them, died; and of those confined to bed, I do not know if a single individual survived for any considerable time."* Hippocrates also recognized that the disease was more common in the winter and that the outcome was slightly better for victims who could walk compared to those confined to bed although eventually all succumbed to death[10].

The term 'tubercle' was coined by *Franciseus Sylvius (1614–1672)*. The term 'tuberculosis' was introduced by *Laurent Bayle (1774–1816)*. *Frascatorius (1483–1553)* hypothesized that the disease was transmitted by air-borne living particles named 'contagium vivium'[11]. In a series of

D.H. Parikh et al. (eds.), *Pediatric Thoracic Surgery*,
DOI: 10.1007/b136543_10, © Springer-Verlag London Limited 2009

11
Lung Abscess

John Hewitson

Introduction

A lung abscess is a localized collection of pus within the lung, in a cavity caused by the destruction of parenchyma. Lung abscesses occur rarely in children, and seldom require surgical intervention. They are classified into *primary* and *secondary*,[1,2] and acute or chronic.[3] A primary abscess is seen in a patient who has no predisposing medical problem, while in a patient with a secondary lung abscess, one or more of the pulmonary defence mechanisms has been compromised by an underlying condition, predisposing to pulmonary infection.[4] An acute abscess is defined arbitrarily as one that has developed in less than 6 weeks. Children with an acute lung abscess are typically ill and febrile, while an inadequately treated abscess may persist as a chronic thick-walled abscess, with low-grade fever and less severe symptoms. Most lung abscesses in children are solitary, although multiple abscesses may be seen with aspiration or hematological spread.

Like many suppurative diseases, the incidence of primary lung abscess in children has risen for obscure reasons.[5] A specific increase in necrotizing pneumococcal pneumonia has been noted in children in communities where pneumococcal vaccination is not widely used.[6–8] An increase in the number of immuno-deficient children due to human immunodeficiency virus (HIV) infection, hematological malignancy, cancer chemotherapy, and organ transplantation has also contributed to an increase in secondary lung abscesses.[8]

In undeveloped countries, in addition to high HIV infection rates, other issues such as malnutrition and various unrelated subtropical diseases may modify the immune response. Also a factor in such communities is the high incidence of pulmonary tuberculosis (TB) and thus of lungs with post-tuberculous damage, which may not be clinically apparent but where pulmonary defences are damaged.

More recently, a growing problem has been the rise in nosocomial infections amongst neonates and immuno-compromised children requiring intensive care.[9,10]

Historical Perspective

Lung abscess has been recognized as a pathological entity since at least the time of Hippocrates, who suggested aspiration from the oropharynx as a likely cause, and described an external drainage as a life-saving procedure.[11] Before the advent of antibiotics death was likely without surgical drainage, and even with external drainage the mortality was high, while chronicity was common among survivors.[12–14]

In 1904, Guillemot gave weight to the theory that aspirated oropharyngeal organisms rather than emboli were the source of pulmonary suppurative disease when he identified, in empyema thoracis, organisms normally found in the mouth.[15] In 1942, Brock[16] added further evidence when he showed that aspirated matter gravitated to dependent portions of the lung, explaining why lung abscesses due to aspiration are commonest in parts of the lung that are dependent when the patient is supine.

In the early nineteenth century, conservative therapy (typically arsenicals and physiotherapy) occasionally resulted in a cure but was usually of little value.[12] Although percutaneous needle aspiration was occasionally tried with success, the favored approach was by external surgical drainage, commonly in two stages, the first stage to stimulate pleurodesis so as to avoid contamination of the pleural space and at the second stage, the actual drainage of the abscess.[12,17] The alternative, pulmonary resection, gradually gained favor after the introduction of the cuffed endotracheal tube together with improved and safer general anesthesia. However, mortality remained high for all approaches.

The introduction of antibiotics had a dramatic impact, and the pendulum of management swung rapidly away from surgery to a conservative approach for most cases.[18,19] There was a short period when bronchoscopic drainage of abscesses was in vogue[20,21] but it proved hazardous, especially in children, because of the risk of sudden flooding of the airways with purulent material.[12] In recent years, the practice of percuteneous drainage has again become popular as a useful tool to both hasten recovery and identify the organism.[19,22,23]

D.H. Parikh et al. (eds.), *Pediatric Thoracic Surgery*,
DOI: 10.1007/b136543_11, © Springer-Verlag London Limited 2009

The use of Fogarty catheters as endobronchial blockers in children has been well described for surgery in the presence of suppurative lung disease.[76,77] More recently the use of a variety of other bronchial blockers have been described, some of them used alongside an endotracheal tube, some through the tube, and some are constructed as part of the tube.[78–80] However, malpositioning of a blocker either initially or through slippage during manipulation or positioning of the patient is a real danger with bronchial blockers.[81] For this reason, and because of the need for very small-size fiberoptic bronchoscopes for proper placement of endobronchial blockers and the limited experience of many anesthesiologists, these techniques have limited application in many units. Intubation of the main bronchus of the contralateral lung has also been described. Although this can work quite well for right lung surgery with direct intubation of the left main bronchus, the intubation of the right main bronch usually blocks the upper lobe bronchus as well.

A safer alternative is the use of the prone position: the patient is positioned prone and slightly head-down (modified Overholt position[82]), the resection being approached through a posterior thoracotomy.[83] This position allows secretions to gravitate to the upper trachea rather than the contralateral lung, and regular suctioning by the anesthetist can remove them. The surgeon should attempt to isolate and clamp the bronchus before the major vessels, to limit the chance of spillage.

Surgical Considerations

By the latter half of the last century, the surgical approach to a problematic lung abscess was commonly resection of the affected lobe.[12,13] In reality, however, resection is seldom necessary in children, especially with the highly effective antibiotic therapy available today, and the remarkable recoverability of a child's lung.[22] Resection is at times appropriate, such as when there is obvious destruction of a lobe with likely residual bronchiectasis, or in special situations with complications such as some cases of pyopneumothorax with uncontrollable bronchopleural fistula. Most such patients have very large or rapidly expanding abscesses and surrounding necrotizing pneumonia with microabscess. Resection is also appropriate in the scenario of a foreign body still obstructing a major bronchus, with distal abscess formation. Such a lobe is certainly destroyed, and the safest way to deal with the foreign body is to remove it along with the lobe. However, in most cases of lung abscess with failed conservative therapy, resection is unnecessary and some type of external drainage will suffice.

After needle aspiration, the least invasive option is a closed-tube pneumonostomy made directly into the abscess cavity across the fused pleura through a small skin incision, with the positioning of a soft drain (e.g., Malecot) in the abscess, the pleural space remaining undisturbed.[18,84] As with percutaneous drainage, postero-anterior and lateral chest radiographs are usually adequate to accurately locate the abscess.

If the abscess contains thick pus mixed with much necrotic tissue debris, then pneumonostomy may be inadequate and open drainage becomes necessary. A mini-thoracotomy is made, also directly over the abscess where the pleura is most likely to be adherent, and a finger-sized hole is made into the abscess by cutting away ("deroofing") a segment of the wall. The contents are gently evacuated, and a soft drain is left in the cavity.[12,18,85]

Slough that is adherent to the wall should not be forcibly removed as it is likely to be viable tissue, and tearing it away can cause excessive bleeding. If the pleura is not adherent at the point of entry or is stripped away during the procedure, pneumothorax and spillage of pus into the pleural space will necessitate the placement of separate pleural drains.

There will invariably be some degree of air leakage from the lung after either procedure, but this is usually minor, the very reason the abscess has not drained adequately internally. The drain is connected to an underwater seal, without suction, for 24–48 h, by which time the cavity has usually collapsed around the drain, the air leak has stopped, and the clinical picture is dramatically improved.

When there is a coexisting empyema or pyopneumothorax requiring open thoracotomy, the abscess should be adequately drained, if necessary by de-roofing as part of the procedure, allowing it to drain freely into the pleural space.[28,86] The adequate drainage of the pleural space and the abscess must take into account presence of a broncho-pleural fistula. The aim of the primary procedure should be to achieve reexpansion of the lung. Decortication may be necessary to achieve this goal of reexpanding the trapped lung and a pedicled muscle flap to contain the bronchopleural fistula. Postoperativley, adequate size of intercostal drains should be strategically placed in the pleural cavity for providing continued drainage. Lobectomy can be considered in difficult and necrotic lung as the best option.[87] Alternatively, after establishing initial adequate drainage, resection may be delayed to a second-stage procedure to allow the sepsis and inflammation to settle, thereby minimising the risks of mediastinal sepsis and the breakdown of the bronchial stump.[88] This topic is covered in empyema chapter.

Rarely a bronchopleural fistula may persist as a chronic problem in patients with extensive parenchymal damage involving larger bronchi. Resection may be indicated in such situation after investigations. However, in the case where the lobe or lung has remained collapsed, expansion can be achieved by decortication and simultaneously managing broncho-pleural fistula through a use of a pedicled muscle flap[89] (Fig. 11.3a, b)

The surgical principle of a chest wall muscle flap is that it must retain its blood supply and have sufficient length to reach the fistula without tension. This requires adequate anatomical knowledge of neurovascular pedicle of the muscle. Most muscles are suitable for the myoplastic flap surgery. In addition, some are large enough to fill the residual intra-thoracic space with minimal functional disability of the arm and shoulder.

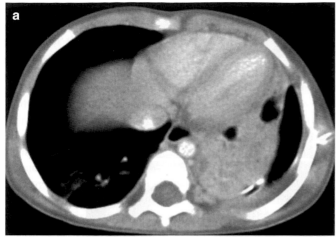

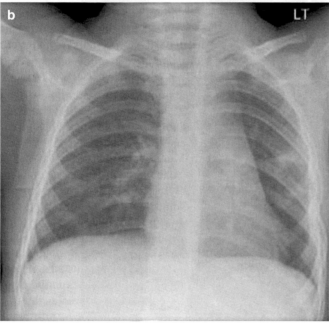

FIG. 11.3. Empyema with broncho-pleural fistula: (a) CT scan demonstrating collapsed left lower lobe with pyopneumothorax and perfusion within the collapsed lung, failure of initial empyema drainage procedure with chest drain continuing to bubble air and draining pus. (b) Follow up chest X-ray a year letter showing a complete resolution and full expansion of the left lower lobe. She was managed with limited decortication and serratus anterior digitation flap onto the bronchopleural fistula

Extra-thoracic muscles require a route of entry when transposed into the thoracic cavity, most often through the bed of a resected piece of the rib or through an appropriate intercostal space.

A lung abscess that is present for longer than 6 weeks is considered "chronic."[3] This implies that the cavity has not drained adequately, has a thickened, fibrous wall, and is therefore likely to be more resistant to conservative measures. However, there may still be a response to prolonged antibiotics and physiotherapy, with the option of external drainage if there is no early response. A chronic abscess that fails to resolve usually requires lobectomy, as the more conservative resection of a lung segment typically encounters inflamed tissues that lead to bleeding and prolonged air leaks.[18,90] However, segmental resection is sometimes possible if the cavity is small and well within the boundaries of a segment as demonstrated by CT scan, and can be safely considered in such cases (Fig. 11.4a–d).[91]

Nosocomial Pneumonia and Lung Abscess

One of the downsides of the antibiotic era has been the growing population of resistant organisms causing infection in hospitalized patients. Nosocomial pneumonia is a leading cause of morbidity and mortality in hospitalized children, with reported mortality ranging from 10 to 20% and higher.[92–96] Prevention of cross-infection through standard measures (handwashing, patient separation, equipment care, sterile techniques for procedures, etc.) is vitally important in limiting the spread of nosocomial infections, though routine use of gloves and gowns for patient contact has not been shown to be additionally helpful.[97] The risks are highest in patients requiring invasive procedures such as endotracheal intubation, catheterisation, invasive monitoring, in post-operative patients, and in immunocompromised patients. Neonates requiring intensive care are particularly vulnerable because of an immature immune system, and inability to adequately clear secretions.[9,10]

Additional reasons that hospitalized patients may be vulnerable to pulmonary infection include lowered levels of consciousness, sedation, and pain that restricts coughing and movement, while many ill children have a generalized lowered immunity.[96] Progression of nosocomial lung infection to lung abscess formation is rare because pulmonary sepsis in hospitalized children is usually detected early and treated with antibiotics before it can be complicated by empyema or lung abscess. However, in an already-sick child progression from a small pneumonic area to abscess formation and/or pleural involvement can happen quickly, especially if pulmonary drainage is compromised by thickened secretions and endotracheal intubation. Further progression to respiratory failure, septicaemia, and multiorgan failure may be just as rapid.[96] The key to preventing these complications is early recognition and adequate antibiotic therapy, which often depends on accurate diagnosis. Thus, any new sign of sepsis in a hospitalized patient must trigger an aggressive search for the site and the organism, with blood culture, sputum or BAL, and urine culture, and other tests as indicated clinically.

Lung abscesses arising in pulmonary contusions following trauma, or through aspiration during or after an elective surgical operation, have a high likelihood of being due to a nosocomial organism with some antibiotic resistance.

The organisms most often associated with nosocomial pneumonia are gram-negative bacilli (chiefly *Acinetobacter baumanii* and *Pseudomonas aeruginosa*), followed by fungi

that this test may not be positive in patients with uncomplicated cysts. The test can be used as monitoring after surgical excision of hydatid disease to indicate presence or absence of other living cysts.

Management

Medical Treatment

The benzimidazole group of compounds (mebendazole, albendazole) was first used to treat hydatid disease in the late 1970s. The effectiveness of these agents depends on the thickness of the pericyst wall and frequently this prevents adequate drug penetration to sterilize the germinal layer. This limits the use of chemotherapy to small (<5cm) non-calcified cysts (Fig. 12.4), unresectable cysts and for residual or recurrent disease after surgery. The duration of treatment ranges from 3–6 months.

Anadol and coworkers studied 376 children with hydatid disease undergoing medical and surgical treatment.[17] The authors found that 72% of pulmonary cysts <9cm diameter responded to treatment with mebendazole or albendazole. Beard also noted favorable results from mebendazole treatment.[19] Most series, however, report limited response to medical therapy for pulmonary hydatid cysts.[16,20]

The effectiveness of medical treatment in preventing recurrence is yet to be evaluated. Recently, preoperative use of praziquantel with albendazole as combination therapy has been recommended to reduce the risk of recurrence and intraoperative anaphylactic reaction in case of accidental spillage. The combined use of albendazole and praziquantel compared with albendazole alone preoperatively has been shown to reduce significantly the number of cysts containing viable parasite.[21]

Conservative Management

Ultrasonographic or CT guided fine-needle aspiration of hydatid cyst contents followed by infusion of 95% ethanol as a scolicide and reaspiration known as PAIR therapy (Puncture, Aspiration, Injection, and reaspiration) has been practiced in some centers but carries significant risk of dissemination, infection, and anaphylactic reaction as a result of cyst puncture and leakage.[22–25] This treatment is not advisable for thoracic hydatids in children.

Surgical Management

- The aim of surgical management is to eradicate the parasite, to prevent intraoperative rupture of a cyst, and obliteration of the residual cavity.
- Capitonnage (folding of the pericystic layer with sutures) with or without partial excision of free portions of pericystic layer is a common practice for obliteration of the residual space cystic space.
- The surgical aim of resection in hydatid disease should be to preserve lung tissue.

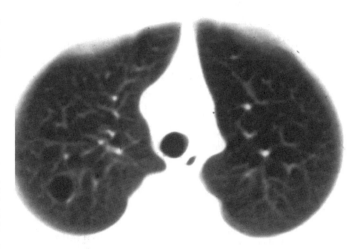

FIG. 12.4. CT scan showing multiple bilateral intraparenchymal thin-walled hydatid cysts managed with cyclical antihelminthics alone

Although small cysts can be eliminated by medical therapy, surgery is still considered the most effective therapy in pulmonary hydatid disease.[17,20,26,27] Indications for surgery include large pulmonary cysts (which rarely respond to medical therapy), recurrence after completion of medical therapy and drug side effects.[28] Pulmonary cysts usually require operation, but occasionally patients with ruptured cyst into the bronchus have been managed without operations. Surgical resection when carried out with parenchyma preserving approach is associated with no recurrence in many series.[20,29,30] Resection with lobectomy is generally reserved for cases when the whole lobe has been affected and destroyed by the hydatid disease or secondary infection.

Essentially, hydatid disease surgery should be uncomplicated and is associated with very low mortality and morbidity. This is especially true in the hands of the experts dealing with this condition regularly.[20,27,31] Giant cysts have slightly higher morbidity than simple cyst intact cysts.[26] Prolonged air leak, postoperative empyema, and pneumonia are the most frequently occurring complications ranging from 10 to 20% of cases.[17,27,32]

Intact Cysts

If the cyst is intact the general principle of surgery is excision without rupture (Fig. 12.5 a–c). At operation, the pleural surface of the cyst is exposed and the adventitial layer incised. The experience of the surgeon and anesthetist are vital to removal of the cyst intact. The anesthetist uses sustained positive pressure ventilation to facilitate delivery of the cyst through the incised pericyst by the surgeon. The laminated membrane should not be grasped directly or it will rupture. Gentle retraction will usually allow the cyst to be mobilized intact. This method of enucleation is effective for small and medium sized cysts. After delivery of the cyst the surrounding lung parenchyma expands and the pericyst collapses. If there is an air leak within the cyst cavity the offending minor bronchus can be suture ligated.

Rupture of a hydatid cyst during removal has serious consequences. Anaphylactic shock, pleural hydatidosis, bronchial contamination with disseminated disease are all well recognized complications.[33] There are a number of techniques to minimize these risks. The surgical field, thoracotomy wound and pleural space should be protected with gauze sponges soaked in iodopovidone, which is scolicidal. Good suction apparatus must be ready for immediate use (some surgeons insist on two suckers).

The risk of cyst rupture increases with cysts over 7–10cm diameter. For large cysts aspiration of the contents and instillation of scolicidal solutions may be a safer option. If this technique is used single lung ventilation or temporary occlusion of the lobar bronchus is imperative to prevent contamination of the bronchial tree with cyst fluid or scolicide. Effective scolicides include:

- 10–20% saline
- 0.5% silver nitrate
- 3% hydrogen peroxide
- 1.5% cetrimide-0.15% chlorhexidine
- 40% cetrimide
- 70–95% ethyl alcohol
- 1% formalin in 0.9% saline
- 10% polyvinylpirrolidone-iodine

The most effective scolicides for intraoperative use are cetrimide or cetrimide/chlorhexidine (Savlon, Novartis UK Limited, UK). Scolicides should be left for around 15 minutes after instillation before attempting to remove the cyst wall. Preoperative treatment with albendazole should be considered if cyst rupture seems likely. The potential advantages are a reduction in cyst wall tension and sterilization of the cyst but this has to be balanced against reports of rupture of large cysts during treatment. In the unfortunate even that cyst spillage does occur albendazole should be continued postoperatively.

Recently minimally invasive techniques have been to treat pulmonary hydatid disease.[34] Although this approach may be associated with reduced postoperative pain and shorter hospital stay, the consequences of cyst rupture cannot be over emphasized. For this reason thoracoscopic techniques should be reserved for dead cysts.[35]

Multiple Pulmonary Cysts

Multifocal pulmonary hydatid disease may occur in children (Fig. 12.6) and this may be associated with involvement of other organs, especially the liver. Multiple unilateral cysts may be resected through a conventional thoracotomy, whereas bilateral disease may require sequential bilateral thoracotomy

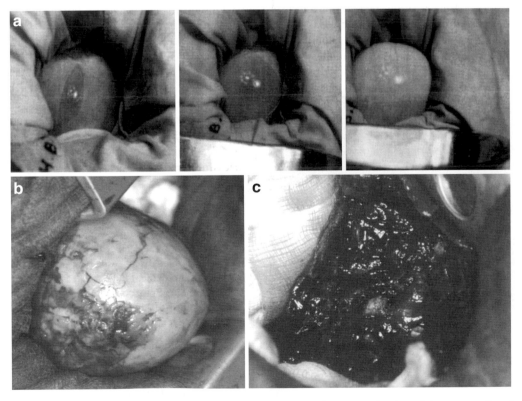

FIG. 12.5. (**a**) Operative pictures of hydatid cysts removal at thoracotomy preventing contamination of the surrounding tissue; (**b**) Infected hydatid cyst in the left lower lobe with empyema; (**c**) Raw surface of the left lower lobe after removal of hydatid cyst. The bronchial leaks are managed and chest drains kept. Postoperative uneventful course and follow up showed no recurrence

or generalized) of pulmonary involvement depends on the etiology, and will only become more extensive while a causative condition persists. On the other hand, *local* progression of the severity of the damage to the airways occurs in spite of resolution of the initial etiology through what has been described as the "vicious cycle" theory.[35] The premise of this generally accepted theory is that the damaged airways can no longer adequately clear secretions due to an impaired mucociliary mechanism, and this "secondary" etiology leads to repeated cycles of infection and inflammation which produce ongoing fibrotic changes in the already-damaged areas.

The histology of bronchiectasis was first outlined by Ogilvie in 1941 and Whitwell in 1952.[36,37] The essential features are destruction of the muscular and elastic tissues of the bronchial wall and their replacement by fibrous tissue. Along with bronchial dilatation there is loss of cilia, with cuboidal and squamous metaplasia, hypertrophy of bronchial glands and lymph nodes, and extensive vascular damage.[31] These changes cripple the airway defenses against bacterial invasion, resulting in the "vicious cycle" of ongoing infection and inflammation (Fig. 13.1a, b).

Temporary dilatation of airways due to increased intraluminal pressure as a result of obstruction, or due to "traction" on the airway walls through collapsed adjacent parenchyma, may be fully recoverable and thus should not be referred to as bronchiectasis, and is sometimes called "pseudobronchiectasis,"[38,39] or "prebronchiectasis"[31] because it might progress to permanent bronchiectasis (Fig. 13.2).

Bronchiectasis after pyogenic or viral infections is frequently limited to basal segments of the lower lobes, and to the middle lobe and lingula. In contrast bronchiectasis associated with congenital and genetic disorders is likely to be more diffuse and bilateral. Bronchiectasis following childhood tuber-

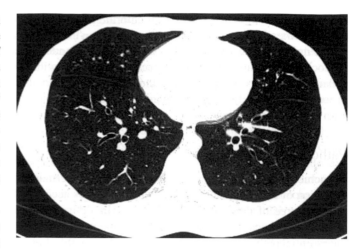

Fig. 13.2. CT scan showing early changes of bronchiectasis being managed by regular clinical followup, medical management, and aggressive physiotherapy.

culosis is typically due to obstruction of airways by external compression with inflamed lymph nodes or by endobronchial granulomatous tissue, and the areas most often affected by this process are the lower lobes.[4]

Bronchiectasis following unrecognized inhaled foreign body is limited to the lobe obstructed by the foreign body (Fig. 13.3a–c).

Extensive disease may lead to pulmonary hypertension, a reflection of the loss of pulmonary vasculature in diseased lung.

A specific middle lobe syndrome is reported when the enlarged peribronchial lymph nodes (usually from TB or other granulomatous disease) cause obstruction to the middle lobe bronchus, infection, and bronchiectasis. However, in reality simple atelectasis of the middle lobe due to the TB

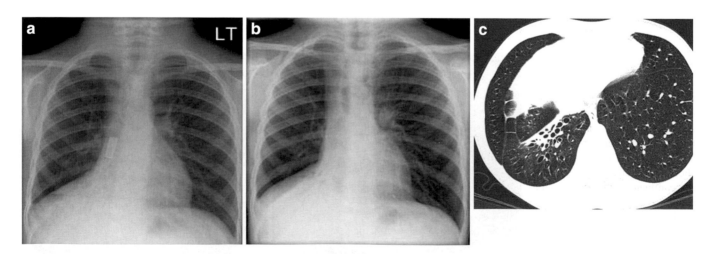

Fig. 13.3. (a–c) A child with inhaled FB – did not report and subsequently chronic collapse of the right lower lobe and functional loss. Follow up after removal of FB failed to re-expand the lobe and has remained the source of recurrent chest infection and shown bronchiectatic changes and no function on ventilatory and perfusion scan. Vegetable foreign bodies such as peanuts tends to cause chemical irritation and are more likely to develop granulations, bronchial stenosis, and bronchiectatic change in the lobe – these children should be followed up after the FB removal and monitored

lymphadenopathy is much more common. In developed nations this "middle lobe syndrome" is most often seen with inappropriately managed bronchial asthma or bronchiolitis with thick tenacious secretions blocking the middle lobe bronchus. If this underlying problem is recognized and adequately managed, the atelectatic or solid lobe generally recovers with no specific treatment. The reason for the middle lobe affection is the acute angle of origin, and the slender and elongated configuration of the right middle lobe bronchus, with poor collateral ventilation from the adjacent lung due to a relatively complete fissure.[40] In pediatric practice, middle lobe syndrome with bronchiectasis requiring lobectomy is rarely encountered.

Clinical Features

The history in many children is vague and nonspecific. In some, there may be a history of an initial causative infection such as measles or whooping cough, or of tuberculosis treatment. Some children have had a productive cough for so long time that they or their parents may consider it normal and report that there are no symptoms of note.

Symptoms are primarily chronic cough productive of purulent sputum, often worst in the morning, as secretions have pooled overnight, though not uncommonly a history is obtained of recurrent acute respiratory infections with productive cough, and relatively symptom-free periods between exacerbations.

Dyspnoea on exertion may be a feature of widespread disease. Chest pain is uncommon, as is hemoptysis. Halitosis can be significant and disconcerting for the patient and relatives in more severe disease. Recurrent fevers and exacerbations of symptoms are frequent, reflecting repeated added infection in damaged areas.

If there is no obvious cause, detailed and specific history must be sought for a possible etiology. If none is found, evaluation for immunodeficiency, cystic fibrosis, chronic aspirations, and other predispositions must be considered according to the clinical picture.

Clinical signs are also characteristically nonspecific. Failure to thrive and malnourishment are common, and auscultation can often define the general extent of the disease. Finger clubbing is variable, but may be seen in about 50% of patients.[30] Distant spread of infection (e.g., brain abscess) or local spread to form a lung abscess or empyema thoracis is seen in about 5% of children with bronchiectasis.[30]

As noted above, symptomatology should dictate treatment, and bronchiectasis can be symptomatically classified into mild, moderate, and severe disease:

- *Mild disease*. Even though there may be obvious damage radiologically, the symptoms are minimal and easily controlled with postural drainage and aggressive antibiotic treatment of any exacerbations.
- *Moderate disease*. Symptoms are significant in terms of interfering with lifestyle, and require careful medical management and perhaps surgery.

- *Severe disease*. Symptoms are not controllable with conservative management, and surgery should be considered if the disease is sufficiently localized to allow resection.

Diagnosis

Investigations

Once the clinical diagnosis of bronchiectasis is suspected, further investigation is necessary to define the extent of the damage. Anatomic localization may help in etiological diagnosis (Fig. 13.4a). Diffuse damage is seen in patients with systemic

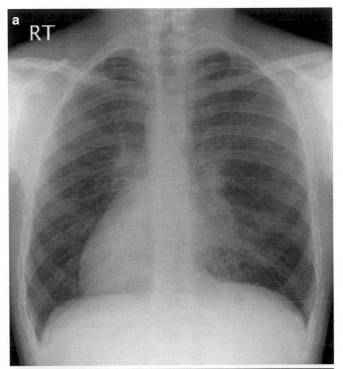

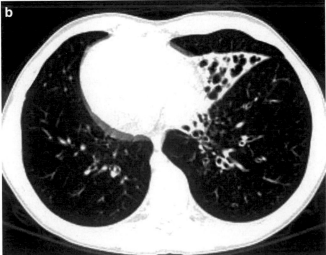

Fig. 13.4. (**a**, **b**) Kartegener's syndrome: Dextrocardia with bronchiectasis in the left lower lobe seen both on chest X-ray and confirmed on CT scan

diseases such as cystic fibrosis, immotile cilia syndrome, immunodeficiency states, and in chronic aspiration. Disease localized to one lobe suggests etiologies, which might obstruct a single bronchus such as foreign body aspiration or nodal compression of an airway.

Chest radiographs are of limited use, and can be normal, or demonstrate nonspecific findings of atelectasis, fibrosis, and pleural thickening.[32,41] The signs suggestive of bronchiectasis are the parallel lines of dilated bronchial walls ("tramlines"), tubular-shaped opacities of pus-filled dilated airways, or ring opacities of cystic spaces ("honeycombing"). Air trapping is possible, as well as compensatory hyperinflation when there is significant loss of volume.

Bronchography was, for many decades, the standard way to assess the disease, but has been gradually supplanted by high resolution CT scanning (HRCT) to determine the presence and exact distribution of bronchiectasis.[41–43] Detailed information about the distribution is particularly important if lung preserving surgery (segmentectomy) is planned rather than lobectomy. HRCT is now considered the benchmark investigation for diagnosis and for delineating the extent of the disease, with findings corresponding well with histological findings after resection[41,44] (Figs. 13.2, 13.3c, 13.4b, 13.5b).

Features of bronchiectasis on CT include the internal diameter of the airways being larger than the adjacent artery ("signet ring" sign), a lack of tapering of the bronchial diameter toward the periphery, and bronchi still visible out near the periphery of the lung. However, simple bronchial wall thickening may be the only clue. It must be remembered that in an acute illness many of these features can be seen as temporary changes, disappearing upon recovery, such that the diagnosis of bronchiectasis must remain a clinical decision rather than a purely radiographic one. However, bronchiectasis remains underdiagnosed in children, as CT scans are delayed either due to lack of facility or due to failure in appreciating the presence of underlying disease clinically.[31]

Upper gastrointestinal contrast study, endoscopy, and PH studies may be indicated to investigate gastroesophageal reflux if this is the suspected cause of bronchiectasis, especially in severely handicapped children (Fig. 13.6a, b).

Magnetic resonance imaging (MRI) has not been particularly useful in the evaluation of bronchiectasis.

Bronchoscopy may be indicated as a diagnostic tool either for certain etiologies or for obtaining bacteriological information. Ventilatory and diffusion studies may reveal more widespread or severe pulmonary involvement than otherwise suspected.

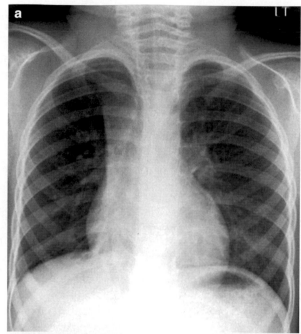

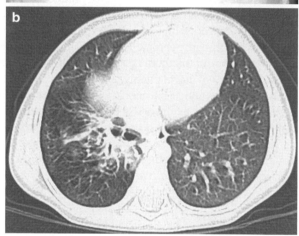

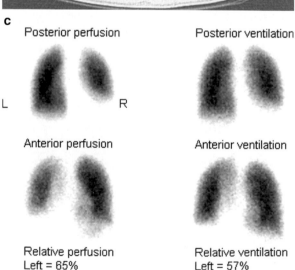

FIG. 13.5. (a–c) Chest X-ray showing collapsed right lower lobe – child presented with recurrent severe hemoptysis and no history suggestive of recurrent chest infections. CT scan: suggested a possibility of a late presenting congenital lung lesion, bronchoscopy, and BAL were nonspecific. V/Q scan: matched ventilation perfusion defect in right lower lobe. The resected right lower lobe showed chronic bronchiectasis. Such instances of bronchiectasis presenting without significant pneumonic illness and not requiring intravenous antibiotics in children are rare

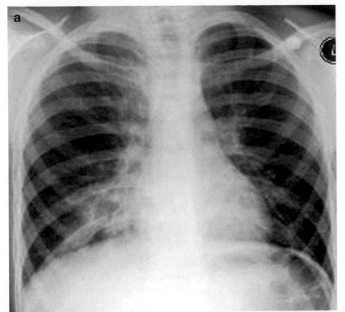

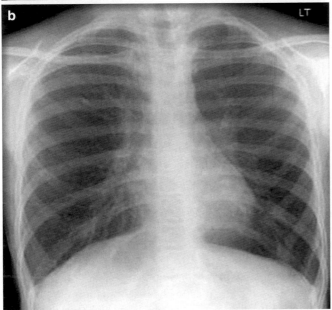

FIG. 13.6. (a, b) A child with proven gastroesophageal reflux and recurrent aspirations is showing early signs of bronchiectasis on chest X-ray. Following fundoplication there is a considerable improvement in clinical and radiological picture (b)

Management

Medical Management

Prevention

It is important for primary care physicians to be aware of the rapidity with which bronchiectasis can follow lower respiratory infection if it is not treated promptly and aggressively, especially in very young or malnourished children.

Measures that help prevent lower respiratory tract infections include appropriate childhood immunization programs, prompt antibiotic treatment, good hygiene and sanitation practices, and good nutrition. When secretions cannot clear efficiently for whatever reason, infection and inflammation may rapidly cause bronchial wall damage. In addition, any obstruction of large airways must be relieved with urgency to prevent the development of distal bronchiectasis.[4]

Management of the Cause

Once the diagnosis of bronchiectasis is made and the underlying etiology has been fully investigated, medical treatment must initially be based on optimizing the treatment of any contributory medical problems. All these children should receive annual influenza and pneumoccocal vaccines.

Management of the Bronchiectasis

The cornerstone of treatment is the promotion of the efficient clearance of secretions through postural drainage and chest physiotherapy.[45] Depending on the etiology, bronchiectasis may remain static and patients can be maintained with mild symptoms or even asymptomatic for long periods, with regular outpatient review and radiological monitoring. Questions have recently been raised about the role of physiotherapy in view of a lack of clear evidence in children,[46] but while there is clearly a need to document its role more clearly, postural drainage techniques remain the accepted basis of long-term management of bronchiectasis. In order for postural drainage to be most effective, both the parents and the child must be specifically trained in the techniques, and a regular daily routine of postural drainage established at home.

Antibiotics for infective exacerbations are another central aspect of treatment. Choice of antibiotic is based on sputum culture if possible, though upper respiratory commensals often confuse the issue. High doses and prolonged courses are preferred because of the danger of further fibrotic airway damage with infective exacerbations. Broad spectrum antibiotics including anaerobic cover (e.g., Amoxycillin and Metronidazole) may be used for several weeks at a time to help clear secretions and bacterial overgrowth. Some physicians advise prophylaxis during winter months and when the child is suffering from a viral infection.

There is suggestive evidence of a small benefit from the use of prolonged or ongoing antibiotics as prophylaxis against exacerbations in children, in a similar way to prophylactic antibiotic usage in transplant and HIV patients, but the evidence is small and there is concern that colonization with resistant organisms may result.[47]

In some cases with deterioration and failure of response, bronchoscopic aspiration and bronchoalveolar lavage may be indicated to obtain specimens for culture and sensitivity.[31,32] Bronchoscopy may also be indicated for persistent segmental atelectasis refractory to physiotherapy, or for the assessment of lesions suspected of obstructing the airway. Bronchoscopy is mandatory preoperatively to assess for anatomical abnormalities, bronchial stricture, and foreign bodies if present.

Other Agents

The mucolytic agents in bronchiectasis have been disappointing, though agents such as aerolized recombinant human deoxyribonuclease are useful in patients with cystic fibrosis.[33]

Bronchodilators may be indicated for associated bronchospasm, and occasionally lung function measurements will show reversible bronchospasm. However, they are not commonly helpful. The role of antiinflammatory therapy is unclear, though popular with some clinicians. Corticosteroids are not advisable.[31,32]

Surgical Management

Principles

- The goal of surgery is to remove all active disease while preserving as much functioning lung parenchyma as possible.
- Localized bronchiectasis is most suitable for surgery.
- Children should "earn" surgery, with recurring or continuing symptoms in spite of adequate medical management.

Surgery is sometimes necessary to address the cause, for example a retained foreign body, but otherwise surgical resection of damaged lung is indicated when conservative measures have failed to control the symptoms adequately. The surgeon must consider several issues when a patient is referred for resection:

1. Has an underlying cause been determined? i.e., Is more investigation required before embarking on resection?
2. Is this bronchial damage permanent? i.e., Should one wait longer to allow an acute process to better heal?
3. Has maximal medical therapy been adequately tried?
4. Do the symptoms truly warrant surgery; Is it interfering with lifestyle and schooling or growth? Or is this simply a radiological diagnosis with minimal symptoms? This is to an extent subjective- and patient-specific, some children coping better than others with similar severity of disease.
5. Finally, what is the anatomical distribution of the disease? Can it be safely resected without significantly compromising pulmonary reserves?

At this stage the extent of the disease should be delineated with HRCT and a decision taken on the safe resectability of the diseased lung. Although it is ideal to resect all diseased portions of lung while preserving all normal lung, it is often necessary to find a compromise. Thus it is sometimes necessary to leave some residual disease in order to spare functioning lung, and similarly some functioning lung will at times be sacrificed. The dependent portions of damaged lung (generally lower lobe areas) are the most important areas to remove. Such "sump" resections may significantly alleviate symptoms and allow the child to grow and function normally, even with residual disease. Upper lobe bronchiectatic damage typically drains well by gravity and is more easily controlled by postural drainage. Significant lung growth continues up to the age of about 8 years, and thus pulmonary function can be expected to improve after resection in younger children. Malnourished children may require only partial resection to improve symptoms sufficiently to allow growth.

Preoperative Preparations

Meticulous preoperative preparation is a key in reducing surgical morbidity. Most children will benefit from intensive in-hospital chest physiotherapy and intravenous administration of appropriate sensitive antibiotics depending on the bacterial cultures obtained at bronchoscopy (with good anaerobic cover, e.g., amoxycillin and metronidazole) for at least a few days prior to surgery in order to reduce the sputum load as much as possible. A good physiotherapist will be able to advice on progress and the surgery should be delayed until the best state has been reached. Occasionally it is apparent that the patient can be returned to a relatively asymptomatic state quite easily, indicating noncompliance with the conservative therapy and postural drainage at home. In other cases, intensive physiotherapy is continued for 2 or 3 weeks as progressive improvement in sputum load is noticed.

Anesthetic Considerations

Prior to endotracheal intubation, a bronchoscopy must be done to clear secretions as far as possible, and to examine the anatomy. Occasionally an unsuspected retained foreign body may be seen at this stage; in such cases the distal airway may contain pus under pressure, and the foreign body should not be disturbed, but rather be removed along with the resected lung at surgery. Releasing the blockage at bronchoscopy can result in catastrophic flooding of the airways with pus.

A major challenge in pulmonary resection in children is protection of the contralateral lung from secretions squeezed out of the resected lung during surgery. Double-lumen tubes may be used to isolate the contralateral lung in larger children (over about 15 kg). However, in the majority of children the airways are too small for conventional double-lumen endotracheal tubes. Other options include right main bronchus intubation for left-sided resections, and bronchial blockade on the side of surgery with a Fogarty catheter. These techniques can be extremely useful in isolating a lung but in the hands of the inexperienced anesthetist are hazardous, as slippage during surgery is possible, potentially leaving an unprotected airway to the contralateral lung.

Various alternative techniques have been proposed for airway management, but the most useful in small children remains that originally described in by Overholt:[48] the patient is positioned prone, slightly head-down, and a posterior thoracotomy is made to approach the lung. Secretions that are squeezed out of the affected lung during surgery will tend to drain downward into the upper trachea where they can be sucked out by the anesthetist, who must suction the airway regularly.

This is a challenging position for the surgeon who must operate through an unfamiliar approach. It is often best to be seated at the side of the patient rather than standing, resisting the temptation to angle the patient away, which would lower the contralateral lung and thereby allow secretions to drain into that lung. In patients with a large secretion load, it is often best to isolate and clamp the bronchus as the first stage of the operation.

Bilateral resections are possible at the same anesthetic, but it is generally better to separate the surgeries by a few weeks.

Good pain control is important postoperatively to allow adequate coughing to clear secretions, and this is best achieved with epidural anesthesia.

Surgical Technical Considerations

Technical aspects of bronchiectasis surgery can be challenging. The surgeon must carefully consider the appropriateness of segmental resections in order to preserve functioning lung if possible, and to this end the preoperative HRCT assessment must be carefully examined.

The inflamed and indurated hilum, usually containing enlarged lymph nodes, can be difficult to dissect. Vessels are painstakingly dissected free, sometimes dissecting under the adventitia to free them. Hemostasis should be ensured by careful ligatures and judicious use of bipolar diathermy. This hilar dissection can cause considerable bleeding in difficult cases. When there is significant hilar lymphadenopathy involving major lobar vessels, the immediate subdivisions within the lung parenchyma may be identified and ligated individually. The bronchus, if inflamed, is vulnerable to tearing or other damage during dissection and needs specific attention. Excessive devascularization or trauma through aggressive dissection or vigorous cautery can predispose to a postoperative fistula. Staple closure of the bronchus, as used routinely to achieve secure closure in adults, is less useful in children due to the bulkiness of the instrument; fine interrupted nonabsorbable sutures are preferable. Typically 3–4 sutures are sufficient to ensure secure closure, which should be tested underwater. Excessive sutures will contribute to devascularization of the cut end, delaying healing and predisposing to fistula formation.

Recently some surgeons have undertaken VATS for the resection of bronchiectatic lobe. The arguments for using minimally invasive surgery are a magnified view and reduced handling/manipulation during surgery. The postoperative pain is less and therefore allows better postoperative lung inflation and reduces the risk of postoperative pneumonia and atelectasis.

Morbidity and Mortality

Complications related to bronchiectasis surgery include prolonged air leak from raw lung surfaces, bronchopleural fistula, and empyema and pneumonia related to intraoperative contamination of normal lung. The reported morbidity and mortality with bronchiectasis surgery is, however, extremely low.

The most serious morbidity relates to spillage of infected material into normal airways causing a postoperative pneumonia.

TABLE 13.2. Patients having resection for bronchiectasis at Red Cross Children's Hospital in 10 years.

Etiology	
Tuberculosis	27
Viral	16
Cystic fibrosis	2
Foreign body	3
Others	24
Total	**72**
Age range	9 months to 12 years
Airway management during surgery	
Prone position	47
Bronchial blocker	6
Double-lumen ET tube	2
None	17
Resections	
Pneumonectomy	39 (15 right, 24 left)
Lobectomy	33 (6 right, 27 left)
Mortality	$1/72 = 1.4\%$
Morbidity	$12/72 = 16.7\%$
Spillage or aspiration to remaining lung	8
Esophageal perforation	1
Pericardial effusion	1
Acute gastric distension, mechanical ventilation	1
Phrenic nerve palsy	1
Recurrent laryngeal nerve palsy	1

This can dangerously compromise pulmonary function, and mechanical ventilation may be required for a period; in severe cases the compromise may prove fatal. However, serious morbidity or mortality is unusual (Table 13.2).

Future Perspective

Better prevention of bronchiectasis depends heavily on the awareness of primary care health personnel and on improved immunization programs. In underdeveloped communities, control of tuberculosis and HIV along with improved social circumstances will have a great impact.

However, it seems unlikely that the predominant causes of bronchiectasis will be significantly reduced in the near future; while the rapid improvement in our ability to accurately detect bronchiectasis in children through new technology seems likely to continue. In some parts of the world, the incidence of tuberculosis and HIV infection among children is still rising, along with the poor getting poorer, so in developing nations we can expect the overall incidence of the disease to increase. This emphasizes the need to improve our understanding of the management options for these children. With the decrease in severe localized bronchiectasis in the developed world there is a danger of loss of surgical skills in dealing with the condition.

residual localized disease in children who will require further immunosuppression.[28, 29] The risks of surgery are substantial in children who are neutropenic, especially if they are requiring mechanical ventilation. The risk of hemorrhage increases as the neutrophil count recovers.

A number of measures are used to reduce the risk of IPA in hospitalized patients. Environmental measures include the use of high-efficiency particulate air (HEPA) filtration systems, cubicles with laminar air flow and scrupulous decontamination of showers and water systems. Prophylactic antifungals are used with variable benefit.

Allergic Bronchopulmonary Aspergillosis

Allergic bronchopulmonary aspergillosis (ABPA) is a hypersensitivity reaction to Aspergillus antigens. This disorder is seen in children with asthma and cystic fibrosis. Children present with fever, wheeze, pleuritic pain and a cough productive of brown sputum and mucous plugs. The chest X-ray shows fleeting pulmonary infiltrates. The total IgE level is very high, specific IgG antibodies and precipitins to Aspergillus are present in serum. ABPA responds rapidly to oral corticosteroids, with relief of bronchospasm and resolution of the infiltrates on chest X-ray.

Chronic Necrotizing Aspergillosis

Chronic necrotizing aspergillosis (CNA) is typically a disease of late adult life which develops on the background to chronic lung disease (e.g. chronic obstructive airways disease, inactive tuberculosis and cystic fibrosis). CNA is an indolent destructive infection. Although the organisms invade the lung parenchyma there is no vascular invasion and distant spread does not occur. The disease is usually confined to the upper lobes or apical segments of the lower lobes. Aspergillomas may form in cavities which develop as a result of CNA. Aspergillus can usually be isolated from sputum or BAL culture or a tissue specimen taken at open lung biopsy. Treatment involves amphotericin B or, more recently, itraconazole. Surgical resection is useful for localized disease or persistent disease despite antifungal therapy.

Pulmonary Candidiasis

Candida infections involving the oropharynx and skin, particularly the diaper region, are very common in infants and children. These infections usually remain superficial and respond readily to treatment with topical antifungal agents. Systemic candida infections are usually seen in patients with impaired cell-mediated immunity, often related to chemotherapy or corticosteroids and HIV infection.

Candida septicemia (candidemia) may occur as a result of direct entry through central venous catheters, invasion of infection from the oropharynx or esophagus, or invasion from the airway. Hematogenous dissemination then occurs with the formation of metastatic microabscesses. Predisposing factors include intravenous catheters, broad spectrum antibiotics, corticosteroid therapy, neutropenia, severe burns, and chemotherapy induced mucositis. When yeasts are isolated from blood or from tissue biopsies a diagnosis is straightforward. Blood cultures, however, often remain negative. Serological tests are available to detect circulating candida antigens and antibodies. Unfortunately, these are often negative in immunocompromised children. False-negatives and false-positive results do occur.

Low birth weight, intravascular catheters and antibiotic drugs are predisposing conditions for systemic candidiasis in neonates. Blood cultures are often positive and there is a high incidence of meningitis. Fungus balls in the ureter or renal pelvis are common and may obstruct the urinary tract. Candida endophthalmitis carries a high risk of blindness because lesions are often localized to the macula.

Pulmonary candidiasis most commonly results from hematogenous dissemination or by bronchial extension in patients with oropharyngeal candidiasis.[30] This results in patchy infiltration of the lungs, which becomes more confluent as the infection progresses. Microabscesses result in hemorrhagic septic infarcts which may break down to form small cavities, although this is usually an agonal event.

Pulmonary candidiasis is difficult to diagnose. The radiographic appearances are non-specific and often complicated by chronic changes from underlying lung disease (e.g. bronchopulmonary dysplasia). However, pulmonary candidiasis does not produce lobar pneumonic changes, large cavitating lesions or pleural effusions.

Treatment of invasive candidiasis requires high dose amphotericin B often in combination with 5- flucytosine. High dose fluconazole and liposomal amphotericin B have also been used with success.

Empiric treatment with amphotericin B should be started in high risk patients with a fever unresponsive to antibiotics. Voriconazole can be used for treatment of fluconazole-resistant candida in children over the age of two. Caspofungin is reserved for infections not responding to fluconazole and amphotericin. Recombinant hematopoietic growth factors have been used to stimulate the immune system.

The risk of life-threatening fungal infection in children undergoing intensive chemotherapy or bone marrow transplantation is so high that prophylactic treatment is used. Nystatin, clotrimazole or miconazole can be used for prevention of oropharyngeal infection. Fluconazole is recommended for prophylaxis against systemic candidiasis.

Actinomycosis

Actinomycosis is a chronic infection caused by the Gram positive bacterium *Actinomyces israelii*. It is rare in children. Actinomycosis is characterized by a granulomatous suppuration which forms sinuses which discharge purulent material containing yellow "sulfur" granules. *Actinomycetes* are part of the normal oral flora. The commonest site for infection is the cervicofacial region and infection typically occurs following oral surgery or in patients with poor dental hygiene. Soft tissue swelling develops in the perimandibular area and sinuses track to the surface and discharge.

Thoracic infection usually occurs as a result of aspiration of oropharyngeal secretions.[31] Occasionally mediastinal infection results from an esophageal perforation, by direct extension from actinomycosis in the neck or abdomen. Pulmonary infection may occur by hematogenous spread from a distant lesion. Thoracic actinomycosis commonly presents as a pulmonary mass, mimicking a tumor. In late cases sinuses may involve the pleura, pericardium, and ultimately discharge to the chest wall.

Management

The diagnosis is made by histological examination of resected tissue and culture from pus, sputum and tissue specimens. The diagnosis is rarely made on admission to hospital and the usual reason for biopsy of pulmonary disease is suspected malignancy.

The treatment of choice is high dose penicillin for 5 weeks. Longer treatment may be necessary if there is bone infection or an empyema. Coinfection with other organisms is common and lack of response to penicillin usually indicates the presence of resistant companion bacteria. Surgery may be required to debride an empyema, drain collections and excise sinus tracks.[32]

Nocardiosis

Nocardia are aerobic Actinomycetes related to *Actinomyces* which cause cutaneous infections in the tropics in immunocompetant individuals. The organisms are ubiquitous saprophytes in soil and decaying vegetable matter. Children in any part of the world with impaired cell-mediated immunity are at risk of disseminated *Nocardia* infections. Disseminated nocardiosis may present with deep abscesses at any site, particularly in the chest and central nervous system (CNS). CNS nocardiosis manifests as a slowly progressive mass lesion, with a host of specific neurologic findings depending on the location of the abscess.[33]

At least 40% of patients with disseminated nocardiosis have pulmonary infection and the clinical presentation may be dominated by the pulmonary symptoms.[34] Clinical manifestations include inflammatory endobronchial lesions or pneumonia, which may be accompanied by cavitation, abscess formation, pleural effusion, and empyema. There are no specific symptoms. Cough and fever are dominant symptoms. There are no specific radiological features.

The diagnosis of nocardiosis is made by identification of organism in tissue fluids, a BAL or tissue specimens. Sulfonamides are the first line antibiotic therapy. Treatment for up to one year is recommended in immunosuppressed children. The indications for surgery are similar to actinomycosis.

Parasitic Infections

Pleuropulmonary Amebiasis

Amebiasis is a parasitic infection caused by *Entamoeba histolytica* and transmitted by fecal-oral spread. Amebiasis is endemic in the Tropics, associated with poor sanitation and poverty. Following ingestion of water contaminated with amebic cysts, trophozoites penetrate the bowel wall and cause a fulminant colitis characterized by profuse bloody diarrhea. Trophozoites are carried in the portal vein to the liver where they form abscesses.

Pleuropulmonary involvement occurs most often as a result of rupture of a liver abscess through the right diaphragm.[35] Rarely, the parasite may infect the lung directly from a primary intestinal lesion by the hematogenous or lymphatic spread. Other factors contributing to pulmonary disease in children are malnutrition and left to right cardiac shunts.[36] Common pleuropulmonary complications include sympathetic effusions, empyema, atelectasis, and lung abscesses.[37] Bronchohepatic fistula is a rare complication characterized by expectoration of "anchovy sauce sputum".

The clinical presentation varies according to the pathology. A child may present with a prolonged fever or blood stained/chocolate color sputum. The child may have right upper quadrant pain referred to the shoulder tip. Typical findings on chest X-ray include the combination of an elevated hemidiaphragm (usually the right), hepatomegaly, and a pleural effusion. The hepatic abscess can be diagnosed by ultrasound, CT or MR scanning. Aspiration of chocolate-colored pus from a pleural or abscess puncture strongly suggests the diagnosis and if examination of the pus under the microscope reveals amebic trophozoites the diagnosis is confirmed. Serological tests are usually strongly positive.[38] Sputum orogastric lavage can be examined for trophozoites. PCR can be used to detect *E. histolytica* DNA in sputum, stool or gastric lavage samples.[39]

Management

Treatment with metronidazole for 15 days combined with pleural drainage is sufficient in most cases. Although surgical drainage is controversial, at times percutaneous drainage of abscesses, empyema and pericardial collections is indicated.[37]

Ascariasis

Ascariasis is an endemic infection in tropical countries caused by the intestinal parasite Ascaris lumbricoides. Transmission is by fecal-oral spread and poor sanitation characterizes regions where infection is prevalent. The adult worm normally resides in the lumen of the human intestine and eggs are passed out in the feces. Ascaria can grow up to 30 cm long and most often cause symptoms because of intestinal obstruction. Larvae can

Lung Resection in the Presence of Chronic Infection

Lung resection in children with chronic suppurative lung disease is technically challenging. The normal anatomical landmarks may be impossible to identify. Consolidated lung surrounding areas of diseased lung may recover although this can be difficult to predict.[61]. Sometimes, it is prudent to undertake a two-stage resection in difficult cases where it may be possible to salvage functioning lung. Preoperative physiotherapy, intravenous antibiotics and bronchoscopic lavage with aspiration of endobronchial secretions are important adjuncts. Protection of the healthy lung is essential and this may involve double lumen endotracheal tubes, bronchus blockers and operating on the child in the prone position.

Indications for lung resection in children with chronic suppurative lung disease include:

- Necrotizing pneumonia with or without empyema [62]
- Bronchiectasis
- Lung abscess
- Recurrent hemoptysis with destroyed lung parenchyma [62]
- Failure of conservative management [63]

Bony Chest Wall Infections

Sternal osteomyelitis may be secondary (following median sternotomy or penetrating injuries) or primary.[64] Primary sternal osteomyelitis is rare, comprising less than 0.3% of all cases of osteomyelitis. *Staphylococcus aureus* is the organism most commonly responsible for both primary and secondary sternal osteomyelitis (PSO, SSO), although *Pseudomonas aeruginosa* is seen in intravenous drug abusers.[65] *Salmonella* may be responsible in children with sickle cell disease. Risk factors for PSO include intravenous drug abuse, blunt trauma, acquired immunodeficiency syndrome and hemoglobinopathies. Sternal osteomyelitis presents with local pain, tenderness, redness, and swelling. PSO may respond to antibiotics alone although surgical debridement is usually necessary.

Tuberculous osteomyelitis of the sternum is rare even in countries where TB is endemic.[66] It accounts for less than 1% of cases of musculoskeletal tuberculosis. Tuberculosis of the sternum may be seen as a late complication of pulmonary tuberculosis, or as reactivation of latent focus formed during hematogenous or lymphatic dissemination of primary tuberculosis. Direct extension from mediastinal lymph nodes has also been described. All TB infections are substantially more common in children infected with HIV. Sternal TB usually presents insidiously as swelling and pain over the bone. The diagnosis is often delayed.

The treatment of tuberculosis of the sternum is based on a combination of adequate antituberculous chemotherapy and surgical debridement. Surgical debridement is necessary when there is a chronic sinus, a large sequestrum or an inadequate response to chemotherapy. The resultant defect may require closure with a muscle flap.

Chest wall sinus formation is an uncommon clinical presentation of osteomyelitis of the rib (Fig. 14.6, 14.7), Pott's disease of the spine, tuberculosis of the rib, and chronic pulmonary infection with actinomycosis[67] and coccidioidomycosis. The authors have also seen a retained foreign body presenting as a chest wall sinus.

References

1. Gupta DK, Sharma S. Management of empyema - Role of a surgeon. J Indian Assoc Pediatr Surg 2005; 10:142–146.
2. Sharma S, Gupta DK. Empyema thoracis – Tubercular and Nontubercular. In: Bhave S. Ed. Textbook of Adolescent Medicine. New Delhi: Jaypee Brothers, 2006: 678–684.
3. Castro AV, Nascimento-Carvalho CM, Ney-Oliveira F, et al. Additional markers to refine the World Health Organization algorithm for diagnosis of pneumonia. Indian Pediatr 2005; 42: 773–781.
4. Ozel SK, Kazez A, Kilic M, et al. Conservative treatment of postpneumonic thoracic empyema in children. Surg Today 2004; 34: 1002–5.
5. Chitkara RK, Krishna G. Parasitic pulmonary eosinophilia. Semin Respir Crit Care Med 2006; 27: 171–84.
6. Stamatis G, Greschuchna D, Freitag L. Indications for surgery and results of 207 thoracotomies in children with diseases of the lung, pleura and mediastinum. Langenbecks Arch Chir Suppl II Verh Dtsch Ges Chir 1990; 845–9.
7. Aboud FC, Verghese AC. Evarts Ambrose Graham, Empyema, and the Dawn of Clinical Understanding of Negative Intrapleural Pressure. Clin Infect Dis 2002; 34: 198–203.
8. Crafoord J, Olin C. Clarence Crafoord –one of the great pioneer surgeons of the century. Lakartidningen 1999; 96: 2627–32 and 2634–7.
9. Cherian SM, Nicks R, Reginald SA. Lord Ernst Ferdinand Sauerbruch: Rise and Fall of the Pioneer of Thoracic Surgery. World J Surg 2001; 25: 1012–1020.
10. Chas. L. Gibson Theodore Tuffier 1857–1929. Ann Surg 1930; 91: 636–637.
11. Naef AP. The mid-century revolution in thoracic and cardiovascular surgery: Part 2 Interact Cardiovasc Thorac Surg 2003; 2: 431–449.
12. Lindskog GE. Bronchiectasis revisited. Yale J Biol Med 1986; 59:41–53.
13. Berdon WE, Willi U. Situs inversus, bronchiectasis, and sinusitis and its relation to immotile cilia: history of the diseases and their discoverers-Manes Kartagener and Bjorn Afzelius. Pediatr Radiol 2004; 34:38–42.
14. Gow KW, Hayes-Jordan AA, Billups CA, et al. Benefits of surgical resection of invasive pulmonary aspergillosis in pediatric patients undergoing treatment for malignancies and immunodeficiency syndromes. J Pediatr Surg 2003; 38:1354–1360.
15. Lupinnetti FM, Behrendt DM, Giller RH, et al. Pulmonary resection for fungal infection in children undergoing bone marrow transplantation. J Thorac Cardiovasc Surg 1992; 104: 684–687.
16. Goodwin RA, Lloyd JE, De Prez RM. Histoplasmosis in normal hosts. Medicine (Baltimore). 1981; 60:231–266.
17. Gugnani HC. Histoplasmosis in Africa: A review. Indian J Chest Dis Allied Sci 2000; 42: 271–7.

18. Shaffer JP, Barson W, Luquette M, et al. Massive haemoptysis as the presenting manifestation in a child with histoplasmosis. Paediatr Pulmonol 1997; 24:57–60.

19. Pate JW, Hammon J. Superior vena cava syndrome due to histoplasmosis in children. Ann Surg 1965; 161:778–785.

20. Crum NF, Lederman ER, Stafford CM, et al. Coccidiodomycosis: A descriptive survey of a reemerging disease. Clinical and current controversies. Medicine (Baltimore) 2004; 83: 149–175.

21. Kafka JA, Catanzaro A. Disseminated Coccidiodomycosis in children J Pediatr 1981; 98: 355–361.

22. Arsura EL, Kilgore WB. Miliary Coccidiodomycosis in the immunocompetent. Chest 2000; 117: 404–409.

23. Rowland VS, Westfall RE, Hinchliffe WA, et al. Acute respiratory failure in miliary Coccidioidomycosis. In: Coccidioidomycosis: Current clinical and diagnostic status. Ajello L Eds. Symposia Specialist. Miami, Florida 1977; 139–155.

24. Cash R, Light RW, George RB. Clinical and roentgenographic manifestations of acute and chronic blastomycosis. Chest 1976; 69: 345–349

25. Sanders JS, Sarosi GA, Nollet DJ, Thompson JI. Exfoliative cytology in the rapid diagnosis of pulmonary blastomycosis Chest 1977; 72: 193–196.

26. Bradsher RW, Rice DC, Abernathy RS. Ketoconazole therapy for endemic blastomycosis. Ann Intern Med 1985; 103: 8729.

27. Soubani AO, Chandrasekar PH. The clinical spectrum of pulmonary aspergillosis. Chest 2002; 121: 1988–1999.

28. Reichenberger F, Habicht J, Kaim A, et al. Lung resection for invasive pulmonary Aspergillosis in neutropenic patients with hematologic diseases. Am J Respir Crit Care Med 1998; 159: 885–890.

29. Matt P, Bernet F, Habicht J, et al. Predicting outcome after invasive pulmonary Aspergillosis in patients with neutropenia. Chest 2004; 126: 1783–8.

30. Kassner EG, Kauffman SL, Yoon JJ, et al. Pulmonary candidiasis in infants: clinical, radiologic, and pathologic features. Am J Roentgenol 1981; 137: 707–716.

31. Mabeza GF, Macfarlane J. Pulmonary actinomycosis. Eur Respir J 2003; 21: 545–551.

32. Endo S, Murayama F, Yamaguchi T, et al. Surgical considerations for pulmonary actinomycosis. Ann Thorac Surg 2002; 74: 185–190.

33. Saubolle MA, Sussland D. Nocardiosis: review of clinical and laboratory experience. J Clin Microbiol 2003; 41: 4497–4501.

34. Hui CH, Au VW, Rowland K, et al. Pulmonary nocardiosis revisited: experience of 35 patients at diagnosis. Respir Med 2003; 97: 709–717.

35. Mbaye PS, Koffi N, Camara P, et al. Pleuropulmonary manifestations of amebiasis. Rev Pneumol Clin 1998; 54:346–52.

36. Shamsuzzaman SM, Hashiguchi Y. Thoracic amebiasis. Clin Chest Med 2002; 23:479–92.

37. Lyche KD, Jensen WA. Pleuropulmonary amebiasis. Semin Respir Infect 1997; 12: 106–12.

38. Rachid H, Alaoui Yazidi A, Loudadssi F, et al. Amoebic infections of the lung and pleura. Rev Mal Respir 2005; 22:1035–7.

39. Hara A, Hirose Y, Mori H, et al. Cytopathologic and genetic diagnosis of pulmonary amebiasis: a case report. Acta Cytol 2004; 48:547–50.

40. Mukerjee CM, Thompson JE. Pulmonary ascariasis. Med J Aust 1979; 2:99–100.

41. Rexroth G, Keller C. Chronic course of eosinophilic pneumonia in infection with ascaris lumbricoides. Pneumologie 1995; 49:77–83.

42. Arene FO, Ibanga E, Asor JE. Epidemiology of paragonimiasis in Cross River basin, Nigeria: prevalence and intensity of infection due to Paragonimus uterobilateralis in Yakurr local government area. Public Health 1998; 112: 119–22.

43. Fischer GW, McGrew GL, Bass JW. Pulmonary paragonimiasis in childhood. A cause of persistent pneumonia and hemoptysis. JAMA 1980; 243:1360–2

44. Weller PF. Parasitic pneumonias. In: Respiratory infections: Diagnosis and management, 3rd ed. Pennington, JE (Ed). Raven Press, New York, 1994, p. 695.

45. Durieu J, Wallaert B, Tonnel AB. Chronic eosinophilic pneumonia or Carrington's disease. Rev Mal Respir 1993; 10: 499–507.

46. Emanuel B, Shulman ST. Lung abscess in infants and children. Clin Pediatr (Phila) 1995; 34: 2–6.

47. Mallick SM, Khan AR, Al-Bassam A. Late presentation of tracheobronchial foreign body aspiration in children. J Trop Pediatr 2005; 51: 145–8.

48. Parikh D, Samuel M. Congenital cystic lung lesions: is surgical resection essential? Pediatr Pulmonol 2005; 40: 533–7.

49. Al-Bassam A, Al-Rabeeah A, Al-Nassar S, et al. Congenital cystic disease of the lung in infants and children (experience with 57 cases). Eur J Pediatr Surg 1999; 9: 364–8.

50. Lejeune C, Deschildre A, Thumerelle C, et al. Pneumothorax revealing cystic adenomatoid malformation of the lung in a 13 year old child. Arch Pediatr 1999; 6: 863–6.

51. Ribet ME, Copin MC, Gosselin BH. Bronchogenic cysts of the lung. Ann Thorac Surg 1996; 61: 1636–40.

52. Aziz D, Langer JC, Tuuha SE, et al. Perinatally diagnosed asymptomatic congenital cystic adenomatoid malformation: to resect or not? J Pediatr Surg 2004; 39: 329–34.

53. Davenport M, Warne SA, Cacciaguerra S, et al. Current outcome of antenatally diagnosed cystic lung disease. J Pediatr Surg 2004; 39: 549–56.

54. Albanese CT, Sydorak RM, Tsao K, Lee H. Thoracoscopic lobectomy for prenatally diagnosed lung lesions. J Pediatr Surg 2003; 38: 553–5.

55. Rothenberg SS. Thoracoscopic lung resection in children. J Pediatr Surg 2000; 35: 271–5.

56. Roggin KK, Breuer CK, Carr SR, et al. The unpredictable character of congenital cystic lung lesions. J Pediatr Surg 2000; 35: 801–5.

57. Sauvat F, Michel JL, Benachi A, et al. Management of asymptomatic neonatal cystic adenomatoid malformation. J Pediatr Surg 2003; 38: 548–52.

58. Parikh DH, Samuel M. Congenital cystic thoracic lesions: Is surgical resection essential. Pediatr Pulmonol 2005; 40: 533–537.

59. Sundararajan L, Parikh D. Evolving experience with video assisted thoracic surgery (VATS) in congenital cystic lung lesions in a British paediatric centre. J Paediatr Surg 2007; 42: 1243–1250.

60. Papagiannopoulos K, Hughes S, Nicholson AG, Goldstraw P. Cystic lung lesions in the pediatric and adult population: surgical experience at the Brompton Hospital. Ann Thorac Surg 2002; 73: 1594–1598.

61. Conlan AA, Moyes DG, Schutz J, et al. Pulmonary resection in the prone position for suppurative lung disease in children. J Thorac Cardiovasc Surg 1986; 92: 890–3.

62. Ayed AK, Al-Rowayeh A. Lung resection in children for infectious pulmonary diseases. Pediatr Surg Int 2005; 21: 604–8.

63. Cowles RA, Lelli JL Jr, Takayasu J, Coran AG. Lung resection in infants and children with pulmonary infections refractory to medical therapy. J Pediatr Surg 2002; 37:643–7.

64. Bryan RT, Noor S, Quaraishi S, et al. Primary sternal osteomyelitis. J Pediatr Orthop B 1999; 8: 125–6.

65. Upadhyaya M, Keil A, Thonell S, et al. Primary sternal osteomyelitis: a case series and review of the litterature. J Pediatr Surg 2005; 40: 1623–1627.

66. Khan SA, Varshney MK, Hasan AS, et al. Tuberculosis of the sternum. J Bone Joint Surg (Br) 2007; 89-B: 817–820.

67. Kobayashi K, Murakami S, Shimizu J, et al. A case of infantile thoracic actinomycosis involving the bronchocu1taneus fistula. Nippon Kyobu Geka Gakkai Zasshi 1994; 42: 442–5.

Section 3
Trauma

15
Thoracic Trauma. General Considerations

Joe Crameri and Kate Ferguson

Introduction

Thoracic injuries are uncommon in children; however, when they occur they are suggestive of a significant mechanism of injury and herald the likelihood of coexisting injuries to other body regions, particularly the head, abdomen, and spine. In a review of children with multiple injuries 25% were associated with thoracic injury.[1] The spectrum of childhood traumatic chest injuries is wide ranging from simple contusion, multiple rib fractures to rare exsanguinating vascular injuries. In general blunt thoracic injuries are far more common than penetrating injuries in the pediatric population. Although isolated thoracic injuries are rarely associated with mortality the presence of a thoracic injury in a pediatric patient is generally associated with significant morbidity and mortality. Those deaths occurring in patients who have suffered thoracic trauma are most often a result of their associated injuries.[2]

Despite the severity of the trauma involved most thoracic injuries in children can be managed conservatively without surgical intervention. This often involves significant respiratory support including analgesia, assisted ventilation and aggressive physiotherapy. Paediatric deaths may occur prehospital and are predominantly secondary to hemorrhagic shock or cardiopulmonary arrest related to a tension pneumothorax. This mortality and morbidity rate can be improved if the patient is transferred to a pediatric center and managed within "the golden hour."

Historical Perspective

Throughout history thoracic injuries and their management have been recorded. Records indicate that the understanding of chest injury physiology by physicians was an important factor making the difference in the management and outcome of this frequently fatal condition. Evidence has been discovered suggesting that Egyptians were managing thoracic injuries with some success more than 5,000 years ago. American Egyptologist Edwin Smith unearthed documentation written prior to 3000 BC recognizing that rib fractures could be managed without surgical intervention.[3] The use of protective armor for the head and chest in wars of ancient times is further evidence that for many centuries it has been recognized that injuries to these regions can be fatal. The management of these battle injuries and the resulting infections were important factors leading to the establishment of thoracic surgery as a specialty in its own right.

The study of wartime history reflects the progression in the management of thoracic injuries. In Crimean war, 6–8% of all wounds were blunt or penetrating thoracic injuries and resulted in a 79% mortality rate. Five years later during the American civil war, the incidence of chest wounds was 8% with 63% mortality. In World War I chest wounds accounted for 2–5% of all injuries with a mortality rate of 25%. This mortality rate was more than halved in the Second World War. Throughout this conflict the incidence of thoracic injuries was still at 8%; however, the mortality dropped to only 12%.[4] The improvement in survival can be attributed to the implementation of rapid evacuations to appropriate field hospitals, a concept originally recommended by Napoleon's surgeon, Larry. The improvements in these survival rates were secondary to better early management of chest wounds, a greater understanding of chest physiology, and the availability of thoracic surgeons in military field hospitals. Although children were rarely the victims of these wars, the lessons learned from these injuries are applicable to civilian road traffic and penetrating injuries sustained by the innocent children of the modern society.

Physiology

Within the thoracic cavity there are a number of functional compartments (air spaces, intrapleural spaces, vasculature, and the mediastinum), each of which requires a specific pressure range in order to function normally. These pressures dictate the pre- and after-load of the heart, the expansion and recoil of the lungs, and therefore the ventilation/perfusion

D.H. Parikh et al. (eds.), *Pediatric Thoracic Surgery*,
DOI: 10.1007/b136543_15, © Springer-Verlag London Limited 2009

relationship. These components are closely related, and therefore a change in the pressure in any one of these regions will affect the others and may potentially result in major physiological compromise. The rationale of management for patients who have sustained a chest injury should be based on an understanding of this anatomical and physiological interplay.

The main objective in the management of pediatric thoracic trauma is to optimize the delivery of oxygen to vital organs.

The subatmospheric intrapleural pressure combined with the contraction of inspiratory muscles, predominantly the diaphragm, allows effective inspiration, alveolar ventilation and subsequent oxygenation of the blood. In chest injuries there can be a disturbance of the mechanics of ventilation along with perfusion/ventilation mismatch and/or cardiovascular injury. These factors can then lead to respiratory compromise and subsequent hypoxemia.

The mechanics of respiration can be affected in a number of ways secondary to chest trauma. Most often this mechanical failure is due to musculoskeletal injuries of the chest wall including loss of chest wall integrity such as that seen in an open pneumothorax (described in the following chapter). Less commonly the mechanics of ventilation can be disturbed by disruption of the tracheobronchial tree by either direct injury or blood accumulation within the airway, thus interfering with the flow of air, and therefore oxygen into the alveoli. Furthermore, chest wall injuries can result in altered effective alveolar ventilation by restricting the lungs' capacity to expand. This restriction may be as a result of a build up of blood or air in the pleural space acting as a space occupying lesion or simply due to splinting secondary to the pain elicited with inspiration.

Hypoxemia in chest trauma may also be from a ventilation–perfusion mismatch. This type of disturbance can result from lung collapse as a sequelae to extrinsic pressure from blood or air within the pleural cavity, herniation of the abdominal contents due to a diaphragmatic rupture, or from intraparenchymal injury as a result of an extensive contusion, a hemorrhage, or the inhalation of gastric contents.

Altered functioning of the cardiovascular system and hemodynamic compromise can also affect the delivery of oxygen to the vital organs. In chest injuries both cardiogenic and hemorrhagic shock may play a role. Hemorrhagic shock means that the effective circulating volume passing through the lungs for oxygenation is reduced, and this can occur in chest trauma as a result of bleeding within the chest from an injury to major thoracic vessels or from external blood loss from other injuries. The cardiogenic shock resulting from chest injuries is secondary to ventricular dysfunction caused by a myocardial contusion, a tension pneumothorax, or a pericardial tamponade, any of which will cause impaired oxygenation.

Despite the seemingly large spectrum of injury types seen in thoracic trauma the resultant morbidity and mortality generally occur via a common pathophysiological pathway – an impairment of oxygen delivery to vital organs. Thus, the primary principle of effective oxygen delivery should be the central focus in the management of any type of chest trauma both in the prehospital and emergency department settings.

The Pediatric Thorax

The thorax of a child differs structurally from that of an adult in several ways. The pediatric chest is more rounded; it has a relatively compliant chest wall and has less developed musculature than that of the adult. The compliance of the chest wall is the most significant of these differences when considering the results of thoracic trauma in children. This increased compliance is due to a more flexible and elastic bony cage. The ribs and sternum of a child can withstand significant deformation from external forces without fracturing. This means that structures within the chest cavity, i.e., lungs and mediastinum, can sustain injuries without an overlying chest wall injury.

Great vessel and mediastinal injuries are far less frequently encountered in the pediatric population than in adults. The reason for this difference is multifactorial. Firstly, the mediastinum in a child is relatively mobile and thus is less susceptible to the rapid acceleration and deceleration forces commonly experienced in traumas. In adults where some mediastinal structures are fixed and others are mobile these types of forces can result in tearing of these structures at the transition points. A further factor contributing to the difference in incidence of great vessel injury is the absence of vascular disease in children. Atherosclerosis and other vascular pathologies commonly seen in adults reduce the elasticity of the muscular vessel walls making them susceptible to tearing or rupture when subjected to shearing forces.

The physiological response to trauma is also different in children when compared with adults. Children generally have far greater cardiovascular and pulmonary reserves than adults and so are less likely to demonstrate compensatory responses until the very late stages of compromise. It is also likely that children will develop gastric distension following any type of trauma due to orophagia (swallowing air). This is a common response to trauma in children and may confound the clinical picture. It is especially relevant in thoracic trauma, as a large degree of gastric distension will reduce respiratory reserves.

Incidence

Thoracic trauma has been reported to comprise 0.2–7.0% of all pediatric trauma internationally (Table 15.1). The ratio of penetrating to blunt injuries varies between countries (Fig. 15.1). In nations such as Australia and the UK where firearms are difficult to access the rate of blunt injuries is significantly higher than that of penetrating injuries. In those countries where firearms are more accessible this difference in reduced.

TABLE 15.1. Thoracic trauma – incidence

Country	Thoracic trauma[1]	Blunt	Penetrating
Turkey[4]	–	60%	40
Ireland (Belfast)[5]	–	91.5%	9.5%
South Africa[6]	0.2%	85.2%	14.8%
USA (Chicago)[7]	–	41%	59%
USA[8]	6%	83%	17%
USA[9]	7%	79%	21%
USA[10]	–	50%	50%
Australia (Sydney)[11]	3.5%	–	–
Australia (Melbourne)	1.7%	94.2%	5.8%

[1]% All pediatric trauma

Mechanisms

The causative mechanisms of injury differ between the blunt and penetrating injury groups. More than half of the blunt thoracic injuries that occur in children are secondary to incidents involving motor vehicles, with the patient having been either a passenger or a pedestrian. The remainder of the blunt injuries

seen is generally due to falls, "other transport" accidents, or, rarely, as a result of nonaccidental injuries (Table 15.2).

Penetrating injuries, however, most commonly result from either stabbing or gunshot wounds (Table 15.3). As mentioned earlier the rates of these vary between countries depending on the accessibility of firearms.

Injury Types

The most frequently encountered thoracic injuries in the pediatric population are pulmonary contusions. These injuries comprise more than 50% of all pediatric thoracic injuries. Other commonly encountered injuries are fractures of the ribs or sternum, and pneumo- and/or hemothoraces (Table 15.4). The patterns of injury will vary depending on the rate of penetrating versus blunt injuries. In areas where penetrating injuries occur more frequently there is a smaller proportion of contusions compared with hemo- or pneumothoraces.

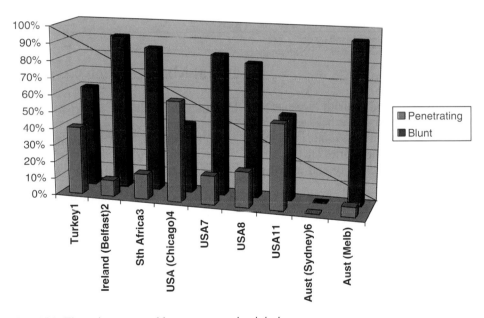

FIG. 15.1. Thoracic trauma – blunt vs penetrating injuries

TABLE 15.2. Thoracic trauma – mechanisms of injury

Country	Passenger	Pedestrian	Other transport	Fall	Sport	Nonaccidental injury	Other
Ireland (Belfast)[12]	2.3%	79%	–	7%	–	–	11.5%
South Africa[6]	5.5%	86%	–	8%	–	–	–
USA (Chicago)[7]	64%		–	18%	–	18%	–
USA[6]	41%	33%	10%	8%	–	–	9%
USA[13]	21.5%	26.5%	18.5%	10%	–	5%	18.5%
USA[10]	25%	44%	8%	6%	8%	–	8%
USA[14]	36%	40%	–	11%	–	9%	4%
Australia (Melbourne)	33.5%	21%	20%	5.5%	15%	–	5.5%

TABLE 16.1.

Mechanism	Percentage
MCA	33.6
Pedestrian	21
M'Bike	10.9
Animal	7.8
Collide	7.8
Fall	5.5
Bicycle	5.5
Other	4.7
Other transport	3.9

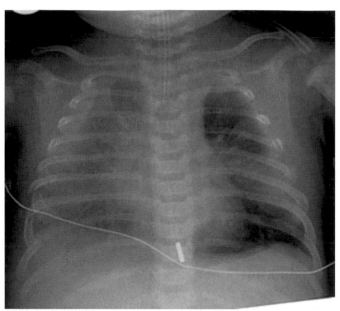

FIG. 16.2. Flail chest

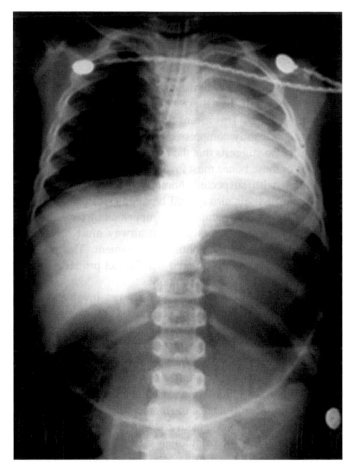

FIG. 16.1. Gastric dilatation

Chest Wall Injury

Rib and Sternal Fractures

Rib and sternal fractures are uncommon in pediatric thoracic trauma. This is because the elasticity and flexibility of the thoracic cage often protects young children from sustaining injuries of the chest wall including flail segments. However, fractures can occur when the injurious forces are great. Because of the severity of the impact required to fracture these bones, these types of injuries are invariably associated with pulmonary contusions and may cause a pneumo- or hemothorax, or a

pulmonary laceration. In one series, 3.2% of children admitted with thoracic injury had rib fractures.[17] It was noted that if they had more than one rib fracture they were more likely to have sustained multisystem trauma.[17] Children with concurrent rib fractures and head injuries have a higher rate of mortality than those with thoracic injury alone. The same study found that while road traffic accidents were the most common cause of chest wall injuries in older children the same injuries in children younger than 3 years old were more commonly due to nonaccidental injuries (NAI).[17] Sternal fractures are rare in children but may be seen secondary to a direct blow such as those encountered in motor vehicle accidents or sporting injuries. Fractures at the angle of the ribs in an infant are highly suggestive of an NAI involving violent compression of the chest.

Flail chest: A flail chest is a very rare event in children but, as with adults, when it does occur it will result in significant ventilatory compromise (Fig. 16.2). In these cases the flail segment can be seen to retract with inspiration and expand with expiration, a phenomenon known as "paradoxical movement." As with other ribs fractures in children a flail chest is always associated with a significant lung contusion and may also indicate an underlying chest wall hemorrhage, lung laceration, or rupture of the alveoli causing a pneumothorax. A flail chest in children reduces venous return due to their relatively mobile mediastinum, which shifts secondary to altered pleural pressures. Diagnosis is often clinically obvious.

Diagnosis

Clinical Examination

- *Inspection*: Chest wall bruising and/or abrasions, respiratory distress, and in the case of a flail chest, abnormal, "paradoxical," chest wall movement

- *Palpation*: Very tender chest wall, decreased expansion, possible subcutaneous emphysema, percussion note may be hyperresonant or dull depending on presence of a pneumo- or hemothorax, respectively
- Auscultation: Normal or decreased air entry

Investigations

CXR is the investigation of choice although it must be recognized that many bony injuries and early pulmonary contusions may not be evident on the initial film. This film should be closely examined for evidence of a pneumo- or hemothorax, or a widened mediastinum. If the clinical suspicion of a chest wall injury is high a repeat CXR is warranted 24–48 h following presentation to allow for the evolution of any parenchymal injuries. A CT scan in selected cases is useful for the diagnosis, and can accurately define the extent and severity of the parenchymal injury.

Serial arterial or venous blood gases may be used to assess the degree of parenchymal injury and the effect on alveolar ventilation. A twelve lead ECG may provide useful information regarding the presence of underlying cardiac injuries in those patients who have suffered an anterior chest wall injury.

Management

Initial management of these patients involves ensuring the presence of a patent airway, fluid resuscitation, supplemental oxygen, and mechanical ventilation if required.

Good analgesia is imperative as the respiratory status will be further compromised by voluntary and involuntary splinting of the chest wall secondary to pain. In presence of inadequate gas exchange, such as that seen with a flail segment, endotracheal intubation and mechanical ventilation may be required to improve oxygenation. In some cases a thoracic epidural may be useful to provide appropriate analgesia and achieve effective ventilation.

In patients able to cooperate chest physiotherapy should play a major role in their recovery and prevent atelectasis. It is important to monitor these patients closely using pulse oximetry and ECG. An underlying pulmonary contusion may not become clinically significant until 24–72 h following the injury and so the aforementioned management should continue for at least this long with a repeat CXR on day 1 or 2. Management of an associated pneumothorax is discussed later.

Complications

Rib and sterna fractures are always associated with some degree of underlying lung injury. In most cases this will be a pulmonary contusion but it may also involve a pneumo- or hemothorax. In some situations these complications may be life-threatening such as a tension pneumothorax or massive hemothorax (see later). Sternal fractures are likely to result in an underlying cardiac contusion, which may precipitate arrhythmias. Mediastinal or intrathoracic structures may be damaged by the sharp edges of the overlying fractured bones.

Pulmonary Contusion

Lung contusion in many series is the most frequently encountered thoracic injury in children.[12,13,18] These types of injuries involve interstitial hemorrhage with edema and collapse of the affected alveoli. In adults a pulmonary contusion is unlikely to occur without overlying bony injury; however, in children, due to the flexibility of the ribs, it is common for pulmonary contusions to occur without evidence of a chest wall injury.

Children who sustain lung contusions may, at initial presentation, appear clinically well. Suspicion should be high for those children in whom there has been a major mechanism of injury, where the patient complains of chest pain or chest wall tenderness, or where there is obvious bruising or abrasions on the chest wall. If any one of these criteria are met the patient should be admitted and observed. Typically pulmonary contusions will evolve over the first 24–72 h following the trauma during which time the patient's clinical status deteriorates and the diagnosis of contusion becomes apparent radiologically. The pathological response to this type of injury is the development of edema and the collection of blood in the alveolar spaces leading to loss of normal lung structure and function. Although pulmonary contusions are generally localized they may lead to atelectasis and consolidation of the adjacent, uninjured air spaces. The clinical sequelae of this is ventilation/perfusion mismatch and thus localized shunting resulting in reduced oxygenation and, potentially, respiratory distress. A blood gas analysis will invariably demonstrate hypoxemia and carbon dioxide retention due to poor gas exchange.

Diagnosis

Clinical Examination

- *Inspection*: Bruising and/or abrasions on the chest wall (anteriorly or posteriorly), increased work of breathing, respiratory distress, decreased oxygen saturation levels
- *Palpation*: Tender chest wall, decreased chest expansion
- *Auscultation*: Reduced breath sounds over affected lung field (may be bilateral)

It should be kept in mind that, as stated earlier, the initial examination of these patients can be unremarkable.

Investigations

CXR is the most appropriate initial investigation in these patients. In the early phase of this type of injury the CXR may appear normal or may demonstrate patchy, diffuse opacities that may be accompanied by a pleural effusion (Fig. 16.3). A number of studies report that using serial arterial blood

A subxiphoid incision is made and the pericardium entered and drained under direct vision. If necessary the incision may be extended to allow for repair of vessels or myocardium as required. If this option is not available however and the patient cannot be stabilized with pericardiocentesis then an emergency room thoracotomy may be necessary. It is widely accepted, however, that this is not the optimal treatment.[46] If the patient can be stabilized but is in a center where pediatric cardiac surgery is not available urgent transfer is required following pericardiocentesis.

Complications

Cardiac tamponade may be complicated by injuries to other structures within the mediastinum. Complications following the management of this injury may include recurrence of the tamponade, infection or mediastinitis. The severity of the tamponade initially may have resulted in myocardial ischemia or infarction causing impaired cardiac function. The reduced systemic blood pressure in the acute presentation may also have caused ischemic injury to other organs including the kidneys or brain.

Myocardial Contusion

This denotes a bruise of the myocardium and is generally secondary to blunt trauma to the anterior chest. The anterior wall of the heart is the most commonly affected region. Myocardial contusion is not commonly reported in children and therefore its true incidence remains unknown. In children the most common etiology for this type of injury is road traffic accidents.[47,48] This type of injury should be suspected in any child with a significant, anterior chest wall injury or a sternal fracture. Occasionally these injuries can result in infarction of the cardiac muscle either due to the direct trauma or secondary to injury of the coronary arteries. This type of injury, similar to pulmonary contusion, may not be clinically evident at initial presentation. The injury tends to evolve over the first 24–48 h following the trauma, and thus the patient's condition may deteriorate over this time.

Diagnosis

Clinical Examination

Early examination may be unremarkable.

- *Inspec*tion: Anterior chest wall bruising, tachypnea, and prolonged capillary refill time.
- Palpation: Anterior chest wall tenderness, tachycardia, and arrhythmias.
- Auscultation: There is generally little to find on auscultation of these patients, unless accompanied by a pericardial effusion (see earlier).

Investigations

Serial 12 lead ECGs are important to monitor for changes similar to those seen in myocardial infarction. Troponin I levels should also be taken at intervals to evaluate damage to the myocardium. An echocardiogram is also useful to determine any impairment of myocardial function (dyskinesis, akinesis). Children with suspected cardiac contusion should be continuously monitored for cardiac dysrhythmias.

Management

These patients require close cardiac monitoring in the ICU with serial ECGs and troponin measurements, and repeat echocardiograms. In most instances this supportive management is all that is required. Blunt myocardial rupture is usually fatal and few victims survive to reach hospital.[49] Delayed sequelae of myocardial contusion include infarction, delayed rupture, rupture of a papillary muscle or the ventricular septum, and valvular dysfunction. They are best evaluated by echocardiography.[48]

Great Vessel Injury

This type of injury when it occurs often results in immediate death by exsanguination, and those who do survive to reach hospital are generally in extremis. In one American study the mortality rate in children with an injury to heart and great vessels was reported to be 75%.[13] Another study suggested that aortic injuries are more likely to be fatal when they occur in children than in adults.[50] This same study concluded that the use of car restraints reduces the deceleration forces acting on the child and therefore the probability of sustaining this type of injury.[50] The thoracic vessels at risk of injury are the aorta (particularly vulnerable at the attachment of ligamentum arteriosum), the vena cavae, the innominate artery and vein, the pulmonary arteries and veins, the azygos vein, the left subclavian artery, and the left common carotid artery. In very rare cases a small wound to the aorta may seal itself temporarily by virtue of its thick muscular wall. Injury to any one of these vessels will be accompanied by a hemothorax and/or pericardial effusion.

Diagnosis

Clinical Examination

- *Insp*ection: Tachypnea, altered level of consciousness, respiratory distress
- Palpation: Tachycardia; unequal upper limb pulses may occur; prolonged capillary refill, possible dull percussion note
- Auscult*ation*: Muffled heart sounds, decreased air entry, and a possible bruit over anterior chest

Investigations

The majority of these patients cannot be stabilized and thus require immediate surgical intervention. For those in whom hemodynamic stability can be achieved an arteriogram is the gold standard investigation. This will localize the injury and assist in guiding the surgical repair. If an initial CXR is completed it should be examined for evidence of a hemothorax, loss of the aortic knuckle, widening of the superior mediastinum, depression of the left main bronchus, or a double contour of the aorta.

Management

This condition needs early recognition and surgical intervention. The surgery will involve repair of the damaged vessel with direct suturing or in some cases with interposition graft. Any hemothorax should be evacuated and intercostal catheters should be inserted for drainage intraoperatively. The use of cardiac bypass is subject to the preference of the surgeon and the site and nature of the vascular injury. The chest drains should be connected to a cell saver or autotransfusion device if available. These types of injuries necessitate aggressive fluid resuscitation including blood transfusions in all cases. The patients will require ICU monitoring, supplemental oxygen and may need ventilatory support. As this management involves major surgical intervention there is a risk of atelectasis and respiratory compromise; therefore, good analgesia and chest physiotherapy are integral to the treatment of these patients. All patients with a vascular injury should be treated with broad spectrum intravenous antibiotics.

Diaphragmatic Rupture

Diaphragmatic injury is a rare but well-recognized injury in the pediatric population that has experienced significant blunt force to the lower chest or abdomen. A sudden, severe rise in intra-abdominal pressure is the most common cause of a rupture of the diaphragm.[51] In children this most often occurs as a result of road traffic accidents either as a passenger wearing a lap-belt restraint or as a pedestrian hit or run over by a vehicle. These ruptures are most commonly left sided and, when the resulting defect is large, abdominal contents may become displaced into the thoracic cavity and cause respiratory compromise. The majority of these injuries, however, are of small to moderate size, and so do not declare themselves in the immediate postinjury period. The smaller tears may present several days following injury with symptoms of bowel obstruction or ischemia.

Diagnosis

Bruising on the abdomen and the mechanism of injury should raise the suspicion of a diaphragmatic injury.

Clinical Examination

- *Inspection*: Increased respiratory effort, tachypnea, decreased chest wall movement, and possibly a scaphoid abdomen and lap-belt bruise mark.
- *Palpation*: Tender abdomen, ipsilateral thorax dull to percussion if displacement of abdominal contents, decreased chest wall expansion.

- *Auscultation*: Decreased breath sounds on affected side; bowel sounds may be heard in thoracic cavity; mediastinal shift may occur.

Investigations

On the chest X-ray the affected hemidiaphragm will be difficult to visualize; there may be evidence of bowel loops in hemithorax and abnormal placement of the tip of the NG tube (Fig. 16.7). Definitive diagnosis can be made with oral contrast studies, which clearly demonstrates bowel in the chest. In cases where the diaphragmatic tear is not large enough to permit passage of abdominal contents the injury may not be evident clinically or on CXR and can therefore go undetected for a prolonged period of time.

Management

Initially these patients will require oxygen supplementation and fluid resuscitation as well as insertion of a nasogastric tube. These injuries require surgical repair of the diaphragm and reduction of the abdominal contents out of the chest. Diaphragmatic tears are best repaired using a laparotomy incision, so that concomitant abdominal injuries can be inspected and managed as required. These patients also warrant investigation for esophageal injuries (see later). Ongoing close monitoring is necessary due to the risk of late bowel perforation secondary to contusions. Analgesia and chest physiotherapy are important in the treatment of these injuries to reduce diaphragmatic splinting and atelectasis.

Complications

Complications may arise from injuries received at the time of the original injury such as bowel contusions and perforations

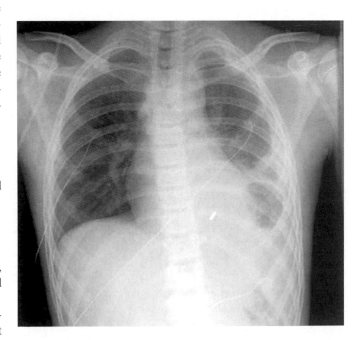

FIG. 16.7. Diaphragmatic rupture

as mentioned earlier. There is also a risk of ischemic injury to the bowel or omentum in those cases where diagnosis is delayed.

Esophageal Injury

Esophageal injury is more commonly associated with a penetrating mechanism rather than a blunt mechanism. However, it is unusual for children to sustain penetrating injuries such as firearm or stab wounds. The most common cause of esophageal injury is iatrogenic during instrumentation of the esophagus such as that seen in dilatations for esophageal strictures. In these situations the perforation most often occurs at the site of the original pathology, e.g., the stricture. Blunt upper abdominal trauma may cause a sudden, massive increase in gastric pressure, forcing gastric contents into the esophagus and thus creating a tear in the wall of the lower esophagus. Violent, forceful vomiting can also result in a sudden rise in gastric pressures with a similar outcome. It is important to have a high index of clinical suspicion for this injury in any child who has received a significant blow to the upper abdomen as delayed recognition is associated with significant morbidity and mortality.

Diagnosis

Clinical Examination

- *Inspection*: Distress, tachypnea, bruising or abrasion to the upper abdomen; fever may be present. Subcuteneous emphysema is seen with perforations.
- Palpation: Tachycardia, decreased chest wall expansion, possible tenderness over the upper abdomen. Intra-abdominal esophageal rupture causes signs of peritonitis with guarding and rigidity.
- Auscultation: Decreased air entry (may be bilateral or unilateral).

Investigations

A chest X-ray may demonstrate a pneumomediastinum, air or fluid in the pleural spaces and/or subcutaneous emphysema.

A CT chest with a water-soluble, oral contrast study will give a definitive diagnosis as well as information regarding the site of the rupture, the compartments with which it communicates, and the size of the leak.

Diagnosis may also be aided by the insertion of an ICC. In some cases of esophageal trauma these catheters may drain gastric fluids from the pleural space.

Management

Many of these injuries can be managed conservatively with good analgesia and close monitoring in an institution with access to pediatric surgeons and anesthetists. These patients should all have a nasogastric tube inserted under radiological guidance and regular chest physiotherapy. Frequent suctioning of the oropharynx may also be required. In cases where there is a significant pneumothorax or a pleural effusion is present insertion of an intercostal catheter may be necessary. These patients are at risk of infection and therefore broadspectrum intravenous antibiotics should be commenced. If the esophageal laceration is large or is not responding to conservative management surgical repair of the injury may be required.

Operative management of these patients is dependent on the timing of the surgery and the severity of the injury. Where possible a primary repair of the injured esophagus is preferable; however, in some cases such as when there has been a delayed diagnosis or massive pleural or mediastinal soiling a two-stage repair is advisable. In these situations proximal diversion should be carried out to avoid continued contamination of the mediastinum and to allow effective control of any infection. These patients will also require the formation of a gastrostomy for feeding until the definitive repair can be performed. Regardless of the operative path taken a mediastinal drain should be inserted intraoperatively to assist in controlling the potential infective complications.

Complications

Esophageal injuries may be complicated by concomitant injuries or by a pneumo- or hemothorax. Leakage of saliva and/or gastric contents may result in an empyema or mediastinitis either of which could lead to potentially lifethreatening sepsis; therefore, broad spectrum antibiotics are commenced early in the treatment of esophageal injuries. Careful, long-term follow-up is essential after the repair or reconstruction of an injured esophagus as strictures are an almost inevitable consequence of these injuries. In addition, all patients who have suffered an esophageal injury should be adequately covered for gastroesophageal reflux with proton pump inhibitors.

References

1. Roux P, Fisher RM. Chest injuries in children: An analysis of 100 cases of blunt chest trauma from motor vehicle accidents, J Pediatr Surg 1992; 27(5): 551–555
2. Inci I, Ozcelik C, Ozgur N, Eren N, Ozgen G. Penetrating chest injuries in children: A review of 94 cases, J Pediatr Surg 1996; 31(5): 673–676
3. Walker PJ, Cass DT. Paediatric trauma: Urban epidemiology and an analysis of methods for assessing the severity of trauma in 598 injured children, Aust N Z J Surg 1987; 15(10): 715–722
4. Cooper A, Barlow B, DiScala C, String D. Mortality and truncal injury: The pediatric perspective, J Pediatr Surg 1994; 29(1): 33–38

5. Peterson R, Tiwary A, Kissoon N, Tepas J, Ceithams E, Pieper P, Arnp-C. Pediatric penetrating thoracic trauma: A five-year experience, Pediatr Emerg Care 1994; 10(3): 129–131

6. Bliss D, Silen M. Pediatric thoracic trauma, Crit Care Med 2002; 30(11) supp: S409–S415

7. Adesunkanmi AR, Oginni LM, Oyelami AO, Badru OS. Epidemiology of childhood injury, J Trauma Injury Infect Crit Care 1998; 44(3): 506–512

8. Ceran S, Sunam SS, Aribas OK, Gormus N, Solak H. Chest trauma in children, Eur J Cardiothorac Surg 2002; 21: 57–59

9. Smyth BT. Chest trauma in children, J Pediatr Surg 1979; 14 (1): 41–47

10. Meller JL, Little AG, Shermeta DW. Thoracic trauma in children, Pediatrics 1984; 74: 813–819

11. Sinclair M, Moore T. Major surgery for abdominal and thoracic trauma in childhood and adolescence, J Pediatric Surg 1974; 9(2): 155–162

12. Nakayama D, Ramenofsky M, Rowe M. Chest injuries in childhood, Ann Surg 1989; 210(6): 770–775

13. Peclet M, Newman K, Eichelberger M, Gotschall C, Garcia V, Bowman L. Thoracic trauma in children: An indicator of increased mortality, J Pediatr Surg 1990; 25(9): 961–966

14. Trupka A, Waydhas C, Hallfeldt KK, Nast-Kolb D, Pfeifer KJ, Schweiberer L. Value of thoracic computed tomography in the first assessment of severely injured patients with blunt chest trauma: Results of a prospective study. J Trauma 1997; 43(3): 405–411

15. Renton J, Kincaid S, Ehrlich PF. Should helical CT scanning of the thoracic cavity replace the conventional chest X-ray as a primary assessment tool in pediatric trauma? An efficacy and cost analysis. J Pediatr Surg 2003; 38(5): 793–797

16. Frush DP, Donnelly LF, Rosen NS. Computed tomography and radiation risks: What pediatric health care providers should know. Pediatrics, 2003; 112: 951–957

17. Garcia VF, et al. Rib fractures in children: A marker for severe trauma. J Trauma 1990; 30: 695–700

18. Roux P, Fisher RM. Chest injury in children: An analysis of 100 cases of blunt chest trauma from motor vehicle accidents. J Pediatr Surg 1992; 27: 551–555

19. Kharisch SJ, Vinci RJ, et al. The routine use of radiography and arterial blood gases in the evaluation of blunt trauma in children. Ann Emerg Med 1994; 23: 212–215

20. Al-Saigh A, Fazili FM, Allam AR. Chest trauma in children: A local experience. Ann Saudi Med 1999; 19(2): 106–109

21. Elmali M, Baydin A, Selim Nural M, Arslan B, Ceyhan M, Gürmen N. Lung parenchymal injury and its frequency in blunt thoracic trauma: The diagnostic value of chest radiography and thoracic CT. Diagn Interv Radiol 2007; 13: 179–182

22. Sivit CJ, Taylor GA, Eichelberger MR. Chest injury in children with blunt abdominal trauma: Evaluation with CT. Radiology 1989; 171: 815–818

23. Donnelly LF, Klosterman LA. Subpleural sparing: A CT finding of lung contusion in children. Radiology 1997; 204: 385–387

24. Dallessio JJ, Markley MA, Lohe A, Kuluz JW, Oiticica C, McLaughlin GE. Management of a traumatic pulmonary pseudocyst using high-frequency oscillatory ventilation. Case report. J Trauma Injury Critic Care1995; 39(6): 1188–1190

25. Smith DW, Frankel LR, Derish MT, Moody RR, Black LE III, Chipps BE, Mathers LH. High-frequency jet ventilation in children with the adult respiratory distress syndrome complicated by pulmonary barotrauma. Pediatr Pulmonol 1993; 15(5): 279–286

26. Frame SB, Marshall WJ, Clifford TG. Synchronised independent lung ventilation in the management of pediatric unilateral lung contusion: Case report. J Trauma 1989; 29: 395–397

27. Hammer GB. Differential lung ventilation in infants and children with pulmonary hyperinflation. Paediatr Anaesth 2003; 13: 373–374

28. Wolf H, Pajenda G, Steiner B, Mousavi M, Vécsei V. Extracorporeal life support in traumatology – Review of 9 patients between 1997 and 2003. Osteo Trauma Care 2006; 14: 10–15

29. Peitzman AB. Thoracic injury, In: The trauma Manual, Peitzman Andrew (ed). Lippincott, Williams and Wilkins, Philadelphia, PA, 2002; 207–235

30. Haxhija EQ, Nöres H, Schober P, Höllwarth ME. Lung contusion-lacerations after blunt thoracic trauma in children. Pediatr Surg Int 2004; 20(6): 412–417

31. Sulc J, Bruthans J, Dlask K, Cvachovec K, Andrlik M, Kofranek J. Serial evaluation of pulmonary function long-term after lung contusion. Chest 2005; 128(4): 351S

32. Jones KW. Thoracic trauma. Surg Clin North Am 1980; 60: 957

33. Guernsey JM, Blaisdell FW. Pulmonary injury, In: Cervicothoracic Trauma, Blaisdell FW, Trunkey DD (eds), Theime, New York, 1986

34. Allshouse MJ, Eichelberger MJ. Patterns of thoracic injury, In: Pediatric Trauma: Prevention Acute care and Rehabilitation, Eichelberger MR (ed). Mosby Year Book, St Louis, Baltimore, MD, 1993; 437–448

35. Wagner RB, Crawford WO, Schrimpf PP. Classification of parenchymal injuries in the lung. Radiology 1988: 167: 77–82

36. Chon SH, Lee CB, Kim H, Chung WS, Kim YH. Diagnosis and prognosis of traumatic pulmonary psuedocysts: A review of 12 cases. Eur J Cardiothorac Surg 2006; 29: 819–823

37. Melloni G, Cremona G, Ciriaco P, Panserra M, Caretta A, Negri G, Zannini P. Diagnosis and treatment of traumatic pulmonary pseudocysts. J Trauma 2003; 54: 737–743

38. Kato R, Horonouchi H, Maenaka Y. Traumatic pulmonary pseudocyst: Report of 12 cases. J Thorac Cardiovasc Surg 1989; 97: 309–312

39. Blaisdell FW. Pneumothorax and haemothorax. In. Blaisdell FW, Trunkey DD (eds), Cervicothoracic Trauma. Theime, New York, 1986

40. Reynolds M. Pulmonary, esophageal and diaphragmatic injuries. In: Management of Paediatric Trauma, Buntain WL (ed). WB Saunders, Philadelphia, PA, 1995; 238–247

41. Eichelberger MR, Anderson KD. Sequelae of thoracic injury in children. In: Pediatric Trauma Care, Eichelberger MR, Pratsch GL (eds). Aspen, Rockville, MD, 1988; 59–68

42. Gorenstein L, Blair GR, Shandling B. The prognosis of traumatic asphyxia in childhood. J Pediatr Surg 1986; 21: 753–756

43. Heller JA, Donahoo JS. Traumatic asphyxia in children: Pathophysiology and management. J Trauma 1971; 11: 453–457

44. Williams JS, Minken JS, Adams JT. Traumatic asphyxia reappraised. Ann Surg 1968; 167: 384–382

45. Galladay ES, Donahoo JS, Heller JA. Special problems of cardiac injuries in infants and children. J Trauma 1979; 19: 526–531

46. Miller FB, Bond SJ, Shumate CR, et al. Diagnostic pericardial window: A safe alternative to exploratory thoracotomy for suspected heart injury. Arch Surg 1987; 122: 605–609
47. Langer JC, Winthrop AL, Wesson DE, et al. Diagnosis and incidence of cardiac injury in children with blunt thoracic trauma. J Pediatr Surg 1989; 24: 1091–1094
48. Tellelz DW, Harden WD, Tekehaski M et al. Blunt cardiac injury in Children. J Pediatr Surg 1987; 22: 1123–1128
49. Hurley EJ, Mayfield W. Cardiac injury, In: Cervicothoracic Trauma, Blaisdell FW, Trunkey DD (eds), Theime, New York, 1986
50. Eddy AC, Rusch VW, Fligner CL, et al. The epidemiology of traumatic rupture of aorta in children: A 13-year review. J Trauma 1990; 30: 989–992
51. Adeymi SD, Stephens CA. Traumatic diaphragmatic hernia in children. Can J Surg 1981; 24: 355–359

17
Penetrating Thoracic Trauma

Joe Crameri and Kate Ferguson

Introduction

Penetrating thoracic injuries are a rare event within the pediatric population. As previously discussed thoracic trauma comprises only 0.2–7% of all trauma in children.[1-7] The proportion of penetrating injuries within this group varies greatly worldwide ranging from 3 to 60%.[1,4,5,8-12] Although infrequent, when these injuries do occur they often result in significant patient compromise and have a reported mortality rate of up to 33%.[5,11-13] It should be noted, however, that it is possible to sustain minor penetrating chest trauma that is superficial and does not enter the chest cavity. Stabbings and gunshot wounds overwhelmingly cause the majority of these injuries at 15–74.4 and 12.5–69%, respectively.[1,2,4,5,7,9,10,12,13] Less commonly penetrating chest wounds occur secondary to road traffic accidents and falls. The nature and depth of the injury depends upon the etiology and anatomical location of the injury and the force and direction of the injurious agent.

The experience of the Royal Children's Hospital in Melbourne is similar to that reported earlier. In the 5-year period between 2000 and 2005 this hospital received 138 admissions for thoracic trauma comprising 1.7% of all trauma admissions. Of these only 5.8% were penetrating injuries, with stabbings being the most common mechanism at 55%. Our experience deviates from those of other countries in that we had no children admitted with firearm-related injuries.

As described in the previous chapter there are a number of functional compartments within the thoracic cavity (air spaces, intrapleural spaces, vasculature, mediastinum), each of which requires a specific pressure range to function normally. These pressures dictate the pre- and after-load of the heart, the expansion and recoil of the lungs, and therefore the ventilation/perfusion relationship. These components are closely related, and therefore a change in the pressure in any one of these regions will affect the others and may potentially result in major physiological compromise.

All penetrating chest traumas should be subjected to a rapid initial assessment to ensure that the patient has an adequate airway and to identify any respiratory compromise. Rarely will thoracic trauma result in obstruction of the upper airway; however, in these cases such compromise must be dealt with first. The majority of the injuries encountered will impact primarily on the patient's respiration and ventilation. Adequate intravenous access should be achieved early and blood should be sent for a full blood count, cross match, and blood gas analysis. A chest X-ray (CXR) is important and should be completed in the basic trauma series. If the patient is hemodynamically stable a CT chest may be undertaken to gain further information regarding the extent of any injury. In those cases where the initial assessment suggests the presence of a pneumothorax, a chest drain should be inserted in order to improve ventilation. A sucking, open chest wound is another indication for the immediate insertion of an intercostal catheter prior to any investigations being carried out.

All of these patients will require supplemental oxygen and close monitoring, good analgesia, insertion of a nasogastric tube, and regular chest physiotherapy. Most will require surgical exploration and many may need a period of ventilatory support. All patients who sustain a penetrating injury also need to have their tetanus immunization status assessed and should be commenced on intravenous antibiotics.

Further management of these patients will be determined by their clinical status and the experience of the managing clinician (Fig. 17.1). In most cases where the patient is stable and has a normal chest X-ray it is reasonable to observe them for 12–24 h. If stability is maintained over this time period it is generally safe to discharge the patient. In a stable patient with an abnormal X-ray, intervention such as insertion of an intercostal catheter and close observation in an ICU or HDU should be undertaken. This admission should be in an institution where pediatric surgeons and anesthetists are available.

In patients who have persistent, large-volume output via the ICC and in patients who are hemodynamically unstable, aggressive fluid resuscitation and close monitoring is important. If the patient does not respond to these measures surgical intervention is indicated. This will involve either thoracotomy

D.H. Parikh et al. (eds.), *Pediatric Thoracic Surgery*,
DOI: 10.1007/b136543_17, © Springer-Verlag London Limited 2009

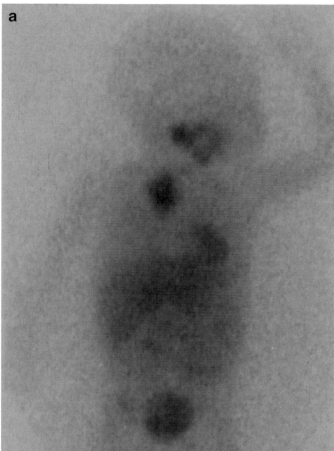

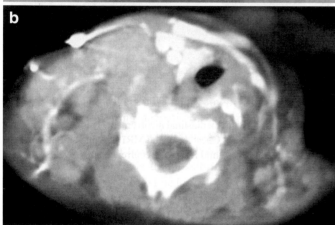

FIG. 19.4. (a) MIBG scan showing persistent uptake in a child with a large cervico-thoracic tumor after chemotherapy. (b) CT angiogram from the same patient showing involvement of the subclavian, vertebral and carotid arteries. The tumor was excised using a modified Dartevelle approach. The child received postoperative chemotherapy and remains recurrence free after 5 years

could be stage 1 or 3 depending on the surgeon involved. The incongruity of this lead a recent conference (Whistler, Canada, September 2005), to propose a new staging system, the International Neuroblastoma Risk Group Staging System (INRGSS) based on age, N-myc status and histology and on pre-treatment imaging criteria (IDRFs),

TABLE 19.2. International neuroblastoma staging system[31]

Stage 1	Localized tumor is confined to the organ of origin; complete resection with or without microscopic residual tumor; ipsilateral and contralateral lymph nodes are microscopically negative
Stage 2a	This involves a localized tumor with incomplete gross resection; ipsilateral and contralateral lymph nodes are microscopically negative
Stage 2b	This involves a unilateral tumor with incomplete or complete gross resection; ipsilateral lymph nodes are positive; contralateral lymph nodes are microscopically negative
Stage 3	In this stage, tumor crosses the midline with or without regional lymph node involvement, unilateral tumor is associated with positive contralateral lymph nodes, or a midline tumor is found with positive bilateral lymph nodes
Stage 4	Distant metastases are present
Stage 4s	This occurs in infants with a localized tumor that does not cross midline, with metastatic disease confined to the liver, skin, and bone marrow (<10% tumor cells in bone marrow)

TABLE 19.3. Image defined risk factors associated with cervical and thoracic tumors

Neck	Tumor encasing vertebral or carotid artery
	Tumor encasing brachial plexus roots
	Tumor crossing the midline
Thorax	Tumor encasing the trachea or principle bronchus
	Tumor encasing the origin and branches of the subclavian vessels
	Thoraco-abdominal tumor encasing the thoracic aorta

the INRGSS is a true pre-treatment stage and more objective than the previous reliance on surgical assessment of respectability [32].

Disease Staging

"Disease Staging" before "Prognostic Factors" "The International Neuroblastoma Staging System (INSS) is shown in Table 19.2. This staging system is based on surgical as well as pathological findings. The main criticism of the INSS staging system is that it describes the post-surgical stage. Thus the same tumor could be stage 1 or 3 depending on the surgeon involved. This incongruity lead a recent conference (Whistler, Canada, September 2005) to propose a new staging system - the International Neuroblastoma Risk Group Staging System (INRGSS) based on age, N-myc status, histology and pre-treatment imaging criteria (imaging-derived risk factors - IDRFs). Imaging-defined risk factors for cervical and thoracic neuroblastomas are shown in Table 19.3. The INRGSS is a true pre-treatment stage and more objective than the previous INSS which relied on surgical assessment of resectability [32]."

"Infants less than one year of age have a good prognosis. They present with lower stage disease and N-Myc amplification is rare.[33,34,35] Less than 5% of all neuroblastomas present in adolescents (aged 10–18 years at diagnosis). Although the primary tumour site and disease stage is similar to younger children, adolescents may present with metastases to unusual sites including the brain, lungs and pleura. N-myc amplification is relatively uncommon but survival rates are worse when adolescents are treated with the standard childhood protocols[36], suggesting that other biological factors are important in this age group."

Tumour stage

Tumour-stage at diagnosis is an important independent prognostic factor (see table)[16]. One exception to this rule is the strange clinical presentation of stage 4s disease first described by D'Angio in 1971[37]. Stage 4s disease occurs, by definition, in infant less than 1 year of age, with a small localised primary and metastases to the liver, skin and bone marrow. Virtually all of these tumours virtually all eventually regress without treatment. However, the rapid progression of hepatic metastases can compromise breathing and thus treatment may be required either in the form of abdominal decompression with a patch or chemotherapy. stage 4s thoracic tumors occasionally require chemotherapy to reduce pressure symptoms caused by compression of the surrounding structures.

Tumour site

The site of the primary has been reported by a prospective POG study to be an independent favourable risk factor even after correction for age and stage[3,16,38,39]. Thoracic site in particular appears to be a good prognostic factor although this is related to favourable histology and lower incidence of N-Myc amplification.[16,40,41] Haberle reviewed 113 thoracic tumours for the German Neuroblastoma group between 1989 and 1995 and found that the incidence of stage 4 disease for thoracic primaries was 24.8% compared with 44.4% for nonthoracic neuroblastoma. Adams et al reviewed 96 primary thoracic neuroblastomas and found that they had an improved prognosis even after correcting for age and stage[3].

Patients with neuroblastoma dumbbell type tumours with intra-spinal extension are reported to have better (97%) than average survival and the majority (66%) enjoy complete neurological recovery[29].

Antenatal diagnosis

Approximately 20% of neuroblastomas are diagnosed either antenatally or in the first 3 months of life[42,43]. More than 90% are of adrenal origin and cystic in nature. Thoracic primaries comprise only a small fraction of this group. The majority of these tumours are asymptomatic. However, on rare occasions, maternal and/or foetal compromise may be observed. Foetal hydrops may result from compression of the great vessels, placental metastases or high-output heart failure. More than 80% of these tumours are stage 1 or 2 and in excess of 90% have favourable biology. Given the reputation of tumours in this group to demonstrate spontaneous regression or maturation, a strategy of expectant observation should be adopted.[42,43]

Mass screening

A Mass screening of infants for neuroblastoma by measurements of urinary excretion of VMA and HVA on a spot urine sample was first introdused in Japan in 1974 and subsequently implemented in Canada, Germany and Austria, mass screening programmes have been based on spot measurement of urinary excretion of VMA and HVA in infants. The age at screening was 6 months in Japan but varied in other countries. Approximately 10% of screen-detected lesions were thoracic. It is now clear that screening results in a doubling of the incidence of neuroblastoma without decreasing the incidence of advanced-stage disease in older children or decreasing the mortality from neuroblastoma[44,45]. Spontaneous regression has been reported in 60%–73% of these lesions[45]. Hence, all screening studies have now been suspended[46].

Differential diagnosis

Neuroblastoma must be differentiated from other neurogenic and non-neurogenic tumours arising within the posterior mediastinum (Table 19.1). A variety of benign conditions may cause a mass lesion within the posterior mediastinum, particularly extralobar pulmonary sequestration and foregut duplication cysts. Tumors presenting with paraneoplastic syndromes may be confused with unrelated medical conditions.

Management options

An Overview of Treatment Strategies

Treatment of children with malignant disease requires a multidisciplinary team (MDT) approach. The biological behaviour of neuroblastomas means that age, radiological stage, pathology and cytogenetics must all be considered prior to reaching a definitive decision about treatment. There is no place for heroic surgery without the consent of the MDT but it also self evident from this statement that the surgical oncologist has a central role in determining treatment. Furthermore, this is not surgery to be attempted on an occasional basis as decisions

TABLE 19.4. Risk stratification used by SIOP

	Patient/tumor characteristics
Low risk	• Infants below 1 year of age • Stage 1 or 2 tumors that can be treated with complete resection alone • Stage 4 s
Intermediate risk	• Children over the age of 1 year with unresectable stage 2 and 3 *without* adverse biological features
High risk	• Children over the age of 1 year with stage 2 or 3 disease *with* N-myc amplification • Stage 4 disease

roblastoma fully. Bone marrow aspiration or trephine biopsy are rarely sufficient to make a diagnosis alone as up to 17% of trephine biopsies provide inadequate samples.[67,68]

Tumor Resection

The decision to attempt resection of a neuroblastoma is made by the MDT on the basis of the relationship of the tumor to adjacent vital structures (i.e., operability), the age of the child, disease stage and biology (Table 19.3). Although cross-sectional imaging helps plan surgery it is usually only possible to determine resectability accurately at operation. Resections are described as complete (removal of all visible tumor, including lymph nodes, even if resection margins contain microscopic tumor), near-complete and incomplete (macroscopic residual tumor following excision).[32]

The pre-operative work-up must be meticulous as these operations are long and difficult. Resection of large tumors incurs significant morbidity and even mortality. It is important to schedule surgery after the bone marrow has recovered the effects of chemotherapy so that the platelet and white cell count have returned to normal. This is usually two weeks after the last course of chemotherapy. Blood should be taken to check the full blood count, coagulation, serum biochemistry and cross match 2 - 4 units of blood.

Prior to operation the imaging should be reviewed to assess tracheal and superior vena caval compression. Although these risks are significantly greater with anterior mediastinal masses they are also seen with posterior mediastinal tumors. Anesthetic considerations include adequate venous access to allow rapid transfusion, central venous pressure monitoring and arterial access to allow blood sampling and continuous arterial pressure monitoring. The need for a double lumen endotracheal tube or a bronchial blocker to allow single lung ventilation should be discussed preoperatively. This is not necessary for most posterior mediastinal tumors. Good post-operative analgesia is essential. How this is achieved is dependant on the skills of the anesthetist and the local hospital policy. In our unit we use thoracic epidurals for postoperative analgesia for at least 48 hours after thoracotomy. They provides very good analgesia and allow early mobilization while avoiding the potential respiratory depressant effects of opiates.

The usual access for open surgical excision of a thoracic neuroblastoma is a posterolateral thoracotomy. Stage 1 and 2 tumors, even high up at the apex of the thorax, can usually be dissected off the chest wall via a high lateral thoracotomy using traction on the tumour and a combination of sharp and blunt dissection. Tumors low in the posterior mediastinum may extend below the diaphragm although they can usually be removed through a thoracotomy providing the anatomy can be defined clearly. However, a thoraco-abdominal approach or a separate laparotomy may be necessary. Tumors extending across the midline into the opposite paravertebral space may require bilateral thoracotomies either under the same anesthetic or at a later stage.

Once the chest is opened and the pathology confirmed the pleura should be incised around the tumor. This provides entry to plane in which the tumor may be dissected off the chest wall. The anatomy is often markedly distorted and it is important to differentiate vessels feeding the tumor from vessels to normal structures which have been displaced and must be preserved. The tumour should be separated from the sympathetic chain by sharp dissection to avoid diathermy injury to the stellate ganglion and segmental intercostal nerves.

Stage 3 and 4 tumors frequently encase major blood vessels. Experience has shown that these tumors do not usually invade the vessel wall but remain outside the subadventitial layer. In the abdomen the principle is to identify the major vessels early before they enter the tumour and then follow them by careful dissection. Once the vessels are free the tumor can be removed piecemeal.[50,51] Of particular concern in the thoracic inlet are the vessels that supply the head, neck and arm and the thoracic duct. As discussed above incomplete resection of thoracic neuroblastomas does not jeopardize the prognosis. Consequently there is no need to take excessive risks during surgery. In this context, tumor extending into an intervertebral foramen can be transected without attempting complete clearance.

All relevant lymph nodes should be sampled at thoracotomy if possible. The Pediatric Oncology Group study reported that although lymph node biopsies were only obtained in 41% of patients undergoing thoracotomy, 36% of those biopsied contained tumor.[3]

The Dartevelle Approach

Cervicothoracic tumors frequently encase the major vessels in the root of the neck and are technically demanding because of restricted access. Dartevelle described a trap-door incision with resection of the medial third of the clavicle to provide access to remove Pancoast tumors in adults. Modifications of this incision provide good exposure for neuroblastomas in the thoracic inlet.[69,70]

A number of modifications have been made to Dartevelle's approach. We prefer the Nazari modification,[71,72] whereby the clavicle is divided to provide exposure and then repaired at the end of the operation. Resection of medial third of clavicle reduces the shoulder girdle mobility and long term results in children may not be acceptable.[73]

The child is placed supine on the operating table with a roll under the shoulders to extend the neck. An L-shaped anterior incision is made and the medial half of the clavicle divided (Fig. 19.5). This allows excellent exposure of the thoracic inlet. The scaleneus anterior muscle is divided to expose the deeper vessels and the tumor. The sternocleidomastoid muscle is retracted medially. The tumor is dissected free from the internal jugular vein and brachiocephalic confluence followed by clearance from the arteries. The neuroblastoma is generally closely associated with the carotid and subclavian arteries and sharp dissection in the adventitial plane of these vessels may be necessary to achieve complete clearance. The phrenic

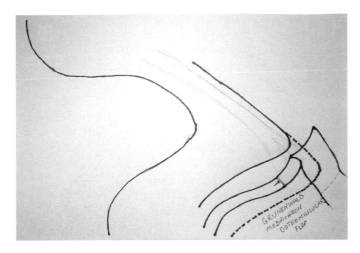

FIG. 19.5. Modifications of Dartevelle's approach to the thoracic inlet. The incision in the neck is taken laterally either above or below the clavicle. The clavicle can be divided at the junction of the middle and medial thirds leaving the sternomastoid attachment intact. Retraction then provides good expose of the tumor. The Grunenwald approach involves division of the manubrium and raising an osteomuscular flap lifting the clavicle along with sternoclavicular joint and the sternocleidomastoid muscle laterally

and vagus nerves are identified and preserved. Once the tumor resection is complete both ends of the clavicle are approximated with long-lasting absorbable sutures. This approach gives good cosmetic results without long term impairment of shoulder joint mobility and stability.

The Grunenwald modification involves division of the manubrium and, if necessary the upper sternum. The sternum then fractures transversely into the ipsilateral thorax allowing elevation of the clavicle, sternoclavicular joint and part of the manubrium to expose the deeper structures (Fig. 19.5).[73,74,75] After the tumor has been resected the sternum is wired together. No one approach is perfect for all cervicothoracic tumors and the surgeon should be familiar with all these modifications[72]. Additionally, if the tumor has an intrathoracic component the thoracic cavity can be exposed by disarticulating the first and second ribs at the costo-chondral junction[75].

situation is perfect and therefore surgeon should be familiar with other modifications and exposure in this area[72]. Additionally, if the tumour has an intra-thoracic component, the thoracic cavity can be exposed by disarticulating first and second ribs at the costo-chondral junction[75]. We recommend our technique as it is useful in most situation in achieving good exposure and complete resection of neuroblastoma with minimal postoperative morbidity.

Minimally invasive resection

Successful thoracoscopic resection of apical and supradiaphragmatic mediastinal neuroblastomas has been reported. Small (≤ 6 cm), stage 1 lesions with favourable histology have been resected with no complications other than minor tumour spillage, resulting in disease free survival without the need for adjuvant therapy[64]. A retrospective comparison of thoracoscopic and open approaches to resection found similar local control and disease-free survival at a mean follow-up of 25 months but the former was associated with a significantly shorter hospital stay[76]. With careful case selection, the major advantages of this approach are the avoidance of a thoracotomy and the enhanced surgical precision afforded by improved visualization[38].

Complications of surgery

The study by Haberle et al. reported postoperative complications in 34 of 195 procedures performed in 104 patients with thoracic tumors, including 6 biopsies.[4] Horner's syndrome (n=14) was the most frequent complication, followed by pulmonary complications (n=13), chylothorax (n=4), other neurologic complications (n=4) and scoliosis (n=1).

Four chylothoraces were noted in 104 tumor resections.[4] Mediastinal neuroblastoma and a 'congenital' chylothorax has been reported in a newborn suggesting that the latter may result from lymphatic obstruction due to the tumor[77]. Chylothorax resulting from surgical resection should be managed in a stepwise fashion starting with chest-tube drainage and a diet containing medium chain triglyceride fats. If the chylothorax fails to resolve a trial of total parenteral nutrition is appropriate. Ligation of the lymphatic pathways is difficult and should be the last resort Neurological complications are uncommon but ischemic injury to the mid-thoracic spinal cord can occur after excision of dumbbell tumors. Permanent paraplegia has been reported is a result.[28]

Survival

The overall survival for thoracic neuroblastomas is much better than for abdominal or pelvic disease, Survival rates of 77%[4], 88%[3] and 100%[41] By way of comparison, the current survival rate for children with high risk non-thoracic neuroblastoma is approximately 15%[1].

Future perspective

The unique biological behavior of neuroblastomas means that conventional descriptions of local, regional and distant spread are of little relevance to the management of this disease. However, the management of high-risk neuroblastoma is still difficult. The role surgery, in particular, needs to be assessed objectively by a multicenter randomized controlled study. The role of post-operative chemotherapy for children unfavorable histology neuroblastoma needs refining.

What is clear for thoracic neuroblastomas is that the prognosis is good and surgery should be performed with the intention of minimizing morbidity. Further developments in minimally invasive surgery are consistent with this aim.

Clinical Presentation

Children with parenchymal lung tumors are usually asymptomatic. When lung tumors do produce symptoms in children these include cough, haemoptysis, fever, recurrent pneumonitis, and symptoms similar to inhaled foreign body causing partial bronchial obstruction. Respiratory compromise may be a symptom associated with generalized infiltration, secondary infection, or collapse of the lung distal to an obstruction. Chest pain is rare and may indicate pleural or chest wall involvement. Large tumors may cause dysphagia and superior vena caval obstruction.

Diagnosis

Radiology

Plain chest X-ray: Chest X-ray is the primary investigation for suspected lung disease (Fig. 20.1a).

CT Scan: Spiral CT scan delineates lung tumors accurately. Intravenous (IV) contrast must be administered to determine vascularity of the tumor. It can occasionally distinguish infective pathology from a tumor. Some pleuropulmonary tumors present with clinical features and radiology suggestive of empyema thoracis. In these cases, a CT scan with IV contrast can be a most useful investigation to differentiate tumor from empyema thus avoiding operative morbidity.[7] A CT scan is mandatory for all pulmonary lesions as well as metastatic disease. CT will define nodules accurately and frequently identifies other deeper and smaller lesions (Fig. 20.1b).

MRI Scan: The anatomical location and extent of most benign and malignant soft tissue lesions are better defined with this radiological investigation. In difficult cases it may be necessary to have both CT and MR scans to ascertain suitability for resection. It is useful to document the anatomical extent of a pulmonary lesion if minimally invasive surgery is contemplated. In addition, MR will assist complete excision of the tumor with adequate margins.

Angiography: This investigation is occasionally useful to clarify the arterial supply to a tumor, although increasingly this information can be obtained using CT or MR. The interventional radiologist can help reduce vascularity prior to resection by embolising major arterial feeders. This preoperative intervention is especially useful for arterio-venous malformations of the lung.

Bone Scan: The isotope scan is useful to identify bony metastasis.

Bronchoscopy: Endobronchial tumors can be detected and biopsied using bronchoscopic techniques. Distal inaccessible endobronchial lesions may be identified by broncho-alveolar lavage or brush biopsy by cytological means.

Biopsy: When imaging and other diagnostic modalities are not able to distinguish between benign and malignant lesions diagnostic biopsy becomes essential. The type of biopsy (excisional, incisional, or needle biopsy) depends upon the location of the tumor, the differential diagnosis and local expertise.

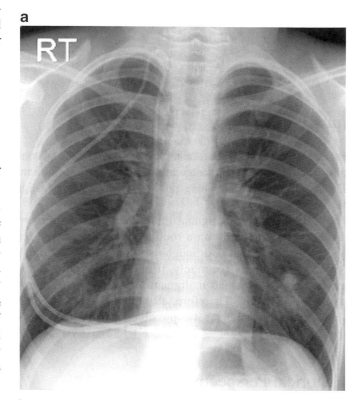

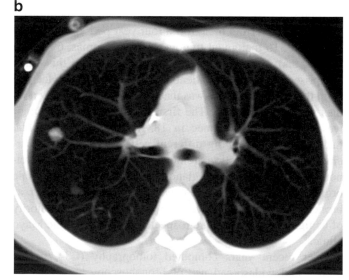

FIG. 20.1. (**a**) Chest X-ray showing an osteogenic sarcoma metastasis in the left lower lobe. (**b**) CT scan showing a small nodule in the right upper lobe. CT is more sensitive than plain films for detecting metastases

Benign Tracheo-Bronchial Tumors

Tracheo-bronchial tumors in children are rare and of variable behavior.

Juvenile papillomatosis: The lesion follows human papilloma virus infection transmitted to the child from the mother. Lesions are usually limited to larynx but in approximately 5% of cases, there may be extensive involvement of the trachea, bronchi, and lung parenchyma.[8] Laryngeal papilloma typically present with hoarseness of the voice, stridor, breathlessness, and hemoptysis. Laryngeal papillomas are best managed by CO_2 laser resection. Repeated resection is required, although spontaneous regression is recognized later in childhood.[9] Distal spread is ominous and parenchymal involvement is usually lethal either as a result of respiratory failure or due to malignant transformation (Fig. 20.2).

Mucous gland adenoma: This is an extremely rare bronchial gland tumor producing an adenomatous lesion within the bronchus. Tumors are usually solitary and produce partial bronchial obstruction causing either distal emphysematous change or chronic lobar collapse. The symptoms and signs may resemble foreign body inhalation in a child. Biopsy is required to distinguish adenomas from inflammatory polyps (Fig. 20.3). Complete resection is curative.

Pleomorphic mixed adenoma: The pleomorphic mixed tumor of the bronchus is similar to the pleomorphic adenoma of the salivary gland. Local recurrence is common if resection is incomplete. Consequently, these lesions can be considered malignant. Pleomorphic adenomas can be polypoid or sessile and develop in the large airways. Rarely they present with acute severe airway obstruction and require emergency management.[10]

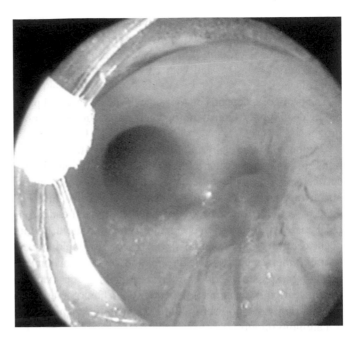

FIG. 20.3. Endo-bronchial obstructive lesion in a three-year-old girl with chronic collapse of the lung. The polypoid lesion is inspected carefully before biopsy to avoid intra-bronchial bleeding

Microscopically pleomorphic adenomas demonstrate epithelial and stromal components with varying degree of differentiation. The epithelial cells are arranged as tubules. Mitoses are infrequent. Wide local excision is required for the adequate management of this tumor.[11]

Malignant Tracheo-Bronchial Tumors

Carcinoid Tumors

Pulmonary carcinoid tumors were historically classified as benign bronchial adenomas. In the light of recent evidence, all carcinoid tumors are considered part of a spectrum of malignant neoplasms along with large cell neuroendocrine carcinomas and small cell carcinomas.[12–14] These tumors generally present in adolescents and comprise 80% of endobronchial lesions in children.[9,15] Carcinoid tumors arise from endobronchial stem cells with neuroendocrine differentiation and enlarge as either an endobronchial lesion or an infiltrative peribronchial mass.[16]

Neuroendocrine tumors of the lung are classified into typical and atypical carcinoid tumors, according to strict pathological criteria.[17,18] The distinction between well differentiated "typical" carcinoid tumors and atypical carcinoid tumors with a more aggressive behavior can be difficult. Atypical carcinoid tumors show increased mitotic activity, cellularity, and invariably have areas of necrosis.

Carcinoid tumors invariably present with symptoms and signs of bronchial obstruction with wheeze, recurrent pneumonia and

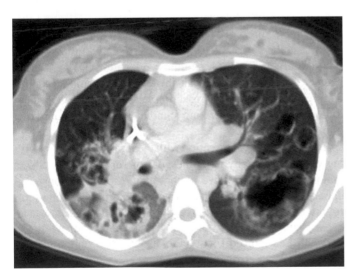

FIG. 20.2. CT scan showing a destructive parenchymal lesion caused by respiratory papillomatosis. The child was initially treated by regular laser ablation of laryngo-tracheo-bronchial polyps. Later metaplasia resulted in an incurable squamous cell carcinoma

in very young children. Type II PPB is mixed solid and cystic, and Type III PPB is a predominantly solid variety identified in older children. Cystic tumors have been identified in preexisting congenital cystic lung lesions and may change into more malignant solid lesions if inadequately managed.[50–52] Although congenital cystic adenomatoid malformation (CCAM) of the lung and PPB are clearly associated with each other, it is unclear whether CCAM progresses to pleuropulmonary blastoma. A few cases of antenatally diagnosed cystic lung lesions resected have been found to contain PPB.[53] Solid areas have also been detected within air filled cysts during followed up, prior to the pathological diagnosis of PPB.[44] Histologically, PPB demonstrates a diffuse proliferation of undifferentiated blastemal cells and contains areas of chondroblastic foci with a stroriform or alveolar pattern and lipoblastic differentiation. Accordingly, PPB may stain with a variety immunohistochemical markers depending upon the composition of the tumor cells, including vimentin, alpha-1 antitrypsin, alpha-1 antichymotrypsin, lysozyme, KP1, desmin, and S100.[46]

Respiratory symptoms such as cough, fever, and chest pain are often the presenting features of PPB.[44] The chest radiograph may suggest pneumonia or a pleural effusion. Pneumothoraces have been seen in younger patients. PPB has been mistakenly diagnosed as an empyema thoracis.[7]

Combination chemotherapy should be given to PPB to improve the outcome prior to surgery.[54] Complete resection and chemotherapy can produce a good long-term outcome. In one study, gender, side, tumor size, preexisting lung cysts, and extent of surgical resection did not affect survival.[55] However, total resection of the tumor did result in significantly better survival.[55]

Pleuropulmonary blastoma is an aggressive malignancy with a 5-year survival rates of 42% for patients with type II and III even after multimodal therapy. There is no statistical difference in survival between the three subtypes. However, type I was found to be readily resectable than type II and III

tumors. Mediastinal and pleural involvement correlated with a poor outcome. Distant metastasis, specifically to the central nervous system and bone, are associated with a dismal outlook.

Rhabdomyosarcoma of the Lung

Rhabdomyosarcoma of the lung is a rare tumor. Previously, some PPB's were mistakenly diagnosed as rhabdomyosarcoma, especially within preexisting cystic lung lesions.[56,57] Rhabdomyosarcomas may be endobronchial, mediastinal, pulmonary, or pleural in origin.[58]

Other Malignant Parenchymal Tumors

Malignant fibrous histiocytomas are rare tumors in children. Complete surgical resection produces good results.[59] Leiomyosarcomas and peripheral nerve sheath tumors are also encountered very rarely.[2,60] Lymphoma, posttransplant lymphoproliferative disorders and Langerhans' cell histiocytosis are other rare tumors encountered by the pediatric thoracic surgeon.

Metastatic Lung Tumors

Metastatic tumors are much more common than primary lung tumors in children. Resection of lung metastases is a well-established treatment of children with malignancies. There are several published series about the outcome following metastasectomy. However, most of the published series include both adult and pediatric patients.[61,62] Few studies show the outcome after resections in children.[63,64]

The commonest tumors presenting with pulmonary metastases amenable to surgical resection are osteogenic sarcoma (Fig. 20.5a, b), Wilm's tumor (Fig. 20.6a, b), malignant germ

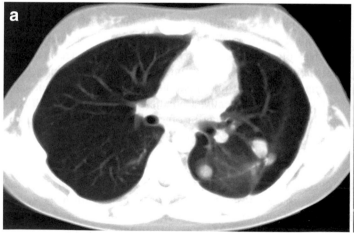
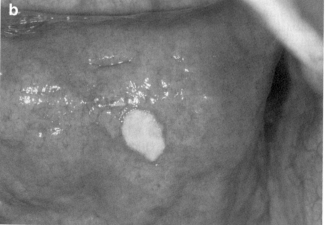

FIG. 20.5. (a) CT scan showing multiple bilateral osteosarcoma metastases. The metastases were resected through sequential bilateral thoracotomies. (b) Operative photograph showing a large osteogenic sarcoma metastasis

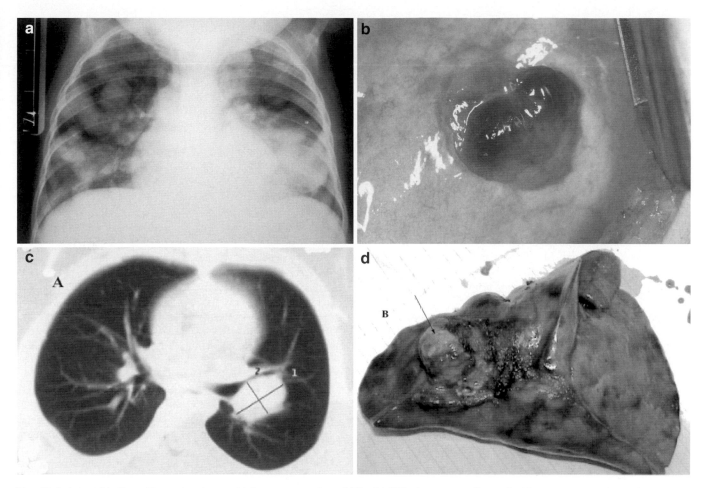

FIG. 20.6. (**a** and **b**) Chest X-ray showing multiple metastases in a child with Wilm's tumor at diagnosis. The response to chemotherapy was very good although a single metastasis persisted and was resected. (**c** and **d**) CT scan showing a soft tissue sarcoma metastasis near the hilum requiring resection by lobectomy. The child remains well more than five years after resection

cell tumors, and soft tissue sarcomas (Fig. 20.6c, d). Regular surveillance following treatment of the primary tumor has allowed early detection of metastatic disease. Computed tomography allows detection of lesions too small to detect on a routine chest X-ray (Fig. 20.1a, b). It is important to appreciate that not all pulmonary lesions detected in this manner are metastases. Benign lesions have also been identified.[65]

Lung metastases may be the only sign of recurrence. Management of pulmonary metastases involves control of the primary tumor and metastasectomy. Survival can be improved significantly by complete resection of metastases.[64,66–70] Data on reoperative metastatectomy is scarce but Temeck et al. reported median survivals of 2.25, 3.6, and 0.96 years in children with metastatic sarcoma after the second, third, and fourth explorations.[67] Survival in this study was not influenced by the type of primary tumor, sex, histology, maximum size, or chemotherapy. Resectability was the most important criterion influencing the survival. Other adult studies have reported similar results with slightly longer disease free intervals.[61,71] In patients with metastatic osteosarcoma,

complete resection is essential to achieve long-term survival and repeat resections are needed in about 44% of patients (Fig. 20.5a, b).[62,66] Adjuvant chemotherapy or radiotherapy has been coupled with surgery to reduce the early relapse rate.[69] Early relapse after metastatectomy is associated with a poor prognosis.

Bilateral metastatectomy can be performed either by sequential posterio-lateral thoracotomy or though a median sternotomy.[72,73] Sequential bilateral thoracotomy with a gap of two weeks between operations is reasonably well tolerated in the paediatric patient. Recovery following sternotomy, including redo sternotomy is more rapid, particularly in children walking with crutches.

The role of VATS in the management of pulmonary metastases is controversial. VATS relies entirely on CT to identify metastases as palpation of invisible lesions is not possible. We frequently detect additional metastases by palpation not identified on CT scanning. VAT wedge resection is feasible and safe, but in one series three out of seven patients had early recurrences within 6 months.[74]

Conclusions and Future Perspectives

All pulmonary nodules in children should be considered as malignant until proved otherwise by histopathology. Prognosis depends on the tumor type and biology. However, complete surgical resection with a clear margin is the crucial factor determining survival for both metastatic and primary lung tumors.

References

1. Cohen MC, Kaschula RO. Primary pulmonary tumours in childhood: a review of 31 years of experience and the literature. Pediatr Pulmonol 1992; 14(4): 222–232.
2. Hartman GE, Shochat SJ. Primary pulmonary neoplasms of childhood: a review. Ann Thorac Surg 1983; 36(1): 108–119.
3. Hancock BJ. Childhood pulmonary neoplasms. J Pediatr Surg 1993; 28(9): 1133–1136.
4. Steele JD. The solitary pulmonary nodule: report of a cooperative study of resected asymptomatic solitary pulmonary nodules in males. J Thorac Cardiovasc Surg 1963; 46: 21.
5. Laennec RTH. Traite de L'Auscultation Mediate et des Maladies des Poumons et du Coeur. 3rd Ed. Chaud, Paris, 1831.
6. Arrigononi MG, Woolner LD, Bernatz PE, et al. Benign tumours of the lung: a ten year surgical experience. J Thorac Cardiovasc Surg 1970; 60: 589.
7. Sharif K, Alton H, Clarke J, Desai M, Morland B, Parikh D. Paediatric thoracic tumours presenting as empyema. Pediatr Surg Int 2006; 22(12): 1009–1014.
8. Somers GR, et al. Juvenile laryngreal papilloma in a pediatric population: a clinicopathological study. Pediatr Pathol Lab Med 1997; 17(1): 53–64.
9. Stocker J. The Respiratory Tract. In Stocker J, Dehner L (eds.) Paediatric Pathology. Lippincot, Williams & Wilkins: Philadelphia 2001; 445–517.
10. Baghai-Wadji M, Sianati H, Nikpour S, et al. Pleomorphic adenoma of the trachea in an 8 year old boy: a case report. J Pediatr Surg 2006; 41(8): e23–e26.
11. Ko JM, Jung JI, Park SH, et al. Benign tumours of tracheobronchial tree: CT-pathologic correlation. AJR 2006; 186: 1304–1313.
12. Travis WD, Rush W, Flieder DB, et al. Survival analysis of 200 pulmonary neuroendocrine tumors with clarification for atypical carcinoid and its separation from typical carcinoid. Am J Surg Pathol 1998; 22: 934–944.
13. Davilla DG, Dunn WF, Tazelaar HD, et al. Bronchial carcinoid tumours. Mayo Clin Proc 1993; 68: 795–803.
14. Sheppard MN. Neuroendocrine differentiation in lung tumours. Thorax 1991; 46: 843–850.
15. Wang LT, Wilkins EW Jr., Bode HH. Bronchial carcinoid tumours in pediatric patients. Chest 1993; 103(5): 1426–1431.
16. Andrassy RJ, Feldman RW, Stanford W. Bronchial carcinoid tumors in children and adolescents. J Pediatr Surg 1997; 12(4): 513–517.
17. Travis WD, Sobin LH. Histologic typing of lung and pleural tumours: International histologic classification of tumours (no.1) Springer-Verlag: New York, 1999.
18. Travis LD, Linnila RI, Tsokos MG, et al. Neuroendocrine tumours of the lung with proposed criteria for large-cell neuroendocrine carcinoma: an ultrastructural, immunohistochemical and flow cytometric study of 35 cases. Am J Surg Pathol 1991; 15: 529–553.
19. Thomas CF, Tazelaar HD, Jett JR. Typical and atypical pulmonary carcinoids. Chest 2001; 119: 1143–1150.
20. McCaughan BC, Martini M, Bains MS. Bronchial carcinoids: review of 124 cases. Thorac Cardiovasc Surg 1985; 89: 8–17.
21. Akiba T, Naruke T, Kondo H, et al. Carcinoid tumour of the lung: Clinicaopathological study of 32 cases. Jpn J Clin Oncol 1992; 22: 92–95.
22. Harpole DH Jr, Feldman JM, Buchanan S, et al. Bronchial carcinoid tumours: a retrospective analysis of 126 patients Ann Thorac Surg 1992; 54: 50–54.
23. Torre M, Barberis M, Barbieri B, et al. Typical and atypical bronchial carcinoids. Respir Med 1989; 83: 305–308.
24. Picard E, Udassin R, Ramu N, et al Pulmonary fibrosarcoma in childhood: fiber-optic bronchoscopic diagnosis and review of the literature. Pediatr Pulmonol 1999; 27(5): 347–350.
25. Pettinato G, Manivel JC, Saldana MJ, Peyser J, Dehner LP. Primary bronchopulmonary fibrosarcoma of childhood and adolescence: reassessment of a low-grade malignancy. Clinicopathologic study of five cases and review of the literature. Hum Pathol 1989; 20(5): 463–471.
26. Lal DR, Clark I, Shalkow J, et al. Primary epithelial lung malignancy in the pediatric population. Pediatr Blood Cancer 2005; 45(5): 683–686.
27. Granata C, Gambini C, Balducci T, et al. Bronchoalveolar carcinoma arising in congenital cystic adenomatoid malformation in a child: a case report and review on malignancies originating in congenital cystic adenomatoid malformation. Pediatr Pulmonol 1998; 25(1): 62–66.
28. Ramos SG, Barbosa GH, Tavora FR, et al. Bronchioalveolar carcinoma arising in a congenital pulmonary airway malformation in a child: case report with an update of this association. J Pediatr Surg 2007; 42(5): E1–E4.
29. Bacci G. Secondary malignancy in 597 patients with Ewing's sarcoma of bone treated at a single institution with adjuvant and neoadjuvant chemotherapy between 1972 and 1999. J Pediatr Hematol Oncol 2005; 27(10): 517–520.
30. Laberge JM, Puligandla P, Flageole H. Asymptomatic congenital lung malformations. Semin Pediatr Surg 2005; 14(1): 16–33.
31. Sundarajan L, Parikh DH. Evolving experience with video-assisted thoracic surgery in congenital cystic lung lesions in a British pediatric centre. J Pediatr Surg 2007; 42:1243–1250.
32. Ota H, Langston C, Honda T, Katsuyama T, et al. Histochemical analysis of mucous cells of congenital adenomatoid malformation of the lung: insights into the carcinogenesis of pulmonary adenocarcinoma expressing gastric mucins. Am J Clin Pathol 1998; 110(4): 450–455.
33. Ohye RG, Cohen D, Caldwell S, et al. Pediatric bronchoalveolar carcinoma: a favourable pediatric malignancy? J Pediatr Surg 1998; 33(5): 730–732.
34. Bahadori M, Liebow A. Plasma cell granulomas of the lung. Cancer 1973; 31:191–208.
35. Su LD. Inflammatory myofibroblastic tumour: cytogenic evidence supporting a clonal origin. Mod Pathol 1998; 11(4): 364–368.
36. Shapiro MP, Gale ME, Carter BL. Variable CT appearance of plasma cell granuloma of the lung. J Comput Assst Tomogr 1987; 11(1): 49–51.
37. Hedlund GL, Aggressive manifestations of inflammatory pulmonary psedotumour in children. Pediatr Radiol 1999; 29(2): 112–116.

38. Lee HJ, Kim JS, Choi YS, et al. Treatment of inflammatory myofibroblastic tumour of the chest: the extent of resection. Ann Thorac Surg 2007; 84(7): 221–224.

39. Applebaum H, Kieran M, Cripe T, et al. The rational for non-steroidal anti-inflammatory drug therapy for inflammatory myofibroblastic tumours: A Children's Oncology Group study. J Pediatr Surg 2005; 40(6): 999–1003.

40. Weinberg PB, Bromberg PA, Askin PB. 'Recurrence' of a plasma cell granuloma 11 years after initial resection. South Med J 1987; 80: 519–521.

41. Carney JA. Gastric stromal sarcoma, pulmonary chondroma, and extra-adrenal paraganglioma (Carney's Triad): natural history, adrenocortical component, possible familial occurrence. Mayo Clin Proc 1999; 76(6): 550–552.

42. Siegelman SS, Khouri NF, Scott WW, et al. Pulmonary Hamartoma: CT findings. Radiology 1986; 160: 313.

43. Meade JB, Whitwell F, Bickford BJ, et al. Primary haemangiopericytoma of lung. Thorax 1974; 29: 1.

44. Priest JR, McDermott MB, Bhatia S, et al. Pleuropulmonary blastoma: A clinicopathologic study of 50 cases. Cancer 1997; 80(1): 147–161.

45. Manivel JC, Priest JR, Watterson J, et al. Pleuropulmonary Blastoma: the so called pulmonary blastoma of childhood. Cancer 1988; 62: 1516–1526.

46. Hachitanda Y, Aoyama C, Sato JK, Shimada H. Pleuropulmonary blastoma of childhood: a tumour of divergent differentiation. Am J Surg Pathol 1993; 17: 382–391.

47. Denher LP, Watterson J, Priest J, et al. Pleuropulmonary blastoma. A unique intrathoracic pulmonary neoplasm of childhood. Perspect Pediatr Pathol 1995; 18: 214–226.

48. Priest JR, Watterson J, Strong L, et al. Pleuropulmonary blastoma: a marker for familial disease. J Pediatr 1996; 128(2): 220–224.

49. Priest JR, et al. Type I pleuropulmonary blastoma: A report from the International Pleuropulmonary Blastoma registry. J Clin Oncol 2006; 24(27): 4492–4498.

50. Murphy JJ, Blair GK, Fraser GC, et al. Rhabdomyosarcoma arising within congenital pulmonary cysts: report of three cases. J Pediatr Surg 1992; 27: 1364–1367.

51. Krous HF, Sexauer CL, Embryonal rhabdomyosarcoma arising within a congenital bronchogenic cyst in a child. J Pediatr Surg 1981; 16:506–508.

52. Valderrama E, Saluja G, Shende A, et al. Pulmonary blastoma: report of two cases in children. Am J Surg Pathol 1978; 2:415–422.

53. Miniati DN, Chintagumpala M, Langston C, et al. Prenatal presentation and outcome of children with pleuropulmonary blastoma. J Pediatr Surg 2006; 41(1): 66–71.

54. Hill DA, Jarzembowski JA, Priest JR, et al. Type I pleuropulmonary blastoma: pathology and biology of 51 cases from the international pleuropulmonary blastoma registry. Am J Surg Pathol 2008; 32(2): 282–295.

55. Indolfi P, Bisogno G, Casale F, et al. Prognostic factors in pleuropulmonary blastoma. Pediatr Blood Cancer 2007; 48: 318–323.

56. Murphy JJ, Blair GK, Fraser GC, et al. Rhabdomyosarcoma arising within congenital pulmonary cysts: report of three cases. J Pediatr Surg 1992; 27(10): 1364–1367.

57. Pleuropulmonary blastoma registry. www.ppbregistry.org/2006.

58. Schiavetti A, Dominici C, Matrunola M, et al. Primary pulmonary rhabdomyosarcoma in childhood: clinico-biologic features in two cases with review of the literature. Med Pediatr Oncol 1996; 26(3): 201–207.

59. Keel SB Bacha E, Mark EJ. Primary pulmonary sarcoma: a clinicopathologic study of 26 cases. Mod Pathol 1999; 12(12): 1124–1131

60. Daw NC, Billups CA, Pappo AS, et al. Malignant fibrous histiocytoma and other fibrohistiocytic tumors in pediatric patients: The St. Jude Children's Research Hospital experience. Cancer 2003; 97(11): 2839–2847.

61. Choong PF, Pritchard DJ, Rock MG, Sim FH, Frassica FJ. Survival after pulmonary metastasectomy in soft tissue sarcoma. Prognostic factors in 214 patients. Acta Orthop Scand 1995;66(6): 561–568.

62. Duffaud F, Digue L, Mercier C, Dales JP, Baciuchka-Palmaro M, Volot F, Thomas P, Favre R. Recurrences following primary osteosarcoma in adolescents and adults previously treated with chemotherapy. Eur J Cancer 2003; 39(14): 2050–2057.

63. Karnak I, Emin Senocak M, Kutluk T, Tanyel FC, Buyukpamukcu N, Pulmonary metastases in children: an analysis of surgical spectrum. Eur J Pediatr Surg 2002; 12(3): 151–158.

64. Abel RM, Brown J, Moreland B, Parikh D. Pulmonary metastasectomy for paediatric solid tumours. Pediatr Surg Int 2004; 20: 630–632.

65. Cohen M, Smith WL, Weetman R, Provisor A. Pulmonary pseudometastases in children with malignant tumours. Radiology 1981; 141(2): 371–374.

66. van Geel AN, Pastorino U, Jauch KW, et al. Surgical treatment of lung metastases: the european organization for research and treatment of cancer-soft tissue and bone sarcoma group study of 255 patients. Cancer 1996 15; 77(4):675–682.

67. Temeck BK, Wexler LH, Steinberg SM, et al. Reoperative pulmonary metastasectomy for sarcomatous pediatric histologies. Ann Thorac Surg 1998 66(3): 908–12; discussion 913.

68. Pogrebniak HW, Roth JA,, Steinberg M, Rosenberg SA, Pass HI. Reoperative pulmonary resection in patients with metastases from soft tissue sarcoma. Ann Thorac Surg 1991; 52: 197–203.

69. Maniwa Y, Kanki M, Okita Y: Importance of the control of lung recurrence soon after surgery of pulmonary metastases. Am J Surg 2000; 179(2):122–125.

70. Saeter G, Hoie J, Stenwig AE, Johansson AK, Hannisdal E, Solheim OP. Systemic relapse of patients with osteogenic sarcoma. Prognostic factors for long term survival. Cancer 1995; 75(5):1084–1093.

71. Kawai A, Fukuma H, Beppu Y, et al. Pulmonary resection for metastatic soft tissue sarcomas. Clin Orthop 1995; 310: 188–193.

72. Antunes M, Bernardo J, Salete M, Prieto D, Eugenio L, Tavares P: Excision of pulmonary metastases of osteogenic sarcoma of the limbs. Eur J Cardiothorac Surg 1999; 15: 590–596.

73. Black CT: Current recommendations for the resection of pulmonary metastases of paediatric malignancies. Pediatr Pulmonol (suppl) 1997; 16: 81.

74. Yim AP, Lin J, Chan AT, Li CK, Ho JK. Video-assisted thoracoscopic wedge resections of pulmonary metastatic osteosarcoma: should it be performed? Aust N Z J Surg. 1995; 65(10): 737–739.

21
Chest Wall Tumors

Khalid Sharif and Dakshesh H. Parikh

Introduction

Chest wall tumors in children include a whole range of primary neoplasm arising from different components of the chest wall or secondary tumors invading the chest wall and originating from the adjacent structures such as breast, pleura, mediastinum, and lung. In addition, metastatic tumors also present diagnostic and therapeutic challenges to a pediatric thoracic surgeon. Chest wall tumors both benign and malignant are rare in children. In many of these tumors, complete surgical resection is frequently the only modality of oncological management. Furthermore, reconstruction of the wide chest wall defects poses a surgical challenge in a child.

Primary tumors of the chest wall arising from bony and soft tissue skeleton account for less than 2% of the primary body tumors in children.[1] Soft tissue tumors of the chest wall are common compared with skeletal bony tumors. Overall reported incidence of solid childhood soft tissue tumors is 1.8%, and majority of these tumors are mesenchymal in origin and can have malignant behavior.[2] Most common primary malignant chest wall tumor reported in children is primitive neuroectodermal tumor (PNET),[3] followed by rhabdomyosarcoma (RMS) and other rarer soft tissue sarcoma namely liposarcoma and fibrosarcoma. Various nomenclature in the literature has been used describing essentially same kind of soft tissue sarcoma; Ewing's sarcoma, primitive neuroectodermal and Askin's tumor[4] due to lack of distinction among these lesions with regards to their neuroectodermal differentiation. Recently, pathologists' have grouped them as a single entity as malignant small round cell tumors (MSRCT).[5] This tumor poses significant diagnostic challenge and requires number of immunohistochemical stains to differentiate it from other tumors.

Historic Perspective

Thoracic wall tumors in ancient history are reported to be fatal, and therefore, very little progress was made in both understanding and management of this condition. Furthermore, the pioneer thoracic surgeons of nineteenth and early twentieth century were involved in the management of War injuries and epidemics of infectious diseases namely tuberculosis.[6] Both nineteenth and twentieth century brought the development of chemotherapy and radiotherapy in childhood tumors. The success of surgical resection of the chest wall tumor became a reality only in twentieth century. The mortality rate from the resection of these tumors improved with better understanding of respiratory physiology, anesthesia, and good postoperative intensive care management. There have been only case reports initially successfully resecting the chest wall tumors. Some of the initial series have included only lesions arising from the bone.

Basic Science/Pathogenesis

Chest wall tumors can be classified differently according to the tumor behavior, tumor type, tissue of origin. Commonly its classification is based on tumor type: benign and malignant. Pathology is described under the heading of individual tumor.

In recent years, it has become evident that soft tissue tumors constitute more than 50% of the chest wall lesions. Thoracic sarcomas in children present special problems with histologic diagnosis, total resection of tumor, and local control. Common sarcomas seen in this region includes Ewing's sarcoma or primitive neuroectodermal tumor (PNET), chondrosarcoma, malignant fibrous histiocytoma, osteosarcoma, synovial sarcoma, and fibrosarcoma.

Malignant small round cell tumor is the predominant lesion reported in all the reported series of pediatric chest wall lesions.[5,7] These tumor are osseous in origin and traditionally been referred as Ewing's sarcomas. In 1979, Askin et al. identified a group of chest wall tumor arising from soft tissue that were characterized by high incidence of local recurrence, lower risk of dissemination, and neuro-

D.H. Parikh et al. (eds.), *Pediatric Thoracic Surgery*,
DOI: 10.1007/b136543_21, © Springer-Verlag London Limited 2009

epithelial derivation on electron microscopy.[8] Linnoila et al. demonstrated that these tumors were positive for neuron specific enolase (NSE) on immunohistology and 2/3 of the tumor cell expressed neurosecretory granules characteristic of neuronal differentiation. Subsequently, these tumors were also shown to contain PAS (periodic acid-Schiff) positive material (glycogen) similar to that reported in Ewing's sarcoma.

Clinical Features

Most frequent presentation of these tumors in children is a palpable mass suddenly noticed and reportedly growing by a parent.[1,9] Chest wall tumors are generally slow-growing and initially asymptomatic. Pain and inflammatory changes on the skin surface of a rapidly expanding tumor can be the presenting features of some tumors and can be mistaken with abscess. This presenting feature is not uncommon and clinician is advised to be vigilant in presence of associated fever, malaise, leukocytosis, and raised ESR. In a series, primitive neuroectodermal tumors and pleuro-pulmonary blastoma have presented as empyema thoracis.[10] Acute or chronic respiratory distress may be associated with chest wall tumors depending upon their site and involvement of the respiratory tract or associated pleural effusion. Clinical symptoms and signs should be adequately assessed and investigated appropriately, to reach the diagnosis.

Diagnosis

Investigations

Chest wall tumors can be a diagnostic dilemma both clinically as well as after investigations. Routine hematological and biochemical investigations are performed for basic preoperative considerations. Any abnormalities in association with any inter-current illness/infection can be misleading and can falsely give an impression of an infective process.[10] Liver function test and serum alkaline phosphates level should also be performed in all cases. Preoperative lung function test and cardiac assessment is useful for anesthesia and postoperative management of these cases.

Radiology

Radiological investigations are vital in identifying the tissue of origin, extent of the disease, and presence of metastasis. Initial plain chest X-ray is a useful guide to the next appropriate investigation. Chest X-ray can reveal the bony tumor with its local extent, pulmonary metastasis, and associated pleural effusion. Ultrasound if performed for the superficial tumors can only differentiate solid from cystic

lesion, show its vascularity and therefore of value in soft tissue hamartomas, hemangiomatous and lymphagiomatous lesions.

Further radiological investigations using computed tomography (CT scan) or magnetic resonance imaging (MRI) are essential to determine the nature and extent of the tumor. CT scan, in addition, is useful for pulmonary metastasis while MRI helps delineate soft tissue and muscular involvement. Both these scans are complimentary in difficult cases of chest wall tumors.[11] These investigations are essential in initial evaluation of the chest wall tumor as well as for the subsequent monitoring. As majority of chest wall lesions are potentially malignant, it is important to rule out metastatic disease. Bone scan is useful in bony lesion to determine its extent locally as well as identifies the involvement of other bones and bony distant metastasis.

Biopsy

Once a lesion is suspected to be a tumor, steps are taken to obtain tissue for the diagnosis, as further management is dependent on the exact pathological diagnosis. Type of biopsy varies according to the site, size, and type of the lesion. Fine-needle aspiration (FNA) biopsy has proved to be a cost-effective technique, with low complication risks and high diagnostic value in distinguishing neoplastic vs. non-neoplastic lesions in many organs. FNA biopsy for both metastatic and primary bone tumors is easy, reliable and can achieve accurate tissue diagnosis. As FNA does not require any surgical incisions as required for open biopsy, this procedure plays an important role in triaging and managing bone lesions with minimum risk or morbidity.[12] False-positive results have major therapeutic implications; this is usually due to inadequate sampling or misclassification with regard to the exact subtype of malignant tumor. However, the advantages have to be weighed against the limitations of this procedure.

Excision biopsy is generally recommended for all rib tumors and small lesions, which can be excised without leaving any need for reconstruction. Incision or true-cut needle biopsy is advisable for soft tissue and unresectable tumors. It is important to place the biopsy incision appropriately so that it can be excised along with future resection of the tumor. Adequate non-necrotic tissue sample is essential to achieve histological diagnosis. The biopsy specimen taken both from the peripheral and inner core of the tumor should be sent fresh for histological, cytogenetic, and biological tumor studies. Incision biopsy from the rib tumors can on occasion result in a sampling error particularly in tumors such as chondrosarcomas where well-differentiated benign areas are encountered giving a diagnosis of chondroma.[13] The management decision based on wrong pathological diagnosis will carry disastrous consequences.

Benign Chest Wall Tumors

Benign rib tumors	Chondroma
	Osteochondroma
	Fibrous dysplasia
	Eosinophilic granuloma/Histiocytosis X
	Mesenchymal hamartoma
	Chondromatous hamartoma
	Osteoblastoma
Benign soft tissue tumors	Desmoid tumors
	Myofibromatosis
	Lipoblastomatosis
	Giant cell fibroblastoma
	Hamartomas like lipoma, lymphangioma, hemengioma, neurogenic tumors
	Arteriovenous malformations

Benign Rib Tumors

- *Slow growing rib tumors causing pain should be resected to confirm diagnosis*
- *Wide excision biopsy should be performed for all benign rib tumors both for diagnosis and resection as it is difficult to differentiate slow growing malignant tumors*

Primary rib and bony tumors of the chest wall should also include both neoplastic and non-neoplastic conditions such as cysts, infections, and fibromatosis. Although these swellings of the bony chest wall have different etiology, they usually have common symptomatology and radiological appearances. Therefore, care should be taken in differentiating these conditions if possible preoperatively so that appropriate management can be instituted.

Osteochondroma

Osteochondroma is the most under reported but the most common benign bony tumor and accounts for almost half of all rib tumors.[14] These neoplasms generally manifest itself in childhood and remain asymptomatic. Most of the time they continue to grow during growth spurt until skeletal maturity. Pain and asymmetry of the chest wall (bony protuberance) are the commonest presenting features; however, pain in the previously asymptomatic tumor is suggestive of malignant degeneration. Characteristically, these tumors arise from a metaphyseal region of the rib with a varying thickness of cartilaginous cap. Usually there is a rim of calcification in the periphery of the tumor as well as stippled calcification within the tumor.[15]

It is advisable to resect all oestochondromas in children after puberty especially previously asymptomatic tumor presenting with pain and tumors with a sudden increase in size.[16–18]

Chondroma

Chondroma are slow growing nontender tumors reported in all the age groups and occurs commonly in the anterior costochondral margins[19,20] (Fig. 21.1). Clinical and radiological features

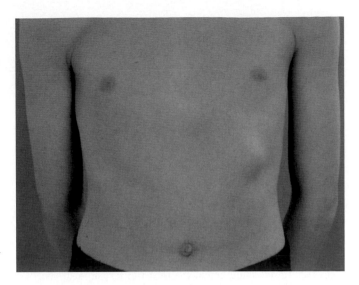

FIG. 21.1. Swelling at the anterior costochondral margin: this is an usual site for chondral tumor. This should be treated with wide excision biopsy as histologically they are difficult to differentiate from chondrosarcoma

of chondroma and chondrosarcoma are similar and are seen as expansile lesions causing thinning of the bony cortex.

Chondroma is grossly a lobulated lesion characterized histologically by lobules of hyaline cartilage. Histologically, it is difficult to differentiate chondroma from chondrosarcoma. Therefore, all chondroma should be considered as low-grade malignant tumor and should be resected with an excision margin of two centimeters.[21] The long-term results are reported to be excellent with wide excision and reconstruction.[22]

Fibrous Dysplasia

Fibrous dysplasia is a cystic expansile non-neoplastic lesion. It is characterized as a developmental anomaly of medullary cavity of the rib. The fibrous replacement of the medullary canal is characteristic of the fibrous dysplasia and is reported as a solitary slowly growing nontender lesion in the posterior-lateral aspect of the rib. In Albright's syndrome, multiple bony cysts, skin pigmentations, and precaucious sexual maturity is reported. Fibrous dysplasia is generally diagnosed incidentally on a routine chest X-ray. Cystic lesion with thinning of the cortex with a central ground glass appearance and no calcification is seen on plain radiographs. The excised lesion on histology shows bony trabaculations with some calcification and fibrous replacement of the medullary cavity.[23–25]

Local excision is curative and generally carried out only for painful enlarging lesions causing diagnostic dilemma. Mostly conservative management is indicated in asymptomatic lesions.[23]

Eosinophilic Granuloma/Histocytosis X

This neoplasm is an expansile lesion of the rib involving the reticulo-endothelial system usually containing a mixed eosinophilic and histiocytic infiltrates. This tumor is commonly

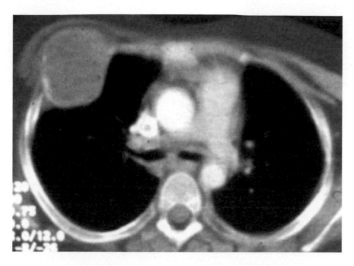

FIG. 21.2. Eosinophilic granuloma of a rib: Expansile lesion of a rib with areas of calcification like egg-shall. This tumor is often confused with osteogenic carcinoma. As the diagnosis is uncertain a wide excision with reconstruction is recommended

seen between 5 and 15 years of age. Three types reported are eosionophilic granuloma, Letterer-Siwe disease, and Hand-Schuller-Christian disease.

Eosinophilic granuloma is limited only to the bone involvement.[20] Letterer-Siwe and Hand-Schuller-Christian disease presents with systemic features of fever, malaise, weight loss and signs of lymphadenopathy, while splenomegaly leukocytosis with eosinophilia and anemia. Letterer-Siwe disease is typically reported in infancy, while Hand-Schuller-Christian disease presents in later childhood. Radiologically all have similar appearances showing (a) expansile bony lesion in the posterior-lateral aspect of the rib cage, (b) uneven destruction of the bony cortex seen as scalloping, (c) new periosteal bone formation. This tumor is frequently confused with Ewing's sarcoma and osteomyelitis (Fig. 21.2).

The excision biopsy of a lesion is indicated for diagnosis and probably results in a cure in a solitary eosionophilic granuloma. The systemic diseases have chronic course and require management with corticosteroids and chemotherapy.

Mesenchymal Hamartoma

Mesenchymal hamartoma is a rare lesion seen in infancy and is usually identified at birth.[26] This benign lesion has also been incorrectly described in the literature as "mesenchymoma." Histologically, it is a focal overgrowth of normal skeletal elements. Among these proliferating skeletal elements are the areas similar to aneurysmal bone cyst.[27,28]

These lesions generally are well circumscribed, compressing but not invading the surrounding structures.[26] Radiologically, it presents as a mineralized extrapleural mass involving one or more ribs. These lesions arise within the rib, which can be detected with CT or MRI (Schlesinger). MRI can differentiate between cartilaginous and blood filled aneurysmal components.[29] This distinction is useful in planning the surgi-

cal management. In the past, surgical excisions was advocated that had invariably resulted in significant bleeding and long term scoliosis. Current advice is to manage these lesions conservatively, and surgery should be reserved for symptomatic lesions as malignancy has never been reported.[30]

Chondromatous Hamartoma

Chondromatous hamartoma of the chest wall is an extremely rare, benign lesion that usually occurs in early infancy. It typically arises in the rib cage and produces a large mass. It is composed of a varying admixture of hyaline cartilage that has features resembling growth plate cartilage, fascicles of spindle cells, woven bone, and hemorrhagic cysts. Surgical excision in these hamartoma is usually curative. Sometime these lesions are multifocal and can also involve sternum and can recur locally after resection.[19]

Osteoblastoma

Osteoblastoma is a rare, benign, bone-forming tumor of the chest wall described under sternal tumors.

Osteoid Osteoma

Osteoid osteoma is a relatively common benign osteogenic tumor reported mainly in children and young adults.[31] The clinical hallmark of the lesion is local pain, typically more severe at night, which often promptly responds to aspirin and other nonsteroidal antiinflammatory drugs. Other possible symptoms include growth disturbances, bone deformity, and painful scoliosis. Osteoid osteoma is commonly seen in male and generally less than 2 cm in greatest dimension. Symptomatic lesion requires local resection and is generally curative.

Benign Soft Tissue Tumors

Number of hamartomatous lesions involving chest wall have been described in early infancy and childhood. These are not considered in this chapter as their presentation and management is similar to those present elsewhere in the body. In particular, lymphangioma, hemangioma, lipoblastoma, and fibroblatic tumors have predeliction to the chest wall and may extend into the neck and anterior mediastinum and can present with acute respiratory distress.

Fibroblastic-Myofibroblastic Tumors

Soft tissue benign mesenchymal tumors are histologically diverse group of tumors. One of the category involves fibroblastic and/or myofibroblastic derivatives with uncertain behavior and is known to have many variants resulting in a considerable confusion in the literature. It is realized that the myofibroblast is the predominant cell in many of the so-called fibromatoses tumors described in the literature.[32] In a large study examining

108 cases of soft tissue tumors of fibroblastic-myofibroblastic tumors from patients of all age groups (neonates to 20 years of age) over 25 year period demonstrated and classified various variants of these tumors.[32] *Infantile myofibromatosis* was the commonest tumor encountered in early infancy of which 15% were recorded as having multiple lesions.[33,34] Surgeons are generally involved for the biopsy of these tumors as most infantile peripheral tumors undergo spontaneous regression and are managed conservatively.[35] Children with infantile myofibromatosis of visceral origin may have complicated outcome including death.

The *desmoid fibromatosis tumor* is the second most common tumor in this group of tumors. Desmoid tumors are rare soft tissue neoplasm derived from fascial or musculoaponeurotic structures. These tumors typically presents in the third decade; however, 20–30% of cases have been reported in children.[36] Chest wall desmoids account for approximately 20% of all patients with desmoid tumors.[37] Desmoid tumor is more commonly seen in girls possibly due to hormonal influence (oestrogen). Isolated desmoid is possibly related to abnormalities in the connective tissue synthesis as it is seen to be arising from connective tissue of fascias, aponeurosis, or inter-muscular striae.

Multifocal nature of these lesions is distressing in children and can result in significant morbidity and is usually a presenting feature of familial polyposis coli or Gardener's syndrome.[38] Thirty-three to 38% of patients with Gardner's syndrome develop desmoid tumors but only 2% of patients with desmoid tumor have Gardner's syndrome and its other associated pathology (familial adenomatous polyposis, osteomas, and other soft tissue neoplasms).[39] These tumors are locally recurring benign tumors in almost 60% of cases especially if inadequately excised.[40] It is documented that although recurring, these tumors do not change the histological appearances or metastasise. Although mortality is rare, one series reported 8% of cases in the series died due to locally uncontrollable and unresectable tumors.[41]

Desmoid tumors were usually identified as noninflammatory asymptomatic masses; and can be symptomatic because of its pressure effect on the adjoining normal structures. These are slow growing tumors that can extend into the pleural cavity and can be extensive displacing mediastinal structures before its symptomatic presentation. Patients with these lesions are often asymptomatic and thus commonly present with lesions greater than 10 cm in size. It is usually present as a poorly circumscribed mass with little or no pain. MRI is mandatory to define the extent so that adequate excision and simultaneous chest wall reconstruction can be planned (Fig. 21.3a–d).

Grossly the desmoid tumor arises from the muscle and fascia and extends along the tissue planes. The tumor is white, firm to hard in consistency, and locally infiltrative (Fig. 21.4). It is usually limited to a single group of muscle but when multifocal can have morbid course and have been known to be associated with mortality. Histologically, the tumor shows uniform small spindle-shaped cells infiltrating the tissue, typically described as fibroblastic cells with well-differentiated abundant collagen. These tumors are difficult to distinguish from low-grade fibrosarcoma. Microscopically, tumor does not show any mitotic activity or cytological aspect of malignancy. Electronic microscopy shows fibroblastic or myofibroblastic proliferation with intracellular collagen fibrillae. This fibrillae are normally synthesized in the extracellular space from precursors secreted by the cells. The presence of these mature fibrillae outside cytoplasm is characteristic of desmoid tumors and this aspect is exceptionally observed in fibroblastic cancers, mesenchymatous tumors or inflammatory process.

These tumors are histologically benign but may behave aggressively at the local level with multiple recurrences after incomplete resection is common. The treatment of these neoplasms is to achieve wide surgical resection with negative margins for the presence of tumor. These wide resections may not be entirely feasible in chest wall; however, when feasible this should be performed in association with chest wall reconstruction. Chest wall reconstruction in children is performed with either prosthetic material and/or autologous tissue. In difficult places where wide excision is not feasible enucleation of the tumor followed by radiation therapy is considered. Some of the tumors may have hormonal influence and may respond to Tomoxifen decreasing both size and symptoms.[42] In some tumors, use of antiinflammatory medication such as ibuprofen has also showed some therapeutic benefit.

There may be recurrence in as many as 75% of patients. Neither adjuvant radiotherapy nor chemotherapy have been shown to reduce the rate of recurrence.[37] Recurrence should also be treated with surgical resection because patients who undergo complete surgical resection of recurrence are as likely to remain disease free after resection as patients who present with primary disease.

Lipoblastomatosis/Liposarcoma

Lipoblastomatosis is a tumor of brown fat and is seen in infancy. Lipoblstomatosis is diffuse lobulated, spreads along the tissue planes and locally recurring tumor.[43] Lipoma is rare in children and should never be clinically diagnosed. The lipoblstoma can be clinically indistiguatiable from lymphangioma as both tend to have similar consistency. Ultrasonography in these cases only differentiates the consistency of the tumor between water filled and solid soft tissue tumors. MRI is a preferred investigation and is extremely useful in both distinction and extent of the tumor. The invasive nature of this tumor into the veins has been reported as a rare event.[44] The distinction between lipoblastomatosis and liposarcoma is histologically difficult; however, cytogenetically is feasible. Cytogenetic studies show a chracteristic rearrangement of chromosome 8 (der pter [8]q13:q21.1qter]) in lipoblastoma, whereas liposarcoma is characterized by a translocation (t[12;16][q13;p11]).[45–49] It is important that clinician be wary of the diagnosis of a simple lipoma in a young infant and tissue should be sent fresh for cytogenetic studies to exclude the diagnosis of lipoblastoma

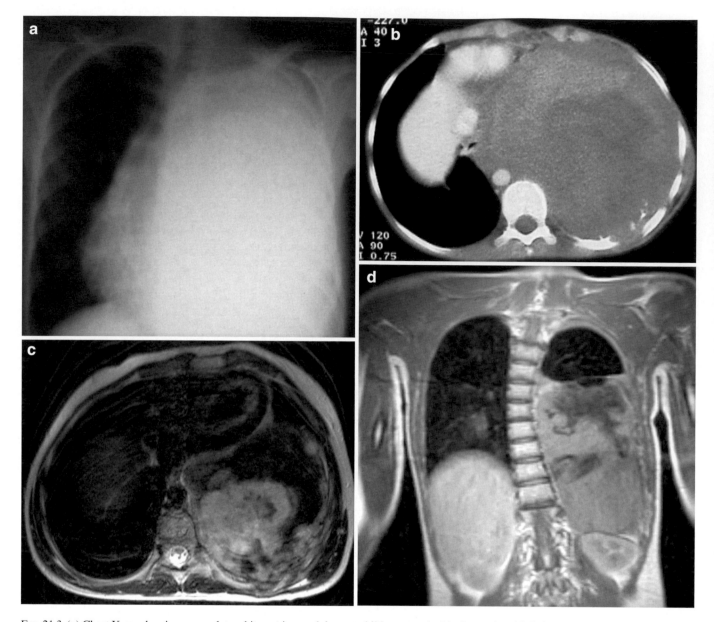

FIG. 21.3. (a) Chest X-ray showing a complete white out in an adolescent child presented with chest pain with little or no respiratory compromise. (b) CT scan showing a very large tumor with central necrosis and mediastinal shift. Biopsy diagnosed this to be a benign myofibroblastic (Desmoid) tumor. Preoperative chemotherapy reduced this tumor to some extent. (c, d) MRI showed the extent of the tumor and muscle infiltration; extensive resection of the chest wall was performed with reconstruction. He had subsequent resection for recurrence once

and liposarcoma.[50] These are usually locally recurring tumors; complete excision is advisable but difficult in certain instances as the tumor can be identified in various tissue planes. Medical management has no value in the management of these tumors both for primary and recurring lesions.

Giant Cell Fibroblastoma

This rare soft tissue tumor occurs predominantly in the first two decades of life. The typical clinical presentation is a solitary, usually 2–6 cm in size, nontender mass of blue-greyish color, which is mostly located on the back, anterior chest wall, thigh, or groin. The histology shows a loose infiltrate of predominantly bland spindle cells in dermis and subcutis. Characteristic elements of the tumor are large angiectoid branching spaces lacking any endo- or epithelium, and relatively small multinucleated cells (floret cells). The recurrence rate is high if the tumor is not excised with adequate margins. Metastases are not reported. It is of preeminent importance to differentiate this rare benign tumor from sarcomas, to avoid an inappropriately aggressive therapy.[51]

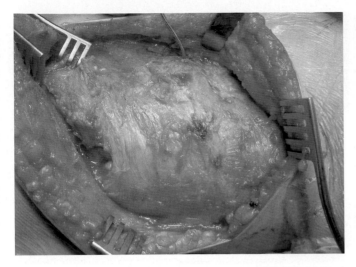

FIG. 21.4. Operative picture of a desmoid tumor of the chest wall: hard in consistency and locally infiltrative

Malignant Chest Wall Tumors

Malignant bony tumors	Chondrosarcoma
	Osteogenic sarcoma
	Ewing's sarcoma (MSRCT)
Malignant soft tissue tumors	Premitive neuroectodermal tumors
	Rhabdomyosarcoma
	Congenital fibrosarcoma
	Liposacoma/lipoblastomatosis
	Neurofibrosarcoma

Malignant Bony Tumors

- *Prompt diagnosis and management with wide excision results in a favorable outcome*

These are generally slow growing tumors of the chest wall except osteogenic sarcoma and Ewing's sarcoma. These are rare in children; however, can be encountered after puberty.

Chondrosarcoma

Chondrosarcoma are reported in children[14] usually occurring at the costochondral arch or the sternum on the anterior chest wall. The commonest reported incidence of these tumors is in third or fourth decade of life and is more frequent in men. As in adults this is a locally invasive slowly growing tumor and usually presents with pain in a previously asymptomatic mass. It is known to recur locally and may have late metastasis. Chondrosarcoma typically arises within the medullary cavity of the bone to form an expansile, glistening mass that frequently erodes the cortex. Microscopically, this tumor closely resembles features seen in chondroma and only showing obvious malignant cellular changes in some undifferentiated tumors. Well-differentiated chondrosarcoma is indistinguishable from chondroma. Microscopically chondrosarcoma vary considerable in appearance. Well-differentiated lesions show only minimal cytologic atypia whereas at the other extreme they may be composed of highly pleomorphic chondroblasts with frequent mitotic figures. Multinucleate cells are present, as are two or more chondroblast lying in lacunae.

Radiologically, the tumor shows destroyed cortex containing mottled type calcification within the tumor. The tumor edges can be poorly defined. Computed tomography helps to define the extent of the tumor. Definitive sarcomatous diagnosis of the rib tumor can only be made histologically. Misdiagnosis as chondroma is not uncommon in differentiated chondrosarcoma resulting in inadequate excision. Therefore, as previously mentioned, all chondral tumors of the ribs should be managed with a wide resectional biopsy rather than incisional or needle biopsies.

Chondrosarcoma respond very poorly to any form of chemotherapy or radiotherapy. The outcome of these tumors is dependant upon initial wide excision, which results in cure, prevents local recurrences, and distant metastasis.[16] The survival and prognosis is related to tumor grade, its size and location.[16] Local recurrences occur due to inadequate excision. Sometime tumor cannot be excised completely with adequate margins due to its size and location.[52]

Malignant Small Round Cell Tumors (MSRCT)

Premitive Neuroectodermal Tumor (PNET) and Mesenchymal Sarcoma

Ewings sarcoma and Askin's Tumor

In 1979, Askin et al.[8] described a malignant small-cell sarcomatous tumor (Askin tumor) in the soft tissues of the chest wall, occasionally in bone and rarely from the periphery of the lung. This neoplasm is now recognized as MSRCT or a type of primitive neuroectodermal tumor (PNET) probably developing from embryonal neural crest cells.[44] This neoplasm histologically should be distinguished from other undifferentiated, small-round-cell tumors such as undifferentiated neuroblastoma, embryonal rhabdomyosarcoma, and lymphoma.[44]

Ewing's sarcoma primarily arising from rib cage is a tumor of childhood with median age of 13–16 years. Boys are twice commonly affected than the girls. Up to 6.5% of Ewing's sarcoma is reported in chest wall. A painful enlarging mass is common presenting feature in association with fever, general malaise, anemia, leukocytosis, and increased sedimentation rate (ESR).

X-ray shows mottled destruction containing both lytic and bony regeneration (Fig. 21.5a). Although not pathognomic, this tumor occasionally show onion-skin appearance on the tumor surface due to subperiosteal new bone formation. Radiating spicules of the bone formation is also seen on the surface. Both clinically and radiologically, this tumor is difficult to differentiate from osteomyelitis and osteogenic

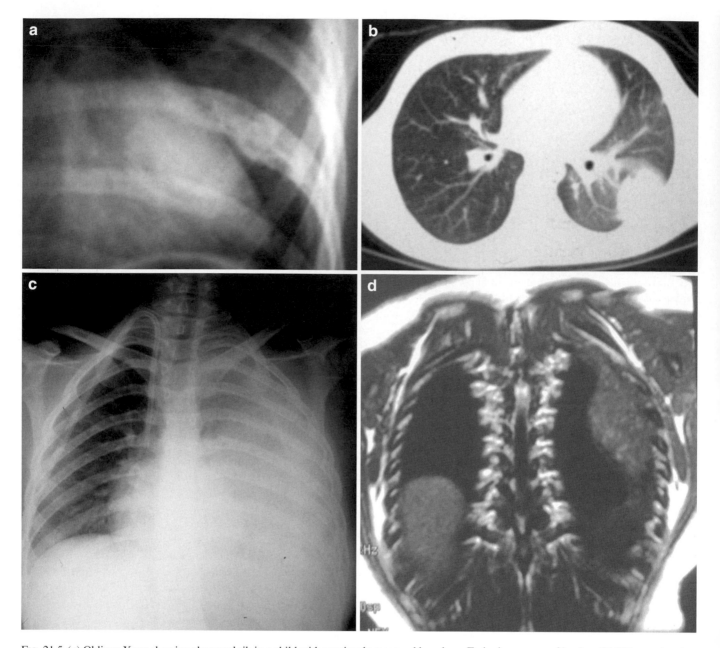

FIG. 21.5. (a) Oblique X ray showing abnormal rib in a child with previously managed long bone Ewing's sarcoma of her leg. (b) CT scan showing the extent of intra-thoracic extension but no other metastasis. The metastasis was excised with chest wall reconstruction. (c) Chest X-ray in an adolescent child with an extensive tumor confirmed on biopsy as PNET. (d) MRI scan showing the residual tumor with infiltration into the ribs and intercostal muscle, lungs were not involved. The resection was carried out with a reasonable margin and reconstruction carried out

sarcoma. CT scan as well as MRI is useful in determining the extent of the tumor; however, areas of hemorrhage and necrosis in large tumors can give the heterogeneous appearance. MRI is informative for determining invasion of chest wall muscle, whereas CT scan is preferred for detecting small pulmonary metastases (Fig. 21.5b–d) Neither imaging technique is adequate for predicting invasion of adjacent lung.[53]

Gross examination of these tumors generally reveal round, ovoid, multinodular or lobulated mass, which can be circumscribed but rarely encapsulated. Cut surface of these tumors show typical grayish-white appearance with granular to glistening texture with areas of hemorrhage and necrosis.

Histopathologically, three basic patterns can be easily defined under low magnification namely: (a) compact sheets of cells, (b) a nesting arrangement of cells with an intervening fibro-vascular stroma, and (c) Serpiginous bands of cells with necrosis. Usually one of the patterns predominates in an individual neoplasm; it is not uncommon to find all three patterns in the same neoplasm. The tumor is seen extending into the adjacent tissue with rounded or lobulated edges. Although the classic Homer Wright pseudo-rosettes are not identified in these tumors, in nearly 50% cellular profile resembling pseudo-rosettes are described. The PAS negative cell profiles are arranged around an acidophilic focus of hyaline or fibrous nature rather than a neurofibrillary composition. The tumor cells measuring $10-14\,\mu m$ in diameter, and containing very little faint blue cytoplasm and a relatively large nucleus with coarse but evenly dispersed chromatin. The cells may show moderate amount of mitotic activity. Ewing sarcomas are composed of sheets of primitive cells with small, fairly uniform nuclei, and only scant cytoplasm. Cytoplasmic glycogen is detected at periodic acid–Schiff (PAS) staining, a feature used to differentiate Ewing sarcoma from primitive neuroectodermal tumors. Electron microscopy shows round or elliptical nuclei with one to four nucleoli. Most cells are generally polygonal and has small to moderate number of variable shaped and sized mitochondria, which are generally segregated to one end of cell.

Histologically, both these tumors are cellular with overlapping features and show neuroectodermal differentiation. These two entities are now considered as one under heading of MSRCT or PNET as chemotherapy regimen for these are similar. In addition, cytogenetic investigations have also shown similar balanced translocation between chromosome 11 and 12 [t(11:22)(q24;q12)] in both these tumors.[54,55] Translocation points of these two tumors have now been mapped and are similar. Both tumors contain high contents of protein products of *mic-2* gene.

It is an extremely aggressive tumor with frequent metastatic spread and local recurrence. Usually this tumor spread through a hematogenous route mainly to lungs and bones. Hence, it is important to achieve control of both local and systemic micrometastasis. Traditionally, local control of this tumor was achieved by radiotherapy or by surgery. However, radiotherapy dose to achieve the local control is very high. Favorable local control rates of 80–85% have been reported with doses of 50–65 Gy. An attempted reduction in the radiation dose has resulted in increased incidence of local recurrence. Aria et al. has reported that reducing the radiation dose to 30–36 Gy without surgical resection in patients with good chemotherapy response has resulted in relatively high local relapse rate of 68%.[56]

These tumors are best treated with multiple modalities with local resection of the entire involved rib with partial resections of the ribs on either side of the tumor.[5,57] The postoperative radiation to the tumor bed is given to mop up residual malignant cells. In a series, good surgical resection with local radiation gave local control in 93% of cases.[58] Chemotherapy is given to control distant disease and has been shown to improve survival rates.[58,59] Preoperative chemotherapy has shown to result in significant reduction in tumor size. This may improve the outcome by achieving complete and wider tumor resection. As ribs are expendable it is possible to remove the entire rib from vertebra to costochondral junction. In lesions located laterally or interiorly on the chest wall, it is possible to leave the posterior portion of the rib. This might help in the reduction of long-term scoliosis. There is risk associated with this approach as Ewing's Sarcoma can have skip lesions in the marrow. It is possible to rule out this possibility with preoperative bone scan or with the help of MRI.

In the nonrandomized trial improved survival was reported by surgical wide resection; however, the critics believe that this difference is due to patient selection as larger tumors were excluded from surgery and given radiotherapy.[60] Tumors less than 8 cm in diameter and 100 mL in volume has been reported to have a better response 78% 3-year survival compared with 17% relapse free survival among tumors larger than 100 mL.[60] Similarly, extra osseous metastasis is also reported to be associated with increased risk of distant metastasis and poor survival rates. Many series have used radiotherapy after surgical resection to improve outcome.[61,62] Dose required is highly controversial.

Osteosarcoma

Osteogenic sarcoma of the bony thorax is significantly rare in children. However, it has been reported in teenagers and young adults. Most tumors present with a rapidly enlarging mass which is often reported as painful. Tumor usually extended into the surrounding soft tissues and appears lobulated. These tumors radiologically show destroyed cortex with ill-defined edges or margins. It also shows calcifications at right angles to the edges described as sunburst and a triangular area of periosteal new bone formation at the edges (Codman's Triangle). Histologically, eosionophillic tumor has a glassy appearance and contains osteoid matrix interspersed with the osteoblastic cells and foci of fibroblastic and chondroblastic cells. Osteosarcoma typically elevates the periosteum and microscopically hallmark of osteosarcoma is formation of osteoid by the malignant mesenchymal cell. The amount of osteoid varies considerably in different tumors. Other mesenchymal elements particularly cartilage may also be present.

Management plan for these tumors are similar to commonly reported sites within long bones of the limbs i.e., incisional biopsy to confirm the diagnosis followed by chemotherapy. Secondary surgical wide resection including the entire length of the rib or sternum with adjacent soft tissue is indicated to reduce local recurrence and produce long-term survival. Survival is directly related to complete surgical resection with clear margins and absence of metastatic disease. Improved survival is associated with a good initial response to preoperative chemotherapy and unifocal nature of osteosarcoma; however, when associated with Paget's disease it has poor outcome.

Rhabdomyosarcoma

Rhabdomyosarcoma is a common tumor of infancy and childhood contributing up to 15% of all solid tumors in children. Although this tumor can occur in any age group but generally have two age peaks; the early peak at two to five years and late peak around puberty to19 years of age. In the first Inter

Rhabdomyosarcoma Study (IRS-1), its incidence in the trunk region was reported in 7.4% of cases. Of these 50% involved the chest wall, one third involved the paraspinous region, and one sixth involved the abdominal wall.[63] The tumor mass is rapidly enlarging and usually deep-seated arising from the striated muscle tissue of the chest wall. It is generally not painful but can appear red and inflamed mistakenly diagnosed as an abscess especially in presence of tumor necrosis or hemorrhage.

Histologically, the most common subtype of rhabdomyosarcoma reported in the chest wall is alveolar followed by embryonal subtype. The alveolar subtype histologically resembles pulmonary alveoli and is commonly seen in the tumors arising from striated muscles of trunk and limbs. Pleomorphic rhabdomyosarcoma containing large, elongated cells with many nuclei or giant nuclei is uncommon in children. Mixed rhabdomyosarcoma where both embryonal and alveolar components are present and for the purposes of therapy, they are described according to its predominant component. Alveolar subtype has relatively poor prognosis

Principles of management of the chest wall rhabdomyosarcoma follow the same guidelines as for rhabdomyosarcoma in other locations. Treatment of rhabdomyosarcoma involves combination of chemotherapy and surgery, and may require radiotherapy. Most tumors respond to Vincristin, Adriamycin and Cyclophosphmide. Despite combination therapy, the alveolar subtype tends to have higher recurrence rate than other histological subtype. Rarely after initial biopsy and subsequent chemotherapy complete remission have been known to occur. Surgery plays a vital role if complete remission cannot be achieved with chemotherapy alone. Resection of the residual tumor with clear margin usually results in a good outcome. Debulking and mutilating surgery should be avoided. It is generally advisable to reduce the tumor size with preoperative chemotherapy in a bulky tumor so as to achieve complete resection (Fig. 21.6). Radical surgery in this chemo-sensitive tumor has no specific role unless tumor is found to be unresponsive. Radiotherapy is considered for residual, recurrences and metastatic disease.

Survival was reported to be correlated with stage of tumor at presentation. Generally, chest wall rhabdomyosarcoma tends to have poor prognosis than in the other areas.[63–65] Factors contributing to this difference in prognosis may include higher proportion having alveolar sarcoma, advanced stage at presentation, difficulties in local resection and early relapse compared with other sites.[65–67] Patients in stage IV (metastasis) had the poorest survival. Overall five year disease free survival in children is 65% as reported by IRS III. Local disease control on the chest wall is fraught with many difficulties especially when relapse occur. Chest wall irradiation inevitably results in the long-term pulmonary fibrosis. This leads to restrictive chest wall movements thus causing decreased lung capacity, alterations in lung growth, and decreased diffusion capacity. Radiation and surgery both results in restrictive defects secondary to altered development of the thoracic cavity and scoliosis.[68]

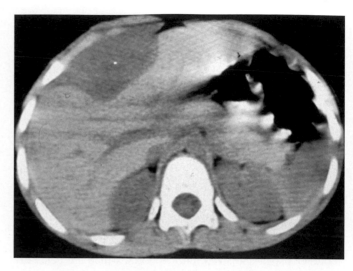

FIG. 21.6. CT scan showing internal extent of a rhabdomyosarcoma: This 3-year old child presented with an increasing swelling on right-side of his chest wall in mid-clavicular line. The tumor did not respond well with intensive course of chemotherapy, subsequent resection of the residual tumor and reconstruction of the chest wall and diaphragm was carried out. Local recurrence as well as distance metastasis resulted in an inevitable outcome in this alveolar rhabdomyosarcoma

Congenital-Infantile Fibrosarcoma

This tumor can present itself at birth, and majority described in first three months of life. Unlike juvenile fibromatosis this tumor demonstrates dense cellularity and mitotic activity but is less anaplastic than usual fibrosarcoma. It is, therefore, important to differentiate it from mesenchymal hamartoma and fibroblastomatosis. This is usually a chemosentitive tumor. Large/giant fibrosarcomas in infancy respond very well to chemotherapy, with significant reduction in tumor size. The preoperative chemotherapy makes the surgical resection possible with minimal morbidity. Chemothearpy protocols used in the management of fibrosarcoma include Vincristine (V), actinomycin-D (A), and cyclophosphamide (C) VAC or Adriamycin (D) in conjunction with VAC (Adria-VAC). Complete resolution of tumor has been reported with Adria-VAC protocol. Surgical resection is indicated in most instances of the residual tumor. Local recurrences have been reported with rare instances of metastasis.[33,69]

Neurofibrosarcoma

Neurofibrosarcoma commonly occurs in the intercostal nerve and typically a disease of an adult life. This tumor is commonly associated with von Recklinghousen's disease. It is generally a well-encapsulated tumor with spindle-shaped cells spreading along the nerve sheath. MRI scan is the investigation of choice to determine both the nature and extent of the tumor. Surgery with wide excision is recommended as like many sarcoma both chemotherapy and radiotherapy is not effective.

Lymphoma

Lymphomas are malignant neoplasm of cells native to lymphoid tissue (i.e., lymphocyte, histiocytes, their precursors, and derivatives). Lymphomas are broadly divided into Hodgkin disease and Non-Hodgkin's lymphoma (NHL). NHL is common in childhood. These tumors can arise in lymphoid tissue anywhere in the body with a small percentage reported to arise in the chest wall.

The American form of Burkitt's lymphoma is a high-grade malignancy, which usually involves the abdomen in children and young adults. Burkitt's lymphoma primarily originating from the soft tissue is rarely reported. The tumor affecting the chest wall usually presents as a chest wall mass.[70] Radiological characteristics include a mass, originating from the soft tissue of the chest wall without any contiguous pleural and lung parenchyma disease. Histopathology can resemble that of a Burkitt's lymphoma.

Another rare and recently described lymphoma affecting the chest wall is Ki-1-positive anaplastic large cell lymphoma (Ki-1 ALCL). This pleomorphic types of lymphoma affects mostly children and adolescents and is sometimes mistaken for carcinoma or sarcoma. Clinically, it can present either with pneumonia-like symptoms or multiple subcutaneous masses in the chest wall. Fine-needle aspiration cytology smears generally show characteristic dissociated cells with abundant, lightly basophilic, vacuolated cytoplasm; oval, round or lobulated nuclei; and binucleate, trinucleate, and multinucleate cells with a wreath like arrangement of nuclei.[71] Most of the tumor cells express immunocytologic reactivity to CD 30. Cytogenetic studies of tumor cell show characteristic abnormal karyotype including a der(17)t(1;17) (q11;p11).[72]

Differential Diagnosis

The differential diagnosis of chest wall mass in children includes infections and chest wall deformities.

Infection

Usual infections that can cause chest wall lesions include tuberculosis and actinomycosis. Rarely chest wall neoplasm can mimic empyema thoracis[10]; therefore, a high degree of caution is advised.

Chest Wall Deformity

Commonest chest wall deformities seen in pediatric population includes pectus excavatum, pectus carinatum, and other rib anomalies such as bifid ribs. These lesions can also be confused with tumors as the costochondral margins become prominent in excavatum and projected sternum can be mistaken as a tumor. Radiological investigations are usually helpful in differentiating these lesions.

Management

The chest wall tumors are managed in the similar fashion as tumors of others parts of body. Initial therapeutic intervention is usually to confirm the diagnosis. Once the diagnosis is confirmed the primary resection is achieved in benign or small, localized malignant lesion. In majority of the malignant tumors, confirmation of diagnosis is followed by chemotherapy. Preoperative chemotherapy usually not only reduces the size of the tumor, but also makes it less vascular and less friable thus allowing adequate surgical excision with clear margins. Chemotherapy regimen varies with the type of tumor and is not discussed in this chapter.

Surgical Management

- *Adequate resection and dependable immediate reconstruction are the essential requirement of a successful outcome*
- *Tumor excision should not be carried out unless surgeon feels confident of closing the chest wall defect*

Surgical resection is considered to be the most important modality in the management of these lesions particularly for MSRCT, osteosarcoma, and chondrosarcoma. It is important to mark the incision appropriately to allow preservation of overlying skin and muscle flap, if possible. In majority of cases, resection of one or more ribs is required.

Particular surgical challenge is the reconstruction of chest wall following complete surgical resection of tumor leaving behind a large surgical defect. The goals for chest wall resection and reconstruction as laid down by Grosfeld et al.[73] include complete removal of tumor, restoration of adequate protection of the thoracic vertebra, restoration of physiological function providing adequate lung and chest wall growth, and an acceptable chest wall appearance. Vast experience in chest wall reconstruction has been reported using various techniques after wide excision of adult chest wall tumors.

Various techniques have been reported for reconstruction of chest wall. These include use of prosthetic material. Various types of prosthetic material used include Marlex mesh (Bard Vascular System Division, Billerica, MA) and Gore-tex tissue patch (W.L. Gore and associates, Inc, Flagstaff, AZ). Major deterrent to the use of these prosthetic materials in the young infants and young children is that they will restrict the chest wall growth on the side and inevitable scoliosis. The defect closed by viable tissue using pedicle grafts may leave behind functional disability as well as unsightly scars.

Chest Wall Reconstruction

Chest wall reconstruction remains a surgical challenge in children especially if wide resection is carried out and especially when the long-term outlook of many tumors has improved in recent years. The challenges of reconstruction in children have different implications and considerations then adults as growth and development continues; loss of function when muscular flaps are used, and wide resections carry a significant risk of scoliosis and respiratory morbidity. Surgically, it is a major procedure, it carries a potentially life-threatening complications both intra and postoperatively.

Over the years various flaps have been available to surgeons to reconstruct the chest wall.[74,75] The understanding of the blood supply of the muscles namely latissimus dorsi, pectoralis major, serratus anterior, rectus abdominis, and external oblique; have resulted in more aggressive chest wall tumor resections and immediate reconstructions. Preoperative evaluations before performing this major procedure should be thorough, as it will allow detection and appropriate management of correctable problems.

Important considerations of chest wall reconstructions:

1. Children at high risk of developing postoperative complications should be evaluated preoperatively by a good clinical history and physical examinations, respiratory and cardiac assessments, radiographic and laboratory examinations.
2. Surgeon undertaking the chest wall tumor resection should be confident of closing the chest wall defect effectively.
3. Combined team approach achieves a safe outcome in association with plastic surgeons, anesthetists, and postoperative care in consultation with intensive care colleagues, respiratory physicians, and physiotherapists.
4. It is essential to ascertain that reconstruction would support the underlying organs and effectively support the respiration.
5. The type of reconstruction is dictated by the location, depth of the chest wall defect, its size, local condition such as previous radiation injury and infection.
6. Preoperative CT scan and or MRI help to determine the extent of the resection and possible deeper unknown problems with lung and mediastinum.

Skeletal Reconstruction

Skeletal reconstruction is carried out if full thickness defect is likely to produce paradoxical movements. The defect site and size are the important factors in surgical reconstruction of the chest wall. Large defects are generally reconstructed using prosthetic materials such as Prolene mesh, Marlex mesh or Gortex soft tissue patch, Collagen-coated Vicryl mesh,[76] metals and absorbable newer material produced from pigs or bovine collagen.[77] The material placed under adequate tension to bridge the defect improves the rigidity of the reconstruction. Soft-tissue patch of Gortex is used by the author successfully in number of large chest wall reconstruction. The patch is kept on the pleural surface and attached to the surrounding rib margins of the defect by suturing it through drill holes in the rib margins. The Gortex graft is stretched to bridge the defect in the chest wall so as to achieve tension and rigidity (Fig. 21.7). This patch has an additional advantage of not allowing air or fluid across into the thoracic cavity. The pros-

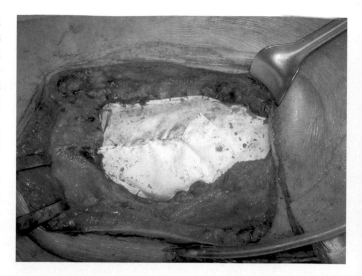

FIG. 21.7. The Gortex reconstruction of the chest wall defect after excision of a chest wall tumor: large chest wall reconstruction by attaching the patch on the pleural surface and drilling holes in the rib margins on each side to attach the graft to achieve tension and rigidity

thetic material is not advisable if there is local infection and possibility of the contamination of the prosthetic graft. In this situation, the use of muscular flap is a preferred option.

Soft Tissue Reconstruction

Autogenous tissue on the pedicle graft is generally a preferred option for the soft tissue reconstruction. Muscles provide a good cover over the chest wall when the skeletal reconstruction is not needed or not advisable. Muscle transposition using latissimus dorsi, pectoralis major, rectus abdominis, or serratus anterior are preferred options depending on the site and size of the defect. Myocutaneous flaps should be considered in case skin cover is required in addition to the soft tissue cover.[78] Plastic surgeon's help is essential in case of complex requirement and flap requirement that will survive and produce a dependable outcome. Free muscle flap with microvascular anastomosis is also useful in difficult circumstances.[79]

Long-Term Complications

Scoliosis

This is the common and well-established complication following excision of large chest wall tumors.[80,81] The severity of the curve is directly related to the number of the ribs resected. Resection of the posterior segment of the ribs produces more scoliosis than resection of anterior segment. Similarly resection of lower ribs produces a greater curve than does resection of upper ribs. The convexity of the curve is generally toward the resected side unless there is marked pleural thickening from radiation or empyema.

Scoliosis progresses with advancing age until child reach the full skeletal maturity. This may require further surgical correction of scoliosis with either insertion of Harrington rod or the use of rib expansion devices. If the chest wall is irradiated following surgery, it may accentuate the severity of scoliosis due to impaired growth on the resected side.

Restrictive Pulmonary Function

Pulmonary functions may be affected following management of chest wall tumors due to restrictive chest wall movement.[73]

Secondary Tumors

Chemotherapy with alkylating agents and radiotherapy increases the risk of secondary osseous sarcomas. This risk increases if radiotherapy dose is greater than 60 Gy; therefore, attempts have been made to reduce the radiation dose less than 60. Acute monocytic leukemia has also been reported.[73]

Sternal Tumors

Primary tumors involving the sternum are extremely rare in children and are reported along with adult tumors. Literature indicates that the adult sternal tumors are frequently reported as malignant originating from the cartilage.[82] However, the majority of childhood sternal tumors are essentially benign and clinically present with asymptomatic swelling.[83] Some of the childhood tumors are locally aggressive and possibility of malignancy should be considered if they were shown to be fast growing and associated with pain. Secondary tumors of the sternum after mediastinal irradiation have been reported and are more difficult to manage due to radiation-induced fibrosis.

Anterior chest wall tumors including sternum is a challenging surgery both for complete resection and simultaneous reconstruction so that stabilization can be achieved. The rib and sternal tumor behave in similar manner, and therefore, the description is limited to only specific sternal tumors.

Pediatric Sternal Tumors

Benign lesions	Malignant lesions
Enchondroma	Chondrosarcoma[84]
Osteoblastoma	Osteosarcoma[85]
Osteochondroma	Rhabdomyosarcoma[86]
Aneurysmal bone cyst	Plamacytoma[87]
Eosinophilic granuloma	Ewing's sarcoma[88]
Nonossifying fibroma	Clear cell sarcoma
Chondromyxoid fibroma[89]	Hodgkin's lymphoma[90]
Inflammatory pseudotumor[91]	Metastatic sternal tumors

Enchondroma

The sternum is an unusual location for an Enchondroma. These tumors, however, are commonly reported in the bones of hands and feet and constitute 11% of all bone tumors.[92] Majority of enchondroma are diagnosed incidentally while some present with pathologic fracture. Mineralization within the tumor varies and if minimal may underestimate the size of the lesion. Sternal lesions are generally difficult to diagnose on plain X-rays but cones down lateral view can be more informative. CT scan is helpful in identifying the subtle calcification in the matrix of the tumor. The available evidence suggests that these are developmental defect rather than a true neoplasm.[82] Histologically these tumors has multilobular growth pattern. Generally, they are composed of islands of cartilage separated by hypocellular collagen fibers with minimum ossification.

Wide resection is suggested in the management of any sternal lesion. However, radical resection for this benign lesion in childhood is not warranted.[82]

Osteoblastoma

Benign osteoblastoma is a rare bony tumor (less than 1% of all bone tumors) that has been reported in a variety of skeletal locations including in the ribs, but rarely in the sternum. It is a tumor of adolescent age group reported between 15 and 20 years of age and affecting males twice more commonly than females. Osteoblastoma has a distinct predilection for axial skeletal, particularly posterior elements of the vertebral column. This tumor can be locally invasive. Clinically insidious onset swelling presents with a dull aching pain, usually progressive in intensity; rarely can be asymptomatic and discovered incidentally. Tenderness on physical examination is a consistent finding. Radiologically osteoblastoma lesion is larger than osteoid osteoma (>2 cm in diameter) and well circumscribed. Osteoblastoma is usually radiopaque but occasionally have radiolucent appearance compared with the surrounding bone. Histologically, it shows similarity to osteoid osteoma. New solid bone formation is a feature of osteoblastoma, which helps differentiate from osteosarcoma.[93] Although commonly these are benign lesions, malignant transformation has been reported in a small percentage of osteoblastoma (1%).[94]

Osteoblastoma is a locally aggressive tumor. Moreover, reportedly it has a 10–21% local recurrence rate and therefore wide resections (en-block resection) of the sternum with reconstruction of the chest wall is recommended.[94–98] Reconstruction of the chest wall can be carried out either with the help of bone graft or a synthetic material. Postoperative radiotherapy is not indicated. A case of an isolated benign osteoblastoma in the sternum of an 11-year-old boy has been described with an affective chest wall reconstruction technique.[94,99] The technique involves resection of the tumor and the reconstruction of the defect with a marlex mesh and methyle methacrylate plate, and covering this material with mobilized pectoralis major.[94]

Clinical Features

Most childhood sternal tumors are benign, slow-growing and present as asymptomatic swellings. These swellings should be

Section 5
Esophagus

22
Congenital Malformations

Spencer Beasley

Introduction

Esophageal atresia presents some of the greatest technical hurdles that the pediatric surgeon has to face. Little more than 60 years ago esophageal atresia was considered a uniformly fatal condition. Now, survival is almost guaranteed and determined by associated abnormalities rather than the esophageal atresia itself. The focus of attention has shifted from survival to minimization of morbidity. Nevertheless, with all its variations, subtleties, technical difficulties, and the long-term implications, esophageal atresia continues to challenge the pediatric surgeon.

Historical Perspective

William Durston is believed to have provided the first description of esophageal atresia over 300 years ago in "a narrative of a monstrous birth."[1,2] After that there were several anecdotal reports until the association of esophageal atresia with other structural abnormalities was recognized by Thomas Hill in 1840.[3] In 1861 Hirschsprung brought together a series of 14 cases. A more complete account of the embryology and clinical diagnosis, including associated anomalies was provided by Morrell McKenzie in 1880.[4] Up until this time, accounts of esophageal atresia had been observational rather than interventional. The first attempt to repair esophageal atresia was by Charles Steel in 1888 when he pushed a metal probe introduced through a gastrotomy up into the lower esophageal segment while another bougie was pushed downward from above. He assumed that the esophagus was blocked by a membrane but his procedure failed and autopsy revealed a gap between the proximal and distal segments.[5] Permanent gastrostomies were performed from 1899 and it was not until the 1930s that definitive repair along the lines currently employed (i.e., division of the tracheoesophageal fistula and esophageal anastomosis) was attempted. Thomas Lanman probably performed the first definitive repair in 1936 although the first to appear in the literature was a case operated in 1938 by Robert Shaw.[6]

Lanman subsequently reported that all 30 operative cases in his series died, but added that "the successful operative treatment of a patient with this anomaly is only a question of time."

The first successful primary repair of esophageal atresia was achieved by Cameron Haight in 1941. His five previous attempts at primary repair all failed.[7] By the mid to late 1940s definitive surgery for esophageal atresia was being performed throughout the world including in infants under 1.5 kg.[8] The first survivor in the Southern Hemisphere was operated in New Plymouth, a small rural hospital in New Zealand in 1948,[9] and the first Australian survivor was treated at the Royal Children's Hospital, Melbourne, the following year.[2] Over subsequent decades, deliberate staged repairs, gastrostomies, cervical esophagostomies, and chest drains all became less common. Even in the very premature infant, early primary definitive repair became routine.

By the early 1990s a few surgeons were performing thoracoscopic mobilization of the esophagus,[10] but it was not until 1999 that Rothenberg reported the first successful complete repair of esophageal atresia thoracoscopically.[11] Since then, the technique has become routine in some centers,[12,13] and has even been applied to the H-type tracheoesophageal fistula.[14]

Basic Science/Pathogenesis

Embryogenesis of Esophageal Atresia

Tracheoesophageal Separation

In general terms, the normal changes that occur during early foregut differentiation into the trachea anteriorly and esophagus posteriorly are well described, although the exact mechanism of separation of the two structures is controversial. Many morphological descriptions have been proffered over the years, each reflecting subtle differences in interpretation of sequential histological observations, microdissections, or scanning electron microscopy images. For example, evidence for an ascending tracheoesophageal septum separating the trachea from the esophagus has been conflicting.[15] Similarly, the

D.H. Parikh et al. (eds.), *Pediatric Thoracic Surgery*,
DOI: 10.1007/b136543_22, © Springer-Verlag London Limited 2009

esophageal atresia appear to be sporadic, with a recurrence rate of between 0.5 and 2%[66,72] for parents with one affected child, and the empirical risk for an affected child born to an affected parent is 3–4%.[72]

Antenatal Diagnosis

The diagnosis of esophageal atresia is being made with increasing frequency on routine antenatal ultrasonography. The likelihood of esophageal atresia being present is increased when there are maternal polyhydramnios or other abnormalities identified on ultrasonography that are known to be associated with esophageal atresia; these include congenital heart disease, urinary tract abnormalities (e.g., hydronephrosis), and other abnormalities of the VATER association.

Specific ultrasonographic features suggestive of esophageal atresia include a distended upper esophageal pouch, a small stomach, or abnormal swallowing.[73,74] The dilated upper esophageal pouch may vary in volume according to fetal swallowing.[74] A blind upper pouch can be seen on multiplanar ultrasonography from 23-weeks gestation.[73] Demonstration of a patent esophagus may be achieved using a high-resolution linear transducer in fetuses with suspected esophageal atresia.[75] Magnetic resonance imaging has been used to confirm esophageal atresia where ultrasonography is equivocal.[76]

Postnatal Diagnosis

Clinical Features

The classical clinical presentation of an infant with esophageal atresia is of an abnormally "mucousy" infant who is drooling excessive amounts of saliva (Fig. 22.7). There may be a history of maternal polyhydramnios and the infant is often born prematurely (Fig. 22.8).

If the diagnosis is not recognized at birth and feeding is commenced, the child may start choking or gagging, develop respiratory distress, aspirate or even become cyanotic; this should immediately alert the clinician to the correct diagnosis. Clinicians should be aware that some very premature infants with esophageal atresia may not appear to secrete much saliva.

Confirmation of Esophageal Atresia

The diagnosis of esophageal atresia is confirmed when a 10G orogastric tube cannot be passed through the mouth into the stomach. The catheter becomes arrested at about 10 cm from the gums (Fig. 22.9). Although some surgeons routinely obtain a plain X-ray of the chest to show where the tip of the catheter lies this is not essential for the diagnosis.

Fluid aspirated from the catheter does not turn blue litmus paper pink as the upper pouch contains saliva alone. If the esophagus is intact and the catheter enters the stomach aspiration of gastric juice would turn the litmus paper pink.

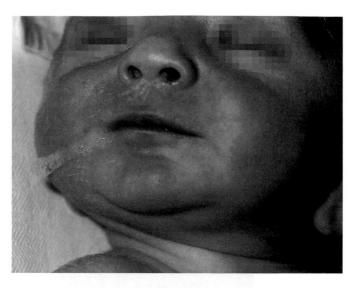

FIG. 22.7. At birth an infant with esophageal atresia typically appears to salivate excessively ("mucousy baby") because saliva accumulates in the blind upper esophageal pouch

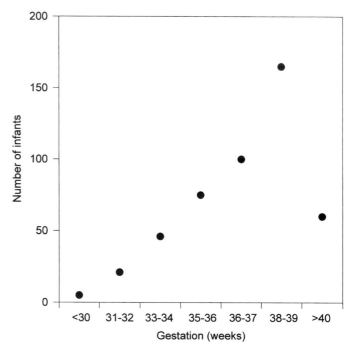

FIG. 22.8. Prematurity is common in infants born with esophageal atresia

A small caliber orogastric tube should not be used because it may curl in the upper pouch giving a misleading impression of esophageal continuity (Fig. 22.10). The catheter is introduced through the mouth rather than the nose to avoid injury to the nasal passages, which are small in the newborn infant. Rarely the oral tube may be passed inadvertently into the trachea and through the fistula into the stomach also giving a false impression of an intact esophagus.[77]

plain ab
"double
fistula ir
be evide

Urinary

The repo
ageal at
abnorma
esis, dup
(e.g., vo
tion). H
1% of i
is fatal,
Patients
often la
the esop
raphy sl
passed t

Mana

Anten

When a
tal ultra
pediatri
the nat
the par
support
birth al
birth. 1
an orog
surgica
knowle
is it of

Preop

The in
heater
upper
A peri
matche
biotics
given
  The
may ii
tantly,
disten
imped
tion a
of eso
plete a

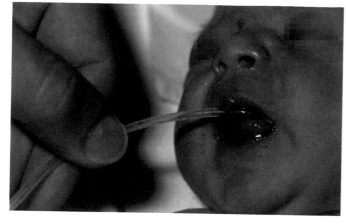

FIG. 22.9. Clinical diagnosis of esophageal atresia is made when a stiff 10G catheter cannot be introduced beyond about 10 cm from the gums

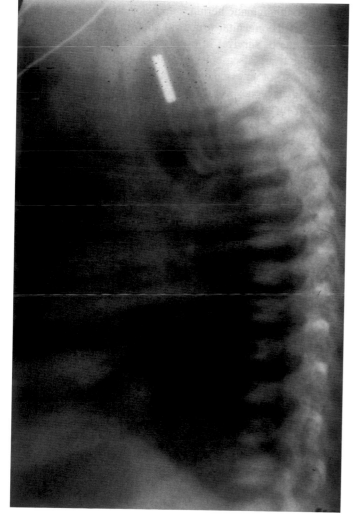

FIG. 22.10. A misleading impression of esophageal continuity can be gained if a small caliber tube is used because it is likely to curl up in the upper esophageal pouch

Traumatic introduction of a suction catheter through the mucosa of the posterior wall of the pharynx may give the impression of esophageal atresia when the infant develops copious drooling of saliva and the tube cannot be advanced into the stomach. This is most likely to be seen in premature babies who have required intensive resuscitation.[78,79] The level of obstruction is lower in the chest on a contrast esophagram than would be seen in esophageal atresia.

Routine passage of an orogastric tube into the stomach of all babies at birth is no longer performed because of the potential risks to the baby of traumatically induced apnea by inadvertent injury to the larynx, even though it would enable a diagnosis of esophageal atresia to be made in all babies before a feed is administered. Mediastinal ultrasonography with installation of saliva into the upper pouch,[80] CT scan of the chest,[81] and three-dimensional volume reformatted "transparency" CT images[82] have been used to confirm the diagnosis, but their role, if any, is yet to be established.

Determination of the Type of Esophageal Atresia

About 85% of infants with esophageal atresia have a distal tracheoesophageal fistula (Fig. 22.11). The presence of a distal tracheoesophageal fistula can be confirmed by the demonstration of gas in the bowel below the diaphragm (Fig. 22.12). Therefore, the combination of inability to pass a catheter through

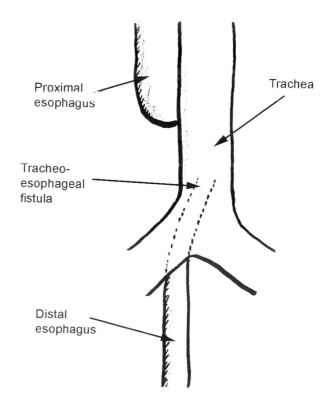

FIG. 22.11. Esophageal atresia with a distal tracheoesophageal fistula. This anatomical variant accounts for approximately 85% of all esophageal atresia and tracheoesophageal fistula cases

A pseudodiverticulum can occur following leakage from the anastomosis but usually heals satisfactorily without long-term mechanical complications. This should be distinguished from ballooning at the site of a circular myotomy, which also produces a diverticulum.[133]

Esophageal Stricture

An anastomotic stricture is the most common reason for further surgery to the esophagus after repair of esophageal atresia.[144] The factors that influence stricture formation are similar to those that produce anastomotic leakage, with the addition of gastroesophageal reflux as a potent cause of stricture formation. The combination of gastro-esophageal reflux and delayed esophageal clearance (because of esophageal dysmotility) means that the acid may bathe the vulnerable region of the anastomosis for prolonged periods, increasing the likelihood of an anastomotic stricture.

Patients with a stricture develop feeding difficulties and dysphagia. As babies they may appear to be "slow feeders" and have excessive regurgitation, with or without cyanotic spells. Older children may present with foreign body impaction of food in the esophagus, particularly in the 2–5-year age group. The diagnosis can be confirmed by either endoscopy or Barium swallow. Endoscopy is used as the first investigation when the child presents with foreign body impaction.

Radial balloon dilatation under fluoroscopic control is probably the most effective and safest technique of dilatation of an anastomotic stricture.[146] One or two dilatations may be all that is required to treat patients with mild narrowing of the esophagus.

Patients with associated gastroesophageal reflux should be placed on an H_2-receptor antagonist or proton pump inhibitor. If these fail or are not tolerated, consideration should be given to performing a fundoplication at which time a further dilatation of the stricture may be required.

Recurrent Tracheoesophageal Fistula

A recurrent tracheoesophageal fistula remains a severe and potentially dangerous complication of esophageal atresia. Its incidence has now declined to under 2%. It is believed that many recurrent fistulae are caused by an anastomotic leakage that results in infection in the area of the repair, particularly when the site of tracheal closure is very close to the anastomosis.

Recurrent fistulae may appear in the early postoperative period, or several years after surgery. They can present with a range of symptoms including coughing, gagging, choking, cyanosis, apnea, dying spellings, and recurrent chest infections. Usually, however, the child simply coughs and splutters with each feed.

The diagnosis is confirmed on bronchoscopy or cineradiographic tube esophagography with the patient prone

(Fig. 22.28). The recurrent fistula usually arises from the pouch of the original fistula.

Spontaneous closure is unlikely to occur. The fistula should be divided when the child is in optimal respiratory and general condition, and this may necessitate a period of total parenteral nutrition. Gastrostomy is now rarely indicated. The conventional approach is through the original right fourth interspace using a transpleural approach. The passage of a fine ureteric catheter through the fistula immediately prior to the thoracotomy may facilitate its localization during the operative repair.

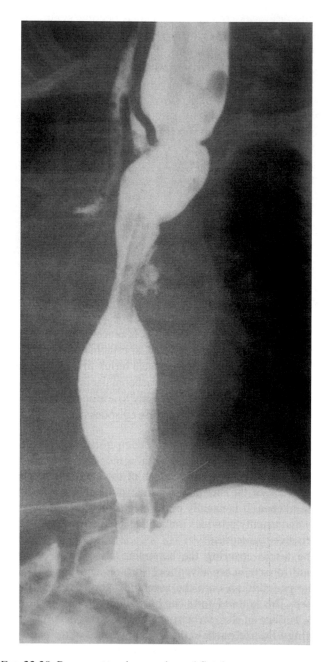

FIG. 22.28. Recurrent tracheoesophageal fistula

There are a number of reports of endoscopic obliteration of recurrent tracheoesophageal fistulae using diathermy obliteration,[147] tissue adhesive,[146] and a combination of a tissue adhesive and sclerosing agent[148] of a coated self-expanding plastic stent.[149] It has been suggested that these techniques may have special application in regions where additional surgery has an unacceptably high morbidity or where parents are reluctant to allow their child to undergo further surgery.[148]

Gastroesophageal Reflux and Esophageal Dysmotility

Gastroesophageal reflux can be troublesome for two reasons:

1. It may lead to aspiration of gastric contents
2. Prolonged exposure of the esophageal mucosa to acid may lead to an anastomotic stricture and Barrett's esophagus

There is a tendency for gastroesophageal reflux to improve with age, but despite this it must be taken more seriously than in the otherwise normal infant. The availability of effective H_2-receptor antagonists and proton pump inhibitors has dramatically reduced the need for early fundoplication. Antireflux surgery is now reserved for those with ongoing episodes of aspiration or recurrent chest infection, or for those in whom medication is not tolerated or has failed.

Laparoscopic antireflux surgery in esophageal atresia has largely replaced open fundoplication.[150] Postoperative pH monitoring identifies most, but not all, infants who will go on to develop esophagitis or require an antireflux procedure.[151]

About 30% of children have short-term dysphagia following fundoplication probably because the increased resistance at the gastroesophageal junction unmasks the preexisting esophageal dysmotility (poor peristalsis and delayed esophageal clearance) that is usual in esophageal atresia. The long-term effects of gastroesophageal reflux into an abnormal esophagus that has poor motility and delayed clearance are discussed in more detail later.

Rare and Unusual Variants

The Congenital "H" Fistula

The isolated tracheoesophageal fistula ("H" fistula) without atresia accounts for about 4% of congenital esophageal anomalies (Fig. 22.29). It presents with entirely different symptoms from esophageal atresia because the esophagus is patent. It is included in discussion of esophageal atresia because of its presumed common etiology.

Figure 22.29 shows the oblique passage of the fistula that runs from the trachea in a caudal direction to the esophagus. The symptoms it produces relate to abnormal passage of air through the fistula from the trachea to the esophagus (and

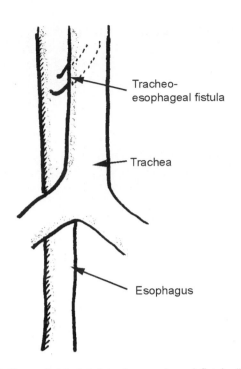

FIG. 22.29. Congenital isolated tracheoesophageal fistula ("H" fistula) without esophageal atresia

stomach) and of esophageal contents, which may include saliva, gastric juice, and milk, into the trachea.

Diagnosis

It usually presents in the first few days of life with choking on feeds and unexplained cyanotic spells.[152] Choking attacks may be associated with abdominal distension.

Older infants may present with recurrent bouts of pneumonia, usually involving the right upper lobe, and unexplained intermittent bouts of abdominal distension. Less common features include a hoarse cry and failure to thrive. Some children are months or years old before the diagnosis is recognized.

Investigation

An isolated tracheoesophageal fistula can be diagnosed radiologically or by endoscopy. Video-esophagography (Fig. 22.30 involves introduction of a tube into the mid-esophagus, with the infant lying prone, with injection of contrast as the tube is slowly withdrawn.[153] Familiarity with the technique is important, as a standard barium swallow will miss an H-fistula in 25% of occasions.[154]

The fistula can be seen readily on bronchoscopy as an abnormal opening on the posterior wall of the trachea. Sometimes bronchoscopy is performed immediately prior to the surgery to divide the fistula so that a catheter can be introduced through the fistula to aid in its identification at open surgical exploration.[155]

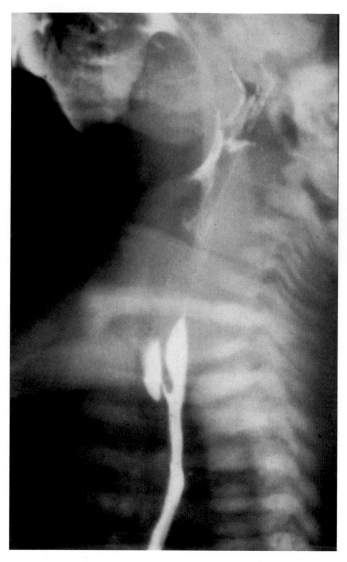

FIG. 22.30. A congenital "H" fistula can be demonstrated by video-esophagography with the infant prone

Operative Management

Almost all H-fistulae can be approached through a right supraclavicular incision.[154,156] The sternomastoid muscle is retracted posteriorly, although division of its sternal head may improve the exposure. The incision is deepened antero-medial to the carotid sheath. The trachea is recognized by palpating its rings. The fistula is found in the groove between the trachea and esophagus, and on its external surface it looks surprisingly short and broad. It is not necessary to dissect completely around the esophagus or to control it with a vessel loop as this increases the risk of damage to the recurrent laryngeal nerve. However, a sling placed around the fistula itself may help its dissection

and division. The fistula should be transfixed and divided rather than ligated alone, to reduce the likelihood of recurrence of the fistula. Placement of muscular flaps between the divided ends of the fistula may also decrease the recurrence rate but is probably not required as a routine. Drainage of the wound is not necessary and gastrostomy is not used. The anesthetist should always inspect the vocal cords to confirm their movement at the completion of the operation. Oral feeds are commenced the next day.

Complications

The main complications of the procedure are recurrent laryngeal nerve palsy, either unilateral or bilateral and recurrence of the fistula.[154] Leakage at the site of closure is rare, but may result in mediastinitis, or a recurrent fistula. Other complications are rare and include injury to the esophagus producing mediastinitis or an esophagocutaneous fistula. Pneumothorax and tracheal obstruction can be avoided with good surgical technique. Postoperative aspiration and pneumonia have also been reported.

Other Rare Variants

A large number of rare variants of esophageal atresia have been reported.[157,158] It is not necessary to list (or learn) them all; rather, the surgeon should be aware that bizarre variants do occur, and may be encountered unexpectedly at the time of surgery. The exact anatomy of the variant should be defined, and the abnormality corrected following normal surgical principles.

Congenital Lower Esophageal Stenosis

An encircling "cartilaginous" rest within the wall of the lower esophagus is a rare but well-recognized condition that occurs in 1:25–50,000 births.[159,160] It may produce obstructive symptoms and often occurs in association with esophageal atresia. Between 5 and 14% of infants born with esophageal atresia will also have a congenital stenosis of the esophagus.[161] Less common variants of this lesion also occur (Table 22.8), but all are believed to have a common etiology.

The lesion usually becomes symptomatic at the time of introduction of solid foods, or suddenly when foreign body impaction of the esophagus occurs.

TABLE 22.8. Classification of congenital stenosis of the lower esophagus.

Encircling cartilaginous "rest", i.e., tracheobronchial remnant in esophageal wall (most common)
Fibromuscular thickening (idiopathic muscular hypertrophy)
Membranous web or diaphragm (extremely rare)

Contrast radiology demonstrates an abrupt and fixed narrowing, which, in esophageal atresia, may be difficult to distinguish from a low esophageal stricture secondary to esophagitis and gastroesophageal reflux. High-frequency catheter probe endoscopic ultrasonography can demonstrate the hyperechoic cartilage at the site of esophageal narrowing.[162] The narrowing persists despite attempts at radial balloon dilatation, and definitive treatment involves resection of the affected esophageal segment and end-to-end esophagoesophagostomy.

Prognosis and Long-Term Outcomes

Predictors of Outcome

Over the last 60 years there has been a dramatic improvement in the survival rate of repaired esophageal atresia (Fig. 22.31). Nowadays, all patients with esophageal atresia are expected to survive almost irrespective of their gestation, provided there are no major concomitant congenital malformations.[163] There has been a steady decline in overall mortality due to esophageal atresia throughout the world until about 1985.[163–166] In the early years much of the mortality was the result of respiratory failure, inadequate resuscitation, pneumonia, hyaline membrane disease, and other complications of prematurity. Another major cause of mortality was from complications of the surgery itself, particularly those related to anastomotic dehiscence and poor nutrition. Recognition of this led to the Waterson classification,[167] which used to be valuable in identifying risk factors and in predicting outcome in infants with esophageal atresia. However, it is no longer relevant because mortality is now largely determined by the type of severity of concomitant congenital abnormalities alone.[163]

Definitive repair of an esophageal atresia may not be appropriate in patients with an identifiable concomitant congenital abnormality that is known to be lethal or associated with an extremely poor prognosis.

Esophageal Function

The most common long-term problem is dysphagia. It occurs in almost half of all patients.[168] Likewise, gastroesophageal reflux occurs in about 48%.[168] It is likely that all patients have a degree of esophageal dysmotility and poor peristalsis, but it appears to improve with age, or alternatively, patients' eating habits are modified to better accommodate it.

Foreign body impaction is most likely to occur under the age of 5 years, after which time it becomes relatively infrequent. However, most children and adults with esophageal atresia will have their meals with a glass of water and deliberately chew their food well.

Growth

Early studies suggested that growth might be impaired in survivors of esophageal atresia.[169] Other studies have confirmed that some children exhibit early physical developmental retardation but that height and weight eventually become normal.[168,170] By adulthood both height and weight centiles after repair of esophageal atresia follow a normal distribution.[171]

Risk of Esophageal Malignancy After Repair of Esophageal Atresia

Now that some of the older survivors of esophageal atresia are reaching their sixth decade some of the potential long-term sequelae of the condition are becoming evident. There have been three reports of esophageal adenocarcinoma following repair of esophageal atresia.[172–174] Two of these patients were in their 20's and two had areas of Barrett's epithelium identified. It is accepted that gastroesophageal reflux and esophagitis are more common in patients after repair of esophageal atresia than in the general population,[175–177] with a concomitant increase in the incidence of Barrett's esophagus, a known precursor of adenocarcinoma.[177] Esophageal atresia patients appear to be particularly vulnerable to the adverse effects of gastroesophageal reflux because of their esophageal dysmotility and poor esophageal clearance, which means that the time the esophageal mucosa is exposed to acid from reflux is prolonged. Squamous cell carcinoma after repair of esophageal atresia has also been reported.[178] There are two other situations in which malignancy may occur in esophageal atresia patients (Table 22.9). During esophageal replacement surgery using

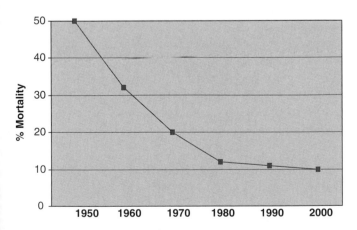

FIG. 22.31. Survival in esophageal atresia, showing the steady improvement in outcome with the passing of each decade. The residual mortality of about 10% is due to congenital abnormalities such as hypoplastic left heart, bilateral renal agenesis, and Trisomy 18

TABLE 22.9. Factors contributing to esophageal malignancy after repair of esophageal atresia.

Combination of gastroesophageal reflux and esophageal dysmotility (poor esophageal clearance of reflux acid) leading to Barrett's epithelium
Retained esophageal segment after oesophageal replacement
Squamous cell carcinoma in skin tube conduits

TABLE 22.10. Esophageal atresia support groups.

Name of group	Country	Contact
International Esophageal Atresia Team		www.tefuater.org/ieat.html
Esophageal Atresia Research Axillary (OARA)	Australia	Holsom@ozemail.com.au
Speiserohrenmi Bbildungen (KEKS)	Germany	Info@keks.org or www.keks.org
Tracheoesophageal Fistula Support Newsletter (CHEW)	UK	Info@tofs.org.uk or www. tofs.org.uk
The VATER Connection	USA	www.vaterconnection.org
EA/TEF Family Support	USA	www.eatef.org
KEKS	Austria	Wagner.c@utanet.at
VOKS	Netherlands	Info@voks.nl
NFO	Norway	www.nfoe.homepage.com
Esofagus Gruppen	Sweden	Rmt@magotarm.sw
KEKS	Switzerland	Keka@datacom.ch

colon or stomach many surgeons have left the distal esophageal remnant in situ. However, it is now recognized that gastric mucosa can replace the normal squamous epithelium in these esophageal remnants, resulting in chronic inflammation and a Barrett's esophagus.[179] It is for this reason that it is recommended that the esophageal remnant should be completely excised, ideally at the time of esophageal replacement, or later if there is radiological evidence of esophagitis or ulceration, or if symptoms occur.[179,180]

A technique that used to be employed to gain gastrointestinal continuity following cervical esophagostomy involved creating an antithoracic tubularized bipedicle skin flap.[181,182] Squamous cell carcinoma is common in these conduits,[183] and they should be removed before adulthood.

At this stage we do not have accurate information on the relative risk of developing an esophageal malignancy after esophageal atresia repair, but it is likely to be increased. Clinicians need to be aware of the possibility that these patients may develop esophageal malignancy at a young age. It is yet to be determined whether the availability of proton pump inhibitors reduces this risk. In older patients, the role of regular endoscopy to assess the esophageal epithelium is yet to be established.

Quality of Life

Almost all adult patients enjoy a normal lifestyle, comparable to that of healthy adults in the general population.[168,169,184] Studies have not identified any differences in overall physical and mental health, and perhaps surprisingly, concomitant congenital abnormalities have not been found to influence generic quality of life. However, about one-third of patients report that the esophageal atresia had some negative effects on their lives, predominantly related to dysphagia (23%).[184]

Parent Support Groups

Details of some of the parent support groups for families who have a child with esophageal atresia are shown in Table 22.10. Many of these groups commenced in the 1980s. Some of them have extended their influence well beyond their own borders. For example, the German group KEKS has helped families in a number of war-torn countries and has brought families and babies born with esophageal atresia to Europe and cared for them in KEKS houses.

The International Esophageal Atresia team is made up of parents of esophageal atresia survivors who have children born with esophageal atresia and or tracheoesophageal fistula. They have joined together with other groups from around the world to offer information and support to families who are affected by esophageal atresia and the VATER association. Support groups can alleviate the isolation parents may feel,[168] and can provide practical assistance and emotional support to families in need. Some groups, e.g., AORA and CHEW, have been influential in setting up a number of major research studies.

References

1. Durston W. A narrative of a monstrous birth in Plymouth. Philos Trans R Soc 1670–1671; 5: 2096–2098.
2. Myers NA. The history of oesophageal atresia and tracheo-oesophageal fistula 1670–1984. Prog Pediatr Surg 1986; 20: 106–157.
3. Hill TP. Congenital malformation. Boston Med Surg J 1840; 21: 320–321.
4. MacKenzie M. Malformation of the esophagus. Arch Laryngol 1880; 1: 301–315.
5. Steele C. Case of deficient oesophagus. Lancet 1888; 2: 764.
6. Shaw R. Surgical correction of congenital atresia of the esophagus with tracheo-oesophageal fistula. J Thorac Surg 1939; 9: 213–219.

7. Haight C, Towsley H. Congenital atresia of the esophagus with tracheoesophageal fistula: extrapleural ligation of fistula and end-to-end anastomosis of esophageal segments. Surg Gynecol Obstet 1943; 76: 672–688.

8. Longmire WP. Congenital atresia and tracheoesophageal fistula. Arch Surg 1947; 55: 330.

9. Myers NA. Oesophageal atresia: the first survival in the Southern Hemisphere. Aust N Z J Surg 1992; 62: 973–974.

10. Allal H. Operative treatment of an oesophageal atresia by thoracoscopic assistance. Presented at the International Congress of Paediatric Surgery and Paediatric Radiology, combined meeting of the World Federation of Association of Pediatric Surgeons, Australasian Association of Paediatric Surgeons and Australasian Society for Paediatric Imaging, Melbourne Australia, 1995.

11. Lobe TE, Rothenberg S, Waldschmidt J, et al. Thoracoscopic repair of esophageal atresia in an infant: a surgical first. Pediatr Endosurg Innovat Tech 1999; 3: 141–148.

12. Holcomb GW, Rothenberg SS, Bax KM, et al. Thoracoscopic repair of esophageal atresia and tracheoesophageal fistula: a multi-institutional analysis. Ann Surg 2005; 242: 422–428.

13. Rothenberg SS. Thoracoscopic repair of esophageal atresia and tracheo-esophageal fistula. Semin Pediatr Surg 2005; 14: 2–7.

14. Allal H, Montes-Tapia F, Andina G, et al.Thoracoscopic repair of H-type tracheoesophageal fistula in the newborn: a technical case report. J Pediatr Surg 2004; 39: 1568–1570.

15. Zaw-Tun HA. The tracheo-esophageal septum – fact or fantasy? Origin and development of the respiratory primordium and esophagus. Acta Anat 1982; 114: 1–21.

16. O'Rahilly R, Muller F. Respiratory and alimentary relations in staged human embryos: new embryological data and congenital abnormalities. Ann Otol Rhinol Laryngol 1984; 93: 421–429.

17. Sutliff KS, Hutchins GM. Separation of the respiratory and digestive tracts in human embryos: crucial role of the tracheo oesophageal sulcus. Anat Rec 1994; 238: 237–247.

18. Qi BQ, Beasley SW. Preliminary evidence that cell death may contribute to separation of the trachea from the primitive foregut in the rat embryo. J Pediatr Surg 1998; 33: 1660–1665.

19. Williams AK, Qi BQ, Beasley SW. Demonstration of abnormal notochord development by three-dimensional reconstructive imaging in the rat model of esophageal atresia. Pediatr Surg Int 2001; 17: 21–24.

20. Qi BQ, Beasley SW. Stages of normal tracheo bronchial development in rat embryos: resolution of a controversy. Dev Growth Differ 2000; 42: 145–153.

21. Beasley SW, Diez-Pardo J, Qi BQ, et al. The contribution of the Adriamycin induced rat model of the VATER association to our understanding of congenital abnormalities and their embryogenesis. Pediatr Surg Int 2000; 16: 465–472.

22. Beasley SW. Embryology. In: Oesophageal Atresia, Beasley SW, Myers NA, Auldist AW (eds). Chapman & Hall Medical, London, 991; 31–43.

23. Schmitz J. Ueber die Formale Genese der Oesophagus-missbildungen. Virch Arch Pathol Anat Physiol 1923; 247: 278–293.

24. Fluss Z, Poppen KJ. Embryogenesis of tracheoesophageal fistula and esophageal atresia; a hypothesis based on associated vascular anomalies. AMA Arch Pathol 1951; 52: 168–181.

25. Broman CN. The genesis of intestinal atresia. Surg Forum 1956; 7: 393–396.

26. Piekarski DH, Stephens FD. The association and embryogenesis of tracheo-oesophageal and anorectal anomalies. In: Anorectal Malformations and Associated Disease, Progress in Paediatric Surgery, Vol 9, Rickham PP, Hecker WC, Prevot J, (eds). University Park Press, Baltimore, 1986; 63–76.

27. Kreuter E. Die angeborenen Verschliessungen und Gerengungen des Darmkanals im Lichte der Entwicklungsgeschichte. Deutsch Z Chir 1905; 79: 1–89.

28. Moore KL, Persaud TVN. The developing human. Clinically orientated embryology, 5th Edn, WB Saunders, Philadelphia, PA, 1993; 53–69.

29. Borycki AG, Mendham L, Emerson CPJr. Control of somite patterning by sonic hedgehog and its downstream signal response genes. Development 1998; 125: 774–790.

30. Qi BQ, Beasley S. Relationship of the notochord to foregut development in the fetal rat model of oesophageal atresia. J Pediatr Surg 1999; 34: 1593–1598.

31. Possoegel AK, Diez-Pardo JA, Morrales C, Tovar JA. Notochord involvement in experimental esophageal atresia. Pediatr Surg Int 1999; 15: 201–205.

32. Arsic D, Qi BQ, Beasley SW. Hedgehog in the human: a possible explanation for the VATER association. J Pediatr Child Health 2002; 38: 117–121.

33. Vleesch Dubois VN, Qi BQ, Beasley SW, Williams AK. Abnormal branching and regression of the notochord and its relationship to foregut abnormalities. Eur J Pediatr Surg 2002; 12: 83–89.

34. Beasley SW, Williams AK, Qi BQ, Vleesch Dubois VN. The development of the proximal oesophageal pouch in the Adriamycin rat model of oesophageal atresia with tracheo-oesophageal fistula. Pediatr Surg Int 2004; 20: 548–550.

35. Crisera CA, Connelly PR, Marmureanu AR, et al. Esophageal atresia with tracheo-esophageal fistula: suggested mechanism in faulty organogenesis. J Pediatr Surg 1999; 34: 204–208.

36. Qi BQ, Merei J, Farmer P, et al. The vagus and recurrent laryngeal nerves in the rodent experimental model of oesophageal atresia. J Pediatr Surg 1997; 32: 1580–1586.

37. Wicking C, Smyth I, Bale A. The hedgehog signalling pathway in tumorogenesis and development. Oncogene 1999; 18: 7844–7851.

38. Litingtung Y, Lei L, Westphal H, Chiang C. Sonic hedgehog is essential to foregut development. Nat Genet 1998; 20: 58–61.

39. Arsic D, Keenan J, Quan BQ, Beasley SW. Differences in the levels of Sonic hedgehog protein during early foregut development caused by exposure to Adriamycin gives clues to the role of Shh gene in oesophageal atresia. Pediatr Surg Int 2003; 19: 463–466.

40. Arsic D, Cameron V, Ellmers L, et al. Adriamycin disruption of the Shh-Gli pathway is associated with abnormalities of foregut development. J Pediatr Surg 2004; 39: 1747–1753.

41. Spilde T, Bhatia A, Ostlie D, et al. A role for sonic hedgehog signalling in the pathogenesis of human tracheoesophageal fistula. J Pediatr Surg 2003; 38: 465–468.

42. Pepicelli CV, Lewis PM, McMahon AP. Sonic hedgehog regulates branching morphogenesis in the mammalian lung. Curr Biol 1998; 8: 1083–1086.

43. Odent S, Atti-Bitach T, Blayau M, et al. Expression of the sonic hedgehog (SHH) gene during early human development and phenotypic expression of new mutations causing holoprosencephaly. Hum Mol Genet 1999; 8: 1683–1689.

44. Brunner HG, van Bokhoven H. Genetic players in esophageal atresia and tracheoesophageal fistula. Curr Opin Genet Dev 2005; 15: 341–347.

45. Hokama R, Myers NA, Kent M, et al. Esophageal atresia with tracheo esophageal fistula: a histopathological study. Pediatr Surg Int 1986; 1: 117–121.

46. Gardner E, Gray DJ, O'Rahilly R. Anatomy, 4th Edn. WB Saunders, Philadephia, PA, 1975; 280–281.

47. Romeo G, Zuccarello B, Proietto F, et al. Disorders of esophageal motor activity in atresia of the esophagus. J Pediatr Surg 1987; 22: 120–124.

48. Kirkpatrick JA, Cresson SL, Pilling GP. The motor activity of the esophagus in association with esophageal atresia and tracheoesophageal fistula. Am J Roentgenol Radium Ther Nucl Med 1961; 86: 884–887.

49. Johnston PW, Hastings N. Congenital tracheoesophageal fistula without esophageal atresia. Am J Surg 1966; 112: 233–240.

50. Haller JA, Brooker AF, Talbert JL. Esophageal function following resection. Studies in newborn puppies. Ann Thorac Surg 1966; 2: 180–187.

51. Burgess JN, Carlson HC, Ellis FJ. Esophageal function after successful repair of esophageal atresia and tracheo-esophageal fistula. A manometric and cine-fluorographic study. J Thorac Cardiovasc Surg 1968; 56: 667–673.

52. Laks H, Wilkinson RH, Shuster SR. Long-term results following correction of esophageal atresia with tracheoesophageal fistula: a clinical and cinefluorographic study. J Pediatr Surg 1972; 7: 591–597.

53. Kawahara H, Kubota A, Okuyama H, et al. The usefulness of videomanometry for studying pediatric esophageal motor disease. J Pediatr Surg 2004; 39: 1754–1757.

54. Tomaselli V, Volpi ML, Dell'Agnola CA, et al. Long-term evaluation of esophageal function in patients treated at birth for esophageal atresia. Pediatr Surg Int 2003; 19: 40–43.

55. Hörmann M, Pokieser P, Scharitzer M, et al. Videofluoroscopy of deglutition in children after repair of esophageal atresia. Acta Radiol 2002; 43: 507–510.

56. Orringer MB, Kirsh MM, Sloan H. Long-term esophageal function following repair of esophageal atresia. Ann Surg 1977; 186: 436–443.

57. Jolley SG, Johnson DG, Roberts CC, Herbst JJ. Patterns of gastro-esophageal reflux in children following repair of esophageal atresia and distal tracheo-esophageal fistula. J Pediatr Surg 1980; 15: 857–862.

58. Shepard R, Fenn S, Sieber WK. Evaluation of esophageal function in post-operative esophageal atresia and tracheoesophageal fistula. Surgery 1967; 59: 608–617.

59. Desjardins JG, Stephens CA, Moes C. Results of surgical treatment of congenital tracheo-esophageal fistula with a note on cinefluorographic findings. Ann Surg 1964; 160: 41–145.

60. Beasley SW. Anatomy. In: Oesophageal Atresia, Beasley SW, Myers NA, Auldist AW (eds). Chapman & Hall Medical, London, 1991; 45–58.

61. Lister J. The blood supply to the oesophagus in relation to oesophageal atresia. Arch Dis Child 1964; 39: 131–137.

62. Wailoo MP, Emery JL. The trachea in children with tracheo-oesophageal fistula. Histopathology 1979; 3: 329–338.

63. Qi BQ, Merei J, Farmer P, et al. Tracheomalacia with esophageal atresia and tracheo-esophageal fistula in fetal rats. J Pediatr Surg 1997; 32: 1575–1579.

64. Davies MR, Cywes S. The flaccid trachea and tracheooesophageal congenital anomalies. J Pediatr Surg 1978; 13: 363–367.

65. Beasley SW, Qi BQ. Understanding tracheomalacia. J Paediatr Child Health 1998; 34: 209–210.

66. Bankier A, Brady J, Myers NA. Epidemiology and genetics. In: Oesophageal Atresia, Beasley SW, Myers NA, Auldist AW (eds). Chapman & Hall Medical, London, 1991; 19–29.

67. Myers NA. Oesophageal atresia: the epitome of modern surgery. Ann R Coll Surg 1974; 54: 277–287.

68. Torfs CP, Curry CU, Bateson TF. Population-based study of tracheoesophageal fistula and esophageal atresia. Teratology 1995; 52: 220–232.

69. Orford J, Glasson M, Beasley SW, et al. Oesophageal atresia in twins. Pediatr Surg Int 2000; 16: 541–545.

70. Beasley SW, Allen M, Myers N. The effect of Down syndrome and other chromosomal abnormalities on survival and management in oesophageal atresia. Pediatr Surg Int 1997; 12: 550–551.

71. Harris J, Källén B, Robert E. Descriptive epidemiology of alimentary tract atresia. Teratology 1995; 52: 15–29.

72. Pletcher BA, Friedes JS, Breg WR, Touloukian RJ. Familial occurrence of esophageal atresia with and without tracheoesophageal fistula: report of two unusual kindreds. Am J Med Genet 1991; 39: 380–384.

73. Shulman A, Mazkereth R, Zalel Y, et al. Prenatal identification of esophageal atresia: the role of ultrasonography for evaluation of functional anatomy. Prenat Diag 2002; 22: 669–674.

74. Centini G, Rosignoli L, Kenanidis A, Petraglia F. Prenatal diagnosis of esophageal atresia with the pouch sign. Ultrasound Obstet Gynecol 2003; 21: 494–497.

75. Malinger G, Levine A, Rotmensch S. The fetal esophagus: anatomical and physiological ultrasonographic characterisation using a high-resolution linear transducer. Ultrasound Obstet Gynecol 2004; 24: 500–505.

76. Matsuoka S, Takeuchi K, Yamanaka Y, et al. Comparison of magnetic resonance imaging and ultrasonography in the prenatal diagnosis of congenital thoracic abnormalities. Fetal Diagn Ther 2003; 18: 447–453.

77. Celayir AC, Erdo an E. An infrequent cause of misdiagnosis in esophageal atresia. J Pediatr Surg 2003; 38: 1389.

78. Cohen RC, Myers NA. Traumatic oesophageal pseudodiverticulum. Aust Paediatr J 1987; 23: 125–127.

79. Barlev DM, Nagourney BA, Saintonge R. Traumatic retropharyngeal emphysema as a cause for severe respiratory distress in a newborn. Pediatr Radiol 2003; 33: 429–432.

80. Gassner I, Geley TE. Sonographic evaluation of oesophageal atresia and tracheo-oesophageal fistula. Pediatr Radiol 2005; 35: 159–164.

81. Ratan SK, Varshney A, Mullick S, et al. Evaluation of neonates with esophageal atresia using chest CT scan. Pediatr Surg Int 2004; 20: 757–761.

82. Soye JA, Yarr J, Dick AC, Paterson A. Multidetector-row computed tomography three-dimensional volume reformatted 'transparency' images to define an upper pouch fistula in oesophageal atresia. Pediatr Radiol 2005; 35: 624–626.

83. Benjamin B. Endoscopy in esophageal atresia and tracheo-esophageal fistula. Ann Otol Rhinol Laryngol 1981; 90; 376–382.

84. Kosloske AM, Jewell PF, Cartwright KC. Crucial bronchoscopic findings in esophageal atresia and tracheoesophageal fistula. J Pediatr Surg 1988; 23: 466–470.

85. Pigna A, Gentili A, Landuzzi V, et al. Bronchoscopy in newborns with esophageal atresia. Pediatr Med Chir 2002; 24: 297–301.

86. Atzori P, Lacobelli BD, Bottero S, et al. Preoperative tracheobronchoscopy in newborns with esophageal atresia: does it matter? J Pediatr Surg 2006; 41: 1054–1057.

87. Bardakjian TM, Schneider A. Association of anophthalmia and esophageal atresia: four new cases identified by the anophthalmia/microphthalmia clinical registry. Am J Med Genet A 2005; 132A: 54–56.

88. Hill CJ, Pilz DT, Harper PS, et al. Anophthalmia-esophageal-genital syndrome: a further case to define the phenotype. Am J Med Genet A 2005; 132A: 57–59.

89. Messina M, Ferrucci E, Buonocore G, et al. Association of microphthalmia and esophageal atresia: description of a patient and review of the literature. Am J Med Genet A 2003; 119A: 184–187.

90. van Dooren M, Tibboel D, Torfs C. The co-occurrence of congenital diaphragmatic hernia, esophageal atresia/tracheoesophageal fistula, and lung hypoplasia. Birth Defects Res A Clin Mol Teratol 2005; 73: 53–57.

91. Mee RBB, Beasley SW, Auldist AW, Myers NA. Influence of congenital heart disease on the management of oesophageal atresia. Pediatr Surg Int 1992; 7: 90–93.

92. Tönz M, Köhli S, Kaiser G. Oesophageal atresia: what has changed in the last 3 decades? Pediatr Surg Int 2004; 20: 768–772.

93. Beasley SW, Myers NA. Mortality. In: Oesophageal Atresia, Beasley SW, Myers NA, Auldist AW (eds). Chapman & Hall Medical, London, 1991; 361–367.

94. Diaz LK, Akpek EA, Dinavahi R, Andropoulos DB. Tracheoesophageal fistula and associated congenital heart disease: implications for anesthetic management and survival. Paediatr Anaesth 2005; 15: 862–869.

95. Phelan E, Kelly JH, Beasley SW. Urinary tract abnormalities. In: Oesophageal Atresia, Beasley SW, Myers NA, Auldist AW (eds). Chapman & Hall Medical, London, 1991; 241–248.

96. Holder TM, Cloud, DT, Lewis JE, Pilling GP. Esophageal atresia and tracheoesophageal fistula: a survey of its members by the Surgical Section of the American Academy of Pediatrics. Pediatrics 1964; 34: 542–549.

97. Louhimo I, Lindahl H. Esophageal atresia: primary results of 500 consecutively treated patients. J Pediatr Surg 1983; 18: 217–229.

98. Beasley SW, Phelan E, Kelly JH, et al. Urinary tract abnormalities in association with oesophageal atresia: frequency, significance and influence on management. Pediatr Surg Int 1992; 7: 94–96.

99. Kalish RB, Chasen ST, Rosenzweig L, Chervenak FA. Esophageal atresia and tracheoesophageal fistula: the impact of prenatal suspicion on neonatal outcome in a tertiary care center. J Perinat Med 2003; 31: 111–114.

100. Bax KM, van Der Zee DC. Feasibility of thoracoscopic repair of esophageal atresia with distal fistula. J Pediatr Surg 2002; 37: 192–196.

101. Rothenberg SS. Thoracoscopic repair of tracheoesophageal fistula in newborns. J Pediatr Surg 2002; 37: 869–872.

102. Nguyen T, Zainabadi K, Bui T, et al. Thoracoscopic repair of esophageal atresia and tracheoesophageal fistula: lessons learned. J Laparoendosc Adv Surg Tech A 2006; 16: 174–178.

103. Krosnar S, Baxter A. Thoracoscopic repair of esophageal atresia with tracheoesophageal fistula: anesthetic and intensive care management of a series of eight neonates. Paediatr Anaesth 2005; 15: 541–546.

104. Tsao K, Lee H. Extrapleural thoracoscopic repair of esophageal atresia with tracheoesophageal fistula. Pediatr Surg Int 2005; 21: 308–310.

105. Rothenberg SS. Esophageal atresia and tracheoesophageal fistula. In: Operative Endoscopy and Endoscopic Surgery in Infants and Children, Najmaldin A, Rothenberg S, Crabbe D, Beasley S (eds). Hodder Arnold, London, 2005; 89–97.

106. Koivusalo A, Turunen P, Rintala RJ, et al. Is routine dilatation after repair of esophageal atresia with distal fistula better than dilatation when symptoms arise? Comparison of results of two European pediatric surgical centers. J Pediatr Surg 2004; 39: 1643–1647.

107. Rickham PP. Infants with esophageal atresia weighing under three pounds. J Pediatr Surg 1981; 16: 595–598.

108. Mackinlay GA, Burtles R. Oesophageal atresia: paralysis and ventilation in the management of the wide gap. Pediatr Surg Int 1987; 2: 10–12.

109. Davies MR, Beale PG. Protection of oesophageal anastomosis following uncomplicated repair of common-type oesophageal atresia by non-reversal of anaesthesia and graded withdrawal of respiratory support. Pediatr Surg Int 1991; 6: 98–100.

110. Al-Salem AH, Qaisaruddin S, Srair HA, et al. Elective, postoperative ventilation in the management of esophageal atresia and tracheoesophageal fistula. Pediatr Surg Int 1997; 12: 261–263.

111. Lyall P, Bao-Quan Q, Beasley SW. The effect of neck flexion on oesophageal tension in the pig and its relevance to repaired oesophageal atresia. Pediatr Surg Int 2001; 17: 193–195.

112. Beasley SW. Does postoperative ventilation have an effect on the integrity of the anastomosis in repaired oesophageal atresia? J Paediatr Child Health 1999; 35: 120–122.

113. Lou CC, Lin JN, Wang CR. Evaluation of oesophageal atresia without fistula by three-dimensional computed tomography. Eur J Pediatr 2002; 161: 578–580.

114. Beasley SW. Oesophageal atresia without fistula. In: Oesophageal Atresia, Beasley SW, Myers NA, Auldist AW (eds). Chapman & Hall Medical, London, 1991; 137–159.

115. Schärli AF. Esophageal reconstruction in very long atresia by elongation of the lesser curvature. Pediatr Surg Int 1992; 7: 101–105.

116. Rao KL, Menon P, Samujh R, et al. Fundal tube esophagoplasty for esophageal reconstruction in atresia. J Pediatr Surg 2003; 38: 1723–1725.

117. Spitz L. Gastric replacement of the oesophagus. In: Rob and Smith's Operative Surgery: Paediatric Surgery, 4th edn, Spitz LV, Nixon HH (eds). Butterworths, London, 1998; 142–145.

118. Hirschl RB, Yardeni D, Oldham K, et al. Gastric transposition for esophageal replacement in children: experience with 41 consecutive cases with special emphasis on esophageal atresia. Ann Surg 2002; 236: 531–539.

119. Spitz L. Gastric transposition via the mediastinal route for infants with long-gap esophageal atresia. J Pediatr Surg 1984; 19: 149–154.

120. Ure BM, Jesch NK, Sümpelmann R, Nustede R. Laparoscopically assisted gastric pull-up for long gap esophageal atresia. J Pediatr Surg 2003; 38: 1661–1662.

121. Ludman L, Spitz L. Quality of life after gastric transposition for oesophageal atresia. J Pediatr Surg 2003; 38: 53–57.

122. Heimlich JH, Winfield JM. The use of a gastric tube to replace or bypass the oesophagus. Surgery 1955; 35: 459–551.

123. Gavriliu D. Aspects of Oesophageal Surgery and Current Problems in Surgery. Yearbook Medical Publishers, Chicago, 1975; 36–64.

124. McCollum MO, Rangel SJ, Blair GK, et al. Primary reversed gastric tube reconstruction in long gap esophageal atesia. J Pediatr Surg 2003; 38: 957–962.

125. Borgnon J, Tounian P, Auber F, et al. Esophageal replacement in children by an isoperistaltic gastric tube: a 12-year experience. Pediatr Surg Int 2004; 20; 829–833.

126. Ring WS, Varco RL, L'Heureaux PR. Esophageal replacement with jejunum in children: an 18 to 33 year follow up. J Thorac Cardiovasc Surg 1982; 83: 918–927.

127. Foker JE, Ring WS, Varco RL. Technique of jejunal interposition for esophageal replacement. J Thorac Cardiovasc Surg 1982; 83: 928–933.

128. Jones BM, Gustavson EH. Free jejnal transfer for reconstruction of the cervical esophagus in children: a report of two cases. Br J Plast Surg 1983; 36: 162–167.

129. Oesch I, Bettex M. Small bowel esophagoplasty without vascular micro-anastomosis: a preliminary report. J Pediatr Surg1987; 22: 877–879.

130. Bax NM, Van Renterghem KM. Ileal pedicle grafting for esophageal replacement in children. Pediatr Surg Int 2005; 21: 369–372.

131. Simms MH, Brearley S, Watson D, Roberts KD. Reconstruction of the oesophagus using a free jejunal graft in complicated atresia. Pediatr Surg Int 1989; 4: 159–161.

132. Najmaldin A, Watanabe Y, Heine RG, et al. Effect of level of circular myotomy on oesophageal function in a piglet model. Pediatr Surg Int 1995; 10: 529–533.

133. Taylor RG, Myers NA. Management of a post-Livaditis-procedure oesophageal diverticulum. Pediatr Surg Int 1989; 4: 238–240.

134. Gough MH. Esophageal atresia – use of an anterior flap in the difficult anastomosis. J Pediatr Surg 1980; 15: 310–311.

135. Foker JE, Kendall TC, Catton K, Khan KM. A flexible approach to achieve a true primary repair for all infants with esophageal atresia. Semin Pediatr Surg 2005; 14: 8–15.

136. Skarsgard ED. Dynamic esophageal lengthening for long gap esophageal atresia: experience with two cases. J Pediatr Surg 2004; 39: 1712–1714.

137. Bowkett B, Beasley SW, Myers NA. The frequency, significance, and management of a right aortic arch in association with esophageal atresia. Pediatr Surg Int 1999; 15: 28–31.

138. Dave S, Shi EC. The management of combined oesophageal and duodenal atresia. Pediatr Surg Int 2004; 20; 689–691.

139. Maoate K, Myers NA, Beasley SW. Gastric perforation in infants with oesophageal atresia and distal tracheo-oesophageal fistula. Pediatr Surg Int 1999; 15: 24–27.

140. Spitz L, Phelan PD. Tracheomalacia. In: Oesophageal Atresia, Beasley SW, Myers NA, Auldist AW (eds). Chapman & Hall Medical, London; 331–340.

141. Weber TR, Keller MS, Fiore A. Aortic suspension (aortopexy) for severe tracheomalacia in infants and children. Am J Surg 2002; 184: 573–577.

142. Kiely EM, Spitz L, Brereton RJ. Management of tracheomalacia by aortopexy. Pediatr Surg Int 1987; 2: 13–15.

143. Spitz L. Dacron patch aortopexy. Prog Paediatr Surg 1986; 19: 117–119.

144. Myers NA, Beasley SW, Auldist AW. Secondary oesophageal surgery following repair of oesophageal atresia with distal tracheo-oesophageal fistula. Pediatr Surg Int 1990; 25: 773–777.

145. D'Urzo C, Buonuomo V, Rando G, Pintus C. Major anastomotic dehiscence after repair of esophageal atresia: conservative management or reoperation? Dis Esophagus 2005; 18: 120–123.

146. Pampino HJ. Endoscopic closure of tracheo-oesophageal fistula. Z Kinderchir 1979; 27: 90–93.

147. Rangecroft L, Bush GH, Lister J, et al. Endoscopic diathermy obliteration of recurrent tracheoesophageal fistulae. J Pediatr Surg 1984; 19: 41–43.

148. Al-Samarrai AY, Jessen K, Haque K. Endoscopic obliteration of a recurrent tracheoesophageal fistula. J Pediatr Surg 1987; 22: 993.

149. Adler DG, Pleskow DK. Closure of a benign tracheoesophageal fistula by using a coated, self-expanding plastic stent in a patient with a history of esophageal atresia. Gastrointest Endosc 2005; 61: 765–768.

150. Esposito C, Langer JC, Schaarschmidt K, et al. Laparoscopic antireflux procedures in the management of gastroesophageal reflux following esophageal atresia repair. J Pediatr Gastroenterol Nutr 2005; 40: 349–351.

151. Koivusalo A, Pakarinen M, Rintala RJ, Lindahl H. Does postoperative pH monitoring predict complicated gastroesophageal reflux in patients with esophageal atresia? Pediatr Surg Int 2004; 20: 670–674.

152. Karnak I, Senocak ME, Hiçsönmez A, Büyükpamukçu N. The diagnosis and treatment of H-type tracheoesophageal fistula. J Pediatr Surg 1997; 32: 1670–1674.

153. Beasley SW, Myers NA. Diagnosis of congenital tracheoesophageal fistula. J Pediatr Surg 1988; 23: 415–417.

154. Kent M, Myers NA, Beasley SW. Tracheo-oesophageal fistula – the "H" fistula. In: Oesophageal Atresia, Beasley SW, Myers NA, Auldist AW (eds). Chapman & Hall Medical, London; 193–207.

155. Garcia NM, Thompson JW, Shaul DB. Definitive localization of isolated tracheoesophageal fistula using bronchoscopy and esophagoscopy for guide wire placement. J Pediatr Surg 1998; 33: 1645–1647.

156. Ko BA, Frederic R, DiTirro PA, et al. Simplified access for division of the low cervical/high thoracic H-type tracheoesophageal fistula. J Pediatr Surg 2000; 35: 1621–1622.

157. Kluth D. Atlas of esophageal atresia. J Pediatr Surg 1976; 11: 901–919.

158. Burren CP, Beasley SW. Oesophageal septum and intramural distal tracheo-oesophageal fistula. Pediatr Surg Int 1990; 5: 198–199.

159. Nihoul- Fékété C, Backer A, Lortat-Jacob, Pellerin D. Congenital esophageal stenosis. Pediatr Surg Int 1987; 2: 86–92.

160. Valerio D, Jones PF, Stewart AM. Congenital oesophageal stenosis. Arch Dis Child 1977; 52: 414–416.

161. Vasudevan SA, Kerendi F, Lee H, Ricketts RR. Management of congenital esophageal stenosis. J Pediatr Surg 2002; 37: 1024–1026.

162. Usui N, Kamata S, Kawahara H, et al. Usefulness of endoscopic ultrasonography in the diagnosis of congenital esophageal stenosis. J Pediatr Surg 2002; 37: 1744–1746.

163. Beasley SW, Myers NA. Trends in mortality in oesophageal atresia. Pediatr Surg Int 1992; 7: 86–89.

164. Konkin DE, O'hali WA, Webber EM, Blair GK. Outcomes in esophageal atresia and tracheoesophageal fistula. J Pediatr Surg 2003; 38: 1726–1729.

165. Bishop PJ, Klein MD, Philippart AI, et al. Transpleural repair of esophageal atresia without a primary gastrostomy: 240 patients treated between 1951 and 1983. J Pediatr Surg 1985; 20: 823–828.

166. Beasley SW, Shann FA, Myers NA, Auldist AW. Developments in the management of oesophageal atresia and/or tracheo-oesophageal fistula. Med J Aust 1989; 150: 501–503.

167. Waterston DJ, Carter RE, Aberdeen E. Oesophageal atresia: tracheo-oesophageal fistula. A study of survival in 218 infants. Lancet 1962; 1: 819–822.

168. Little DC, Rescorla FJ, Grosfeld JL, et al. Long-term analysis of children with esophageal atresia and tracheoesophageal fistula. J Pediatr Surg 2003; 38: 852–856.

169. Andrassy RJ, Patterson RS, Ashley J, et al. Long-term nutritional assessment of patients with esophageal atresia and/or tracheoesophageal fistula. J Pediatr Surg 1983; 18: 431–435.

170. Rickman PP. Infants with esophageal atresia weighing under three pounds. J Pediatr Surg 1981; 16: 595–598.

171. Chetcuti P, Myers NA, Phelan PD, Beasley SW. Adults who survived repair of congenital oesophageal atresia and tracheo-oesophageal fistula. Brit Med J 1988; 297: 344–346.

172. Adzick NS, Fisher JH, Winter HS, et al. Esophageal adenocarcinoma 20 years after esophageal atresia repair. J Pediatr Surg 1989; 24: 741–744.

173. Alfaro L, Bermas H, Fenoglio M, et al. Are patients who have had a tracheoesophageal fistula repair during infancy at risk for esophageal adenocarcinoma during adulthood? J Pediatr Surg 2005; 40: 719–720.

174. Pultrum BB, Bijleveld CM, de Langen ZJ, Plukker JT. Development of an adenocarcinoma of the esophagus 22 years after primary repair of a congenital atresia. J Pediatr Surg 2005; 40: e1–e4.

175. Krug E, Bergmeijer JH, Dees J, et al. Gastroesophageal reflux and Barrett's esophagus in adults born with esophageal atresia. Am J Gastroenterol 1999; 94: 2825–2828.

176. Deurloo JA, Ekkelkamp S, Bartelsman JF, et al. Gastroesophageal reflux: prevalence in adults older than 28 years after correction of esophageal atresia. Ann Surg 2003; 238: 686–689.

177. Deurloo JA, Ekkelkamp S, Taminiau JA, et al. Esophagitis and Barrett esophagus after correction of esophageal atresia. J Pediatr Surg 2005; 40: 1227–1231.

178. Deurloo JA, van Lanschot JJ, Drillenburg P, Aronson DC. Esophageal squamous cell carcinoma 38 years after primary repair of esophageal atresia. J Pediatr Surg 2001; 36: 629–630.

179. Shamberger RC, Eraklis AJ, Kozakewich HP, Hendren WH. Fate of the distal esophageal remnant following esophageal replacement. J Pediatr Surg 1988; 23: 1210–1214.

180. Qureshi R, Norton R. Squamous cell carcinoma in esophageal remnant after 24 years: lessons learnt from esophageal bypass surgery. Dis Esophagus 2000; 13: 245–247.

181. Sauerbruch F. Osophago-dermato-jejuno-gastostomie. In: Chirurgie der Brustorgane. Springer, Berlin, 1925; 568–570.

182. Linder F, Linder M. Krebsige entartung im hauselaugh einer osophagoplastik [Cancerous degeneration in a skin tube of esophagoplasty]. Thoraxchir Vask Chir 1968; 16: 48–55.

183. LaQuaglia MP, Gray M, Schuster SR. Esophageal atresia and ante-thoracic skin tube esophageal conduits: squamous cell carcinoma in the conduit 44 years following surgery. J Pediatr Surg 1987; 22: 44–47.

184. Deurloo JA, Ekkelkamp S, Hartman EE, et al. Quality of life in adult survivors of correction of esophageal atresia. Arch Surg 2005; 140: 976–980.

185. Said M, Mekki M, Golli M, et al. Balloon dilatation of anastomotic strictures secondary to surgical repair of oesophageal atresia. Br J Radiol 2003; 76: 26–31.

23
Esophageal Stricture

Philip Morreau

Introduction

An intact esophagus is a prerequisite for normal feeding. Delay in restoration of esophageal function in early life hinders development of a normal feeding pattern which may have long term consequences. Esophageal strictures in children are rare and should be managed in specialist centers.

Esophageal strictures in children are rarely neoplastic, in contrast to adults. Congenital malformations and gastroesophageal reflux (GER) are the commonest cause of esophageal strictures in children. In some parts of the world caustic strictures are still common.

The natural instinct of the surgeon is to conserve the native esophagus. For most conditions causing esophageal strictures this is correct. However, a considered approach must be taken and for some children repeated operations on a useless esophagus causes only misery to the child and family.[1] The esophagus may still join the mouth to the stomach but the child will not swallow and family life has disintegrated as a result of countless months spent in hospital. The surgeon needs to be aware of this and recognize that there are times when esophageal replacement is the best course of action. The complex subject of esophageal replacement is covered in detail in chapter 24.

Historical Perspective

The earliest written accounts of esophageal surgery come from the Egyptian document the "Smith Surgical Papyrus" unearthed by Edwin Smith in 1862. The papyrus describes management of "a gapping wound with penetrating injury to the gullet".[2] The first esophageal dilatation was carried out by Thomas Willis in 1674 using a cork-tipped whale bone. In 1868 Kussmaul inserted a lighted tube into the esophagus for diagnosis by extending the patient's neck with the help of a sword swallowing entertainer.[3] In nineteenth century, the esophagus was still considered a surgical challenge because of the mortality associated with esophageal resection.

Consequently most surgeons avoided tackling the obstruction and performed an ante-thoracic esophageal replacement.[4] Skin-lined tubes were created in the subcutaneous tissues of the anterior chest wall to connect the cervical esophagus to the stomach. Subsequently intestine was used as an esophageal substitute although an ante-thoracic or retrosternal route was taken to avoid the posterior mediastinum and resection of the stricture.[5] Successful operations for gastroesophageal reflux (GER) appeared in the middle of the last century. Thal described a technique involving incision of a distal esophageal stricture with suture of a serosal fundal patch to the defect.[6]

The development of fiberoptic endoscopes revolutionized the management of esophageal strictures. Safe, accurate endoscopic assessment became possible. Disposable balloon dilators became available in the early 1970's and this opened a new era in the treatment of esophageal strictures.

Etiology

Esophageal strictures in children may be congenital or acquired. Congenital esophageal strictures comprise esophageal webs, areas of fibromuscular dysplasia, and stenoses due to tracheobronchial remnants.[7, 8] Acquired lesions are most commonly postoperative at the site of an anastomosis, secondary to trauma such as alkali burns, or the consequence of gastroesophageal reflux (GER). Less common causes for an acquired stricture include long standing foreign body impaction and following the treatment of esophageal varices by injection sclerotherapy. Aberrations of the great vessels within the chest such as vascular rings or retroesophageal left subclavian artery may mimic an esophageal stricture as may an intramural leiomyoma or a duplication cyst. An alternative classification is to subdivide the causes into extrinsic compression, intramural lesions and abnormality within the lumen itself.

The common causes of esophageal strictures encountered in children are shown in Table 23.1.

D.H. Parikh et al. (eds.), *Pediatric Thoracic Surgery*,
DOI: 10.1007/b136543_23, © Springer-Verlag London Limited 2009

TABLE 23.1. Esophageal strictures.

Congenital strictures	Acquired Strictures
Congenital webs	Corrosive ingestion
Areas of fibromuscular dysplasia	Acid/alkali and household chemicals
Tracheobronchial remnants	Iatrogenic
Collagen diseases	Postanastomosis
Epidermolysis bullosa	Postinstrumental disruption
Congenital lesions causing obstruction	Sclerotherapy for varices
(not stricture)	Peptic esophagitis and stricture
Leiomyoma	Eosinophilic esophagitis
Duplication cysts	Schatzki's ring
Vascular ring	Traumatic strictures
	Foreign body impaction
	Acquired webs

Congenital Lesions

Congenital esophageal stenoses are rare. It is estimated that the incidence is between 1:25000 and 1:50000 live births with either sex equally affected. Congenital strictures due to tracheobronchial remnants are commonly associated with esophageal atresia (9, 10).

Clinical Features and Diagnosis

Children with congenital esophageal strictures typically present with dysphagia and vomiting at the time solids are first introduced into the diet. Neglected cases present with failure to thrive and recurrent respiratory symptoms from aspiration. Frequently there is a delay in diagnosis.[11]

A Barium swallow will reveal a narrowing. The location of the stricture may give a clue to the cause (Fig. 23.1). Strictures related to tracheobronchial remnants usually occur in the distal esophagus and show as a localized narrowing close to the cardia. Fibromuscular disease typically results in a more tapered narrowing compared with the abrupt narrowing of a tracheobronchial remnant but these differences are subtle and not universal. Strictures from esophageal webs and fibromuscular dysplasia may be more proximal but there is overlap in the appearances and position of all three entities and the radiological findings alone is not diagnostic.

The histological findings in tracheobronchial remnants are those of mature or immature cartilage and seromucinous bronchial glands along with ciliated epithelium. Fibromuscular hyperplasia is associated with proliferation of smooth muscle and varying degrees of fibrosis in the muscular wall of the esophagus. An esophageal web comprises a thin membrane of squamous epithelium.

Differentiation of congenital strictures from inflammatory strictures due to GER may be difficult. The endoscopic appearance, mucosal biopsy findings and the response to dilatation are all important. Tracheobronchial remnants show as an abrupt distal narrowing with no esophagitis that does not yield to dilatation. Endoesophageal ultrasound is a more recent method for the differentiation of tracheobronchial

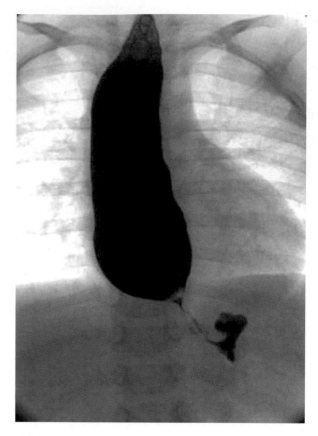

FIG. 23.1. Contrast swallow showing a dilated esophagus with a stricture at the lower end in an infant. Endoscopy ruled out peptic esophagitis. The stricture proved unresponsive to balloon dilatation. A cartilaginous ring was found at the gastroesophageal junction and this was confirmed histologically

remnants from other causes of esophageal stricture but use in children is still very limited.[7, 11]

Management

Strictures due to tracheobronchial remnants invariably require resection whereas esophageal webs respond well to dilation alone. Strictures caused by fibromuscular dysplasia will dilate but the response if usually temporary. The pragmatic approach is to dilate the stricture and assess the response. A stricture that will not respond to dilatation or early recurrence of symptoms following 2–3 dilatations constitute indications for resection. Failure to appreciate this risks perforation due to the unyielding nature of the stenosis and frustration on the part of the surgeon.[8, 12]

The operative approach for resection of an esophageal stricture is via the chest or the abdomen, depending on the location of the stenosis. A segmental resection of 1–2.5 cm esophagus followed by immediate anastomosis is the procedure of choice.[9] At the time of surgery the esophagus is encircled and the abnormality inspected and palpated. A balloon dilator in the lumen of the esophagus may assist identification of the stenosis as the external appearances are often normal. If there is still difficulty identifying the stricture intraoperative endoscopy can be very useful. Enucleation of a tracheobronchial remnant from the esophageal wall has been described as has a myotomy in strictures due to fibromuscular dysplasia.[13] Specific post operative complications include anastomotic leakage, recurrent stenosis and GER if the sphincter mechanism has been disrupted.

Acquired Lesions

Peptic Stricture

Gastroesophageal reflux (GER) is very common in infancy and generally resolves spontaneously. Not all GER is benign and recognized complications include hemorrhage, stricture formation, recurrent respiratory symptoms, Barrett's change and ultimately carcinoma. First line treatment is medical and surgical management is reserved for failed medical therapy and complications of GER. Severe peptic esophageal disease with stricture is now relatively uncommon.

Pathogenesis

Untreated acid reflux into the lower esophagus initially results in inflammatory changes confined to the mucosa. In chronic peptic esophagitis deeper structural damage takes place with destruction of the muscular fibers and replacement by fibrosis. The lower esophageal sphincter (LES) can be destroyed in the process and both circumferential and longitudinal contraction of the esophagus occurs. A hiatus hernia can result if there is significant shortening of the esophagus. Microscopically, the mucosa and submucosa are infiltrated with chronic inflammatory cells. Fibrosis appears in the muscle layer. Periesophagitis, mucosal ulceration and increased vascularization as a result of chronic inflammation may cause recurrent bleeding.

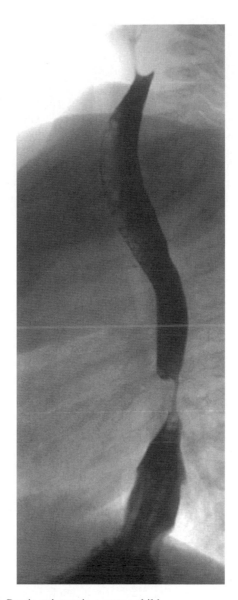

FIG. 23.2. Peptic stricture in a young child

Clinical Features and Diagnosis

Dysphagia, vomiting, slow feeding, failure to thrive, and sometimes respiratory symptoms due to aspiration are the usual symptoms in a child with an esophageal stricture. Dysphagia is usually of insidious onset and progressive in nature. In most cases failure to thrive is subtle and not associated with significant protein caloric malnutrition. Anemia is invariably present due to recurrent bleeding from esophagitis. Food bolus impaction can occur but is relatively uncommon in children with peptic strictures alone. Dysphagia is hard to appreciate in infancy when the diet is predominantly milk.

A stricture is usually identified first on an upper GI contrast study or during an upper GI endoscopy (Fig. 23.2). The contrast study will also provide useful information about gastric emptying and intestinal rotation. The majority of peptic strictures are in the distal third of the esophagus although strictures

in the proximal third may also occur. Endoscopy is mandatory and biopsies should be taken to support the diagnosis and look for Barrett's epithelial changes. The magnitude of the reflux can be confirmed with an ambulatory 24 hour pH study.

Management

Proton pump inhibitors should be started as soon as a peptic stricture is diagnosed although this is not adequate treatment alone.[14] Intralesional steroid injection (triamcinolone) may improve the response of the stricture to dilation.[15] However, a peptic esophageal stricture is generally considered to be an absolute indication for antireflux surgery to give long term disease control.[14,16] Indefinite treatment with proton pump inhibitors might be considered an alternative to surgery but data on the long term efficacy and safety of this medication is only available for up to 2 years in children and 11 years in adults.[17]

Schatzki's Rings

Schatzki and Gray described mucosal rings in the lower esophagus rings on contrast swallow[18]. These are seen endoscopically just above the squamo-columnar junction of the esophagus. Histologically a Schatzki ring shows infiltration of chronic inflammatory cells within the submucosa with little changes in the mucosa or the muscular layers. Manometric studies in adults suggest a second area of high pressure in the region of the ring, separate from the LES.[19] Many authors have noted an association between Schatzki rings and GER and a small hiatus hernia although a causal relation is disputed by others.[20]

Pain during swallowing is the predominant feature of a Schatzki ring. Symptoms usually resolve with proton pump inhibitors. Occasionally dilatation and rarely antireflux surgery are necessary.

Eosinophilic esophagitis

Eosinophilic esophagitis (EE) is reported with increasing frequency in the western world.[21] Eosinophilic esophagitis is reported in young children with dysphagia. Food bolus impaction is also well recognized.[22] This condition is also reported after repair of esophageal atresia.[23]

The diagnosis of eosinophilic esophagitis is confirmed by examination of an esophageal biopsy. [24, 25, 26, 27] The characteristic histological feature is a dense eosinophilic infiltrate (more than 20 eosinophils per high power field).[28] The esophageal mucosa often has a granular appearance visible at endoscopy. Erythema, whitening, ulceration (29) and linear furrowing are also recognized endoscopic signs.[30] Sometimes the endoscopic appearance is normal and the diagnosis is made only on microscopic examination.

Management

Topical steroids provide effective symptomatic relief from eosinophilic esophagitis. Fluticasone swallowed from an asthma inhaler is a convenient method for delivering this. [31] Hypoallergenic elemental milk formulas and oral steroids are also effective.[27, 32, 33]. Eosinophilic esophagitis generally responds poorly to standard antireflux medications. Liacouras et al. demonstrated, in a prospective study of 20 patients with EE, histological improvement with a four-week course of oral methylprednisolone.[33] Faubion et al reported success with inhaled corticosteroids. [28] Sodium cromoglycate is effective in some children although no controlled series are available.[34] Esophageal perforation has been reported with an increased frequency following diagnostic endoscopy and dilatation in children with EE.[35, 36]

Post-anastomotic strictures

Primary repair of esophageal atresia stands out as one of the major advances in pediatric surgery in the twentieth century. Survival is now the norm although anastomotic strictures are reported in as many as 50% of the survivors.[37]

The occurrence of a stricture at the anastomosis remains a troublesome surgical problem (Fig.23.3). Contributory factors include tension at the anastomosis, mucosal ischemia, GER, and impaired esophageal motility.

Management

Infants with an anastomotic narrowing should be started on proton pump inhibitors, and the stricture dilated. Many would suggest that acid suppression therapy should be started prophylactically in all infants recovering from esophageal atresia repair. Once a stricture is discovered dilatation is usually necessary and may need to be repeated. Intralesional injection of triamcinolone may facilitate management of refractory strictures. In general the response to dilatation and medical control of GER is excellent.[37, 38, 39, 40] Recurrent stenosis should be managed by laparoscopic fundoplication.

Dystrophic Epidermolysis Bullosa and Esophageal Stricture

Children with epidermolysis bullosa (EB) present with a wide variety of upper gastrointestinal symptoms. The incidence of EB is 1:300,000 live births and the condition is a genetically inherited abnormality of collagen. There are various subtypes of EB including simple disease, junctional EB, and dystrophic EB. Mucosal lesions are mainly seen in junctional and dystrophic EB. Esophageal involvement is found most commonly in dystrophic EB.[41, 42] The genetic defect in EB makes the mucosa vulnerable to repeated friction injury during swallowing of food boluses, causing oral blisters, dysphagia, esophageal stricture, microstomia, pyrosis, dental caries, and lingual adhesions.[43]There is a spectrum of esophageal involvement varying from erosions to ulceration and stricture formation.

Clinical Features and Diagnosis

Painful swallowing in a child with EB suggests mucosal disease with ulceration, although pain may also occur from esophageal spasm. Dysphagia caused by a stricture is a chronic progressive condition. Anemia is common in children with EB, in part because of an inadequate diet. Food bolus impaction, recurrent pulmonary aspiration, spontaneous esophageal perforation and hemorrhage are all reported complications of esophageal strictures in children with EB.

The commonest site for an esophageal stricture in children with EB is at the level of the cricopharyngeus (Fig. 23.4). Less frequently strictures occur in mid-esophagus and at the gastroesophageal junction.[42] Upper GI endoscopy is contraindicated because of the risk of mucosal trauma and a contrast swallow is the investigation of choice. This investigation may

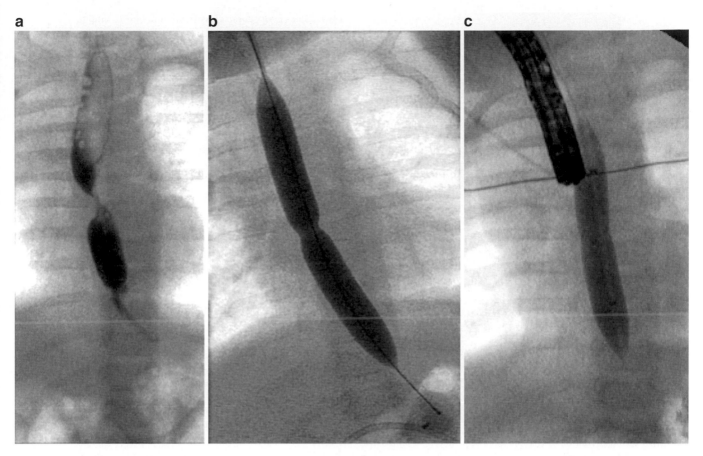

FIG. 23.3. Anastomotic stricture after long gap esophageal atresia repair by delayed primary anastomosis. Figures (**a**), (**b**) and (**c**) show the stricture before, during and after balloon dilatation. Note radioopaque contrast medium in the balloon in figure (**b**). Contrast medium and the fiberoptic endoscope are visible in figure (**c**), which confirms that the esophagus is intact post-dilatation

also show GER, mucosal edema, esophageal spasm and areas of ulceration. Pseudo-diverticula involving the esophagus have also been reported.[44, 45]

Management

The prognosis for children with EB complicated by esophageal stricture has improved substantially as a result of better general care, particularly attention to nutrition.[46, 47] Prior to the development of balloon dilators the management of esophageal strictures in these children was controversial and generally unsatisfactory. The risks of exacerbating the stricture by endoscopy and bouginage were recognized with the result that esophageal replacement was considered the only option.[48, 49, 50] Bouginage is contraindicated in EB because the tangential shearing forces cause detachment of the mucosa and further scarring. Flexible endoscopy is best avoided for the same reason.

Balloon dilatation is now the treatment of choice for esophageal strictures complicating EB.[51] A guidewire should be negotiated through the stricture under fluoroscopic control and then an appropriate sized balloon catheter used for dilatation.

The balloon is kept inflated for as short a time as possible and deflated immediately the stricture is fully dilated. The inflation time should not exceed 5 seconds to minimize injury to intact mucosa adjacent to the stricture. Balloon dilatation is well tolerated in children with EB. It can be performed safely, repeatedly with minimal injury to the intact esophagus and pharynx and with a short hospital stay.[52]

High dose corticosteroids have been recommended by some authors to reduce edema and may reduce the recurrence rate.[53] Phenytoin may reduce the risk of skin blistering and it has been used to reduce the risk of esophageal structure.[54]

Esophageal dilatation requires general anesthesia and great care must be taken to avoid iatrogenic skin damage. Conventional adhesive tape used to secure intravenous lines and endotracheal tube cannot be used, nor can conventional EKG electrodes.[55]

Esophageal replacement is now rarely necessary in children with EB. Indications for esophageal replacement are restricted to recalcitrant strictures unresponsive to serial dilatation and esophageal perforation with mediastinitis.[56]

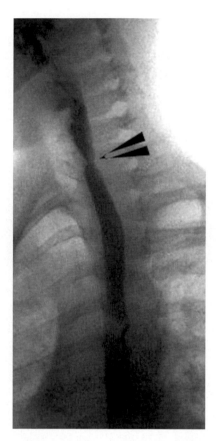

FIG. 23.4. Stricture in the upper esophagus in a child with epidermolysis bullosa and dysphagia

Corrosive strictures

Worldwide caustic strictures remain the commonest cause of esophageal stricture in children. The majority occur in children are under the age of five and boys are more often affected than girls.[57, 58] In the western world caustic strictures are now uncommon as a result of child-proof containers and home safety education. Regrettably this is not the case in developing countries. [59, 60] A number of household agents cause esophageal burns including caustic soda, battery acid, kitchen detergents, potassium permanganate, potassium chloride, sodium benzoate, aspirin, iodine, paint strippers, Clinitest tablets and hair dye products.

Pathogenesis

Ingestion of alkali causes liquifactive necrosis with deep penetration of the tissues whereas acid causes coagulative necrosis which is relatively more superficial. The lips, mouth, pharynx, epiglottis, larynx, and upper gastrointestinal tract are all commonly damaged as a result of caustic ingestion. The corrosive effect will vary depending upon the chemical composition of the caustic agent, the amount taken and the contact time. Household dishwashing machine detergents are often granular and typically cause injury to the oropharynx. Damage to the esophagus results in intense inflammation, infection and later fibrosis.

TABLE 23.2. Endoscopic classification of caustic injury.

Stage I: mucosal damage with redness
Stage II: ulceration, focal necrosis, and petechiae; sometimes changes can be seen extending into the muscle layers
Stage III: extensive necrosis and bleeding, with black or brown circumferential mucosal discoloration
Stage IV: complete carbonization of the mucosa

Full thickness necrosis may occur with perforation of the esophagus or stomach and, rarely, fistulation into the airway or aorta. The severity of a caustic injury can be classified based on endoscopic evaluation (Table 23.2). This has been used to predict the likelihood of stricture formation.[61]

Clinical features and Diagnosis

Any child presenting after accidental ingestion of a corrosive should be assumed to have an esophageal injury. Most children will be drooling saliva and burns around the lips may be evident although their absence does not exclude a significant esophageal injury. Endoscopy should be performed within the first 48 hours, providing the general condition of the child is satisfactory and there is no suggestion of perforation.[62] Cervical surgical emphysema, mediastinal air, mediastinal widening and a pleural effusion are all radiological signs on a chest X-ray that suggest perforation.

At endoscopy the nature of the injury is determined. The depth of the injury, the length of esophagus involved and the presence of circumferential burn injury should be noted. Using the scoring system in Table 23.2 the severity of the injury can be assessed. The stomach should also be examined because caustic injury may involve the stomach and pylorus in severe cases. If minimal injury is present the child is allowed to feed following recovery from the anesthetic.

An upper gastro-intestinal contrast swallow should be arranged in all children with endoscopic abnormalities. The examination should be performed at around 3–4 weeks post injury because this corresponds to the most likely time of stricture formation.[63] The study may show a stricture has already developed. An area of esophagus which atonic or spastic and indistensible is likely to stricture.[64,65] Repeat endoscopy should be performed in these children and dilations planned if necessary.

Management

The immediate management of a child with a caustic injury to the esophagus starts with assessment of the airway, breathing and circulation. The chemical nature of the substance ingested should be ascertained. Aspiration of corrosive agents may damage the larynx and airway as well as producing a chemical pneumonitis. Any suggestion of airway involvement should be confirmed by early airway endoscopy. Because of the potential for glottic edema endotracheal intubation and mechanical ventilation should be instituted early.

Caustic injuries are very painful and adequate analgesia with opiates is essential. The use of systemic steroids does not prevent stricture formation.[66]

A nasogastric tube can be inserted at the time of the first endoscopy. This allows enteral feeding to be resumed before the child is willing to swallow by mouth. The tube also maintains a track through the esophagus which may facilitate subsequent dilatation. Alternatively a Stamm gastrostomy can be opened. Care should be taken when siting the gastrotomy to avoid the greater curve which would make future esophageal replacement more difficult. Gastroesophageal reflux is common in children with caustic strictures and this exacerbates the esophageal damage. Control of GER with proton pump inhibitors prolongs the response to dilatation.[67,68]

The majority of caustic strictures can be managed by esophageal dilation (Fig.23.5). Relative contraindications to dilatation include a stricture > 5 cm long, a stricture which is markedly tortuosity and friable. Occasionally it is impossible to negotiate a stricture from above and in this situation retrograde dilatation through a gastrostomy is usually successful. Retrograde dilatation can be facilitated by leaving a string through the stricture.[60]

The stricture is gradually dilated at weekly and then fortnightly intervals until the caliber of the esophagus stabilizes. The frequency of dilatation can then be reduced although usually it is necessary to persist with dilatations for 6–12 months before deciding on the success or failure of this plan. There is anecdotal evidence that injection of a long-acting steroid (triamcinolone) into the stricture prior to balloon dilation reduces the recurrence rate. [68,69,70] Topical Mitomycin-C may also have a role in the management of difficult strictures.[71] The likely mode of action of both agents is suppression of granulation tissue and fibrosis.

There is little consensus regarding when to abandon dilatation in favor of esophageal replacement. Setting a time limit alone is overly simplistic. The frequency of dilatation,

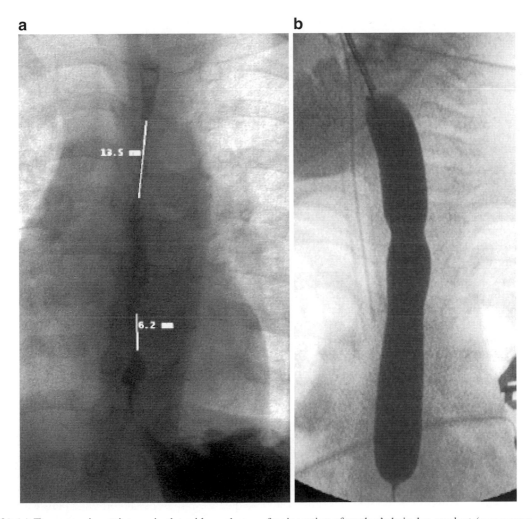

FIG. 23.5. (a, b) (a) Two corrosive strictures in the mid-esophagus after ingestion of mother's hair dye product (measurements correspond to the length of each stricture).(b) Balloon dilatation showing a minor residual waist at the site of one of the stricture. Despite a guide wire perforation, which was treated conservatively, the strictures responded to repeated dilatations and intralesional steroid injections. The child is now tolerating a normal diet

progress, appearance and caliber of the esophagus, the impact of repeated hospitalization on the child and family and the occurrence of complications should all be considered. The most common acute complication is perforation which occurs in 1–18% cases.[1, 63] If perforation is suspected following dilatation a chest X-ray should be performed immediately and intravenous fluids and antibiotics started. A contrast swallow will be diagnostic. The perforation may seal with conservative management if it is small and the esophagus is in relatively good condition but often the perforation has to be repaired surgically. Guide wire perforation can usually be managed conservatively.

Esophageal Dilation

Bouginage

The traditional method of dilating an esophageal stricture is by bouginage. A variety of dilators are available (mercury loaded tip, gum elastic) in varying sizes. Passage of a bougie achieves dilatation with a tangential force. The main difficulty with bouginage is negotiating the dilator into the stricture and occasionally it may be necessary to do this with a retrograde approach via a gastrostomy. Bouginage is an effective, quick, cheap and, in experienced hands, safe method of managing esophageal strictures.

Bouginage in children requires general anesthesia. The esophagus is intubated with a rigid esophagoscope and the stricture identified. A lubricated bougie is gently passed through the stricture under direct vision. The diameter of the stricture can be calibrated using the largest bougie which will pass through the stricture without resistance. This should be recorded each time dilatation is performed. It is wise to limit the dilatation in one sitting to a dilator a maximum of three sizes larger than the dilator used to calibrate the stricture. This minimizes the risk of perforation. Minimal pressure should be applied to the dilator.

Techniques then evolved by first establishing the lumen using a guide wire, and confirming this with the image intensifier, before the passage of a dilator. Excellent results can be obtained (63).

Balloon dilation

Balloon dilatation has now replaced bouginage as the method of choice for esophageal dilatation in many centers. Balloon dilatation has several merits. A flexible guide wire is negotiated through the stricture using fluoroscopic control. The guide wire remains in place throughout the dilatation which avoids the risk of creating a false passage with the dilator. A balloon dilator applies a radial force to the stricture which, theoretically, should be more efficient. Progress of the dilatation can be monitored fluoroscopically. The principle disadvantage of balloon dilatation is the absence of tactile feedback during dilatation. Large series now attest to the safety of balloon dilatation in children.[72, 73, 74]

Balloon dilatation can be performed in the X-ray department. However, most surgeons prefer to perform the procedure in the operating room with a mobile image intensifier. The esophagus is inspected with a flexible endoscope. Once the stricture is encountered an appropriate sized balloon catheter is selected and passed through the working channel of the endoscope and across the stricture. The position of the guide wire and balloon is confirmed radiologically and visually with the endoscope. The balloon is inflated with a 50:50 mixture of water soluble contrast and saline using a Levene inflating syringe with a threaded plunger and a pressure gauge fitted (Fig. 24.3b, c). Balloon inflation is observed both by direct vision and radiologically. A waist appears in the balloon as it is inflated which confirms the stricture is engaged. As the balloon is inflated to its rated pressure the stricture is dilated. Successful dilatation is achieved when the waist on the balloon is abolished. The balloon should remain inflated for 60 seconds before deflation. Incremental dilatation with balloons of increasing size is safer than using a single large dilator. After dilatation the stricture is inspected with the endoscope to exclude perforation.

The instrument channel in small pediatric endoscopes is too small to accommodate a balloon catheter. An alternative approach is to cannulate the stricture with a guide wire passed through the endoscope. The endoscope is then withdrawn over the guide wire, which remains in place. This necessitates using a guide wire which is 260 cm long. The balloon dilator is then threaded over the guidewire. The endoscope can be inserted alongside the guidewire and balloon to provide visual confirmation but it is quite acceptable to rely on fluoroscopic guidance.

Although the esophagus is examined with the endoscope after dilation it is wise to perform a chest X-ray and water-soluble contrast study post operatively if there is any suspicion of perforation. As with bouginage, esophageal balloon dilatation should take place in a progressive fashion. Dilatation should advance in increments of no more than 2 mm. The diameter of the normal esophagus is equal to the diameter of the owner's thumb.[74]

Summary

Congenital strictures of the esophagus tend to be associated with other congenital anomalies of the esophagus and gastrointestinal tract. Acquired lesions are more common, especially in developing countries where caustic ingestion remains the most likely cause. The rapidity with which a child presents with obstructive symptoms depends on age and consistency of the diet. Respiratory symptoms and failure to thrive often predominate in infancy. A contrast swallow is the investigation of first choice. Treatment is tailored to the cause. Dilatation, stricture resection and fundoplication are all effective and safe operative procedures which will restore esophageal function.

References

1. Hamaza AF, Adelhay S, Sheif H, et al. Caustic oesophageal strictures in children: 30 year's experience. J Pediatr Surg 2003; 38: 276–281.

2. Breasted JH. The Edwin Smith Surgical Papyrus. University of Chicago Oriental institute publications. University of Chicago Press, Chicago, Il. 1930; 46: 312–316.

3. Mark G. Gastroenterology and nutrition. Gastroenterologic endoscopy in children: Past, present and future. Curr Op Pediatr 2001; 13: 429–434.

4. Othersen HB, Parker EF, Smith CD. The Surgical Management of Esophageal Stricture in Children: A Century of Progress. Ann Surg 1988; 207: 590–596.

5. Ochsner A, Owens N. Antethoracic oesophagoplasty for impermeable stricture of the oesophagus. Ann Surg 1934; 100: 1055–1091.

6. Thal AP, Hatafuku T, Kurtzman R. New operation for distal esophageal stricture. Arch Surg 1965; 90: 464–472.

7. Nihoul-Fekete C, de Bracker A, Lortat-Jacob S, et al. Congenital esophageal stenosis: a review of 20 cases. Pediatr Surg Int 1987; 2: 86–92.

8. Ibrahim A, Al Malki TA, Hamaza AF, Bahnassy AF. Congenital esophageal stenosis associated with esophageal atresia: new concepts. Pediatr Surg Int 2007; 23: 533–537.

9. Yeung CK, Spitz L, Brereton R, et al. Congenital esophageal stenosis due to tracheobronchial remnants: a rare but important association with esophageal atresia. J Pediatr Surg 1992; 27: 852–855

10. Zhao L, Hsieh WS, Hsu WM. Congenital esophageal stenosis due to tracheobronchial remnants. J Pediatr Surg 2004; 39: 1183–1187

11. Usui N, Kamata S, Kawahara H, et al. Usefulness of endoscopic ultrasound in the diagnosis of congenital esophageal stenosis. J Pediatr Surg 2002; 37: 1744–1746

12. Amae S, Tio M, Kamiyama T, et al. Clinical characteristics and management of congenital esophageal stenosis: a report of 14 cases. J Pediatr Surg 2003; 38: 565–570.

13. Takamizawa S, Tsugawa C, Mouri N, et al. Congenital Esophageal stenosis: therapeutic strategy based on etiology. J Pediatr Surg 2002; 37: 197–201

14. Numanoglu A, Millar AJW, Brown RA, et al. Gastroesophageal reflux strictures in children, management and outcome. Pediatr Surg Int 2005; 21, 631–634.

15. Berenson G, Wyllie R, Caulfield M, et al. Intralesional steroids in the treatment of refractory esophageal strictures. J Pediatr Gastroenterol Nutr 1994; 18: 250–252.

16. Tovar JA, Luis AL, Encinas JL, et al. Pediatric Surgeons and gastroesophageal reflux. J Pediatr Surg 2007; 42: 277–283

17. Hassel E. Decisions in diagnosing and managing chronic gastroesophageal reflux disease in Children. J Pediatr 2005; 146: S3–12.

18. Schatzki R, Gray JE. Dysphagia due to a diaphragm like localised narrowing in the lower oesophagus: "lower oesophageal ring". Am J Roentgenol 1953; 70: 911–922.

19. Jeyasingham, K. Benign strictures of the esophagus. In: General Thoracic Surgery, 4th edition. Shields T (ed). Williams & Wilkins, Philadelphia, PA, 1994; 1594–1611.

20. Goyal RK, Bauer JL, Spiro HM. The nature and location of lower esophageal rings. N Engl J Med 1971; 284: 1175–1180.

21. Noel RJ, Rothenberg ME. Eosinophilic esophagitis. Curr Opin Pediatr 2005; 17: 690–694.

22. Desai TK, Stecevic V, Chang CH, et al. Association of eosinophilic inflammation with esophageal food impaction in adults. Gastrointest Endosc 2005; 61: 795–801.

23. Batres AL, Liacouras C, Schnaufer L, Mascarenhas MR. Eosinophilic esophagitis associated with anastomotic strictures after esophageal atresia repair. J Pediatr Gastroenterol Nutr 2002; 35: 224–226.

24. Potter JW, Saeian K, Staff D, et al. Eosinophilic esophagitis in adults: an emerging problem with unique esophageal features. Gastrointest Endosc 2004; 59: 355–361.

25. Croese J, Fairley SK, Masson JW, et al. Clinical and endoscopic features of eosinophilic esophagitis in adults. Gastrointest Endosc 2003; 58: 516–22.

26. Parfitt JR, Gregor JC, Suskin NG, et al. Eosinophilic esophagitis in adults: distinguishing features from gastroesophageal reflux disease: a study of 41 patients. Mod Pathol 2006; 19: 90–96.

27. Liacouras C, Markowitz J. Eosinophilic esophagitis: A subset of eosinophilic gastroenteritis. Curr Gastroenterol Rep 1999; 1: 253–258.

28. Faubion WJ, Perrault J, Burgart L, et al. Treatment of eosinophilic esophagitis with inhaled corticosteroids. J Pediatr Gastroenterol Nutr 1998; 27: 118–119.

29. Orenstein S, Shalaby T, Lorenzo CD, et al. The spectrum of pediatric eosinophilic esophagitis beyond infancy: a clinical series of 30 children. Am J Gastroenterol 2000; 95: 1422–1430.

30. Gupta SK, Fitzgerald JF, Chong SK, et al. Vertical lines in distal esophageal mucosa (VLEM): a true endoscopic manifestation of esophagitis in children? Gastrointest Endosc 1997; 45: 485–489.

31. Noel RJ, Putnam PE, Collins MH, et al. Clinical and immunopathologic effects of swallowed fluticasone for eosinophilic esophagitis. Clin Gastroenterol Hepatol 2004; 2: 568–575.

32. Kelly K, Lazenby A, Rowe P, et al. Eosinophilic esophagitis attributed to gastroesophageal reflux: improvement with an amino acid-based formula. Gastroenterology 1995; 109: 1503–1512.

33. Liacouras C, Wenner W, Brown K, et al. Primary eosinophilic esophagitis in children: successful treatment with oral corticosteroids. J Pediatr Gastroenterol Nutr 1998; 26: 380–5.

34. Perez-Millan A, Martin-Lorente JL, Lopez-Morante A, et al. Subserosal eosinophilic gastroenteritis treated efficaciously with sodium cromoglycate. Dig Dis Sci 1997; 42: 342–344.

35. Straumann A, Rossi L, Simon HU, et al. Fragility of the esophageal mucosa: a pathognomonic endoscopic sign of primary eosinophilic esophagitis? Gastrointest Endosc 2003; 57: 407–412.

36. Kaplan M, Mutlu EA, Jakate S, et al. Endoscopy in eosinophilic esophagitis: "feline" esophagus and perforation risk. Clin Gastroenterol Hepatol 2003; 1: 433–437.

37. Konkin DE, O'Hali WA, Webber EM, et al. Outcomes in esophageal atresia and tracheo esophageal fistula J Pediatr Surg 2003; 38: 1726–1729.

38. Bregmeijer JHJJ, Tibboel D, Hazebroek FWJ. Nissen fundoplication in the management of gastroesophageal reflux occurring after repair of esophageal atresia. J Pediatr Surg 2000; 35: 573–576

39. Wheatley MJ, Coran AG, Wesley JR. Efficacy of the Nissen fundoplication in the management of gastroesophageal reflux following esophageal atresia repair. J Pediatr Surg 1993; 28: 53–55.

40. Myers NA, Beasley SW, Auldist AW, et al. Secondary esophageal surgery following repair of esophageal atresia with distal tracheo esophageal fistula: long term results following repair of esophageal atresia by end to end anastomosis and ligation of tracheo-esophageal fistula. J Pediatr Surg 1990; 25: 773–777.

41. Lin AN, Carter DM. Epidermolysis bullosa: when the skin falls apart. J Pediatr 1989; 112: 349–355.

42. Orlando RC, Bonzymski EM, Brignnaman RA, et al. Epidermolysis bullosa: gastrointestinal manifestations. Ann Intern Med 1974; 81: 203–206.

43. Travis SPL, McGrath JA. Turnball AJ, et al. Oral and gastrointestinal manifestations of epidermolysis bullosa. Lancet 1992; 340: 1505–1506.

44. Agha FP, Francis JR, Ellis CN. Esophageal involvement in epidermolysis bullosa dystrophica: clinical and roentgenographic manifestations. Gastrointest Radiol 1983; 8: 11–17.

45. Hahn AL. Esophageal epidermolysis bullosa dystrophica? Ann Intern Med 1975; 82: 427.

46. Haynes L, Atherton DJ, Ade-Ajayi N, et al. Gastrostomy and growth in dystrophic epidermolysis Bullosa. Br J Dermatol 1996; 134: 872–879.

47. Kay M, Wyllie R. Endoscopic dilatation of esophageal stricture in recessive epidermolysis bullosa: new equipment, new technique. J Pediatr Gastroenterol Nutr 2002; 34: 515–518.

48. Schuman BM, Arciniegas E. The management of esophageal complications of epidermolysis bullosa. Am J Dig Dis 1972; 17: 875–80.

49. Fonkalsrud EW, Ament ME. Surgical management of esophageal stricture due to recessive dystrophic epidermolysis bullosa. J Pediatr Surg 1977; 12: 221–226.

50. Harmel RP Jr. Esophageal replacement in two siblings with epidermolysis bullosa. J Pediatr Surg 1986; 21: 175–176.

51. Fujimoto T, Lane GJ, Miyano T, at al. Esophageal strictures in children with recessive dystrophic epidermolysis bullosa: experience with balloon dilatation in nine cases. J Pediatr Gastroenterol Nutr 1998; 27: 524–529.

52. Castillo RO, Davies YK, Lin Y-C, et al. Management of oesophageal stricture in children with recessive dystrophic epidermolysis bullosa. J Pediatr Gastroenterol Nutr 2002; 34: 535–541.

53. Katz J, Gryboski J, Rosenbaum HM, Spine HM. Dysphagia in children with epidermolysis bullosa. Gastroenterology 1967: 52: 259–262.

54. Feurle GE, Weidauer H, Baldauf G, et al. Management of oesophageal stenosis in recessive dystrophic epidermolysis bullosa. Gastroenterology 1984; 87: 1376–1380.

55. Culpepper TL. Anesthetic implications in epidermolysis bullosa dystrophica. AANA J 2001; 69: 114–118.

56. Demirogllari B, Sonmez K, Turkyilmaz Z, et al. Colon interposition for esophageal stenosis in a patient with epidermolysis bullosa. J Pediatr Surg 2001; 36: 1861–1863.

57. Spitz L, Lakhoo K. Caustic ingestions. Arch Dis Child 1993; 68: 157–158.

58. Fyfe AH, Auldist AW. Corrosive ingestion in children. Z Kinderchir 1984; 39, 229–233.

59. Gupta DK, Srinivas M, Dave S, Lall A. An epidemiological survey on corrosive esophageal strictures in children. J Indian Assoc Pediatr Surg 2003; 8: 80–85.

60. Cywes S. Corrosive strictures of the oesophagus in children. Pediatr Surg Int 1993; 8: 8–13.

61. Di Constanzo J, Noirclerc M. New therapeutic approach to corrosive burns of the upper gastro-intestinal tract. Gut 1980; 21: 370–375.

62. Dogan Y, Erkan T, Cokugas FC, Kutlu T. Caustic Gastroesophageal lesions in childhood: an analysis of 473 Cases. Clin Pediatr 2006; 45: 435–438.

63. Kukkady A. Pease PWB. Long-term dilatation of caustic strictures of the esophagus. Pediatr Surg Int 2002; 18: 486–490.

64. Franken EA. Caustic damage of the gastrointestinal tract: Roentgen features. AM J Roentgenol 1973; 118: 77–85.

65. Kuhn JR, Tunell WP. The role of cineesophagography in caustic esophageal injury. Am J Surg 1983; 146: 108–111.

66. Anderson KD, Rouse TM, Randolph JG. A controlled trial of corticosteroids in children with corrosive injury of the esophagus. N Engl J Med 1990; 323: 637–640.

67. Said A, Burst DJ, Gaumnitz EA, Reichelderfer M. Predictors of early recurrence of benign esophageal strictures. Am J Gastroenterol 2003; 98: 1252–1256.

68. Rodreiguez-Baez N, Anderson JM. Management of esophageal strictures in children. Curr Treat Op Gastroenterol 2003; 6: 414–425.

69. Engin A, Sabite K, Bilge T, et al. Intralesional steroid injection in benign esophageal strictures resistant to bougie dilation. J Gastroenterol Hepatol 2004; 19: 1388–1391.

70. Kochar R. Usefulness of intralesional triamcinolone in treatment of benign of esophageal strictures. Gastrointest Endosc 2002; 56: 829–834.

71. Kumar A, Bhatnagar V. Topical application of mitomycin-C in corrosive esophageal strictures. J Indian Assoc Pediatr Surg 2005; 10: 25–27.

72. Lan LCL, Wong KKY, Lin SCL, et al. Endoscopic balloon dilatation of esophageal strictures in infants and children;17 years experience and a literature review. J Pediatr Surg 2003; 38: 1712–1715.

73. Tam PKH, Sprigg A, Cudmore RE, et al. Endoscopy-guided balloon dilatation of esophageal strictures and anastomotic strictures after esophageal replacement in children J Pediatr Surg 1991; 26: 1101–1103.

74. London RL, Trotman BW, Di Marino AJ, et al. Dilation of severe esophageal strictures by an inflatable balloon catheter. Gastroenterology 1981; 80: 173–175.

24
Esophageal Replacement

Juan Carlos Pattillo and Alex W. Auldist

Introduction

It is well established that there is no better conduit than the native esophagus[1] but there are some conditions in which the native esophagus cannot be preserved and needs to be replaced. The main indications for esophageal replacement in the pediatric population are *long-gap esophageal atresia* (LGEA) and severe *esophageal strictures*. There are several options for replacement depending on the organ (i.e., stomach, colon, jejunum) and the route used (i.e., subcutaneous, retrosternal, transhiatal).

The ideal esophageal replacement

- Allows normal swallowing
- Does not become redundant and tortuous
- Does not cause respiratory embarrassment
- Technically simple to perform
- Low morbidity and possible in small children/infants
- Minimal GER in the conduit and low risk of future malignancy

---

In most patients with *esophageal atresia* (EA) it is possible to preserve the native esophagus and perform a primary anastomosis.[2] But the group of patients with EA without a distal tracheoesophageal fistula (8% pure EA and 2% EA with proximal tracheoesophageal fistula) shares the common features of a small stomach and small distal esophageal stump, which may preclude a primary anastomosis. The initial surgery of these patients is done during the first days of life. At this stage a laparotomy and gastrostomy are performed. Through an upper abdominal incision the stomach is accessed and the lower esophageal pouch is assessed under fluoroscopy introducing metal dilators. The gastrostomy should be placed distally and away from the greater curve to facilitate surgery at a later stage; it can be difficult in these patients due to a small stomach. The presence of a proximal tracheoesophageal fistula should be recognized before or at the beginning of the surgery with a contrast study of the upper esophagus and endoscopic examination. If a proximal fistula is demonstrated it should be divided, generally through a neck incision. Cervical esophagostomies are avoided whenever possible and reserved as a salvage option in a patient with catastrophic complications. The patients are kept on intermittent or continuous oroesophageal sump suction and bolus feeds through the gastrostomy.

All patients with LGEA are assessed for possible primary anastomosis. In those with a very meager lower esophagus, that is about one-third of the patients, a primary replacement is considered sometime in the first 3 months, depending on prematurity. This waiting period is important to allow the stomach to grow. But esophageal replacement surgery should not be delayed unnecessarily as delay may harm the patients' ability to develop a normal swallowing mechanism.

Indications for esophageal substitution in esophageal atresia

- Long-gap esophageal atresia (LGEA) (Fig. 24.1)
- Extreme prematurity unsuitable for delayed primary anastomosis
- EA + TEF long gap (rare)
- Failed anastomosis leading to esophagostomy
- Major after EA repair leak with anastomotic disruption
- Nonfunctioning aperistaltic esophagus due to overzealous attempts to preserve native esophagus
- Failed previous esophageal substitutes

Esophageal strictures are a less common indication for esophageal replacement. They can be congenital, caustic, or peptic in origin. Most of them can be treated conservatively with repetitive dilatations, medical therapy, and antireflux surgery when indicated. When the medical treatment fails, more radical procedures can be done with preservation of the native esophagus (i.e., resection of the stricture and anastomosis). There are a small number of patients who will need an esophageal replacement.

Esophageal replacement has occasionally been used in other rare conditions in children such as large benign tumors,[3] scleroderma,[4] epidermolysis bullosa,[5-8] diffuse candidiasis,[9,10] herpes virus infections,[10] etc.

D.H. Parikh et al. (eds.), *Pediatric Thoracic Surgery*,
DOI: 10.1007/b136543_24, © Springer-Verlag London Limited 2009

opened, the right gastric artery is identified and preserved, and the left gastric artery is divided. The distal esophageal stump is now freed. The body and fundus of the stomach are now completely mobilized, and the distal esophagus can be excised and oversewn. To achieve further length the second portion of the duodenum is mobilized. Pyloroplasty can be done at this stage, though this is still controvertial.[88] The highest part of the fundus is identified and stay sutures are placed.

The advocates of this technique usually perform a cervical esophagostomy at the first operation, which is now mobilized, taking care not to damage the recurrent laryngeal nerve. The virtual space between the trachea and the prevertebral fascia is opened by blunt dissection. The same is done from the abdomen through the bed of the esophagus, developing the plane behind the heart and anterior to the prevertebral fascia. In a case with extensive adhesions (i.e., caustic injury) or previous surgery, a thoracotomy may be needed to complete the resection of the esophagus and the tunnel is created under direct vision. Alternativelly, the retrosternal space can be used for the pull-up.

A large hemostat is placed from the neck and the stay sutures are pulled. Particular care must be taken not to twist the stomach during this maneuver.

The gastroesophageal anastomosis is completed in the neck. A large nasogastric tube is left in the stomach through the anastomosis and the cervical wound is closed.

The pylorus is fixed bellow the hiatus. A feeding jejunostomy can be created before the abdominal wound is closed.

Most of these patients require postoperative mechanical ventilation. A contrast study is performed 1 week after the operation and oral feed is commenced.

The gastric pull-up can be assisted with the laparoscope.[89]

Results and Discussion on Gastric Pull-Ups

The main advantage of the gastric pull-up lies in its simplicity. Gastric pull-ups have been used after the failure of other replacement techniques, and, even with previous gastric tubes or antireflux operations, it is possible to mobilize the stomach safely.[38] Gastric pull-ups involve only one anastomosis and hence a theoretical reduced risk of leakage.[90]

One of the major problems with the gastric pull-up is the large amount of space occupied by the stomach in the chest and the risk of compression of intrathoracic organs. The mortality rate in contemporary series is about 5% usually secondary to respiratory failure. The average postoperative mechanical ventilation was 4 days in one series.[38] Despite this, the long-term respiratory function remains acceptable in most of the patients.[90]

The incidence of leakage and stricture is about 20% and is comparable to other replacement techniques (Table 24.2).

Because of the mobilization, essential to complete the pull-up, the stomach is vagotomised and therefore gastric emptying relies on gravity. Gastric emptying is quite variable but there is no good correlation between symptoms and functional studies.[90] Patients frequently complain of heartburn, regurgitation, vomiting, and breathlessness.[93] Dumping is not infrequent with almost every series reporting some cases. Some advocates of the procedure perform a pyloromyoromy or pyloroplasty routinely though this is controversial.[88] In general, patients who have the procedure done primarily are less symptomatic than patients who had previous procedures, including attempted primary esophageal anastomosis.[90,93]

Volvulus of the stomach is a well-described and serious complication of the operation.[94]

Jejunal Transposition

Operative details: A *pedicled jejunum transposition* is performed dividing a loop of bowel distal to the angle of Treitz with preservation of its vascular pedicle. The length of the pedicle is achieved by sacrificing variable length of the distal jejunum. The curvature of the isolated jejunal loop is reasonably straight if the mesentery is divided keeping the first vascular arcade intact. As mentioned earlier, it can be difficult to achieve enough length due to the inferior attachments of these vessels. Secondly, the loss of distal jejunum may create short bowel syndrome. The recent practice is to prepare the jejunum while performing the initial gastrotomy ligating the vessel at the base of the jejunal loop in continuity. This procedure develops improved vascular anastomosis from distal jejunal mesentery and hypertrophy of the vascular arcade, thus improving the blood supply of the isolated jejunal loop when required for interposition. Initial results with this technique are encouraging allowing the replacement of the entire length of the thoracic esophagus without any anastomotic leak or graft necrosis. The isolated loop of jejunum with its pedicle is then pulled up through the mesentery of the transverse colon, posterior to the stomach and through the esophageal

TABLE 24.2. Results of gastric pull-up series published after 1980.

		n	Leak	%	Stricture	%	Reoperations	Death
Atwell[34]	1980	6	1	17	1	17	Reoperations 2 in 1 patient for small bowel obstruction	2
Valente[40]	1987	10	2	20	2	20	1 Revision to colonic replacement	3 (late)
Marujo[91]	1991	21	4	19	3	14	1 Gastric necrosis	1
Hirschl[3]	2002	41	15	37	20	49	0	0
Spitz[38]	2004	173	21	12	34	20	1 For leak, 3 for strictures	9
Tannuri[92]	2007	34	6	18	4	12	1 Graft necrosis, 1 anastomotic dehiscence, 3 volvulus of stomach, 2 leaks	2

hiatus into the mediastinum. During this process the pedicle should not be allowed to be twisted. The jejunum is then anastomosed to the stomach and introduced in the chest through the hiatus where the thoracic anastomosis with the proximal esophagus is completed. A primary jejunojejunal anastomosis is done at the site where the graft was taken. If the jejunum is straightened then the redundancy is minimal in long term and can be an ideal substitute. Experience suggests that it retains the peristaltic activity and has no jejunogastric reflux causing ulceration. However, the technical aspect of the pedicle jejunal graft is demanding and does not produce the same results in all centers. It requires dedicated surgeons to produce consistently good results, unlike other techniques of esophageal substitution, which can reproduce results of other surgeons.

A *free jejunal graft* involves a microsurgical anastomosis between the vascular pedicle of the graft and suitable vessels in the chest. The procedure is then completed as with a pedicled graft. This technique has high rate of failure and carries significant postoperative morbidity and mortality.[51,54]

Discussion on jejunal interpositon: Jejunum interpositions have some theoretical advantages compared with colon interpositions and gastric pull-ups. The jejunum has a similar diameter to the esophagus, and thus there is no compression of mediastinal structures by a space-occupying lesion. The jejunal grafts preserve the peristaltic activity, which contribute to the clearance of the organ and help in prevention of acid injury.[51,54] As with colon interposition, this technique involves three intestinal anastomoses. Leakage and stricture are not uncommon complications (Table 24.3). The precarious blood supply of the jejunum is responsible for some of the serious early complications seen with this technique, including complete necrosis, perforation of the graft, and mediastinitis.[49–51,54] For that reason leakage in free jejuna grafts should be approached earlier and aggressively.[54] The potential advantages of free jejunum grafts are eclipsed by the discouraging complications and long-term results. The pedicled jejunal interposition is less demanding technically and results seem to be better.[53]

Colonic Transposition

Colonic transposition still is the most popular esophageal replacement technique in children despite the severe complications it can have. The viability of the colon is based on the collateral circulation provided by Riolan's arcade.

Operative details: To perform the transposition the abdomen is accessed through an upper abdominal incision. The colon is completely mobilized after division of all the peritoneal attachments from the distal ileum. The mesocolon is lifted and the arterial system is identified assisted by transillumination.

If the *right colon*[95] is to be used, the middle colic vessels are preserved. The right colic artery is identified and occluded with a vascular clamp. The appendix is removed and the distal ileum is prepared for division. After 15 min of occlusion the colon is inspected and the pulsation of the marginal arcade is reassessed. If the colon remains pink and the pulsation through the vessels is satisfactory the right colic artery is divided near its origin. The graft is completed after division of the terminal ileum and transverse colon distal to the middle colic artery. The ileum is anastomosed to the transverse colon to reestablish intestinal continuity. The graft is passed behind the stomach and in front of the left lobe of the liver.

A cervical incision is then performed, the esophageal space accessed, and the retrosternal space opened with blunt dissection. The anterior attachments of the diaphragm are divided from below and the tunnel is completed. The graft is advanced through the retrosternal space taking special care not to twist it. The colon is anastomosed to the anterior wall of the stomach, and the cervical anastomosis between the ileum or colon and the esophagus is completed.

The *transverse colon* and the *left colon* can be used based on the left colic vessels. The complete procedure can be done through a left thoracotomy as described by Waterston,[60] through separate thoracic and abdominal incisions,[96] or through a thoracoabdominal incision.[8] The colon is mobilized and the vascular arcades are identified. Viability is confirmed; the selected loop is divided, and a colocolonic anastomosis is performed. The graft is advanced behind the pancreas and the stomach. The left colon can be placed in the left chest through the diaphragm at the costodiaphragmatic angle or in the mediastinum through the hiatus.[62] After the cervical esophagostomy is freed the coloesophageal anastomosis is completed.

Pyloroplasty or pyloromyotomy can be performed to improve gastric emptying.

Results and Discussion on Colonic Transposition

Serious complications of colonic grafts are related to its delicate vascular supply. Arterial obstruction can cause early necrosis of the graft. Venous thrombosis is responsible for low-grade obstruction, necrosis, and late perforations.

TABLE 24.3. Results of jejunal grafts – series published after 1980.

		n	Leaks	%	Strictures	%	Lost grafts	Deaths
Ring et al.[49]	1982	16	4	25	2	13	0	
Saeki et al.[50]	1988	19	3	16	2	11	1	2
Cusick et al.[51]	1993	6	1	17	2	33	1	2
Bax et al.[52,53]	2007	24	5	21	10	42	0	0
Cauchi et al.[54]	2007	8	4	50	4	50	3	1

Chagas disease is a form of achalasia associated with infection with the parasite *Trypanosoma cruzi*. The parasite damages the intramural ganglia of the esophagus. Chagas disease is confined to areas of South America where trypanosomiasis is endemic and there is no evidence to support the infective agent theory for achalasia in other regions of the world. Most attention is now focused on achalasia being an immune-mediated disorder as opposed to a myopathy or vagal neuropathy.[15,16] As the pathogenesis of achalasia remains unclear, management is based on symptomatic relief. Unfortunately this can produce inconsistent and unsatisfactory results.

Clinical Features and Diagnosis

Achalasia of cardia is largely a disease of adult life. Achalasia is known to occur in families and it is seen occasionally in infancy.[17] In pediatric practice most achalasia is reported during adolescence, more often in boys (boys: girls = 2:1). Typical symptoms include dysphagia, vomiting or regurgitation of food, chest pain, and weight loss or failure to thrive. Symptoms often predate the diagnosis by 1–2 years. Adolescents with achalasia usually suffer from halitosis. In children respiratory symptoms consistent with aspiration may occur.[7] Bronchiectasis has also been reported in children with recurrent aspirations especially if achalasia is associated with Down's syndrome.[18] There are usually no specific clinical findings in achalasia.

Radiology and Manometric Studies

The chest x-ray of a child with achalasia may show a widened esophagus and an air fluid level. Further evidence comes from the barium swallow which will show a widened, and at times, tortuous esophagus, narrowing down at the cardia to a bird's beak (Fig. 25.1). The diagnosis is confirmed by esophageal manometry. The characteristic findings on manometry are (1) a high resting pressure within the LES, (2) failure of the LES to relax on swallowing and (3) a variable reduction in the amplitude of peristaltic waves in the body of the esophagus (Fig. 25.2). A normal manometric study will show a wave of high pressure (in the range of 80 mm of Hg) progressing down the body of the esophagus after swallowing with complete relaxation of the lower esophageal sphincter.

Other conditions such as diffuse esophageal spasms (DES) and vigorous achalasia (VA) can be diagnosed using manometry to investigate children with dysphagia. In both conditions repetitive high amplitude peristaltic waves are seen in the body of the esophagus. The lower sphincter does relax in DES but this is not coordinated with the peristaltic wave. Diffuse esophageal spasm is more common than VA and known to be a precursor of achalasia. In VA the lower esophageal sphincter demonstrates a characteristic non-relaxation.

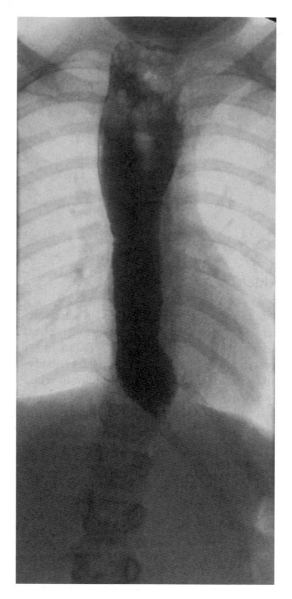

FIG. 25.1. Contrast swallow demonstrating "bird beak" appearance of achalasia with dilatation of the esophagus

Esophageal manometry is difficult in children, particularly young children, because a large degree of cooperation is required. Acceptance can be improved by passing the manometry catheter under general anesthesia the evening prior to the study. Interpretation of the manometric findings in children is also difficult, again because considerable cooperation is required to locate the LES manometrically. The child also has to be willing to swallow when instructed. Unfortunately the results of serial manometric studies may be conflicting in the same patient with achalasia.[19,20]

Endoscopic examination of the esophagus is essential to exclude a stricture. The classical endoscopic findings are a dilated esophagus filled with food debris yet no impediment to passage of the endoscope through the LES. It is common to find evidence of peptic esophagitis in association with achalasia.

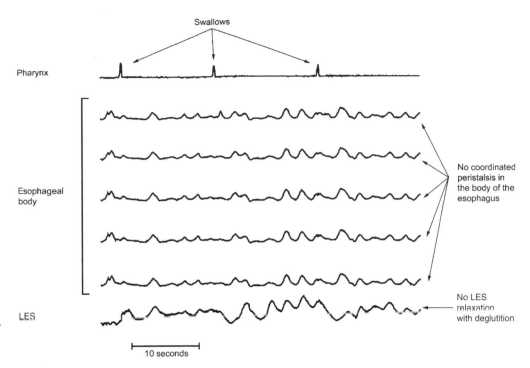

Swallows

Pharynx

Esophageal body

LES

No coordinated peristalsis in the body of the esophagus

No LES relaxation with deglutition

10 seconds

FIG. 25.2. Manometric study showing classical features of achalasia with failure of relaxation of gastroesophageal sphincter and uncoordinated peristalsis in the body of the esophagus

Management

Medical

Calcium channel blockers and anti cholinergic drugs have been used to treat achalasia in adults. They are of minimal benefit to children with achalasia. Systemic side effects frequently become intolerable as the dose is increased

Surgical

Dilatation

Early surgical treatment of achalasia involved regular bougienage. Subsequently dilatation was used to forcibly rupture the sphincter mechanism and overcome the functional obstruction. Balloon dilatation under fluoroscopic control has been used with variable success to treat achalasia. Repeated dilatation is invariably necessary. The use of two dilators in tandem to disrupt the LES has been described and may be more effective than a single dilator.[21]

The success rates for balloon dilatation in adults are well established. The risk of perforation during balloon dilation in the adult literature is quoted at 2–7%, with a death rate of 1–2 %. The procedure compares favorably with cardiomyotomy although a recent publication of long term results in adults gave a 10 year remission rate of only 36%.[22] A recent report concluded that repeat intervention was more likely to be necessary after dilatation than cardiomyotomy, which supports the view that myotomy is the treatment of choice for the fit and young.[23]

Limited data is available in children. Initial success rates up to 90% have been reported.[9,24,25] Long term data is not available for children and one suspects the long term remission rate will be lower than in adults. The risk of perforation seems lower in children but only small numbers are available.[9]

Injection of Botulinum Toxin

Botulinum toxin (BT) has been used to treat achalasia in adults and, more recently, in children. This has been used as the sole treatment although some authors have used it in combination with pneumatic dilatation. Data is now available to show that BT injection is short acting with the benefit unlikely to last more than six months.[26] This is inferior to balloon dilation.[27] Moreover, BT injection is no safer than laparoscopic myotomy.[28] Routine use of BT injection for achalasia is no longer recommended unless life expectancy is short, or the patient is unfit for general anesthesia.

The impact of previous endoscopic treatment on the outcome of subsequent cardiomyotomy remains contentious. Surgeons may comment instinctively that cardiomyotomy is simpler in patients who have not been subjected to previous endoscopic treatment. This finds support in the adult literature with perforation rates of 28% during myotomy reported in group of patients who had previous dilatation, whereas no perforations were reported in the group who had not received previous endoscopic treatment.[29,30]. However, other centers have published data to show that prior treatment by pneumatic dilatation does not affect the surgical technique nor the long term outcome.[31,32]

31. Bessel JR, Lalley CJ, Schloithe A et al. Laparoscopic cardiomyotomy for achalasia: Long term outcomes. ANZ J Surg 2006; 76:558–562.

32. Torquati A, Richards WO, Holzman MD et al. Laparoscopic myotomy for achalasia: Predictors of successful outcomes after 200 cases. Ann Surg 2006; 243:587–593.

33. Ellis FH, Olsen AM, Holman CB. Surgical treatment of cardiospasm. JAMA (1958) 166:29.

34. Pellegrini C, Wetter LA, Patti M. Thorascopic esophagomyotomy. Initial experience with a new approach for the treatment of achalasia. Ann Surg 1992; 216: 291–299.

35. Shimi S, Nathenson LK, Cushieri A. Laparoscopic cardiomyotomy for achalasia. J R Coll Surg Edinb 1991; 36:152–154

36. Patti MG, Pellegrini CA, Horgan S. Minimally invasive surgery for achalasia: an 8 year experience with 168 patients. Ann Surg 1999; 230:587–594

37. Sharp KW, Khaitan L, Sholtz S, et al. 100 consecutive minimally invasive Heller myotomies: Lessons learned. Ann Surg 2002; 235:631–639

38. Richards WO, Torquati A, Holzman MD, et al. Heller myotomy versus Heller myotomy with Dor fundoplication for Achalasia. Ann Surg 2004; 240:405–415.

39. Esposito C, Mendoza-Sagaon M, Roblot-Maigret B, et al. Complications of laparoscopic treatment of oesophageal achalasia in children. J Pediatr Surg 2000; 35: 680–683.

40. Falkenback D, Johansson J, Oberg S et al. Heller's esophageal myotomy with or without a 360 degree floppy Nissen fundoplication for achalasia. Dis Esophagus 2003;16: 284–90

41. Vane DW, Cosby K, West K et al. Late results following esophagomyotomy in children with achalasia. J Pediatr Surg 1988; 23:515–519.

26
Gastro-esophageal Reflux

Alex W. Auldist, Thomas Clarnette, and Naeem Samnakay

Introduction

Gastroesophageal reflux (GER) is the retrograde flow of gastric contents into the oesophagus.[1] It is normal for most people to experience short episodes of GER, especially after meals. In infants, vomiting and regurgitation after feeds is a common event, and one that most infants grow out of.[2] Gastroesophageal reflux disease (GERD) occurs when the spectrum of reflux exceeds the physiological norm, resulting in symptoms and complications.[3] Reflux-associated symptoms include pain, heartburn, failure to thrive, or chronic cough, while reflux-associated complications include esophageal mucosal changes such as inflammation, bleeding, stricture, ulceration, and metaplasia.

The distinction between physiological reflux and pathological reflux in infancy is difficult, partly because of the large proportion of infants with self-limiting vomiting and regurgitation, and partly because of the degree of anxiety expressed by parents of vomiting or irritable infants.

The true prevalence of GERD in children is unknown, because there is no standard definition of GERD worldwide and because of the high prevalence gerd of physiological vomiting and regurgitation in early infancy. Prevalence studies suggest that 50% of infants under 2 months of age have vomiting and regurgitation, rising to 70% by 4 months of age. The prevalence of these symptoms declines after 6 months of age, with only 1–5% of infants over 12 months displaying them.[4,5]

Children with symptoms of reflux beyond age 18 months are thought more likely to have GERD as adults.[1] Older children with GERD present with gerd symptoms more like adults with reflux. It is thought that a significant proportion of adults with GERD will have had symptoms of GERD in childhood.

Historic Perspective

Billard first published a case of esophagitis in a child in ger 1828 in Paris.[6] In 1855, Rokitansky attributed esophagitis to GER.[7] Yet it was not until half a century later in 1906 that Tileston clearly described the symptoms of esophagitis.[8] The term "peptic esophagitis" itself was coined in the German literature in 1934 by Professor Hamperl.[9] Wilkenstein wrote a detailed description of GER in 1935, using the term "esophagitis" in the English literature.[10] In infants, GER was well described in the mid 1900s, as were ger the benefits of postural treatment with nursing infants in the upright position.[11]

Even though the anatomical anomaly of hiatus hernia was well described, it was in 1951 that Professor Phillip Allison attributed GER as an abnormal physiological condition secondary to anatomical defects at the gastroesophageal junction.[12] He devised the transthoracic procedure to reduce the herniated gastric cardia into the peritoneal cavity, to suture it to the phrenocolic ligament to keep it in place, and lightly suture the crura of the hiatus. In 1973, Allison presented a 20-year follow-up of his procedure, which showed a 49% recurrence rate.[13]

Nissen first performed the "complete wrap" in 1955 after initially having tried anterior gastropexy for the management of hiatal hernia and reflux symptoms. He published two cases of the Nissen fundoplication in 1956, calling the procedure "gastroplication."[14] His procedure gained popularity worldwide by the 1970s, and it is the open Nissen fundoplication that has been modified to the laparoscopic approach in this era.

It was Allison's operation that was practised for children with GERD at our institution, The Royal Children's Hospital, Melbourne, until GERD 1972. In this year, the first Nissen fundoplication at our institution was performed in a child in whom a previous Allison procedure had failed. The Nissen fundoplication has since been the antireflux procedure of choice, both laparoscopic and open, at the Royal Children's Hospital, Melbourne.

The medical management of GERD has also evolved dramatically, with refinements in diagnosis and the development of effective pharmacologic agents, from H_2 antagonists as the mainstay of treatment in the last century, to proton pump inhibitors (PPIs) used as the mainstay of treatment currently.

D.H. Parikh et al. (eds.), *Pediatric Thoracic Surgery*,
DOI: 10.1007/b136543_26, © Springer-Verlag London Limited 2009

Basic Science/Pathogenesis

Mechanisms Preventing Reflux

A host of factors combined help create the antireflux barrier at the gastroesophageal junction. These are both anatomical and physiological.

1. The mechanical barrier

   (a) Lower esophageal sphincter (LES)

   The LES is a high-pressure zone at the distal esophagus, readily detected on manometry. It was first described in 1956 as a high-pressure zone.[15] It is not an anatomically identifiable structure as such, but a specialized region of smooth muscle of the esophageal wall that remains in a state of tonic contraction.[16,17] This state of contraction prevents retrograde passage of gastric contents up the esophagus. Ultrasonic anatomical assessment reveals that the smooth muscle fibers are thicker at the LES compared with the rest of the esophagus.[18,19] The LES is thought to span a distance of 4 cm, 2 cm of which is intrathoracic and grasped by the diaphragmatic crura.[17] The distal 2 cm is intraabdominal. Oblique smooth muscle fibers from the stomach also contribute to the LES.[17]

   LES tone at rest is usually greater than 4 mmHg.[2] The LES relaxes during episodes of swallowing, belching, or vomiting. During swallowing, neurologically controlled, timed relaxation of the LES occurs as the wave of peristalsis approaches the distal esophagus, allowing the food bolus through.[17]

   (b) Intraabdominal esophagus

   The success of the LES as a barrier for reflux is a function of pressure, overall length of the LES as well as intraabdominal length of the LES.[20] In an adult, the distal 2 cm of the LES is intraabdominal.[17] Intraabdominal pressure applied to both the stomach and intraabdominal esophagus will by Laplace's law preferentially result in collapse of the soft narrow-lumen intraabdominal esophagus compared with the large-lumen stomach.

   The intraabdominal component of the esophagus is small in the neonate, but lengthens over the subsequent 6 weeks after birth to become an effective component of the antireflux barrier.[21]

   (c) Diaphragmatic pinchcock

   The role of the diaphragmatic crura at the esophageal hiatus in the barrier against reflux was first described in 1958 by Ingelfinger.[22] The esophageal hiatus in the diaphragm is formed mainly from the anatomical right crus of the diaphragm. The anatomical arrangement of the hiatus results in the esophagus being pulled to the right and caudally.[23] The crura at the hiatus encircle the proximal half of the LES. Contraction of the diaphragm results in pinchcock-like compression of the LES by the crura, forming an external sphincter mechanism.[24] The phrenoesophageal membrane attaches the esophagus to the diaphragmatic hiatus, and marks the transition of the intrathoracic esophagus to the intraabdominal part.

(d) Angle of His

The angle of His is the acute angle formed at the junction of the esophagus and gastric fundus. This acute angle, along with the posterolateral position of the gastric fundus, minimizes contact of gastric content with the esophagogastric junction. Loss of the acuteness of the angle of His, as with gastric distension and with stretching the gastric wall after formation of gastrostomy, results in a funnel-like arrangement at the gastroesophageal junction, directing gastric contents that are retropulsed into the funnel and up the esophagus.

(e) Mucosal rosette

In the presence of an acute Angle of His, the mucosa at the gastroesophageal junction forms rosette-like folds, which compress against each other with increased intraabdominal pressure to prevent reflux.[25]

The mechanical factors described earlier are interrelated and work in combination to achieve an integrated functional antireflux barrier. While the mechanisms described in this category are the main antireflux measures, further processes decribed later also help in minimizing damage from reflux that occurs if the mechanical barrier is breached.

2. Lumenal clearance factors

Prompt clearance of refluxate from the esophagus occurs with the assistance of esophageal peristalsis clearing the lumen, as well as the influence of gravity in promoting caudal flow of esophageal contents. Studies show that defective peristalsis is more likely in those with both reflux and esophagitis than in those with reflux alone.[26] Whether the defective peristalsis is secondary to the reflux and mucosal damage, or a primary event, is still unclear.

3. Mucosal protection

There is a poorly formed preepithelial mucosal barrier. Saliva, along with limited mucous from esophageal submucosal glands, helps neutralize acid in the refluxate. Epithelial mechanisms help limit the rate of HCl diffusion into cells, and to buffer acid. Epithelial blood flow helps with prompt removal of H^+ ions and in maintaining the acid–base balance at the epithelial level[27] (Fig. 26.1).

Etiology of GERD

A breakdown of the antireflux mechanisms results in reflux, hence the etiology of GERD is multifactorial. We shall discuss the common causative factors and associations with reflux.

GERD may be classed as primary, or secondary to other problems of the gastrointestinal tract such as gastric outflow obstruction and cow's milk protein intolerance.

While the etiology of primary GERD is multifactorial, the main recognized cause is transient LES relaxations (TLESR), rather than a low basal esophageal sphincter tone, as was previously thought.[2,28,29] TLESRs are unrelated to swallow, and have lower basal pressures and longer duration of relaxation than swallow-associated sphincter relaxations. TLESRs occur more frequently postprandially. A TLESR occurs when LES

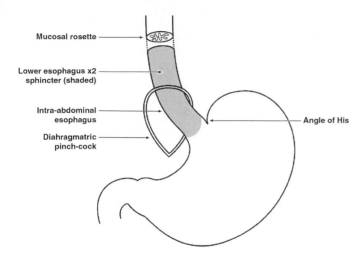

Fig. 26.1. Factors preventing gastroesophageal reflux

Labels: Mucosal rosette; Lower esophagus x2 sphincter (shaded); Intra-abdominal esophagus; Diahragmatic pinch-cock; Angle of His

pressure drops to the level of gastric pressure or 0–2 mmHg for 10 s or more.[2]

There are data to show that LES tone physiology is similar in the neonate, infant, child, and adult, with swallow-associated sphincter relaxations and TLESRs occurring in all age groups in a similar fashion.[30–33]

Associations/Predisposing Factors

Various associations with and predisposing factors to GERD have been recognized.

A genetic association with pediatric GERD is thought to exist on a locus on chromosome 13q14.[34–37]

Both sexes seem equally affected by GERD.

The presence of a hiatus hernia has long been associated with GERD. While hiatus hernia itself was well described by the first half of the twentieth century, it was not until the second half of the twentieth century that Allison attributed functional reflux to the presence of hiatus hernia resulting in breakdown of the mechanical barrier arrangement.[7] This observation led to the development of surgical procedures that addressed both the problem of the hernia as well as the associated reflux.

There is an increased incidence of GERD in children with neurological impairment, and it mainly manifests as vomiting. Various factors are thought to contribute to this increased incidence – general hypotonia, recumbent posturing with loss of the aid of gravity in esophageal clearance, and periods of increased intraabdominal pressure due to factors such as seizures or muscle spasticity. In addition, neurologically impaired children are more likely to require gastrostomy for feeding, as they often have incoordinate swallow mechanisms and are at high risk of aspiration. Creating a gastrostomy alters the anatomy of the stomach, changing the acuity of the angle of His by stretching the anterior wall of the stomach. It is estimated that about 30–50% of children with no significant reflux prior to gastrostomy will have symptomatic reflux and vomit feeds postgastrostomy.[38,39]

In addition, large bolus feeds via the gastrostomy can exacerbate the problem, and changing to continuous lower volume feeds can be helpful in curbing the problem.

Children with tracheoesophageal fistula and esophageal atresia have a high incidence of associated GERD, with 35–58% of TEF/EA patients diagnosed with reflux.[40,41] The incidence of reflux is thought to be even higher in children with pure EA.[42] This association may be due to the inherent maldevelopment and motor dysfunction of the esophagus, perhaps exacerbated by shortening of the intraabdominal component of the esophagus due to tension at the anastomosis.[43,44] GERD in TEF patients causes or exacerbates anastomotic stricturing and makes dilatation of strictures less likely to be successful unless the underlying GERD is treated.[40] It is also thought to exacerbate the effects of coexisting tracheomalacia. The dysmotility of the esophagus in EA is associated with poor clearance of the refluxed fluid with a resultant increase in all the complications of GERD.

Increasingly, obesity is an associated factor predisposing to the development of GERD.

Delayed gastric emptying may predispose to the development of GERD and aggravate its effects. Delayed emptying with distension for excessive time periods may lead to shortening of the intraabdominal component of the esophagus as well as loss of the angle of His due to its incorporation into the distension at the gastroesophageal junction.[45]

Clinical Features

Presentation

The clinical presentation of reflux in the pediatric population varies. The presentation in infants is generally different to that of the older child. Infants present mainly with regurgitation, vomiting, and irritability. One is reliant on the history from parents and caregivers. Most infantile regurgitation and vomiting settle spontaneously after 6 months to 1 year of age. It is difficult to distinguish between physiological regurgitation and pathological reflux in the infant population.

Older children, who are able to describe their problems, present with similar symptoms to adults. Table 26.1 lists the different age-related modes of presentation of GERD.

The presentation and symptoms of GERD in children are related to the effects of reflux on the esophagus, the respiratory tract and the general growth and development of the child. Thus, complications of reflux can be viewed in four main categories:

1. Esophagitis and effects on the esophagus:
   (a) Pain
   In older children and adults, the commonest manifestation of pain is heartburn due to esophageal irritation from the acid refluxate. The pain is typically a burning sensation, often substernal and epigastric. Dysphagia, or pain on swallowing, may also occur. Infants with reflux may also

TABLE 26.1. GERD symptoms.

Infants	
Gastrointestinal	Vomiting
	Failure to thrive
	Feeding difficulty
	Irritability, pain, colic
	Hematemesis
	Anemia
Respiratory	Apneas, blue spells
	Chronic cough
	Stridor
	Recurrent aspiration
	Pneumonia
Neurobehavioral	Sandifer syndrome
	Seizure activity, infant spasms
Older children	
Gastrointestinal	Nausea
	Dysphagia
	Heartburn
	Anemia
	Hematemesis
	Hoarseness
	Esophageal foreign body obstruction
Respiratory	Cough
	Asthma
	Aspiration pneumonia

have pain, but whether this is heartburn is difficult to ascertain in the infant age group.

(b) Hematemesis

Esophageal mucosal inflammation with ulceration can result in hematemesis as the initial manifestation of GERD. The hematemesis is often streaks of blood mixed in the vomitus.

(c) Stricture

Esophagitis may result in chronic fibrosis and luminal stricturing. Food bolus obstruction at the stricture, odynophagia, or dysphagia may thus be the first manifestations of underlying GERD, with no other symptoms of esophagitis being present. In our experience, once the underlying GERD is treated, the stricture heals.

(d) Sandifer syndrome

Sandifer syndrome is an uncommon syndrome of abnormal head, neck, and trunk movements in patients with GERD. The abnormal movements are temporally associated with episodes of reflux. While it has been described mainly in young, neurologically normal male children, there are reports of Sandifer syndrome affecting females, adults, and neurologically impaired children too. The pathophysiological relationship between GERD and these abnormal neurologic movements is yet to be defined.[46] The most likely explanation is that the reflux episodes themselves result in the abnormal posturing, a postulation supported by the fact that these abnormal movements usually abruptly stop after antireflux surgery.[46,47]

(e) Barrett's esophagus

Barrett's esophagus is the presence of metaplastic columnar epithelium in the distal esophagus. It is well established as a complication of esophagitis, present in up to 13% of children with GERD.[48] In children, esophageal stricture is often present with Barrett's esophagus.[48–51] Barrett's esophagus is considered to be a risk factor for esophageal adenocarcinoma. It is associated with progressive dysplasia and the risk of developing adenocarcinoma, occasionally reported in childhood.[52] The management of Barrett's esophagus in childhood is difficult and unclear, and is discussed later in this chapter.

2. Failure to thrive and affects on growth

Infants and children with constant chalasia may fail to thrive due to various reasons. The main reason is loss of caloric intake via the frequent vomitus. Exacerbating this issue is also poor feeding and oral aversion to feeding as the child associates feeding with symptoms such as pain and dysphagia.

3. Respiratory symptoms

It can be extremely difficult to prove a causal relationship between respiratory symptoms and GERD. Respiratory symptoms can range from chronic cough, wheezing and asthma-type symptoms, to aspiration and recurrent pneumonitis. Microaspiration resulting in chronic cough and airway spasm is more common than gross aspiration and aspiration pneumonia. Vagal irritation in the esophageal wall by esophagitis processes may initiate laryngospasm and bronchospasm in the absence of any aspiration via neural reflex arcs. Reflux can be a cause of chronic stridor and hypoxia in infants.[53]

In premature infants, GERD can exacerbate existent respiratory problems and should be suspected and managed if there is deterioration of respiratory status, especially in the presence of other GERD-related symptoms such as regurgitation and failure to thrive.[53,54]

4. Dying spells

GERD is associated in some infants with severe life-threatening apneas (also known as "blue spells" or "dying spells"). Obstructive apneas in response to reflux are thought to occur in about 1% of infants, and are due to laryngeal or airway closure that presumably is triggered in response to reflux.[53] They are an absolute indication for antireflux surgery.

Diagnosis

A good history and examination establishes the clinical circumstances of each individual with suspected GERD. The particular clinical circumstances in turn determine the appropriate selection of investigations to aid diagnosis and management. For example, a contrast study is important in an infant with postfeed vomiting, to rule out distal obstruction, whereas endoscopy is an important investigation in an older child with severe heartburn.

The aim of investigations is to accurately diagnose the presence of GERD, to accurately define the presence of complications, and in some cases (especially in those with respiratory manifestations) to ascertain a causal link between reflux and presenting symptoms.

1. Investigations

(a) Radiology

Contrast study of the esophagus, stomach, and duodenum is very important in the assessment of an infant or child with vomiting or regurgitation. It will help in defining the anatomy of the upper GI tract, and may pick up the presence of hiatus hernia. It will exclude obstructive causes such as pyloric stenosis, malrotation, and antral and duodenal webs. It may identify refluxing contrast, but is not a useful test for quantifying reflux.

(b) Endoscopy and biopsies

Endoscopy and biopsies are most useful in cases where esophagitis is suspected. Biopsies are an integral part of the investigation as it is well documented that endoscopic appearances alone do not correlate with the presence of esophagitis. Mucosal biopsies are highly sensitive and specific for the presence of GERD-related esophagitis.[55] Histologic features of esophagitis include the presence of inflammatory cells and some eosinophils in the epithelium, basal cell hyperplasia to 20% or more of total mucosal thickness, and elongation of stromal papillae into the upper half of the epithelium.[56,57] Biopsies will help differentiate GERD from eosinophilic esophagitis, which is characterized by the presence of large numbers of eosinophils in the mucosa, and which will not respond to the usual treatments for GERD.[58]

Endoscopy will also document and evaluate the presence of strictures, ulceration, and Barrett's esophagus. Endoscopic appearances alone cannot accurately identify the presence of Barrett's esophagus, and biopsies are the key investigation defining its presence. Barrett's esophagus is defined by the presence of metaplastic columnar epithelium. Three types of metaplasia of the distal esophagus are described: cardiac, fundic, and intestinal. The intestinal type carries a significant risk of dysplasia and malignant transformation.

(c) pH studies

These have been in use since the 1970s.[59] Transnasally placed pH probes continuously measure esophageal pH over a period of 24h, which is recorded on a computer to allow analysis. Generally, a pH below 4.0 indicates reflux of gastric content. The duration and quantity of reflux episodes are analyzed. An activity diary during the pH measurement study allows one to correlate reflux episodes with various activities. The total percentage of time that the pH is below 4 is known as the "reflux index," and this is used as a quantification measure for reflux.[60]

pH studies generally are not required in the work-up of children with regurgitatation and endoscopy-diagnosed esophagitis. pH studies are most helpful in diagnosing the presence of reflux where the clinical presentation is unclear, and in eliciting its role in the child's symptom complex. For example, is reflux the underlying cause in a child with recurrent pneumonias, airway disease, or apneas? Is recurrent reflux present in a child with symptoms after fundoplication?

(d) Multichannel impedance

pH studies are unable to detect nonacid reflux and do not detect what has been termed acid rereflux. Acid rereflux is reflux that occurs while the pH probe still reads a pH of under 4.0 after a previous reflux episode.[61,62] It is thought to be a major cause of delayed acid clearance from the esophagus after reflux episodes. Multichannel intraluminal impedence monitoring is a new diagnostic study that detects flow of gastric contents into the esophagus. Electrode pairs throughout the esophagus and stomach measure impedance, which drops from high to low by contact with gastric content. Multichannel impedance monitoring is not yet established in routine clinical practice.

(e) Manometry

Sophisticated pressure transducers and recorders allow measurement of esophageal motility in all age ranges, from premature infants to adults. It is through manometry that we understand the function of the LES, know that its function is similar in all age groups, and that TLESRs are the main underlying cause of reflux. In adults, manometry has shown that increasing severity of reflux correlates with deteriorating esophageal function.[63] Clinically, manometry plays a limited role in the work-up of children with reflux. It may be useful in demonstrating an underlying motility disorder, for example, in children with previous esophageal atresia repair.

(f) What is the role of gastric emptying studies?

There is controversy over the role of delayed gastric emptying in the pathophysiology of GERD. Theoretically, gastric distension from delayed gastric emptying will shorten intraabdominal esophageal length, impairing LES function and promoting reflux with gastric contractions. While it has been shown that up to 40% of children with reflux have evidence of delayed gastric emptying, it has not been confirmed that this proportion is any more than one would find in nonrefluxing children.[64–66] There is evidence to suggest that preoperatively present delayed gastric emptying improves in a proportion after fundoplication.[67] There is evidence that delayed gastric emptying is more commonly present in neurologically impaired children.[68] Is the higher reflux recurrence rate postfundoplication in this group due in some way to the underlying delayed gastric emptying? Studies have not shown a definite benefit from combining pyloric drainage procedures with fundoplication, and the complication rate may be higher if pyloric drainage procedures are routinely performed.[69,70]

Given the limited evidence in this matter, the role of routine gastric emptying studies prior to fundoplication is unclear. Even if delayed gastric emptying is detected, its impact on the outcome after reflux surgery cannot be predicted at present.

2. Differential diagnosis

The differential diagnosis of GERD is broad, and should be a symptom-based differential. In a neonate and infant with vomiting and regurgitation, surgical causes such as pyloric stenosis, pyloric or duodenal atresia, or web and malrotation should be considered. Medical causes for vomiting include sepsis, cow's milk allergy with eosinophilic esophagitis, and metabolic diseases. In the older child with epigastric pain, gastritis and pancreaticobiliary disease may need to be excluded. Hiatus hernia may be present and detectable on chest X-ray. Respiratory symptoms such as chronic cough, apneas, and recurrent pneumonia should trigger the thought of possible underlying GERD as a precipitant or contributor.

Management

Management options for GERD include reassurance, positioning, thickened feeds, pharmacological management, and surgery. Chosen management depends on a range of factors including age of the child, the presenting symptoms and their severity, parental preference and compliance. Treatment of GERD aims to relieve symptoms, heal mucosal damage, and prevent and manage complications of GERD.

1. Medical management

(a) Nonpharmacological management

Parents of most infants with mild degrees of vomiting and regurgitation require reassurance. The odds are in favor of the infant outgrowing the problem. Positioning of the infant has been used for years as part of the management of regurgitation. The sitting position at 60° increases reflux, probably because of increased intragastric pressure in this position, whereas the prone position with 30° head up decreases reflux.[71] With the increased risk of sudden infant death syndorme (SIDS) associated with prone positioning, this is not generally recommended. The left lateral position has been shown to reduce reflux in preterm and term neonates.[72] The effect of pacifier use on reflux is equivocal and depends on positioning of the infant.[73]

Feeds thickened with agents such as carob and rice cereal have been shown to reduce regurgitation in infants.[74,75] Thickened infant formulae are also available on the market, but further data on their clinical efficacy are required.

A recent review of randomized trials on nonpharmacological management of reflux suggested that it generally does not have a proven effect on reflux, even if regurgitation symptoms appear improved.[76]

In older children, dietary recommendations include a lowtfat diet and avoiding foods that exacerbate reflux symptoms, such as chocolate and spicy foods.

(b) Pharmacological management

• Prokinetic agents

Prokinetic agents such as metoclopramide and domperidone are commonly used to help reduce regurgitation by increasing LES tone and increasing esophageal and gastric emptying. However, there are no efficacy data about their use in children. In addition, there are significant side effects, such as tardive dyskinesia.[77] Erythromycin is an analogue of the hormone motilin, which stimulates gastric emptying. It may be of use in infants with GERD who have underlying delayed gastric emptying, but there is no controlled trial data to support this theory. Cisapride was hailed as an effective motility agent, but controlled trial data have not shown a consistent improvement in reflux symptoms, although it has been shown to reduce esophageal acid exposure.[78]

• Proton pump inhibitors

Proton pump inhibitors such as omeprazole, esomeprazole, and pantoprazole have had a major impact on the management of GERD – in adults they are the mainstay of medical management of GERD. Their successful use in adults has led to their use in the pediatric population, often as first line pharmacologic agents. PPIs selectively inhibit gastric acid production by blocking the gastric parietal cell H^+/K^+ ATPase pump. The only way for the cell to recover from this block is to synthesize new H^+/K^+ ATPase pumps, a turnover that is thought to have a half-life of 48 h in adults and likely shorter in children.[3]

Experience with PPIs in children is limited compared with their use in adults. Within the recommended dosage, omeprazole use has been shown to be both safe and effective in children.[79] Studies have shown effective resolution of symptoms of esophagitis with PPI use in children.[79,80] Rapid healing of esophagitis with PPI use in children has also been documented, including severe esophagitis, with one study showing 100% healing of ≥stage 2 esophagitis by 12 weeks of PPI treatment in a cohort of 28 children.[81]

A variety of PPIs are available for clinical use in oral and intravenous preparations. There are no strong clinical data to compare the efficacy between agents.

To date, there have been no serious problems of acid suppression and hypergastrinemia documented secondary to PPI usage in children, but long-term follow-up is needed. Gastric and fundic polyps have been reported in children on PPIs, as well as hyperplasia of parietal cells.[82]

• H_2 receptor antagonists

Enterochromaffin-like cells of the stomach secrete histamine, which binds to the parietal cell H_2 receptor, stimulating gastric acid secretion. H_2 receptor antagonists are competitive inhibitors of histamine at the parietal cell H_2 receptor. H_2 receptor antagonists such as ranitidine have been used successfully in the management of GERD in the pediatric population, with improvements in symptoms and endoscopic erosive esophagitis. Tachyphylaxis does develop quickly with H_2 receptor antagonists.[1] Once again, there is a lack of controlled trials in children looking at efficacy, side effects, and long-term effects of acid suppression.[3] The rise in gastric pH due to H_2 receptor antagonist use in neonates is associated with bacterial overgrowth.[83] With the advent of PPIs, use of H_2 receptor antagonists is given less priority, as PPIs are highly efficient and seem to be at least as safe.

- Other drugs

There is limited experience in infants with antacids such as bicarbonate salts and aluminum- or magnesium-based alkali complexes. They have a rapid onset of action and hence are used for symptom relief from heartburn in the adult population. In infants and toddlers, the use of aluminum-based antacids should be avoided because of the risk of systemic absorption of aluminum and its potential osteo- and neurotoxicity. Magnesium-rich preparations can cause diarrhea and preparations containing sodium carbonate may have excessive sodium content from a nutritional intake perspective. Mucosal coating agent sucralfate contains aluminum and should be avoided in infants.

2. Surgical management

The indications for surgery in children with GERD have changed with time, especially with the advent of the PPIs.

Surgical management is indicated in the following situations:

- Children with life-threatening complications of GERD: apneas and laryngospasm
- Children with failure to thrive from caloric loss due to regurgitation and vomiting despite conservative management
- Children with esophageal stricture with underlying GERD
- Children with EA who have anastomotic strictures in the presence of GERD
- Children with persistent respiratory tract problems secondary to GERD such as aspiration pneumonitis
- Children who have failed to respond to maximal medical therapy, who have significant side effects from medical therapy, who are unable to maintain compliance with medical therapy, or whose parents opt against long-term medical management for GERD

Surgery for reflux is generally thought to have good short- and long-term results and low complication rates.[84,85] In neurologically normal children, the success rate of fundoplication is quoted as >90% with 5-year follow-up, and around 60% for neurologically impaired children at 5-year follow-up.[85]

Laparoscopy is the preferred approach for fundoplication currently, with the three most common techniques being the Nissen (360° wrap), Toupet (180° wrap), and Thal (270° wrap) fundoplications. Other described techniques used in children include the Boix-Ochoa procedure.

Surgery is thought to work by creating a high-pressure zone at the distal esophagus with the wrap. Additionally, any hiatus hernia is repaired, the abdominal component of the esophagus is fixed abdominally, and the Angle of His is recreated.

Laparoscopic Nissen Fundoplication

The technique of choice at our institution is the laparoscopic Nissen fundoplication. This is a direct modification of the open Nissen fundoplication.

Parental consent involves careful discussion about the indication for surgery, the expected short- and long-term outcomes, the potential complications and failure rate, and the small risk of conversion to open fundoplication.

Under general anesthetic, the child is placed at the end of the operating table, in the frog-leg position for infants, or the legs supported in stirrups for older children, with the operator standing between the legs. It is important to ensure that the stirrups are positioned low, so that the knees of the patient do not obstruct operative movement.

A nasogastric tube is placed preoperatively, and a dose of prophylactic antibiotics given (IV caphazolin at our institution). The patient's skin is prepared with antiseptic solution from nipple level to pubis, extending well laterally, especially onto the left side, where a lateral port will be placed. Sterile drapes are placed around the operative field.

An umbilical port is introduced via the Hasson technique, and the peritoneal cavity insufflated with CO_2. A 30° laparoscope is used. All other ports are then placed under vision. Two working ports are placed on either side of the umbilicus; in bigger children, these will be more cranial on the abdomen, in smaller children, more caudal. An epigastric midline port is placed just under the xiphisternum for the liver retractor. We usually prefer to use a ratcheted toothed grasper that clasps the hiatus above the esophagus and lifts up the left lobe of liver. A Nathanson retractor may be used instead of the grasper. A low left lateral port is placed – this allows for an additional instrument to control the positioning of the stomach and esophagus during the procedure.

The patient is positioned with elevation of the head end of the bed. With the liver retracted giving a clear view of the esophageal hiatus, we start off by defining the space between the crus and esophagus on both the left and right sides, divide the overlying peritoneum, and develop this space with gentle blunt dissection. The retroesophageal plane is defined using the two working instruments together and the esophagus lifted, ensuring that the posterior vagus nerve is intact (Fig.

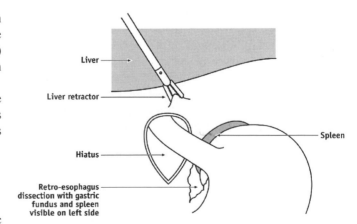

FIG. 26.2. Laparoscopic Nissen fundoplication: retroesophageal dissection

26.2). A retractor placed via the low left port is used to keep the esophagus in a lifted position while the hiatus is inspected. We usually place one or two sutures in the hiatus to secure it, taking care not to tighten the space excessively (Fig. 26.3). A good rule of thumb is to leave enough laxity in the sutured hiatus to allow in the tip of a 5-mm grasper alongside the esophagus.

The fundus is then pulled through from left to right from behind the esophagus (Figs. 26.4 and 26.5). The "shoeshine" maneuver is performed (moving the pulled fundus portion side to side behind the esophagus) to ensure the wrap is not too tight. We rarely have to divide short gastric vessels when they limit mobility of the fundus to achieve an acceptable wrap. We usually place three sutures to fashion

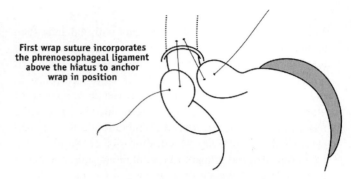

FIG. 26.6. Laparoscopic Nissen fundoplication: the first wrap stitch

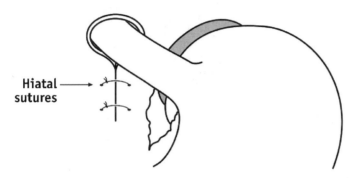

FIG. 26.3. Laparoscopic Nissen fundoplication: hiatal sutures placed

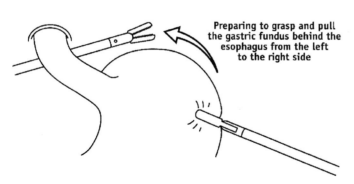

FIG. 26.4. Laparoscopic Nissen fundoplication: preparing to wrap the fundus

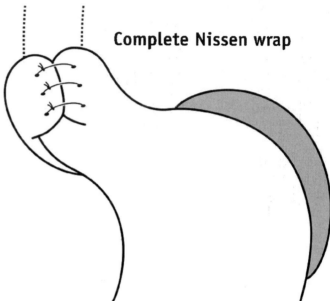

FIG. 26.7. Laparoscopic Nissen fundoplication: completed wrap

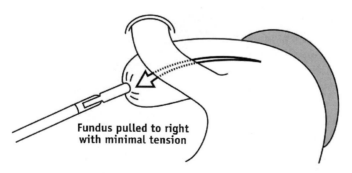

FIG. 26.5. Laparoscopic Nissen fundoplication: the fundus should come across with ease

the complete 360° wrap, the cranial-most suture incorporating the hiatus above the esophagus, to fix the wrap in position (Figs. 26.6 and 26.7).

In children requiring gastrostomy at the same time, a laparoscopic gastrostomy is fashioned after the fundoplication procedure. In most children requiring fundoplication with gastrostomies in situ, it is possible to perform the procedure laparoscopically without taking down the gastrostomy.

Postoperatively, the nasogastric tube is left to free drainage until the following day. Oral intake is graded up from clear fluids to solids over a couple of days. Children are advised to maintain a soft and pureed diet and to avoid chunky foods such as meat and bread for 4–6 weeks.

Previous surgery and adhesions may make the laparoscopic approach difficult, as may the presence of portal hypertension and organomegaly. In neurologically impaired children with limb contractures and scoliosis, positioning for laparoscopic surgery may be difficult and will require some adjustment of port positioning.

Other Antireflux Procedures

Proponents of the Toupet procedure (posterior 270° wrap) (Fig. 26.8) describe it as a better procedure in patients with known preoperative esophageal dysmotility, or for children with previous esophageal atresia repair (this group of children generally also have underlying esophageal dysmotility), as it theoretically is less tight than a complete wrap, minimizing the risk of dysphagia and gas bloat postoperatively.[86]

Proponents of the Thal procedure (Fig. 26.9) claim that the anterior 180° wrap preserves the intraabdominal component of the esophagus and re-creates the angle of His, while allowing a physiological degree of reflux and vomiting to occur.[27]

There are no randomized trials comparing outcomes of these three operative tachniques. A recent European study comparing outcomes of the Thal, Toupet, and Nissen procedures in neurologically normal children in three different centers did not demonstrate much difference in the long-term outcomes and complication rates between the three types of procedure.[87]

The Boix-Ochoa wrap is a modification of the Thal wrap that, in addition to the 180° wrap, includes plicating the remaining fundus to the left hemidiaphragm to re-create the angle of His.[27]

Redo Fundoplication

Redo laparoscopic fundoplication, although technically challenging, has been shown to be a safe and feasible approach for children requiring reoperation for undone or failed wraps.[88,89] The complication and failure rates in short-term follow-up are acceptably low.

Esophagogastric Dissociation

The failure rate of fundoplication in neurologically impaired children is relatively high (12–45%). In severely neurologically impaired children, especially those unable to feed orally and reliant almost completely on enteral feed because of incoordinate swallow, esophagogastric dissociation has been described as a procedure to definitively stop reflux.[90–92] It has been described both as a rescue procedure in neurologically impaired children with failed fundoplications and also as a primary antireflux procedure in a carefully selected group of neurologically impaired children with reflux. The procedure involves disconnecting the gastric cardia from the esophagus, sealing off the gastric cardia, and creating a Roux-en-Y esophagojejunal anastomosis, a feeding gastrostomy, and pyloroplasty to facilitate gastric drainage.[93]

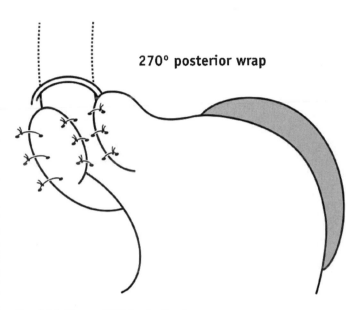

FIG. 26.8. Toupet 270° fundoplication.

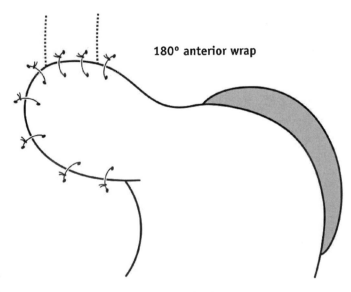

FIG. 26.9. Thal anterior 180° fundoplication.

Complications of Antireflux Surgery

1. Description and incidence

Complications post antireflux surgery are significantly higher in neurologically impaired children than neurologically normal children,[84] thus studies quoting complication and failure rates of antireflux surgery should be analyzed for the proportion of neurologically impaired children in their cohort. Reflux in neurologically impaired children is discussed in more detail later in this chapter.

Large cohort studies have established that the complication and recurrence rates of antireflux procedures have been acceptably low in both neurologically impaired and neurologically normal cohorts.[84] However, there is criticism in the recent literature about the quality of the follow-up studies of surgical outcome, suggesting that the complications and failure rates of antireflux surgery are being underestimated and improperly studied.[94] The argument is really one of balancing the true risks of fundoplication with the remarkable success of PPIs in managing GERD.[94] However, there is no doubt that in many cases with complications of volume reflux, such as failure to thrive from caloric loss from vomiting, antireflux surgery is indicated.

(a) Intraoperative complications:
Conversion to open procedure – Five to ten percent of laparoscopic cases need to be converted to an open procedure. This is usually in the setting of adhesions or intraoperative bleeding.

Pneumothorax – Occurs in 2% of laparoscopic cases when the pneumoperitoneum communicates with the pleural space.

Esophageal or gastric perforation – One percent risk. May be unrecognized at the time and present in the postoperative period. Perforation may occur during division of the gastric vessels, injuring the stomach wall in the process, or during esophageal manipulation.

Bleeding – Uncommon, but bleeding from the liver or spleen may necessitate conversion to open to achieve hemostasis and good vision, and rarely may require transfusion.

(b) Complications in the postoperative period:
Dysphagia – This is worse in the first 4–6 weeks postsurgery when tissue edema is present. It can be a persistent symptom if the wrap is too tight, or if there was an underlying esophageal motility problem. While it has been suggested that Nissen fundoplication has a higher incidence of postoperative dysphagia than partial wraps, there is no definite evidence to back this claim. A recent series showed that dysphagia was reported in 2.9% of cases postoperatively and spontaneously disappeared by 6 months post-op.[87]

Hiatal herniation (from disruption of the crural stitch or lax crural closure) can occur postoperatively. This is usually associated with recurrence of symptoms. It will require surgical correction.

Wrap slippage – To prevent this complication, the cranial most suture of the wrap usually incorporates the phrenoesophageal ligament to keep the wrap in position. If not, the wrap can slip down the body of the stomach, effectively acting as a constricting, obstructing band around the gastric body.

Gas-bloat syndrome – The inability to burp after fundoplication due to the "one-way valve" created by surgery may result in gas bloat in 2–5% patients.[95] Patients should be counseled preoperatively about avoiding predisposing foods such as carbonated drinks.

Failure of fundoplication with recurrent reflux or symptoms requiring reoperation – One large series in children noted that redo fundoplication was required in 3.6% of neurologically normal children and in 11.8% of neurologically impaired children.[84] Subsequent studies have shown a failure rate postfundoplication of between 4 and 44%,[87,96] with the higher end of the scale reflecting rates in neurologically impaired

children. Persistent and forceful retching and vomiting predispose to wrap failure.[94] In one recent series, up to two-thirds of children were reported to be persistently symptomatic or on antireflux medication after antireflux surgery. However, in this series, a high percentage (74%) of children in this series had concomitant medical disorders such as cystic fibrosis or neurodevelopmental delay, which may explain their unusually high rate of failure of antireflux surgery.[97]

2. Diagnosis and management of complications
Intraoperative complications are usually fairly evident as they occur, and can immediately be addressed and corrected. Intraoperative pneumothorax (secondary to intraperitoneal insufflated CO_2 escaping into the pleural cavity) interfering with ventilation may require placement of a chest drain. Gastric or esophageal perforation may not be recognized during the procedure and may present postoperatively with signs of peritonitis or free gas under the diaphragm. A small leak may be managed conservatively with fasting, IV fluids, and antibiotics. A large persistent leak evident on contrast study, or a child with peritonitis, will require operative intervention.

Children may present with dysphagia or regurgitation of food in the immediate postoperative period due to edema and tightness at the wrap. Good preoperative counseling about expecting this phenomenon and avoiding predisposing foods such as bread and meat for 4–6 weeks after surgery is important. A small minority will have persistent dysphagia. For these children, contrast study may show tightness at the wrap or crural closure site. Revision surgery will be required if so. In children whose manometry shows esophageal dysmotility, preoperative consideration may be given to a loose partial wrap, although definitive evidence to say that dysphagia rates are lower after partial wraps is lacking. Dietary advice about avoiding fizzy drinks is also important to minimize the occurrence of gas bloat postoperatively. Patients should be aware that if they develop severe left upper quadrant tightness and discomfort, they should present for medical assistance. The diagnosis may be clinically obvious with visible and palpable tender gastric fullness in the left upper quadrant. Erect CXR will show a large gastric bubble. Nasogastric decompression will usually ease symptoms.

Recurrent reflux will present in a variety of ways, often with the same symptoms that the child had preoperatively. Endoscopy to assess the wrap and presence of esophagitis, contrast study to assess the wrap, and esophageal pH studies will help confirm the diagnosis of recurrent reflux. Redo laparoscopic surgery is generally feasible and effective.[88]

Special Cases

Reflux in Children with Neurological Impairment

Neurologically impaired children have a higher incidence of vomiting and GERD than the general pediatric population.[98] Underlying this increased incidence are factors such as recumbency, hypotonia, scoliosis, spastic quadriplegia, and concomitant seizure disorders. Poor oral intake and incoordinate swallow with subsequent failure to thrive and growth restriction often necessitate the fashioning of a gastrostomy for enteral nutrition, which can further exacerbate vomiting and reflux. The complications of reflux are also more frequent in the neurologically impaired group, mainly esophagitis,[99] but also strictures,[100] Barrett's esophagus,[101] and respiratory complications.[99,100] Medical management may be useful for controlling esophagitis, but volume effects of ongoing vomiting with calorie loss, failure to thrive, and aspiration often require surgical intervention in this group.

The antireflux procedure of choice for neurologically impaired children at our institution is the laparoscopic Nissen fundoplication. Other institutions perform the Thal procedure by choice, under the theoretical premise that the partial wrap allows postoperative physiological burping and vomiting, and is thus less likely to be disrupted than the Nissen.[102] While antireflux surgery has good success rates in controlling symptoms in neurologically impaired children, with high rates of satisfaction with the outcome in parents and caregivers,[103] complication and failure rates are higher than in nonneurologically impaired children.[104]

Parents and carers of neurologically impaired children should be carefully counseled about the high complication (up to 12.8% reported), mortality (up to 20% reported), and failure rates of fundoplication in this group (30–46%).[84,96,105] This is usually manifested as a recurrence of symptoms such as vomiting. In the subgroup of neurologically impaired children who have little or no oral intake, esophagogastric dissociation may be considered as a primary definitive antireflux operation, or as revision surgery if initial fundoplication fails.[90,93]

Whether or not neurologically impaired children undergoing gastrostomy placement for feeding should routinely undergo fundoplication is a point of debate. Routine fundoplication with gastrostomy has been proposed in the past in view of the increased risk of GERD postgastrostomy placement.[106] Our practice is to perform gastrostomy only where indicated, and to perform fundoplication later should symptomatic GERD develop, a position that is well accepted in the literature. Less than half of these children will develop symptomatic reflux,[38,107] and it is generally possible to perform lap fundoplication around preexisting gastrostomies without having to take them down.[108]

Reflux in Children and Adults with Previous Esophageal Atresia Repair

Children with TEF/EA have a high incidence (35–58%) of associated GERD.[40,41] Reflux in these children can result in the usual complications of esophagitis, respiratory complications, and death spells. In addition, reflux exacerbates complications with esophageal anastomoses such as stricture formation.[40] About 50% of affected children respond to medical management of reflux, with the other 50% requiring surgical intervention.[27,40] Good results after antireflux surgery are reported in

this group of children,[109–111] with a 15–18% failure rate noted in the literature.[111,112]

Adults with previous esophageal atresia repair also seem to have a higher incidence of reflux symptoms such as heartburn and a higher incidence of esophagitis and are thought to have a higher risk of Barrett's esophagus than the general population.[113–115] 'Barrett's esophagus denotes specifically the presence of intestinal metaplasia in the esophagus, and is a risk factor for adenocarcinoma. In two studies, gastric epithelium was found on esophageal biopsies in 6–8% of TEF/EA children and young adults on follow-up endoscopy,[116,117] but there is uncertainty about whether this represented true metaplasia or normal gastric mucosa pulled up above the hiatus. One study has showed the presence of true Barrett's esophagus in 6% of adults with previous TEF/EA in their study cohort.[113] Whether this group of patients truly has a higher risk of Barrett's esophagus than the general population is unknown. It is thought that there is not enough evidence at this stage to recommend regular endoscopic screening for this cohort of patients.[115] There are at least three case reports in the literature of adenocarcinoma of the esophagus in young adults with previous TEF/EA repair.[118–120] It may be that regular long-term follow-up of these patients with specific regard to symptoms of reflux and early endoscopy to investigate any new symptoms such as dysphagia is prudent.

Controversies

Barrett's Esophagus in Children with GERD

Barrett's esophagus is the presence of specialized metaplastic columnar epithelium in the lower esophagus replacing the normal stratified squamous epithelium.[121] Mucosal damage to the lower esophagus from GERD is thought to heal abnormally with metaplastic columnar cells replacing squamous ones. The prevalence of Barrett's esophagus is associated with length of GERD symptoms.[122] The diagnosis of Barrett's esophagus is made on endoscopy and biopsy confirming the presence of columnar metaplasia in the distal esophagus.

Barrett's esophagus is a precursor to esophageal adenocarcinoma, the incidence of which is increasing in the Western world. It is estimated that cancer develops in 0.5% of adult patients with Barrett's esophagus per year.[123] Progressive dysplasia in the intestinal metaplasia of the distal esophagus is well documented over a period of years.[124] From these risks has arisen the practice and recommendation of endoscopic screening for patients with Barrett's esophagus in order to detect patients with dysplasia or carcinoma early.

There are many difficulties with endoscopic screening. Up to 40% of patients with Barrett's esophagus have no prior history of GERD symptoms, making it difficult to define the population to screen.[125] Only about 5% of patients with adenocarcinoma were known to have Barrett's esophagus prior to their presentation with cancer.[126] Screening has not been proven to reduce deaths from adenocarcinoma.[121] Detection of dysplasia relies on random endoscopic biopsies from the area of metaplasia, since the presence of dysplasia cannot be grossly identified at endoscopy.[121] Patients in whom high-grade dysplasia is detected on screening biopsies face the difficult options of undergoing further intensive endoscopic surveillance, endoscopic ablation of the dysplastic area, or esophagectomy.

There is some evidence that treatment of patients with Barrett's esophagus with PPIs may result in partial regression of the metaplastic epithelium.[127] Whether or not either medical or surgical antireflux treatment reduces the risk of cancer in Barrett's esophagus is unknown.[121]

Given the earlier uncertainties in managing adult patients with Barrett's esophagus, one can imagine the difficulties in planning management in children with Barrett's esophagus. The prevalence of Barrett's esophagus in adults undergoing endoscopy ranges from 8–12%,[128,129] whereas it is thought to be lower in children. One retrospective study estimated the prevalence of Barrett's esophagus in children undergoing endoscopy to be 2.7%, but it is likely that this is an underestimate.[130,131] If GERD is a risk for Barrett's esophagus, and dysplasia and malignancy in Barrett's esophagus are also a function of time, then logically GERD and Barrett's esophagus spanning from childhood will carry significant risk for esophageal carcinoma. At present though, there is no evidence to support the presumption that this risk is any higher for a child with Barrett's esophagus than for an adult with Barrett's esophagus. There is general agreement that regular endoscopic screening with biopsies should be instituted and maintained for children with known Barrett's esophagus.

Conclusion

GERD can be successfully managed with medications and antireflux surgery, achieving good symptom control. However, the natural history of GERD diagnosed in childhood is as yet unclear, and further research is required in defining the links of childhood-onset GERD to Barrett's esophagus and future risk of malignant change, and on how best to treat children so that these risks are minimized.[1,132]

References

1. Gold, B., Gastroesophageal reflux disease: could intervention in childhood reduce the risk of later complications? Am J Med, 2004. Suppl A: p. 23S–29S.
2. Suwandhi, E., Ton, M.N., and Schwarz, S.M., Gastroesophageal reflux in infancy and childhood. Pediatr Ann, 2006. 35(4): p. 259–66.
3. Vandenplas, Y., Salvatore, S., and Hauser, B. The diagnosis and management of gastro-oesophageal reflux in infants. Early Hum Dev, 2005. 81(12): p. 1011–24.
4. Nelson, S.P., et al., Prevalence of symptoms of gastroesophageal reflux during infancy. A pediatric practice-based survey. Pediatric Practice Research Group. Arch Pediatr Adolesc Med, 1997. 151(6): p. 569–72.
5. Nelson, S.P., et al., One year follow-up of symptoms of gastroesophageal reflux during infancy. Pediatric Practice Research Group. Pediatrics, 1998. 102(6): p. E67.
6. Billard, C., Traite des Maladies des Enfans Nouveaux-Nes et a la Mamelle: Fonde sur de Nouvelles Observations Cliniques et d'Anatomie Pathologique, Faites a l'Hopital des Enfans-Trouves de Paris, dans le Service de M. Baron. 1828, Paris: JB Bailliere.
7. Stylopoulos, N. and Rattner, D.W., The history of hiatal hernia surgery: from Bowditch to laparoscopy. Ann Surg, 2005. 241(1): p. 185–93.
8. Tileston, W., Peptic ulcer of the oesophagus. Am J Med Sci, 1906. 132: p. 240–65.
9. Hamperl, H., Peptische oesophagins. Verh Dtsch Pathol, 1934. 27: p. 208.
10. Winklestein, A., Peptic esophagitis: a new clinical entity. JAMA, 1935. 104: p. 906–9.
11. Carre, I.J., Postural treatment of children with a partial thoracic stomach ('hiatus hernia'). Arch Dis Child, 1960. 35: p. 569–80.
12. Allison, P.R., Reflux esophagitis, sliding hiatal hernia, and the anatomy of repair. Surg Gynecol Obstet, 1951. 92(4): p. 419–31.
13. Allison, P.R., Hiatus hernia: (a 20-year retrospective survey). Ann Surg, 1973. 178(3): p. 273–6.
14. Nissen, R., Eine einfache Operation zur Beeinflussung der Refluxeosophagitis. Schweiz Med Wochenschr., 1956. 86: p. 590–2.
15. Code, C.F., Fyke, F.E., Jr., and Schlegel, J.F., The gastroesophageal sphincter in healthy human beings. Gastroenterologia, 1956. 86(3): p. 135–50.
16. Liebermann-Meffert, D., et al., Muscular equivalent of the lower esophageal sphincter. Gastroenterology, 1979. 76(1): p. 31–8.
17. Mittal, R.K. and Balaban, D.H., The esophagogastric junction. N Engl J Med, 1997. 336(13): p. 924–32.
18. Ziegler, K., et al., Endosonographic appearance of the esophagus in achalasia. Endoscopy, 1990. 22(1): p. 1–4.
19. Liu, J.B., et al., Transnasal US of the esophagus: preliminary morphologic and function studies. Radiology, 1992. 184(3): p. 721–7.
20. DeMeester, T.R., et al., Biology of gastroesophageal reflux disease: pathophysiology relating to medical and surgical treatment. Annu Rev Med, 1999. 50: p. 469–506.
21. Boix-Ochoa, J. and Canals, J., Maturation of the lower esophagus. J Pediatr Surg, 1976. 11(5): p. 749–56.
22. Ingelfinger, F.J., Esophageal motility. Physiol Rev, 1958. 38(4): p. 533–84.
23. Dent, J., Recent views on the pathogenesis of gastro-oesophageal reflux disease. Baillieres Clin Gastroenterol, 1987. 1(4): p. 727–45.
24. Mittal, R.K., et al., Effect of crural myotomy on the incidence and mechanism of gastroesophageal reflux in cats. Gastroenterology, 1993. 105(3): p. 740–7.
25. Altschuler, S.M., et al., Simultaneous reflex inhibition of lower esophageal sphincter and crural diaphragm in cats. Am J Physiol, 1985. 249(5, Part 1): p. G586–G591.
26. Kahrilas, P.J., et al., Esophageal peristaltic dysfunction in peptic esophagitis. Gastroenterology, 1986. 91(4): p. 897–904.
27. Boix-Ochoa, J., Ashcraft, K., Gastroesophageal Reflux, In: Pediatric Surgery, Ashcraft, K.W., editor. 2005, Elsevier Saunders: Philadelphia. p. 383–404.
28. Kawahara, H., Dent, J., and Davidson, G., Mechanisms responsible for gastroesophageal reflux in children. Gastroenterology, 1997. 113(2): p. 399–408.

29. Rudolph, C.D., et al., Guidelines for evaluation and treatment of gastroesophageal reflux in infants and children: recommendations of the North American Society for Pediatric Gastroenterology and Nutrition. J Pediatr Gastroenterol Nutr, 2001. 32 Suppl 2: p. S1–S31.

30. Omari, T.I., et al., Mechanisms of gastro-oesophageal reflux in preterm and term infants with reflux disease. Gut, 2002. 51(4): p. 475–9.

31. Omari, T.I. and Davidson, G.P., Multipoint measurement of intragastric pH in healthy preterm infants. Arch Dis Child Fetal Neonatal Ed, 2003. 88(6): p. F517–F520.

32. Omari, T.I., et al., Mechanisms of gastroesophageal reflux in healthy premature infants. J Pediatr, 1998. 133(5): p. 650–4.

33. Omari, T.I., et al., Characterisation of relaxation of the lower oesophageal sphincter in healthy premature infants. Gut, 1997. 40(3): p. 370–5.

34. Orenstein, S.R., et al., Autosomal dominant infantile gastroesophageal reflux disease: exclusion of a 13q14 locus in five well characterized families. Am J Gastroenterol, 2002. 97(11): p. 2725–32.

35. Hu, F.Z., et al., Fine mapping a gene for pediatric gastroesophageal reflux on human chromosome 13q14. Hum Genet, 2004. 114(6): p. 562–72.

36. Hu, F.Z., et al., Refined localization of a gene for pediatric gastroesophageal reflux makes HTR2A an unlikely candidate gene. Hum Genet, 2000. 107(5): p. 519–25.

37. Hu, F.Z., et al., Mapping of a gene for severe pediatric gastroesophageal reflux to chromosome 13q14. JAMA, 2000. 284(3): p. 325–34.

38. Langer, J.C., et al., Feeding gastrostomy in neurologically impaired children: is an antireflux procedure necessary? J Pediatr Gastroenterol Nutr, 1988. 7(6): p. 837–41.

39. Grunow, J.E., al-Hafidh, A., and Tunell, W.P. Gastroesophageal reflux following percutaneous endoscopic gastrostomy in children. J Pediatr Surg, 1989. 24(1): p. 42–4; discussion 44–5.

40. Kovesi, T. and Rubin, S., Long-term complications of congenital esophageal atresia and/or tracheoesophageal fistula. Chest, 2004. 126(3): p. 915–25.

41. Engum, S.A., et al., Analysis of morbidity and mortality in 227 cases of esophageal atresia and/or tracheoesophageal fistula over two decades. Arch Surg, 1995. 130(5): p. 502–8; discussion 508–9.

42. Lindahl, H. and Rintala, R., Long-term complications in cases of isolated esophageal atresia treated with esophageal anastomosis. J Pediatr Surg, 1995. 30(8): p. 1222–3.

43. Shono, T., et al., Motility function of the esophagus before primary anastomosis in esophageal atresia. J Pediatr Surg, 1993. 28(5): p. 673–6.

44. Romeo, G., et al., Disorders of the esophageal motor activity in atresia of the esophagus. J Pediatr Surg, 1987. 22(2): p. 120–4.

45. Dent, J., et al., Mechanisms of lower oesophageal sphincter incompetence in patients with symptomatic gastrooesophageal reflux. Gut, 1988. 29(8): p. 1020–8.

46. Frankel, E.A., Shalaby, T.M., and Orenstein, S.R., Sandifer syndrome posturing: relation to abdominal wall contractions, gastroesophageal reflux, and fundoplication. Dig Dis Sci, 2006. 51(4): p. 635–40.

47. Bray, P.F., et al., Childhood gastroesophageal reflux. Neurologic and psychiatric syndromes mimicked. JAMA, 1977. 237(13): p. 1342–5.

48. Dahms, B.B. and Rothstein, F.C., Barrett's esophagus in children: a consequence of chronic gastroesophageal reflux. Gastroenterology, 1984. 86(2): p. 318–23.

49. Hassall, E., Weinstein, W.M., and Ament, M.E., Barrett's esophagus in childhood. Gastroenterology, 1985. 89(6): p. 1331–7.

50. Hassall, E., Barrett's esophagus: new definitions and approaches in children. J Pediatr Gastroenterol Nutr, 1993. 16(4): p. 345–64.

51. Hassall, E., Childhood Barrett's esophagus under the microscope. Am J Surg, 1994. 167(3): p. 287–90.

52. Hoeffel, J.C., Nihoul-Fekete, C., and Schmitt, M., Esophageal adenocarcinoma after gastroesophageal reflux in children. J Pediatr, 1989. 115(2): p. 259–61.

53. Orenstein, S.R., An overview of reflux-associated disorders in infants: apnea, laryngospasm, and aspiration. Am J Med, 2001. 111 Suppl 8A: p. 60S–63S.

54. Hrabovsky, E.E. and Mullett, M.D., Gastroesophageal reflux and the premature infant. J Pediatr Surg, 1986. 21(7): p. 583–7.

55. Glassman, M., George, D., and Grill, B., Gastroesophageal reflux in children. Clinical manifestations, diagnosis, and therapy. Gastroenterol Clin North Am, 1995. 24(1): p. 71–98.

56. Black, D.D., et al., Esophagitis in infants. Morphometric histological diagnosis and correlation with measures of gastroesophageal reflux. Gastroenterology, 1990. 98(6): p. 1408–14.

57. Behar, J. and Sheahan, D., Histologic abnormalities in reflux esophagitis. Arch Pathol, 1975. 99(7): p. 387–91.

58. Liacouras, C.A., Eosinophilic esophagitis: treatment in 2005. Curr Opin Gastroenterol, 2006. 22(2): p. 147–52.

59. Hill, J.L., et al., Technique and experience with 24-hour esophageal pH monitoring in children. J Pediatr Surg, 1977. 12(6): p. 877–87.

60. Jolley, S.G., et al., Patterns of postcibal gastroesophageal reflux in symptomatic infants. Am J Surg, 1979. 138(6): p. 946–50.

61. Shay, S.S., Johnson, L.F., and Richter, J.E., Acid rereflux: a review, emphasizing detection by impedance, manometry, and scintigraphy, and the impact on acid clearing pathophysiology as well as interpreting the pH record. Dig Dis Sci, 2003. 48(1): p. 1–9.

62. Shay, S.S., Bomeli, S., and Richter, J., Multichannel intraluminal impedance accurately detects fasting, recumbent reflux events and their clearing. Am J Physiol Gastrointest Liver Physiol, 2002. 283(2): p. G376–G383.

63. Stein, H.J. and DeMeester, T.R., Indications, technique, and clinical use of ambulatory 24-hour esophageal motility monitoring in a surgical practice. Ann Surg, 1993. 217(2): p. 128–37.

64. Euler, A.R. and Byrne, W.J., Gastric emptying times of water in infants and children: comparison of those with and without gastroesophageal reflux. J Pediatr Gastroenterol Nutr, 1983. 2(4): p. 595–8.

65. Jolley, S.G., Leonard, J.C., and Tunell, W.P., Gastric emptying in children with gastroesophageal reflux. I. An estimate of effective gastric emptying. J Pediatr Surg, 1987. 22(10): p. 923–6.

66. Fonkalsrud, E.W., et al., Operative treatment for the gastroesophageal reflux syndrome in children. J Pediatr Surg, 1989. 24(6): p. 525–9.

67. Maddern, G.J. and Jamieson, G.G., Fundoplication enhances gastric emptying. Ann Surg, 1985. 201(3): p. 296–9.

68. Fonkalsrud, E.W. and Ament, M.E., Gastroesophageal reflux in childhood. Curr Probl Surg, 1996. 33(1): p. 1–70.

69. Maxson, R.T., et al., Delayed gastric emptying in neurologically impaired children with gastroesophageal reflux: the role of pyloroplasty. J Pediatr Surg, 1994. 29(6): p. 726–9.

27
Esophageal Foreign Bodies

Tom Clarnette

Introduction

Foreign bodies that lodge in the esophagus are potentially a serious problem that peaks in children between the ages of 6 months and 3 years.[1] The majority of the ingested foreign bodies in children are lodged in the esophagus. Once the foreign body passes beyond the esophagus it usually negotiates itself through the rest of the gastrointestinal tract. Failure to recognize or appropriately manage a foreign body in the esophagus may lead to complications and occasional mortality.

Foreign bodies in the esophagus are ingested in young children by curiosity as they put objects in the mouth. Accidentally ingested foreign bodies are also seen either as food bolus impaction or in older children holding objects between their teeth. The impacted foreign body in the esophagus may be identified in a previously managed or unrecognized esophageal stricture.

Historic Perspective

Kelling has been credited with the invention of the first flexible esophagoscope in 1902.[2] Other prominent surgeons, namely Mikulicz, were also instrumental in the development of a flexible scope using lighting at the end of the scope. However, the beginning of esophagoscopy in late nineteenth century was the result of forward thinking by Professor Adolf Kussmaul, of Freiburg, who passed a hollow tube with a reflected light in the esophagus of a sword swallower.

Initially indirect visualization using a mirror was first described by Bozzini in 1809. Unfortunately, a view beyond the oropharynx could not be obtained. The use of an electrical light source and transmission of light along the cable rather than through a prism formed the basis of the modern endoscope that is in use today.[3]

In the past the diagnosis of an esophageal foreign body was achieved using a stethoscope on the patients back, which detected a gurgling sound resulting from liquid obstruction at the site of the foreign body. In 1875, Duplay used an esophageal resonator, which detected a scratching noise at the site of the esophageal obstruction.[4]

Basic Science/Pathogenesis

Foreign bodies are most likely to lodge where the esophagus is narrow. These areas include the upper esophageal sphincter formed by cricopharyngeaus, the level of the aortic arch (T4) where the esophagus is indented on the left by the aortic arch, and the lower esophageal sphincter at the gastroesophageal junction.

Some series report that, with the exception of sharp objects, foreign bodies lodge at either the upper or lower sphincter in the vast majority of cases. Our experience suggests that the most common site of obstruction for blunt objects is at the level of the thoracic inlet (Fig. 27.1). Small sharp objects, such as fish bones tend to lodge in the tonsillar region.[5] This poses a major problem in places such as China because of their habits of cooking and easting fish on the bone.[6]

The vast majority of esophageal foreign bodies occur in a normal esophagus. However, underlying esophageal pathology should always be considered. The most common cause is an esophageal stricture in conjunction with esophageal dysmotility following repair of esophageal atresia. A foreign body may be the first presentation of peptic stricture of the esophagus. Food bolus impacted at the lower end of the esophagus following fundoplication may indicate that the wrap is too tight.

The most common foreign bodies are coins, which account for up to two-thirds of all esophageal foreign bodies in children.[7] Food bolus is a common cause if there is underlying esophageal narrowing. Other foreign bodies less commonly encountered include needles, hairpins, disc batteries, and bones (usually fish or chicken).

D.H. Parikh et al. (eds.), *Pediatric Thoracic Surgery*,
DOI: 10.1007/b136543_27, © Springer-Verlag London Limited 2009

28
Foreign Bodies in the Airway

David C.G. Crabbe

Introduction

In the USA approximately 300 children die each year from choking. In the UK approximately 24 children die each year. The number of children presenting to emergency rooms with foreign body aspiration (FBAO) is at least 100-fold higher. The majority of deaths from FBAO occur in children under the age of 5. The objects most commonly aspirated are liquids in infants, and food, nuts, candy, small objects, and balloons in older children.

Prevention of FBAO involves a combination of parental education and manufacturing law. In the UK the Consumer Affairs Department of the Department of Trade and Industry monitors accidental injuries from choking in children.[1] Standards relating to the design and safety of toys are regulated by European directive BB/378/EEC and in the USA by Federal law (Consumer Product Safety Commission "small arts regulations").[2,3] This legislation involves testing childrens' toys using a "small parts cylinder" with dimensions that mimic the size of an infant's pharynx (Fig. 28.1). Toys with detachable components less than $2.5\,cm \times 3.2\,cm$ are deemed unsuitable for children under the age of 3.

Considerable effort has been put into first aid and paramedic training to deal with FBAO.[4,5] Algorithms for treatment are centered around basic life support and the Heimlich maneuver (Fig. 28.2).[6,7] Recent advice suggests that the Heimlich maneuver should not be used on infants because of the potential risk of injury to the abdominal viscera.[8-10] Infants should be inverted and foreign bodies disimpacted using chest thrusts.

Historical Perspective

Until the late nineteenth century the only method available to remove foreign bodies from the airway was bronchotomy. The results were generally poor with mortality rates around 25%. Death was either rapid from hypoxia or protracted from bronchiectasis. Killian is credited with successfully removing a bone from the right main stem bronchus of a German farmer in 1897. Jackson amassed considerable experience in the endoscopic removal of foreign bodies in the early twentieth century, describing techniques that are still in use.[11] By 1936, the mortality from an aspirated foreign body had decreased from 24 to 2%. The practical problem of illumination hampered endoscopy until the early 1960s when fiber optic cables became commercially available. The Hopkins rod-lens telescope was introduced by Storz in 1966. Light transmission and viewing angle increased substantially allowing instrument diameter to be reduced without diminishing the quality.

Basic Science and Epidemiology

Children between the ages of 1 and 3 are most at risk of FBAO. Toddlers are naturally inquisitive creatures who frequently place objects in their mouths yet lack the cognitive ability to distinguish edible from inedible objects. Their swallowing mechanism is still relatively immature and they lack the adult dentition for grinding food. Adult supervision of toddlers is a challenging exercise at the best of times, and most episodes of aspiration in children of this age are difficult, if not impossible, to prevent.

Children can aspirate almost anything that they place in their mouths. Toys, or small parts of toys, are frequent culprits, despite the legislation discussed previously. Food is probably aspirated most commonly by children. Peanuts and other nuts or seeds are particularly liable to aspiration. Peanuts tend to lodge in a main bronchus because of their size and smooth surface. Smaller fragments lodge more distally. Peanuts swell as they absorb water and the peanut oil causes a marked inflammatory reaction with mucosal edema. Granulation tissue develops around the nuts within a few days, making extraction progressively more difficult (Fig. 28.3).

FBAO in infants is less common and usually involves liquids. If an infant presents with a solid FBAO parental supervision should be questioned and occasionally this may involve the child protection agencies. FBAO in older

D.H. Parikh et al. (eds.), *Pediatric Thoracic Surgery*,
DOI: 10.1007/b136543_28, © Springer-Verlag London Limited 2009

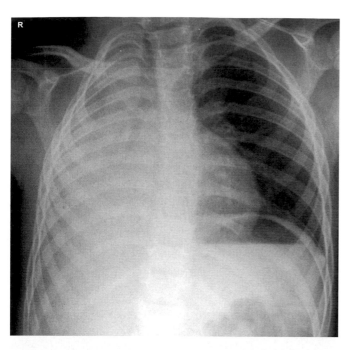

FIG. 28.5. Chest X-ray showing complete collapse of the lung from a foreign body

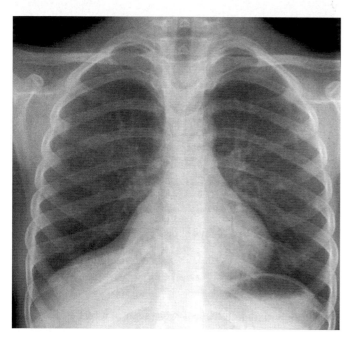

FIG. 28.6. Chest X-ray showing right lower lobe collapse from a foreign body

Management

Immediate Management of Inhaled Foreign Bodies

First-aid management depends on whether the airway is partially or totally obstructed. Coughing, choking, and gagging are involuntary efforts to clear the airway. They indicate partial airway obstruction, and the child may expel the foreign body without further intervention. Immediate assistance is generally unwise – a spontaneous cough is likely to be more effective and safer than any maneuver a rescuer might perform. Blind finger sweeps of the pharynx may unintentionally force a foreign body into the hypopharynx with fatal consequences. Back blows also risk exacerbating the airway obstruction in a conscious child.

If the child is unconscious or has an ineffective cough help is needed quickly. The child will be unable to speak and may be cyanosed and unconsciousness. Inappropriate action may cause injury but inertia may cause death. Help must be summoned. The current American Association of Pediatrics guidelines (1988)[5] and the current UK resuscitation council guidelines (2005)[7] recommend back blows to a child under the age of 1 placed in the prone position as the initial treatment. If this fails the child should be turned into a supine position and chest thrusts administered, similar to external cardiac massage. If this is not successful mouth-to-mouth resuscitation is commenced. For children over the age of 1 year the Heimlich maneuver should be used. If this fails mouth-to-mouth resuscitation should commence. Attempts to retrieve a foreign body from the pharynx digitally should only be performed on an unconscious child if the object is visible.

Definitive Management

Basic resuscitation should be continued in the emergency room for an unconscious child and 100% oxygen administered using bag and mask ventilation if necessary. Desperate attempts to intubate an asphyxiated child in the emergency room in the hope of forcing a foreign body into one or other main bronchus are invariably futile.

Rigid bronchoscopy is the definitive method for removing foreign bodies from the airway. This is not for the tyro. The importance of checking that all the necessary equipment are present and compatible cannot be overestimated. The scrub nurse must be familiar with the equipment and the likely sequence of events. Telescopes and bronchoscopes must be kept warm to minimize condensation, which will fog the endoscopic view. The surgeon and anesthetist should discuss strategy and their relative responsibilities prior to the arrival of the child. Failed retrieval of an inhaled foreign body has the potential to produce complete airway obstruction, with predictable consequences.

General anesthesia is essential with monitoring of EKG, pulse oximetry, capnography, and blood pressure.[29] Intravenous access is mandatory. Inhalational induction is recommended using either sevoflurane or halothane in 100% oxygen. This can take some considerable time when the airway is obstructed.

Spontaneous ventilation is preferable, although occasionally gentle assistance with mask ventilation may be necessary. Spontaneous ventilation is unlikely to cause distal migration of the foreign body and also reduces the risk of air trapping and pneumothorax.

The Stortz ventilating bronchoscopes are the best choice for endoscopic extraction of foreign bodies. These bronchoscopes are available in a full range of sizes but for foreign body extraction the 3.5, 3.7, and 4.0-mm diameter bronchoscopes should be used because optical grasping forceps are available (Fig. 28.7a, b). A wide range of instruments is available to enable retrieval of a foreign body (FB), as well as other therapeutic procedures. Oxygenation and anesthesia are maintained by connecting the anesthetic circuit T-piece to the sidearm of the bronchoscope.

A preliminary examination of the pharynx and larynx should be made with the anesthetic intubating laryngoscope because occasionally foreign bodies can be retrieved from this region using McGill's forceps. The next objective is to assess the airway to confirm or exclude the presence of a foreign body. Great care must be taken to ensure that the lumen of the airway remains in view at all times to avoid pushing a foreign body further down the tracheobronchial tree. Once the foreign body is located the bronchoscope is positioned approximately 2 cm above the obstruction and supported by the surgeon. The optical biopsy forceps is then assembled with the correct telescope and introduced into the bronchoscope. The jaws of the forceps are opened once they emerge from the end of the bronchoscope and the foreign body is grasped under direct vision. In the case of spherical or globular foreign bodies it is important to ensure that the blades of the forceps pass beyond the equator of the object to minimize the risk of fragmentation during retrieval. This is a particular problem with peanuts, which must be grasped with great delicacy. The anesthetist should temporarily suspend ventilation at this point. If the foreign body is small and unlikely to fragment it may be retrieved through the bronchoscope. This is not usually possible in which case the

foreign body and bronchoscope must be withdrawn together. It is easy to loosen the foreign body in the upper trachea or larynx at this stage. After the bronchoscope has been removed the anesthetist should take over control of the airway with a face mask while the retrieved object is inspected.

If the object cannot be grasped through the bronchoscope retrieval with a Fogarty embolectomy catheter may be successful.[30] The Fogarty catheter can be passed down the bronchoscope. The catheter is advanced beyond the foreign body and the balloon is inflated. Traction is exerted on the catheter to withdraw the foreign body (Fig. 28.8). The bronchoscope should be removed at this stage and an anesthetic laryngoscope inserted. As the object appears in the laryngeal inlet it can be grasped with McGill's forceps and retrieved.

Rarely foreign bodies are found in the tracheobronchial tree that are too large for removal through the larynx endoscopically. If this is felt likely then it is safer to remove the foreign body from the airway through a cervical tracheotomy than risk impacting the object in the subglottis during extraction through the larynx.[31] The tracheal incision can then be closed.

It is mandatory to examine the distal airway after removal of a foreign body to exclude additional foreign bodies and to aspirate secretions. Residual foreign body fragments may need to be removed in which case the procedure described earlier above should be repeated.

Fibreoptic bronchoscopy has been used for retrieval of foreign bodies and this may be successful in some instances.[32] However, the range of instruments for foreign body extraction

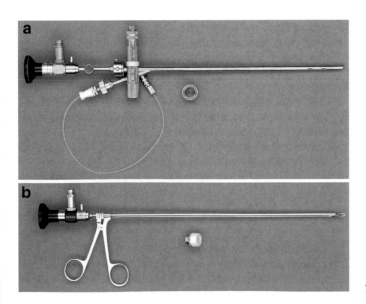

FIG. 28.7. (**a, b**) Storz ventilating bronchoscope and optical grasping forceps

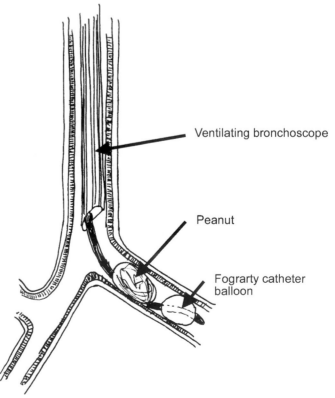

FIG. 28.8. Retrieval of a foreign body using a Fogarty catheter

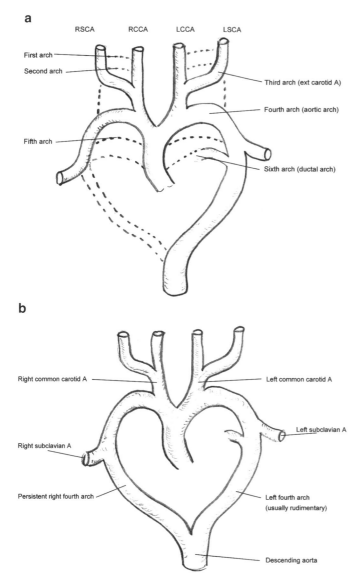

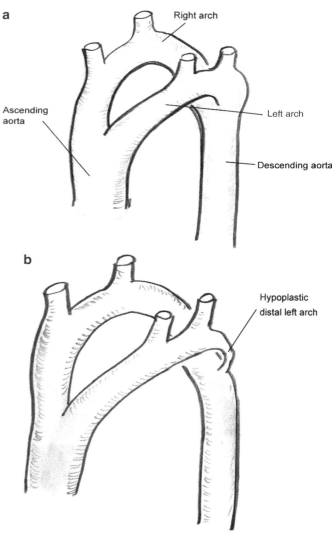

FIG. 29.1. Diagrammatic representation of the paired branchial arches and their relationship to the anatomical appearance at completion of development. (**a**) Normal arrangement. (**b**) Shows the arrangement in a double aortic arch. The *dotted lines* represent embryological structures that normally involute during development. *LSCA* left subclavian artery, *RSCA* right subclavian artery, *LCCA* left common carotid artery, *RCCA* right common carotid artery

FIG. 29.2. Double aortic arch. A common carotid and a subclavian artery arise from each arch. (**a**) Equal dominance of the two arches. (**b**) The commoner situation of dominant right arch with hypoplasia of the distal left arch. This may be only an atretic, fibrous cord

Right aortic arch with left-sided ductus: This is the second commonest vascular ring (25–30%). A right-sided aortic arch, by definition, passes over the right main bronchus (Fig. 29.4). In most right arches the first branch is a left-sided innominate artery, although it may be the left common carotid artery in which case the left subclavian arises anomalously as a fourth branch of the arch (passing behind the esophagus). In fact, in the case of a right arch/left duct vascular ring this is the *commonest* arrangement (70% of cases), with the anomalous left subclavian artery often arising from a diverticulum of Kommerell (Fig. 29.5). The descending thoracic aorta reverts

to its usual position on the left side of the chest. Thus, the indentation in the posterior esophagus is created by the distal right arch crossing back to the left side. If there is an anomalous left subclavian artery, this may also contribute to the posterior impression. The ductal ligament is left sided and runs directly back (over the left main bronchus) to insert into the distal arch (or into the root of the anomalous left subclavian artery) to complete the ring.

A left (i.e., normal) arch with a right-sided ductus is recognized but it is extremely rare and usually only seen in association with complex intracardiac defects. One clue can be that the descending thoracic aorta is right sided despite a left arch. Bilateral ductus ligaments are seen occasionally but the right-sided

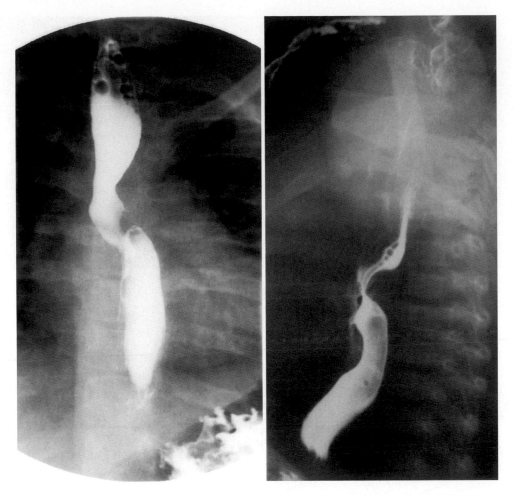

FIG. 29.3. AP and lateral views from a barium swallow showing indentation of the esophagus from a vascular ring (double aortic arch)

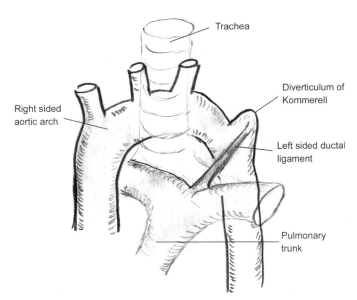

FIG. 29.4. Right-sided arch with left-sided duct ligament. The ligament inserts into a diverticulum of Kommerell, which is probably a remnant of the distal portion of the left aortic arch (fourth branchial arch). The trachea and esophagus are trapped between the arch and the duct ligament

ligament usually arises from the root of the innominate artery and so does not run posteriorly and, consequently, does not create a complete ring.

The diverticulum of Kommerell represents persistence of the posterior remnant of the fourth arch, appearing as an outpouching from the distal arch passing behind the esophagus. It is frequently associated with anomalous origin of the subclavian artery, which arises from the distal end of the diverticulum. The diverticulum is most commonly seen in association with a right-sided arch, and the duct ligament inserts into the apex of the diverticulum, creating the vascular ring. The anomaly clearly demonstrates the spectrum of varying degrees of persistence of a double arch. Less commonly, the diverticulum is seen with a left-sided arch, in which case the duct usually inserts to the left side and there is no vascular ring.

Pulmonary artery sling: This is the third commonest form of vascular ring (15–20%) and differs from the others in two important ways. Firstly, the sling encircles the trachea only and so does not cause esophageal compression. Secondly, and more importantly, it is frequently (50–67% of cases)[8,9] associated with varying degrees of tracheal stenosis including complete tracheal rings – the so-called *sling-ring* anomaly.

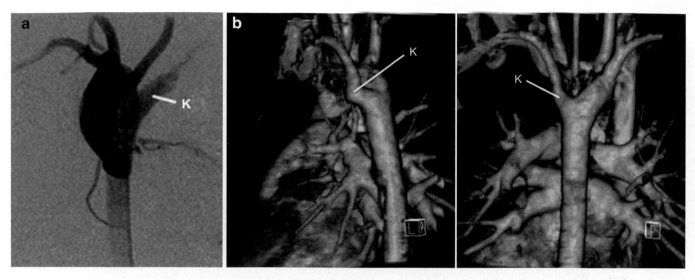

Fig. 29.5. Right-sided arch with aberrant left subclavian arising from a diverticulum of Kommerell. This is shown by both the angiogram (**a**) and on the 3-D reconstructed CT, viewing the aorta and heart from behind (**b**)

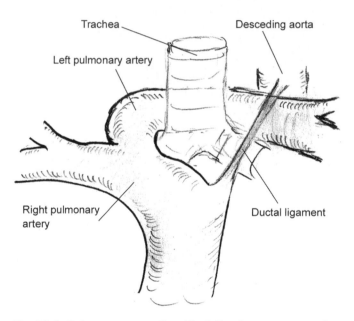

Fig. 29.6. Pulmonary artery sling. The left pulmonary artery arises as the first branch of the right pulmonary artery and then runs behind the trachea toward the hilum of the left lung

The sling is created by anomalous origin of the left pulmonary artery (LPA), which arises as the first branch of the right pulmonary artery. The vessel runs behind the trachea toward the left hilum (Fig. 29.6). The trachea is trapped in the sling created by the LPA. A ductal ligament running from the main pulmonary artery completes the ring. The pathognomonic sign on barium swallow is anterior indentation of the esophagus (caused by the LPA).

Vascular compression syndromes: Symptoms of vascular compression may occur in the absence of a vascular ring. The commonest is *innominate artery compression* of the trachea that occurs due to a relatively anterior position of the innominate artery in association with a narrow thoracic inlet, creating vascular compression of the anterior wall of the trachea ("innominate artery compression syndrome"). Anterior pulsatile indentation is seen on bronchoscopy but the degree of narrowing is usually minor. An *anomalous right subclavian artery* arising from a left arch and passing behind the esophagus will produce a posterior indentation visible at endoscopy and on barium swallow. There is no vascular ring but the posterior course of the artery can occasionally cause a minor degree of dysphagia, usually only in later life when a degree of atherosclerosis decreases the elasticity of the vessel. This is the so-called *dysphagia lusoria* named from the original description of the anomalous right subclavian artery as the *arteria lusoria*.

Clinical Features

Vascular rings produce symptoms related to compression of the trachea and/or esophagus. The commonest presenting symptom of a vascular ring is stridor. Around 50–70% of symptomatic cases present during the first year of life.[10] Early presentation is associated with a tight ring. Children may be misdiagnosed as "asthmatic" or present with recurrent chest infections at which time the airway obstruction is diagnosed.[11] Younger children have a characteristic "seal-bark" cough associated with biphasic stridor. Older children may present with a persistent nonproductive cough, which is due to tracheal irritation. In most cases stridor is due to tracheomalacia from extrinsic compression on the airway at the site of the ring. Vascular rings occasionally cause esophageal symptoms. Infants may suffer from vomiting, failure to thrive, and difficulty in feeding. Older children may present with dysphagia for solids. Vascular ring may be discovered coincidentally on a barium swallow.

Asymptomatic vascular rings require no treatment. Pulmonary artery slings represent a special case because a significant number are associated with congenital tracheal stenosis.

Vascular rings occasionally present in later life, usually with low-grade airway symptoms but occasionally with dysphagia. Delayed presentation usually indicates a vascular ring that has caused minimal airway compression. In later life atherosclerotic changes may decrease the compliance of the vascular ring to a point where it becomes symptomatic.

Diagnosis and Investigations

Clinical examination may reveal inspiratory or biphasic stridor. A plain chest radiograph is not usually diagnostic. There are, however, features that may suggest the diagnosis of a vascular ring. The cardiac silhouette may reveal the knuckles of a double arch on each side of the trachea (Fig. 29.7) or the silhouette of a right arch. Occasionally a very tight double aortic arch will cause air trapping with overinflation of the lungs.

The most useful first-line investigation if a vascular ring is suspected is a barium swallow (Fig. 29.3). Provided good distension of the esophagus is obtained there will be a fixed indentation in the posterior esophagus. Pulsatility may be appreciated on screening. In the case of a pulmonary artery sling anterior indentation of the esophagus may be seen. Computerized tomography, with intravenous contrast, or MR scanning are required to define the vascular anatomy in detail (Fig. 29.8). It is rarely possible to define the anatomy completely using transthoracic echocardiography. Increasingly MR with 3-D reconstruction of the vascular structures and trachea is becoming the preferred method of imaging vascular rings.[12,13]

Angiography (Fig. 29.9) has been largely superseded by CT/MRI although occasionally this may be necessary if there is doubt about which side of the arch is dominant.

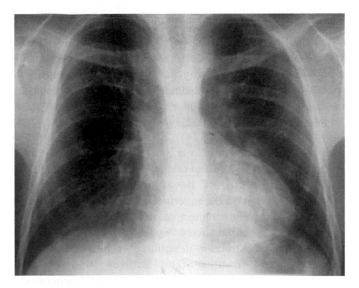

FIG. 29.7. Plain CXR of an adult with double aortic arch

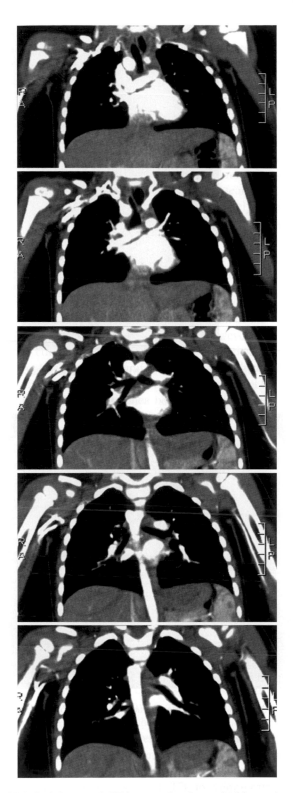

FIG. 29.8. Serial coronal CT images showing a double aortic arch. This series of five frames moves sequentially from anterior to posterior, top to bottom. In the first frame two arches can be seen straddling the trachea – the right arch being dominant and considerably larger than the left. The tracheal compression caused by the ring can be seen in the next frame and the "double-knuckle" appearance of the two arches joining posteriorly can be seen in frames 3 and 4. In the final frame the descending aorta only reaches the left side of the thorax at the level of the diaphragm

Minimally invasive approaches to treat vascular rings are becoming popular. Until recently thoracoscopy was generally reserved for the division of ligamentous structures on the grounds that patent vascular structures are probably approached more safely through open thoracotomy. In 1995 Burke et al. reported a series of eight patients treated by video-assisted thoracoscopic surgery.[18] More recently Al-Bassam and colleagues reported a series of nine children treated successfully using minimally invasive surgery, including two children with double aortic arches.[19]

Outcomes

Surgery is safe and operative mortality is low. Early mortality of 1–2% is reported in the current era.[20,21] The only exception to this is when extensive tracheal surgery is required at the same procedure. Mortality in the region of 10–15% is attributable to the tracheal surgery.[9,22]

There is immediate improvement in stridor in about 85% children following surgery. *Complete* resolution of stridor is unusual and this often persists for several months, depending on the degree of tracheomalacia. Severe symptomatic tracheomalacia, particularly in infants, may necessitate further treatment. Bronchoscopy should be performed to assess the airway and consideration given to aortopexy or tracheopexy if these were not performed at the primary operation. This reinforces the importance of proper assessment of the airway at the time of surgery. The alternative to aortopexy is usually several months of airway support (usually CPAP) until the tracheomalacia regresses.

Complications

Persistent tracheomalacia requiring prolonged ventilatory support is the most serious complication. If the trachea is of normal dimension and all compression has been relieved then the outcome is extremely good, although typically requires at least noninvasive positive pressure airway support for 3–6 months. Other specific complications include injury to the phrenic or recurrent laryngeal nerves with a risk of 2–5%. There is a risk of major bleeding but, as long as care is taken to control the vessels prior to division, this should be a rare occurrence.

Controversies

There is still debate over whether aortopexy/tracheopexy should be performed as a matter of routine at the time of division of the vascular ring. The role of video-assisted thoracic surgery (VATS) in the management of vascular rings is still not defined. Many of the patients are neonates or small infants and, as a result, many surgeons still prefer an open approach. Most vascular rings would be quite suitable for a

VATS approach but thoracoscopic division of major vessels demands considerable expertise with minimally invasive surgery and also a sufficiently large caseload to develop and maintain competence.

Conclusions and Future Perspectives

Vascular rings are a rare group of conditions that are eminently suitable to surgical repair. Long-term results are very good and patients can expect permanent relief of symptoms. The small group of children with pulmonary artery slings associated with complex tracheal anomalies remains the greatest challenge. The prognosis for these unfortunate children depends on the nature of the tracheal anomaly rather than on the vascular ring.

Computerized tomography and magnetic resonance scanning have brought considerable advances in the imaging of vascular rings. Angiography is now rarely necessary. Recognition of the importance of tracheomalacia has led to a more thoughtful approach to assessing the airway pre- and postoperatively and a more liberal approach to concomitant aortopexy.

References

1. Stewart JR, Kincaid OW, Edwards JE. An Atlas of Vascular Rings and Related Malformations of the Aortic Arch System. Thomas, Springfield, IL, 1964.
2. Bayford D. An account of a singular case of obstructed deglutition. Mem Med Soc Lond 1794: 2; 275–280.
3. Gross RE. Surgical relief for tracheal obstruction from a vascular ring. N Eng J Med 1945: 233; 586–590.
4. Potts WJ, Holinger PH, Rosenblum AH. Anomalous pulmonary artery causing obstruction to right main bronchus. Report of a case. JAMA 1954: 155; 1409–1411.
5. McElhinney DB, Clark BJ, Weinberg PM, et al. Association of chromosome 22q11 deletion with isolated anomalies of aortic arch laterality and branching. J Am Coll Cardiol 2001: 37; 2114–2119.
6. Virdi IS, Keeton BR, Shore DF, Monro JL. Surgical management in tetralogy of Fallot and vascular ring. Pediatr Cardiol 1987: 8; 131–134.
7. Kupferschmid JP, Burns SA, Jonas RA, et al. Repair of double aortic arch associated with D-transposition of the great arteries. Ann Thorac Surg 1993: 56; 570–572.
8. Backer CI, Mavroudis C, Dunham ME, Holinger LD. Pulmonary artery sling: Results with median sternotomy, cardiopulmonary bypass and reimplantation. Ann Thorac Surg 1999: 67; 1738–1744.
9. Fiore AC, Brown JW, Weber TR, Turrentine MW. Surgical treatment of pulmonary artery sling and tracheal stenosis. Ann Thorac Surg 2005: 79; 38–46.
10. Bonnard A, Auber F, Fourcade L, et al. Vascular ring abnormalities: A retrospective study of 62 cases. J Pediatr Surg 2003: 38; 539–543.
11. Linna O, Hyrynkangas K, Lanning P, Niemenan P. Central airways stenosis in school-aged children: Differential diagnosis from asthma. Acta Paediatr 2002: 91; 399–402.

12. Haramati LB, Glickstein JS, Issenberg HJ, et al. MR imaging and CT of vascular anomalies and connections in patients with congenital heart disease: Significance in surgical planning. Radiographics 2002: 22; 337–347.

13. Beekman RP, Beek FJ, Hazekamp MG, Meijboom EJ. The value of MRI in diagnosing vascular abnormalities causing stridor. Eur J Pediatr 1997: 156; 516–520.

14. Backer CL, Mavroudis C, Rigsby CK, Holinger LD. Trends in vascular ring surgery. J Thorac Cardiovasc Surg 2005: 129; 1339–1347.

15. Grillo HC, Wright CD, Vlahakes GJ, MacGillvray TE. Management of congenital tracheal stenosis by means of slide tracheoplasty or resection and reconstruction, with long-term follow up of growth after slide tracheoplasty. J Thorac Cardiovasc Surg 2002: 123; 145–152.

16. Backer CL, Mavroudis C, Holinger LD. Repair of congenital tracheal stenosis. Semin Thorac Cardiovasc Surg Pediatr Card Surg Annu 2002: 5; 173–186.

17. De Leon SY, Quinones JA, Pifarre R. Innominate artery reimplantation for displaced innominate artery. J Thorac Cardiovasc Surg 1994: 107; 947–948.

18. Burke RP, Rosenfeld HM, Wernovsky G, Jonas RA. Video-assisted thoracoscopic vascular ring division in infants and children. J Am Coll Cardiol 1995: 25; 943–947.

19. Al-Bassam A, Mallick MS, Al-Qahtani A, et al. Thoracoscopic division of vascular rings in infants and children. J Pediatr Surg 2007: 42; 1357–1361.

20. Backer CL, Ilbawi MN, Idriss FS, De Leon SY. Vascular anomalies causing tracheoesophageal compression. Review of experience in children. J Thorac Cardiovasc Surg 1989: 97; 725–731.

21. Anand R, Dooley KJ, Williams WH, Vincent RN. Follow-up of surgical correction of vascular anomalies causing tracheobronchial compression. Pediatr Cardiol 1994: 15; 58–61.

22. Antón-Pacheco JL, Cano I, Comas J, Galletti L, Polo L, García A, López M, Cabezalí D. Management of congenital tracheal stenosis in infancy. Eur J Cardiothorac Surg 2006: 29; 991–996.

12. Merry C, Spurbeck W, Lobe TE. Resection of foregut-derived duplications by minimal-access surgery. Pediatr Surg Int 1999; 15: 224–6.

13. Partrick DA, Rothenberg SS. Thoracoscopic resection of mediastinal masses in infants and children: an evaluation of technique and results. J Pediatr Surg 2001; 36: 1165–7.

14. Bratu I, Laberge JM, Flageole H, Bouchard S. Foregut duplications: is there an advantage to thoracoscopic resection? J Pediatr Surg 2005; 40: 138–41.

15. Stringer MD, Spitz L, Abel R, et al. Management of alimentary tract duplication in children. Br J Surg 1995; 82: 74–8.

Section 7
Lung Disease

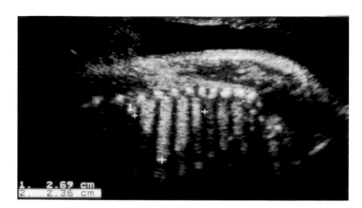

FIG. 32.2. Fetal pulmonary sequestration

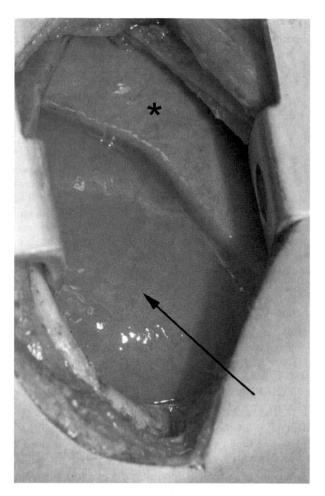

FIG. 32.1. Extra-lobar sequestration (*arrow*) with a separate visceral pleural investment from the lower lobe (*asterisk*)

pores of Kohn and result in recurrent infection. It is rare for an ELS to have any connection with the bronchial tree and consequently infectious complications are rare. The vascular supply for both ILS and ELS generally arises directly from the lower thoracic or upper abdominal aorta.[11] The majority of sequestrations have a single arterial feeder, although up to a third may have multiple vessels. The venous drainage is usually normal to the left atrium but abnormal drainage to the right atrium, vena cava, and azygous vein have all been documented.[11] Both ELS and ILS have been documented in the same patient.

It is not uncommon for other congenital abnormalities to be associated with PS, more with ELS then ILS. These include, but are not restricted to, congenital diaphragmatic hernia, vertebral anomalies, congenital heart disease, pulmonary hypoplasia, and colonic duplication.[2,11] In one series, ELS was associated with CCAM in up to 50% of cases, again suggesting that these conditions are simply a spectrum of a single disease process.[13,14]

Clinical Features

The clinical presentation varies depending on the size, type, and location of the PS. More and more lesions are being detected in the prenatal period by routine ultrasound. They

tend to be echogenic masses, which can be small or occupy the entire thoracic cavity (Fig. 32.2). Larger lesions may cause mediastinal shift and in extreme cases hydrops secondary to vascular compression. A large percentage of these lesions, in some series over 70%, will regress during gestation so postnatal evaluation is essential.[15–17]

Intralobar sequestration is more common than extralobar but rarely diagnosed in early life because most patients are asymptomatic until pulmonary infection occurs. Up to 25% of infants with ELS will present early with feeding difficulties or respiratory distress, or both. Recurrent pneumonia is less uncommon in these infants. Older infants can present with evidence of congestive heart failure because of excessive blood flow through the aberrant artery. Most symptoms from ELS are secondary to a mass affect. PS may be discovered coincidentally in an older asymptomatic patient on a routine chest X-ray. In rare cases, these patients may present with heart failure, secondary to high flow through the anomalous systemic artery, or with hemoptysis.[4]

There are reports of massive hemoptysis occurring in untreated sequestrations.[18–21] There are case reports of a fibrous mesothelioma and carcinoma arising from an ILS.[22,23] However, these appear to be hybrid lesions and may be more consistent with CCAM. This again supports the contention that all congenital lung lesions should be excised.

Diagnosis

Many PSs are now detected antenatally by ultrasound. ELS appears as a well defined echodense homogenous mass, which is separate from the lung. The classic finding is that of a systemic artery coming from the aorta to the lung lesion, which is easily identified with color flow Doppler US (Fig. 32.3). Occasionally, a systemic artery can also be seen in a CCAM as documented by Coran and Stocker in over 50 cases.[13] MRI has also been used in the prenatal period and can help to differentiate between PS, CCAM, and CDH.[24] However, none of these diagnostic methods have proven to be 100% specific.

Postnatal diagnosis is made by a number of modalities. An initial chest X-ray (CXR) can be highly suggestive. This usually

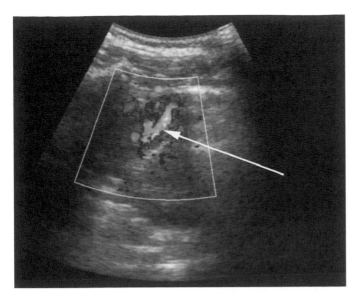

FIG. 32.3. Doppler ultrasound identifying feeding vessel to sequestration (*arrow*)

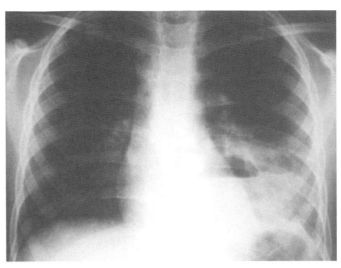

FIG. 32.5. Air-fluid levels within an infected left basal ILS in an eight-year-old child

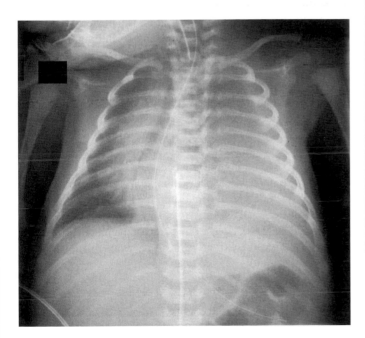

FIG. 32.4. Newborn with a large left ELS causing mediastinal shift and respiratory failure

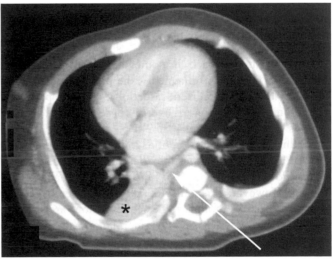

FIG. 32.6. Spiral CT scan showing right basal sequestration (*asterisk*) and feeding vessel (*arrow*)

shows a mass of uniform increased density within the lower thoracic cavity or within the parenchyma of the lobe. There may be a mass effect with mediastinal shift early in the newborn period (Fig. 32.4). Chest X-ray may also show air-fluid levels due to bronchial communication (Fig. 32.5), primarily in cases of ILS. If PS is expected a contrast CT scan is obtained. This can confirm the extralobar mass in cases of ELS and show abnormal parenchyma in cases of ILS. Other findings include large cavitating lesions with air-fluid levels, many small cystic lesions containing fluid or air, or a well-defined cystic mass.

Emphysematous changes may also be present on the periphery of the mass.

Conventional CT does not always demonstrate the systemic artery, especially if the vessels are less then 1 mm. Therefore, a contrast enhanced or helical CT is recommended which can show greater definition and increase the yield of these studies (Fig. 32.6).[25,26] Magnetic resonance imaging (MRI) can show the lesion and identify the aberrant artery especially if an MR angiogram (MRA) is used[27] (Fig. 32.7). Previously angiography was recommended prior to surgery to demonstrate the arterial anatomy and the location of the aberrant systemic artery, but this is no longer necessary with improved CT and MRI. Ultrasound with Doppler can also be used in the postnatal period but most authors agree that CT is more sensitive and specific.[28]

antenatal steroids, postnatal surfactant therapy and improvements in ventilatory management.

Pathogenesis and Basic Science

Respiratory distress syndrome results from the deficiency of surfactant due to immaturity of the lungs. Prematurity is an important contributory factor in the development of RDS, although there are several predisposing factors.[4] Males are more likely to develop RDS than females. Black infants are less likely to develop RDS. Babies born with a poor respiratory effort, bradycardia or poor tone at birth are more likely to develop RDS.[6] Fetal hypoxia causes decreased lung perfusion and damage to the capillaries. This results in leakage of protein rich fluid that inhibits surfactant. The resulting hypoxia and acidosis further reduce surfactant production. Family history of RDS, second twin and hypothermia are other predisposing factors.

Surfactant is a complex substance containing phospholipids and a number of apoproteins that is produced by type II alveolar cells, and lines the alveoli and smallest bronchioles. Surfactant reduces surface tension, thereby increasing lung compliance. Deficiency of surfactant leads to alveolar collapse, decreased lung compliance and reduced functional residual capacity and ventilation-perfusion mismatch. Most babies have some surfactant at birth. The symptoms of RDS worsen when protein rich exudates leaks into the damaged lung, inhibiting surfactant. Alveolar hypoventilation results in hypoxia and acidosis reduce surfactant production and affect pulmonary vascular resistance, cardiac contractility, cardiac output and systemic blood pressure. The lungs remain noncompliant until levels of surfactant begin to rise at around 36–48 hours. Pulmonary arterial pressure (PAP) remains high in babies with RDS up to one week of life.[7] High PAP may result in right to left shunting.

Microscopic examination of the lung in RDS reveals collapse of peripheral airspaces and alveolar epithelial cell necrosis. Hyaline (proteinaceous) membranes are formed on denuded areas and by 24 hours more extensive membrane formation occurs, lining the distended terminal and respiratory bronchioles. There is also a noticeable diffuse interstitial edema with congested capillaries and dilated lymphatics.[8]

Clinical Features

The spectrum of severity varies from a mild form to a severe, fatal form. The diagnostic criteria for RDS are respiratory rate more than 60 per minute, expiratory grunt, sternal and intercostal recessions and cyanosis in air. The disease presents within the first 4 hours of life. In the milder form the disease initially worsens by 24–36 hours and the severity decreases by 36–48 hours as the surfactant synthesis commences. This is often associated with spontaneous diuresis. Some babies may present with alternate periods of shallow, rapid breathing with slow breathing with recessions. This is often associated with apneas and is a sign of respiratory failure. The more mature

babies present with tachypnea, grunting, flaring of the alae nasi and cyanosis needing oxygen. In contrast the immature babies may need positive pressure ventilation from birth.

Diagnosis

Radiological Diagnosis

The chest radiograph (CXR) (Fig. 34.1) helps to establish the diagnosis. The CXR shows diffuse, fine granular opacification of both lung fields with an 'air bronchogram' due to air filled bronchi that stand out against the white opacified lung. The ground glass appearance with an obscured heart border is a classical picture of RDS.

Blood gas estimations help to detect hypoxemia and hypercapnia. This is useful to assess the severity of the lung disease and in further management. In ventilated babies with RDS, it is important to perform blood gases regularly, ideally arterial but capillary blood gas may be done, especially within half an hour after surfactant administration to prevent hypocapnia which is detrimental to the brain.

Differential Diagnosis

There are a number of conditions that have similar clinical features to RDS. Congenital pneumonia, aspiration pneumonia, meconium aspiration syndrome, transient tachypnea of the newborn, pneumothorax, diaphragmatic hernia and

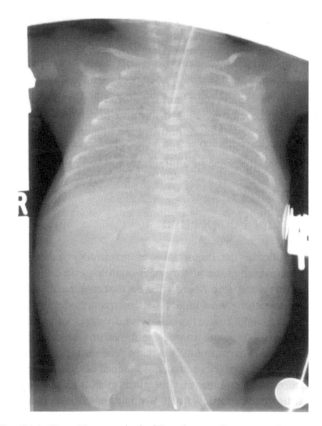

FIG. 34.1. Chest X-ray typical of Respiratory distress syndrome

congenital heart disease are some of them. However the history, presentations and CXR findings vary.

Management

Prenatal Steroids

Antenatal administration of corticosteroids such as dexamethasone or betamethasone significantly reduces the incidence of RDS in preterm neonates.[9] Betamethasone is now preferred because of a lower incidence of periventricular leukomalacia.[10] It should ideally be administered 48 hours prior to delivery but its usefulness has been shown even if administered less than 24 hours.[11] Risk assessment for the administration of steroids to mother in preterm labor has shown negligible risk and improved survival of preterm infants. Increased risk of infection in the mother with prolonged rupture of membranes and diabetic mothers with disturbed glucose homeostasis can be managed effectively. Studies of neonates who received prenatal steroids have shown that they do not suffer from more infective episodes or developmental delay.

Surfactant Replacement

Prophylactic surfactant has been shown to reduce the incidence of pneumothorax, mortality and combined outcome of mortality and chronic lung disease (CLD). Trials comparing prophylactic surfactant versus selective use of surfactant have shown a better outcome in the prophylactic group. There was significant reduction in mortality and a borderline significant reduction in pneumothorax.[12]

Surfactant therapy improves the outcome of infant with RDS. Trials have demonstrated that there is greater early improvement in requirement for ventilatory support, fewer pneumothoraces and fewer deaths with natural surfactant compared to synthetic surfactant.[3] Surfactant administration is associated with reduced oxygen and ventilatory requirement. It has been shown to reduce the incidence of pneumothorax, mortality and combined outcome of chronic lung disease (CLD) and mortality.[12]

Neonatal Intensive Care

The mortality and morbidity among premature infants with RDS is significantly reduced by skilled resuscitation after delivery and subsequent neonatal intensive care management. The management of RDS comprises of supportive management supplemented with surfactant and assisted ventilation to maintain adequate gas exchange. Maintenance of normal temperature, oxygenation and correction of acid base balance is vital as hypothermia, hypoxemia and acidosis can inactivate surfactant. These babies should be handled minimally as if they become hypoxic and their right to left shunt increases, their PaO_2 may fall rapidly. Blood gas measurement should be undertaken regularly with an aim to maintain the arterial PaO_2 in the range of 7–10 kPa (50–75 mmHg). Normal $PaCO_2$ in a newborn baby is between 4.6–5.4 kPa (30–40 mmHg). However in more mature infants and older babies it is acceptable to run higher $PaCO_2$ providing the pH is satisfactory. Hypocapnia should be avoided because it is associated with periventricular leukomalacia.[13] Fluid restriction in initial phase of the management is vital. Very immature infants may require infusion of dopamine to treat hypotension.

Respiratory Support

Progressive hypercapnia is a sign of respiratory failure and constitutes an indication for mechanical ventilation. Acidemia is common in the neonate with RDS. Respiratory acidosis is treated with assisted ventilation. Metabolic acidosis has a number of causes including hypoxia, hypotension, infection and respiratory muscle exhaustion. It is important to identify the cause and treat it according. Correction of a metabolic acidosis with intravenous sodium bicarbonate or trishydroxymethylaminomethane (THAM) is sometimes necessary.

The severity of RDS increases with decreasing gestation. The amount of support required may vary from supplemental oxygen to ventilation. Continuous positive airway pressure (CPAP) improves oxygenation by increasing functional residual capacity through recruitment of collapsed alveoli. It may be used in infants with persistently low PaO_2 below 7 kPa (50–70 mmHg) despite increase in oxygen requirement to 50%.[14] One meta-analysis concluded that the use of CPAP in preterm babies with RDS reduced respiratory failure and mortality.[15] However, there have been other studies to suggest that babies with mild RDS treated with early CPAP did not do as well as the controls.[16] Nevertheless, many centers use nasal CPAP in preference to early intubation and IPPV.[17, 18]

Mechanical ventilation is used in more severe respiratory disease to achieve adequate gas exchange while decreasing the work of breathing. The approach should be one that delivers an appropriate tidal volume while minimizing complications. Ventilatory strategies have evolved using time cycled pressure limited ventilation with an aim to improving survival and minimizing CLD. Other modes of ventilation such as volume controlled and high frequency ventilation are also available although these have not been shown to confer any major benefit over conventional ventilation. In premature infants less than 1000 grams with a patent ductus arteriosus on echocardiogram the outcome may be improved by pharmacological or surgical closure of the ductus.

Pulmonary Air Leak Syndromes

Air leak syndromes encompass a wide-spectrum of diseases that share a common problem. They include pneumothorax, pulmonary interstitial emphysema (PIE) pneumomediastinum, pneumopericardium, pneumoperitoneum and subcutaneous emphysema. Pneumothorax and PIE are the most commonly

to secondary bacterial infection. Persistent pulmonary hypertension (PPH) with right to left shunting complicate matters further.

Clinical Features

The baby presents with signs of respiratory distress such as tachypnea, intercostal recession and grunting. The symptoms may settle within 24 hours or persist for a week. Severe cases need ventilatory support. Depending on the severity of the original perinatal hypoxic insult, the baby may become encephalopathic.

Diagnosis

Meconium aspiration will be evident in the delivery room. Hypoxia may be noted on blood gas analysis. The CXR shows widespread patchy infiltration. Pleural effusion, pneumothorax, patchy atelectasis and emphysema or changes suggestive of PIE may be seen. In severe cases there may be diffuse opacification of both lung fields.

Management

In the immediate period after birth oropharyngeal suction should be performed to clear meconium from the oral cavity. Chest physiotherapy with humidified oxygen may suffice for mild cases. In an asphyxiated baby endotracheal intubation and suctioning of meconium is required. Respiratory support will be required with gentle assisted ventilation. Nasal or endotracheal continuous positive airway pressure support (CPAP) may improve oxygenation. Positive pressure ventilation should be reserved for infants who are unable to maintain an arterial PaO_2 greater than 50 mm of Hg in 100% oxygen. High end expiratory pressure should be avoided to prevent air trapping, lung injury and pneumothorax although moderate levels of PEEP may be needed in some cases. Surfactant therapy is indicated as meconium inactivates surfactant.[66] Inhaled nitric oxide may be required if the baby has PPH and extracorporeal membrane oxygenation (ECMO) is of benefit if other options fail (see chapter 41). Antibiotics should be given to prevent secondary bacterial infection.

Prognosis

Meconium aspiration carries a high risk of respiratory complications and PPH. The mortality is high in severe cases. Prompt obstetric intervention in the event of fetal distress during labor and expert resuscitation at delivery improves the outcome.

Persistent Pulmonary Hypertension of the Newborn

Persistent pulmonary hypertension of the newborn (PPHN) exists when the pulmonary artery pressure (PAP) fails to decline after birth. The condition is characterized by severe hypoxia, relatively mild lung disease and shunting across persistent fetal pathways (the ductus arteriosus and foramen ovale) in the presence of a structurally normal heart. PPHN may be primary or secondary to intrapartum asphyxia, infection or pulmonary hypoplasia.

Pathogenesis and Basic Science

Infants with PPHN may have normal or abnormal pulmonary vascular morphology. PPHN associated with normal pulmonary vascular morphology occurs in response to hypoxia in association with asphyxia, MAS or sepsis. Anatomical abnormalities of the lung and the pulmonary vascular bed are associated with pulmonary hypoplasia (including congenital diaphragmatic hernia and large congenital cystic lung lesions). Maldevelopment of pulmonary vessels and abnormalities of vascular smooth muscle have been identified in the lungs of infants dying from PPHN.[67] Smooth muscle hypertrophy within the walls of arterioles to the level of the intra-acinar vessels that are normally non-muscular causes luminal obstruction. PPHN is associated with chronic intrauterine hypoxia.

Clinical Features and Diagnosis

Infants with PPHN typically present within 12 hours of birth with cyanosis but relatively mild respiratory distress. This often mimics congenital cyanotic heart disease. Infants with PPHN secondary to a respiratory disease will have features of the underlying condition. The second heart sound may be loud on auscultation and a murmur of tricuspid insufficiency may be heard. Arterial blood gas analysis will show a severely reduced pO_2 with a relatively normal pCO_2. There will be a difference in oxygen saturation in the blood between the right radial and umbilical arteries. The chest X-ray in idiopathic PPHN looks relatively normal although reduced pulmonary vascular markings and cardiomegaly may be apparent. In infants with PPHN secondary to lung disease (e.g. MAS) these features should be apparent on chest X-ray. Prompt cardiac assessment with ultrasound is essential to rule out an underlying cardiac anomaly and to assess the degree of pulmonary hypertension.

Management

The main aim in all infants with PPHN is to lower the pulmonary vascular resistance, maintain systemic blood pressure, reversing the right to left shunt. It is important to avoid hypothermia, hypovolemia and hypoglycemia. Acidosis should be corrected. Maintenance of systemic blood pressure is important and adequate ventilation should be established. Vasodilator drugs such as tolazoline, prostacyclin and magnesium sulfate were widely used until the discovery of nitric oxide (NO). Extracorporeal membrane oxygenation is a rescue treatment.

Prognosis

The mortality in babies with PPHN is in the range of 20–40% and neurological handicap ranges from 10–25%.[68, 69]

Chronic Lung Disease

Chronic lung disease (CLD) is a condition that develops in the newborn treated with oxygen and mechanical ventilation for a primary lung disorder. All babies who are oxygen dependent beyond 28 days of life, by definition, have CLD. Two distinct forms of CLD can be recognized: Wilson-Mikity syndrome and bronchopulmonary dysplasia (BPD).

Bronchopulmonary Dysplasia

Bronchopulmonary dysplasia is a chronic lung disease that most affects premature infants who have needed oxygen therapy and mechanical ventilation for respiratory distress syndrome. It may also develop in premature infants who have few signs of lung disease in the early post natal period.[70] Although primarily a disease of the premature infant, BPD may occur in term infants who have needed prolonged ventilatory support.

The exact definition of BPD remains the subject of debate. BPD is generally defined as the presence of chronic respiratory signs, a persistent oxygen requirement, and an abnormal chest X-ray at one month or 36 weeks corrected age. However, there is a growing recognition that CLD occurring after preterm delivery in the surfactant era may have a different clinical course and pathology. This recent, so-called, 'new BPD' is characterized by a disruption of distal lung growth. [70] A more extensive definition has been proposed by a US NIH-sponsored workshop that incorporates many elements of the older definition and attempts to categorize the severity of the CLD.[71]

The overall incidence of BPD is about 20% of ventilated newborns with birth weight less than 1500 grams.[72] However, the incidence varies based on the definition used. Most infants with BPD are born prematurely and 75% of the infants affected weigh less than 1000 g at birth.[73]

Pathogenesis and Basic Science

BPD has a multifactorial etiology. Factors that increase the risk of development of BPD include volutrauma and barotrauma, oxygen toxicity, inflammation, infection and poor nutrition. That ventilator-induced lung injury results in BPD is suggested by studies that show an inverse relationship between hypocarbia and BPD.[74] The association between BPD and oxygen toxicity was first described in 1967. Prolonged exposure to high oxygen concentrations has complex biochemical and microscopic effects on the lungs which relate to increased production of cytotoxic oxygen free radicals which overwhelm the host antioxidant defense mechanisms.[75] Premature babies are more vulnerable to oxygen toxicity as they are deficient in antioxidant enzyme systems.

There is a strong association between patent ductus arteriosus and BPD and the effect is potentiated by infection. Chorioamnionitis may predispose to BPD.[76] PIE has been associated with an increased risk of BPD.[77] Inflammation plays an important role in the pathogenesis of BPD. Oxygen toxicity, barotrauma and volutrauma induce an inflammatory reaction which persists in infants with BPD. Pro-inflammatory cytokines (IL-1β, IL-6 and ICAM-1) present from day one reach a peak during the second week in babies with RDS who proceed to develop BPD. Leukotrienes are also present in high levels in infants with BPD. These mediators cause bronchoconstriction, vasoconstriction, edema and mucous production.[78]

Lung compliance is reduced in babies with BPD due to small airway narrowing, interstitial fibrosis, edema and atelectasis. This results in ventilation perfusion (V/Q) mismatch. Cardiovascular changes associated with BPD include pulmonary hypertension and, potentially, cor pulmonale.

Clinical features

Most babies with BPD are premature. Respiratory signs include tachypnea, shallow breathing, retractions, and a paradoxical breathing pattern. Course rhonchi and wheeze may be apparent on auscultation. A Harrison's sulcus may be present. Rarely, signs of right heart failure may be present. Babies with BPD usually fail to thrive and are at risk of recurrent infection. They may also develop osteopenia.[79] There is a high incidence of feeding problems and gastro esophageal reflux.

Diagnosis

Characteristic abnormalities on chest X-ray in babies with BPD include hyperinflated lung fields, multiple linear interstitial opacities, lung cysts and emphysema.[80] Computed tomography is more sensitive, especially in older babies, and shows multifocal areas of hyperinflation, bronchial wall thickening and linear and triangular subpleural opacities.[81]

Management

Prevention is the key strategy with BPD. The rationale is limitation of disease progression while maintaining adequate gas exchange. Oxygen administration is reduced as quickly as possible to the minimum required. The association of barotrauma or volutrauma with BPD has led to the use of ventilator strategies designed to keep lung injury to the minimum. High tidal volumes are avoided. Peak inspiratory pressures should be kept to the minimum to maintain adequate gas exchange. The results of randomized trials of high frequency oscillatory ventilation and jet ventilation to reduce BPD have yielded inconsistent results.[82, 83] Many centers prefer to minimize mechanical ventilation by the use of nasal CPAP with or without exogenous surfactant and some have reported

38. Hill A, Perlman JM, Volpe JJ. Relationship of pneumothorax to occurrence of intraventricular hemorrhage in premature newborns. Pediatrics 1982; 69:144–149.

39. Kuhn JP. 1990. The pleura. In Essentials of Caffey's Pediatric Diagnosis. Silverman FN and Kuhn JP, eds. Chicago: Year Book, 222–225.

40. Kuhns LR, Bednarek FJ, Wyman ML et al. Diagnosis of pneumothorax or pneumomediastinum in neonates by transillumination. Pediatrics 1975; 56:355–360.

41. Korvenranta H, Kero P. Intraesophageal pressure monitoring in infants with respiratory disorders. Crit Care Med 1983; 11: 276–279.

42. Mcintosh N, Becher JC, Cunningham S et al. Clinical Diagnosis Of Pneumothorax Is Late: Use Of Trend Data And Decision Support Might Allow Preclinical Detection. Pediatr Res 2000; 48:408–415.

43. Soll RF. Prophylactic natural surfactant extract for preventing morbidity and mortality in preterm infants. Cochrane Database Syst Rev. 2000;(2):CD000511. Review.

44. Greenough A, Milner AD, Dimitriou G. Synchronized mechanical ventilation for respiratory support in newborn infants. Cochrane Database Syst Rev. 2004;(4):CD000456. Review.

45. Henderson-Smart DJ, Bhuta T, Cools F et al. Elective high frequency oscillatory ventilation versus conventional ventilation for acute pulmonary dysfunction in preterm infants. Cochrane Database Syst Rev. 2003;(4):CD000104. Review.

46. Bakker JC, Liem M, Wijnands JB et al. Neonatal pneumothorax drainage systems: in vitro evaluation. Eur J Pediatr 1989; 149:58–61.

47. Williams O, Greenough A, Mustfa N et al. Extubation failure due to phrenic nerve injury. Arch Dis Child Fetal Neonatal Ed. 2003; 88:F72–3.

48. Sarkar S, Hussain N, Herson V. Fibrin glue for persistent pneumothorax in neonates. J Perinatol 2003; 23:82–4.

49. Grosfeld JL, Lemons JL, Ballantine TV et al. Emergency thoracotomy for acquired bronchopleural fistula in the premature infant with respiratory distress. J Pediatr Surg 1980; 15: 416–21.

50. Berger JT, Gilhooly J. Fibrin glue treatment of persistent pneumothorax in a premature infant. J Pediatr 1993; 122:958–60.

51. Madansky DL, Lawson EE, Chernick V et al. Pneumothorax and other forms of pulmonary air leak in newborns. Am Rev Respir Dis. 1979; 120:729–.

52. Hook B, Hack M, Morrison S et al. Pneumopericardium in very low birth weight infants. J Perinatol. 1995; 15:27–31.

53. Logaker MT, Laberge JM, Dansereau J et al. Primary fetal hydrothorax: natural history and management. J Pediatr Surg 1989; 24:573–576.

54. Whittle MJ, Gilmore GH, McNay MB et al. Diaphragmatic hernia presenting inutero as unilateral hydrothorax. Perinatl Diagnosis 1989; 9:115–118.

55. Madhavi P, Jameson R, Robinson MJ. Unilateral pleural effusion complicating central venous catherisation. Arch Dis Childh Fetal Neonatal Ed 2000; 82:F248–F249.

56. Booth P, Nicolaides KH, Greenough A et al. Pleuroamnoiotic shunting for fetal chylothorax. Early Hum Dev 1987; 15: 365–367.

57. Hagay Z, Reece A, Roberts A, Hobbins JC et al. Isolated fetal pleural: a prenatal management dilemma. Obstet Gynecol 1993; 18:147–152.

58. Van Aerde J, Campbell AN, Smyth JA, et al. Spontaneous chylothorax in newborns. Am J Dis Child 1984; 138:961–4.

59. Amodio J, Abramson S, Berdon W et al. Iatrogenic causes of large pleural fluid collections in the premature infant: ultrasonic and radiographic findings. Pediatr Radiol. 1987; 17:104–8.

60. Mercer S. Factors involved in chylothorax following repair of congenital posterolateral diaphragmatic hernia. J Pediatr Surg 1986; 21:809–11.

61. Helin RD, Angeles ST, Bhat R. Octreotide therapy for chylothorax in infants and children: A brief review. Pediatr Crit Care Med 2006; 7:576–9.

62. Raju TN, Langenberg P. Pulmonary hemorrhage and exogenous surfactant therapy: a metaanalysis. J Pediatr. 1993; 123:603–10.

63. Cleary JM, Wiswell Te. Meconium stained amniotic fluid and meconium aspiration syndrome: an update. Pediatr Clin N Am 1998; 45:511–529.

64. Zagariya A, Bhat R, Uhal B et al. Cell death and lung cell histology in meconium aspirated newborn rabbit lung. Eur J Pediatr 2000; 59:819–826.

65. Dargaville PA, South M, McDoughall PN. Surfactant and surfactant inhibitors in meconium aspiration syndrome. J Pediatr 2001; 138:113–115.

66. Findlay RD, Taeusch HW, Walther FJ. Surfactant replacement therapy for meconium aspiration syndrome. Pediatrics 1996; 97:48–52.

67. Murphy JD, Rabinovitch M, Goldstein JD, Reid LM. The structural basis of persistent pulmonary hypertension of the newborn infant. J Pediatr 1981; 98:962.

68. Ballard RA, Leonard CH. Development follow-up of infants with persistent pulmonary hypertension of the newborn. Clin Perinatol 1984; 11:737.

69. Sell EJ, Gaines JA, Gluckman C, Williams E. Persistent Fetal Circulation Am J Dis Child 1985; 139:25

70. Kinsella JP, Greenough A, Abman SH. Bronchopulmonary dysplasia. Lancet 2006; 367:1421–31.

71. Jobe AH, Bancalari E. Bronchopulmonary dysplasia. Am J Respir Crit Care Med 2001; 163:1723–9.

72. Avery ME, Tooley WH, Keller JB, et al. Is chronic lung disease in low birth weight infants preventable? A survey of eight centers. Pediatrics 1987; 79:26–30.

73. Rojas MA, Gonzalez A, Bancalari E et al. Changing trends in the epidemiology and pathogenesis of neonatal chronic lung disease. J Pediatr 1995; 126:605–10.

74. Kraybill EN, Runyan DK, Bose CL et al. Risk factors for chronic lung disease in infants with birth weights of 751 to 1000 grams. J Pediatr 1989; 115:115–20.

75. Bonikos DS, Bensch KG, Northway WH Jr. Oxygen toxicity in the newborn. The effect of chronic continuous 100 percent oxygen exposure on the lungs of newborn mice. Am J Pathol. 1976; 85:623–50.

76. Gonzalez A, Sosenko IR, Chandar J et al. Influence of infection on patent ductus arteriosus and chronic lung disease in premature infants weighing 1000 grams or less. J Pediatr 1996; 128:470–8.

77. Cochran DP, Pilling DW, Shaw NJ. The relationship of pulmonary interstitial emphysema to subsequent type of chronic lung disease. Br J Radiol 1994; 67:1155–7.

78. Mirro R, Armstead W, Leffler C. Increased airway leukotriene levels in infants with severe bronchopulmonary dysplasia. Am J Dis Child 1990; 144:160–1.

79. Steichen JJ, Gratton TL, Tsang RC. Osteopenia of prematurity: the cause and possible treatment. J Pediatr 1980; 96: 528–34.

80. U G Rossi and C M Owens. The radiology of chronic lung disease in children. Arch Dis Child 2005; 90: 601–607.

81. Oppenheim C, Mamou-Mani T, Sayegh N et al. Bronchopulmonary dysplasia: value of CT in identifying pulmonary sequelae. Am J Roentgenol 1994; 163:169–72.

82. Courtney SE, Durand DJ, Asselin JM et al. High-frequency oscillatory ventilation versus conventional mechanical ventilation for very-low-birth-weight infants. N Engl J Med 2002; 347:643–52.

83. Johnson AH, Peacock JL, Greenough A et al. High-frequency oscillatory ventilation for the prevention of chronic lung disease of prematurity. N Engl J Med. 2002;347:633–42.

84. Albersheim SG, Solimano AJ, Sharma AK and et al. Randomized, double blind controlled trial of long term diuretic therapy for bronchopulmonary dysplasia. J Pediatr. 1989; 115:615–620.

85. Shah V, Ohlsson A, Halliday HL et al. Early administration of inhaled corticosteroids for preventing chronic lung disease in ventilated very low birth weight preterm neonates. Cochrane Database Syst Rev. 2000;(2):CD001969. Review.

86. Barrington KJ. The adverse neuro-developmental effects of postnatal steroids in the preterm infant: a systematic review of RCTs. BMC Pediatr 2001;1:1.

87. Darlow BA, Graham PJ. Vitamin A supplementation for preventing morbidity and mortality in very low birthweight infants. Cochrane Database Syst Rev. 2002;(4):CD000501. Review.

88. Davis JM, Parad RB, Michele T et al. Pulmonary outcome at 1 year corrected age in premature infants treated at birth with recombinant human CuZn superoxide dismutase. Pediatrics. 2003;111:469–76.

89. Barrington KJ, Finer NN. Inhaled nitric oxide for respiratory failure in preterm infants. Cochrane Database Syst Rev. 2006;(1):CD000509. Review.

90. Halliday HL. Pulmonary disorders and apnea. Campbell AGM, McIntosh N, editors. Forfar and Arneil's Textbook of Pediatrics. Edinburgh: Churchill Livingstone, 1998 175–198.

91. Gross SJ, Iannuzzi DM, et al. Effect of preterm birth on pulmonary function at school age: a prospective controlled study. J Pediatr. 1998; 133:188–92.

92. Holinger LD Etiology of stridor in the neonate, infant, and child. Ann Otol Rhinol Laryngol 1980; 89:397–400.

93. Jacobs IN, Wetmore RF, Tom LW, et al Tracheobronchomalacia in children. Arch Otolaryngol Head Neck Surg 1994; 120:154–158.

94. Doull IJ, Mok Q, Tasker RC. Tracheobronchomalacia in preterm infants with chronic lung disease. Arch Dis Child Fetal Neonatal Ed. 1997; 76:F203–F205.

95. Morrison G. Airway problems. In: Janet M Rennie, editor. Roberton's Textbook of Neonatology. Philadelphia: Elsevier, 2005:603–17.

96. Downing GJ, Kilbride HW. Evaluation of airway complications in high-risk preterm infants; application of flexible fibreoptic airway endoscopy. Pediatrics 1995; 95;567 72.

97. Mok Q, Negus S, McLaren CA, et al. Computed tomography versus bronchography in the diagnosis and management of tracheobronchomalacia in ventilator dependent infants. Arch Dis Child Fetal Neonatal Ed. 2005 90: 290–293.

98. Carden KA, Boiselle PM, Waltz DA, et al. Tracheomalacia and Tracheobronchomalacia in Children and Adults: An In-depth Review. Chest 2005; 127:984–1005.

99. Furman RH, Backer CL, Dunham ME, et al. The use of balloon-expandable metallic stents in the treatment of pediatric tracheomalacia and bronchomalacia. Arch Otolaryngol Head Neck Surg 1999; 125:203–207.

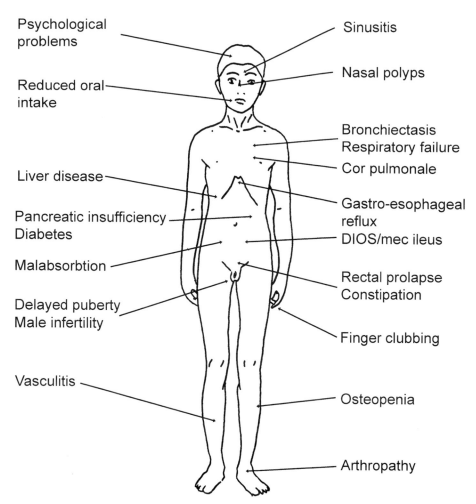

Fig. 35.1. Cystic fibrosis: a multi-system disorder

Labels in figure: Psychological problems; Reduced oral intake; Liver disease; Pancreatic insufficiency Diabetes; Malabsorbtion; Delayed puberty Male infertility; Vasculitis; Sinusitis; Nasal polyps; Bronchiectasis Respiratory failure; Cor pulmonale; Gastro-esophageal reflux; DIOS/mec ileus; Rectal prolapse Constipation; Finger clubbing; Osteopenia; Arthropathy

affected people (see sweat test below). It also accounts for why babies with CF taste salty if their foreheads are licked (eighteenth century folklore relates "Woe is the child who tastes salty from a kiss on the brow, for he is cursed, and soon must die"). The basic problem of thick sticky secretions accounts for many of the clinical effects, with small airways, pancreatic ducts, bile ducts, and the vas deferens all blocked or poorly formed. For example, blocked pancreatic ducts lead to an exocrine insufficiency, hence fat malabsorption, steatorrhoea and failure to thrive. The body's host defence and inflammatory response to infection is also an important part of the pathogenesis, particularly in the lungs.

Diagnosis

Aside from the history and examination, investigations are required to confirm the diagnosis.

Immunoreactive Trypsin

Immunoreactive trypsin (IRT) is released from the pancreas into the small intestine. However in CF, due to pancreatic duct obstruction, IRT is not secreted into the gut, but instead is released into the bloodstream. Hence IRT is usually raised

in affected neonates (two to fivefold) and is even high in children who are pancreatic sufficient. Unfortunately, the test is unreliable in neonates who have had surgery for meconium ileus. The level of IRT falls over the first two months of life, and the test is unreliable after the first 6 weeks. In general, a level $>900\,\mu g/L$ means CF needs excluding. Raised IRT on a Guthrie card forms the starting point of the UK newborn screening programme.

Sweat Test

This is the gold standard for making the diagnosis, and British guidelines for sweat testing are available on http://www.acb.org.uk. It involves collecting a small amount of sweat from the child's forearm or leg using pilocarpine iontophoresis; the macroduct system tends to be used now rather than collection onto preweighed filter paper. With the macroduct, 100 mg of sweat is no longer required, and analysis can be reliably performed on smaller quantities. Sweat testing can be performed once a baby is $>48\,h$ old, although often inadequate samples are obtained in the first few weeks. It is also difficult to obtain enough sweat from children with dry atopic eczema. It is important that the test is carried out in experienced centers to obtain reliable results and tests should be performed in duplicate. The test measures levels of sodium and chloride in the sweat, which are elevated in CF. Although results must be interpreted in the clinical context, the normal range is $Cl^- < 40$ mmol/L (<30 mmol/L in infants); equivocal range is Cl^- 40–60 mmol/L (although in infants, this is likely to be CF); and a level indicative of CF is $Cl^- > 60$ mmol/L. Levels in the equivocal range must be repeated, although if the $Na^+ > Cl^-$ it is more likely to be normal. There are a number of conditions theoretically linked to false-positive sweat test results, although this is rarely seen in practice. False-negative results can occur with malnutrition and rarely (<1%) with certain CF mutations; flucloxacillin has no effect on a sweat test.

DNA Analysis for Genotype

Genetic analysis should be performed in all children with a positive or borderline sweat test. Genotype screening can be tailored for different ethnic populations. It will also form part of the screening programme in infants with elevated IRT. However, there are a number of important limitations to genetic testing. There are at least 1,400 known CFTR mutations. Clearly, it is not feasible to test for all mutations, and so if there is no known mutation within the family, it is only possible to test for the more common mutations. Negative genetic analysis does not therefore exclude CF (although a positive result can be relied upon). Similarly, the isolation of only one mutation does not necessarily confirm carrier status rather than disease. As with all investigations, the results need to be interpreted in the context of the clinical situation.[3]

Fecal Elastase

In patients who are pancreatic insufficient, fecal elastase levels are low. There are degrees of pancreatic insufficiency, and the levels of elastase measured will reflect this. Although a level <200 μg/g stool is abnormal, patients with CF who are pancreatic insufficient, almost always have a level <15 μg/g. Samples should be obtained after 3 days of age in term infants, and after 2 weeks in those born at less than 28 weeks gestation, as the test is unreliable prior to this time.[4] It must be stressed that this is not a diagnostic test for CF, but nevertheless is important additional evidence toward the diagnosis. A false-positive result may be found in infants who are severely malnourished or have an enteropathy.[4]

Neonatal Screening

By 2007 neonatal screening for CF should be universal throughout the UK alongside the programs of Australia and the USA. Screening will detect a significant proportion of cases, and involves initially testing for raised immunoreactive tryspsin (IRT) on the Guthrie card bloodspot taken at 6 days of age. If the sample is positive, then the sample is sent for two stage genetic analysis. As it is not possible to test for every known gene, some children will test positive for IRT, but may only have one, or possibly neither, gene isolated. If there is

any uncertainty, a sweat test will need to be performed to determine if these children are likely to be carriers or to have CF. There are a number of causes of false-positive IRT, which will leave the diagnosis uncertain in a proportion of children until an adequate sweat test is performed. There have been a number of long-term studies looking at the benefits of screening programmes for CF. The most important has been the randomized controlled trial conducted in Wisconsin, USA. The significant findings from Wisconsin have been the improved growth and nutritional status in those children detected by screening.[5] Also, as a result of earlier correction of low plasma vitamin E, improved cognitive function was detected in children aged 7–16 years.[6] However, no differences were seen in lung function at 7 years.[7]

Clinical Presentations

Some of the commoner presentations are outlined in Table 35.1.

Meconium Ileus

Because of reduced fluid secretion into the intestines, babies with CF produce thick viscid meconium, which may lead to intestinal obstruction. This is known as meconium ileus (MI) and around 10–15% of patients with CF present in this manner. However, MI strongly suggests an underlying diagnosis of CF as >90% babies with it have CF, hence all infants must be investigated. All CF infants presenting with MI are pancreatic insufficient. The condition can also occur antenatally and may be first detected as "echogenic bowel" during antenatal ultrasound. Complications of MI include peritonitis, volvulus, atresia, necrosis of the bowel, and perforation.

Presentation is with signs and symptoms suggestive of intestinal obstruction – abdominal distension, bile-stained vomiting, and failure to pass meconium, usually within 48 h of birth. The plain abdominal radiograph will show dilated loops of small bowel (Fig. 35.2a). Calcification in the lower abdominal cavity can indicate sterile perforation that has occurred antenatally. There may also be clinical features of perforation (meconium peritonitis), but since it is sterile the child is not as toxic as in a typical bowel perforation seen in older children. The soap-bubble sign is sometimes seen within

TABLE 35.1. Commonest presentations of CF by age.

Newborn	Neonatal obstruction – meconium ileus
	Prolonged conjugated jaundice
	Newborn screening
	Screening due to family history
Infancy and older children	Failure to thrive with abnormal stools
	Recurrent respiratory infection/symptoms
	Rectal prolapse
	Nasal polyposis
Adults	Infertility
	Bronchiectasis

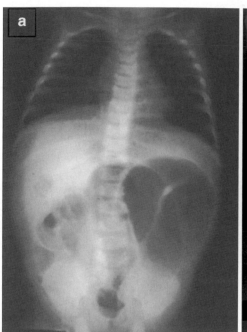 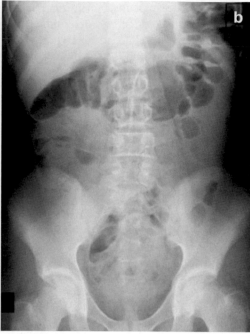

FIG. 35.2. Plain abdominal radiographs of (a) neonatal intestinal obstruction due to meconium ileus, and (b) distal intestinal obstruction syndrome with marked fecal loading

the bowel as a result of small (swallowed) air bubbles mixed with meconium. A contrast enema may show the presence of a microcolon with meconium pellets.

Many uncomplicated cases of meconium ileus can be managed with the administration of water-soluble contrast enemas such as gastrografin. This is administered as a hyperosmolar solution, which draws water into the gut. This influx of fluid can cause significant bowel distension, which may lead in extreme cases to perforation and ischemia of the bowel mucosa. Patients may easily become hypovolaemic due to the considerable fluid shift into the bowel, so all infants must be closely monitored and given intravenous fluids following the enema administration.[8]

More severe cases and those with peritonitis require surgery. Enemas should not be administered in these patients. Surgery may involve intraoperative bowel irrigation via an enterostomy or small bowel resection; it is important to record how much ileum is resected. Primary anastomosis is usually achievable but sometimes a temporary ileostomy is necessary. The stoma is usually closed once the child has reached 5 kg body weight. Occasionally a hemi-colectomy may be required.

Malabsorption and Failure to Thrive

Because of pancreatic insufficiency, infants often develop steatorrhoea with malabsorption. The frequent stools are pale, greasy, loose, and offensive due to fat malabsorption. As a result, there is associated poor weight gain, with reduced muscle mass; wasting is particularly evident in the buttocks and thighs. The malabsorption is corrected with pancreatic enzyme supplementation together with fat soluble vitamins.

The stool consistency and frequency corrects fairly quickly allowing catch-up growth. Once treatment starts, the child's appetite often seems to decrease, but this is because they are no longer ravenously hungry; the babies are usually much more content as well.

If there is inadequate response to the enzyme supplementation, it is worth considering concomitant diagnoses such as coeliac disease or cow's milk protein intolerance. Some of the newly diagnosed infants are sodium depleted, which will also impact adversely on growth. In an infant who is failing to thrive, a random urinary sodium should be measured, and if <20 mmol/L is evidence of total body sodium depletion, supplementation is required.

Recurrent Respiratory Infections

One of the commonest presenting features in infants and young children is that of recurrent chest symptoms. The child may have an overt pneumonia with chest radiographic signs; if this occurs early or more than once the child needs to have CF excluded. More common than actual pneumonia is the presentation of recurrent "chestiness." This is manifested by recurrent acute episodes or a more chronic picture of a persistent cough, sometimes with wheeze. If the child is pancreatic sufficient and is thriving, there is more likelihood the diagnosis is missed or delayed, as many infants have recurrent chest symptoms, which are more usually due to simple viral colds or infantile asthma. A wet cough, particularly if productive of sputum in an older child, must be taken seriously and a sweat test is mandatory. Features such as finger or toe clubbing and chest deformity are also warning signs.

Pseudo-Bartter's Syndrome

This is due to an underlying electrolyte imbalance, causing hypochloraemic, hypokalaemic metabolic alkalosis. Treatment involves electrolyte supplementation to correct the biochemical abnormalities. Depletion of electrolytes through sweat losses can occur in hot weather. Generally, this can be managed by adding extra salt to food. However, in some situations, additional sodium supplementation may be required.[9]

Rectal Prolapse

Infants and young children may first present with a rectal prolapse so any child with this condition must have CF excluded with a sweat test. It is reported to occur in up to 23% of patients with CF and commonly occurs between the ages of 6 months and 3 years. It is usually a manifestation of a loaded bowel and often corrects once enzyme supplementation is started and the diet improves. Most cases respond to manual reduction. If this fails, then treatment with a sclerosing agent may be effective. Surgery is occasionally required if the above measures are unsuccessful, if there is significant pain or bleeding, or if the prolapse is incarcerated. Outcome following surgery is variable, with some patients developing recurrent prolapse.[10]

Rarer Neonatal Presentations

Vitamin E deficiency can lead to hemolytic anemia and other hematological abnormalities can occur.[11] Hypoalbuminaemia due to malnutrition may lead to the presentation of edema, sometimes accompanied by a Kwashiorkor-like skin rash.[12]

Clinical Features and Their Management

Respiratory Disease

CF lung disease is the major cause of morbidity and mortality in CF. It is due to a combination of excessive viscous secretions, poor mucociliary clearance, and chronic bacterial infections with a subsequent excessive neutrophilic inflammatory response. Although children with CF appear to have normal lungs at birth, lung function abnormalities manifest early in life.[13] The lung disease inevitably progresses, but at varying rates in different patients, and bronchiectasis develops (Fig. 35.3). Respiratory function and exercise tolerance fall, and eventually this results in respiratory failure, which is by far the leading cause of death in CF.

Infection and Respiratory Exacerbations

It is beyond the scope of this chapter to outline in detail all aspects of respiratory infections, but this has been recently reviewed.[14] The principle of antibiotic therapy is for long courses with high doses. Prophylactic antibiotics are used as well as suppressive treatment of chronic infection.[15]

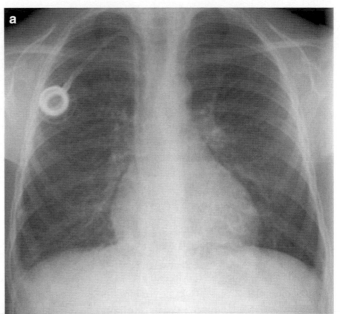

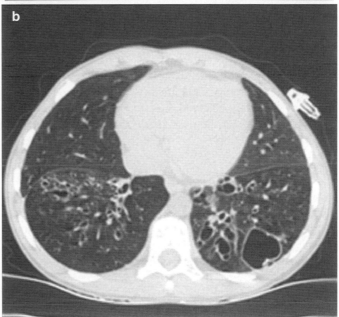

FIG. 35.3. (a) Chest radiograph of an adolescent showing moderately severe lung disease with an indwelling portacath on the right. (b) Chest CT scan of a different child showing severe bilateral cystic bronchiectasis

Exacerbations are treated quickly and antibiotics changed once sensitivities are known. Regular surveillance is importance, culturing cough swabs or sputum. Sometimes bronchoalveolar lavage is necessary in nonsputum producing children. If a child has a general anesthetic it is usual to take the opportunity of obtaining cultures from the lower airways with blind or bronchoscopic lavage.

Respiratory exacerbations occur more frequently as the children get older and their lung disease deteriorates. They are commoner in the winter and can be due to many of the microorganisms outlined below. Symptoms include: increased cough, increased sputum production (which is darker and thicker), breathlessness with reduced exercise tolerance, lethargy and malaise, occasionally chest pain, and occasionally hemoptysis. Reduction in lung function is usual and a significant decline is an absolute drop in FEV_1 of >10% predicted; oxygen saturation may also drop. It is unusual for there to be accompanying pyrexia, and the chest may be clear on auscultation. Sputum or a cough swab should be sent for microbiological analysis. Oral antibiotics will be started immediately and intravenous antibiotics given if there is no response.

Respiratory Viruses

Respiratory viral infections have a significant impact on patients with CF, especially in the autumn and winter, and respiratory viruses may precipitate up to 40% of chest exacerbations. Viruses implicated in causing infections in CF are the same as those that may affect anyone, namely respiratory syncytial virus (RSV), adenovirus, parainfluenza virus types 1–3, influenza A & B, and rhinovirus. Viral infections may lead to increased frequency and duration of hospitalization for respiratory exacerbations, followed by deterioration in clinical status and lung function, which may persist for several months. The viruses that have the greatest impact in CF are RSV and influenza. Respiratory viral infections are also associated with onset of secondary bacterial infections, and the first isolation of a particular organism (particularly *P. aeruginosa*) often follows a viral infection.

Staphylococcus aureus

Methicillin-sensitive *Staphylococcus aureus* (MSSA) is the most common pathogen isolated in sputum of children with CF during the first decade. It is an important pathogen throughout life and often occurs as a coinfecting organism in patients chronically infected with other bacteria. In children, it can be associated with an increase in respiratory symptoms but rarely causes a systemic inflammatory response. There is still some debate as to its pathogenicity, as it can be cultured in sputum without any change in symptoms; and bronchoscopy studies indicate that up to 40% of infants under 3 years have *S. aureus* cultured from bronchoalveolar samples. Some CF centers advocate the use of long-term prophylactic anti-staphylococcal antibiotic treatment, while others treat on the basis of symptoms and positive sputum cultures, usually with flucloxacillin.

Hemophilus influenzae

This occurs reasonably frequently in patients with CF, but there is little evidence to indicate its significance. This organism is pathogenic in non-CF bronchiectasis and chronic obstructive pulmonary disease, so there is no reason to suggest that is not the case in CF. It is often associated with increased symptoms and should be treated when isolated with an oral antibiotic such as co-amoxiclav.

Pseudomonas aeruginosa

This is the most common organism causing chronic lung disease in patients with CF and chronic infection with *P. aeruginosa* is an important predictor of survival in CF and the most important cause of morbidity. Infection usually occurs late in the first decade, or during the second decade of life, and by the third decade, over 80% of people with CF have chronic infection with *P. aeruginosa*. Once this is established in CF airways, it is not possible to permanently eradicate it. At this point the *P. aeruginosa* has established a bacterial-host relationship, which results in a sustained host inflammatory response.[16] When first isolated, an attempt is made to eradicate the organism with oral ciprofloxacin (or two intravenous antibiotics if the child is unwell) and 3 months of nebulised antibiotics (usually colistin). Once established, chronic infection is partially controlled with long-term nebulised antibiotics (colistin or tobramycin).[17] Chest exacerbations are treated with oral antibiotics if minor or at least two weeks of two intravenous antibiotics if more severe.

Stenotrophomonas maltophilia

The prevalence varies considerably from center to center and some have reported prevalence rates of up to 30%. A number of studies have demonstrated that *S. maltophilia* is not a cause of significant adverse morbidity or mortality in CF.[18] However, some patients do become chronically infected, and have chronic symptoms as well as acute exacerbations in a similar way to those seen in *P. aeruginosa* infection. The organism is constitutively multiply antibiotic resistant but cotrimoxazole can be useful.

Burkholderia Cepacia Complex

Since the earlier reports of infection with *Burkholderia cepacia* and its consequences in CF, it has become recognized that *Burkholderia* is a genus containing a number of species that were previously identified as genomovars. All of the members of the *B. cepacia* complex group have been described as causing infection in CF, but the majority are caused by *B. cenocepacia* (previously genomovar III) and *B. multivorans* (previously genomovar II). Infection with *B. cepacia* complex is associated with increased morbidity and reduced survival in CF but the individual response to this infection is very variable and is determined by the species involved and the host response to infection. *B. cenocepacia* is the most highly transmissible member of this complex and is associated with a rapid deterioration and early death in up to one third of patients who acquire the organism (cepacia syndrome).[19] For those patients who do not succumb to an acute cepacia syndrome, subsequent prognosis is still poor. The problem is that *B. cepacia* is almost always multiply resistant and frequently pan-resistant to antibiotics making effective therapy difficult. It is critical that infected patients do not come into contact with other CF patients to avoid cross-infection.

Methicillin-Resistant *Staphylococcus aureus* (MRSA)

S. aureus stains resistant to methicillin and other β-lactam antimicrobials have become an endemic problem in most healthcare facilities in the Western world. MRSA is usually acquired from the hospital environment but there is evidence that strains can be community-acquired. Patient to patient spread has also been well documented. Patients need to be segregated from all CF patients and not attend regular clinics until they have three clear sputum cultures over 6–12 months. Not surprisingly the prevalence of MRSA in CF varies from center to center, but has been reported in up to 23% of centers in North America. Infection with MRSA most frequently occurs in patients with poor lung function and may result in an increase in requirement for antibiotics. However, other studies have not demonstrated any significant deterioration in CF patients infected with this organism. Eradication with topical treatment should be initiated and if it is felt that the MRSA is having a clinical impact, then options include IV vancomycin or teicoplanin or oral linezolid.

Aspergillus Species

Aspergillus is a widely-distributed spore-bearing fungus, and since it can grow at body temperature and the spores are respiratory particle sized (2–4 µm), it can be associated with respiratory disease in humans There are several species but *A. fumigatus* is most often implicated. *Aspergillus* is commonly found in the sputum in CF (variably reported as 1–60%), and it is not always obvious whether it is causing disease or just harmless colonization. *Aspergillus* lung disease may take the form of lung infection, aspergilloma, invasive aspergillosis, or allergic bronchopulmonary aspergillosis (see below). It is the first and last that are most relevant to CF, however. An aspergilloma is a discrete fungal ball (mycetoma) found in an existing cavitatory lung lesion, which commonly causes hemoptysis. It is rare in children with CF but may be more common in adult patients, and is likely to be recognized more often with increased use of chest CT scanning. Invasive aspergillosis occurs when the fungus invades the lung tissue; it is rare and more often associated with congenital or acquired immunodeficiency (including posttransplant). If *Aspergillus* is repeatedly cultured, (and especially if no bacteria are isolated), then in a patient who is symptomatic or chronically deteriorating, treatment with an antifungal agent is prudent. A typical regimen would be oral itraconazole or voriconazole for 1 month.

Non-Tuberculous Mycobacteria

Mycobacterium avium complex (MAC) is the most common non-tuberculous mycobacterial infection in CF, accounting for around 70% of isolates, while the rapid grower *M. abscessus* accounts for 16%. Isolates may cause transient infection or are often present in low numbers, and it is likely NTM are acquired from the environment. Patients with NTM infection compared with case controls do not show any acceleration in decline in lung function[20] but *M. abscessus* seems to be more virulent than MAC or other types of NTM. The diagnosis of clinically significant NTM infection is difficult to make in CF as many features suggesting NTM is pathogenic are found in CF lung disease anyway. NTM are usually resistant to standard anti-tuberculous antibiotics, but there are certain combinations that may be helpful, for example rifampicin, ethambutol, azithromycin, and a fluroquinolone (ciprofloxacin or moxifloxacin) have been shown to be of benefit in CF and non-CF populations. If undertaken, treatment may be required for 6–18 months.

Chest Physiotherapy

Chest physiotherapy should be initiated at the time of diagnosis and becomes part of the daily treatment for patients with CF, even when well. The aim of physiotherapy is airway clearance; it helps the child to bring up pulmonary secretions that would otherwise stay within the lower airways. Children do not tend to expectorate sputum until over 6 years or so, the younger ones swallow the sputum and if large amounts are being produced may vomit mucus. For a young child, physiotherapy is provided by parents or carers. As children become older they are able to take a more active role in their treatment. By introducing physiotherapy in well asymptomatic young children, treatment becomes part of normal routine. Parents and children become skilled in physiotherapy techniques and also develop awareness of when sputum production is increased, heralding a probable exacerbation.[21]

Physiotherapy for infants and young children involves postural drainage, chest percussion, and other manual techniques. Breathing techniques can be employed from around the age of 3 years onwards. For older children, active cycle of breathing techniques (ACBT), which comprise a specific sequence of breathing manoeuvres, may be combined with postural drainage to clear secretions. Adjunctive devices may be helpful in older children if sputum is particularly difficult to expectorate. These include positive expiratory pressure (PEP) masks and Flutter devices. The latter create an intermittent oscillatory positive expiratory pressure, which is transmitted to the airways and aids clearance of secretions. Physiotherapy is the most time-consuming treatment for children and their families and is usually the main area of nonadherence to treatment. Exercise should also be encouraged but is not a substitute for physiotherapy.

Wheeze and Small Airways Disease

Patients with CF may also have bronchial hyperreactivity with wheeze, and respond to bronchodilator therapy and inhaled corticosteroids as per routine asthma management.[22] The presence of atopy to common aeroallergens (excluding aspergillus) and a strong atopic family history may point to concomitant asthma. Treatment is with conventional asthma therapy. Unresponsive wheeze may indicate an alternative diagnosis such as allergic bronchopulmonary aspergillosis (ABPA), tracheobronchomalacia, or gastro-oesophageal reflux, in which case further investigations may be indicated. There are a small group of children with severe small airways disease unresponsive to treatment and they represent a difficult clinical problem.[23]

Bronchodilators

Bronchodilator therapy (salbutamol or terbutaline) should be administered prior to physiotherapy, to aid bronchodilation and airway clearance. Otherwise they are used for acute bronchospasm i.e., when the children become wheezy or have a tight chest with a dry tight cough.

Inhaled Corticosteroids

These may be taken twice daily to control symptomatic wheezing when bronchodilators alone are not sufficient. They have also been used as antiinflammatory therapy to combat lung inflammation, although there is little evidence this is effective in CF.

Long-Acting β_2 Agonists

Some children who have small airways problems despite inhaled corticosteroids may need an inhaled long-acting β_2 agonist (salmeterol or formoterol) in addition.

Other Respiratory Therapies

Mucolytics

It is important to maintain adequate hydration to prevent drying of secretions. If sputum remains particularly viscous and difficult to expectorate, nebulised treatments may be beneficial. The two commonest treatments in use at present are recombinant human deoxyribonuclease (rhDNase) and hypertonic saline.

Recombinant human deoxyribonuclease (rhDNase, Pulmozyme): Dead and dying neutrophils are responsible for 7% of the viscosity of the sputum. rhDNase breaks down neutrophil-specific DNA so can reduce viscosity and aid sputum clearance. It is nebulised, usually once a day or on alternate days. As with all nebulised treatments, it may cause bronchospasm, and therefore a supervised trial dose is given first, with spirometry if possible. Bronchodilator therapy is usually administered prior to treatment. It is expensive, but can be extremely effective.[24]

Hypertonic (7%) saline: This works to draw water into the airway, thus loosening viscous secretions and rehydrating the airway surface liquid. Although it has not been shown to significantly improve lung function, hypertonic saline appears to decrease respiratory exacerbations.[25] Presumably this is through improved mucus clearance. It is much less expensive than rhDNase, but it is poorly tolerated in some children due to the taste, and can cause severe bronchospasm so a bronchodilator should be given prior to treatment. A 3.5% solution may be more acceptable in some children.

Long-Term Azithromycin

The macrolide antibiotic azithromycin can reduce the activity of *Pseudomonas aeruginosa*. Although it does not directly kill the bacteria, it helps break down the mucoid colonies allowing other antibiotics to be more effective. It is likely they also have an antiinflammatory effect. Small but significant improvements in lung function have been demonstrated in patients treated with azithromycin long term.[26] Clinical experience has also shown a reduction in the number of exacerbations the patients experience.

Allergic Bronchopulmonary Aspergillosis

Allergic bronchopulmonary aspergillosis (ABPA) is a hypersensitivity disease of the lung due to an immune response to *A. fumigatus* antigens, which occurs in around 6% of patients with CF in the UK.[27] The diagnosis of ABPA is based on a combination of clinical, biological, and radiological criteria. Diagnosis is, however, difficult as several of the criteria are common manifestations in patients with CF without ABPA.[28] Presenting features include wheeze, worsening cough which may be dry or productive of brown/black plugs of sputum, dyspnoea, chest pain, or malaise. There is usually a reduction in lung function with reduced exercise tolerance.

Features suggestive of the diagnosis are:

- Brown/black plugs in sputum, which may culture *A. fumigatus*
- High serum IgE – in particular an abrupt recent rise to >500 IU/mL or a fourfold increase above baseline IgE. Even more suggestive if this falls with prednisolone therapy.
- High specific IgE aspergillus radioallergosorbent test (RAST) or positive skin prick test to aspergillus antigen
- Positive IgG aspergillus precipitins
- Eosinophilia
- Chest X-ray pulmonary infiltrates >1 cm diameter and segmental collapse
- Reversible bronchoconstriction
- Central bronchiectasis on HRCT scan

Management consists of oral nonenteric coated corticosteroids and an antifungal agent such as itraconazole or voriconazole. The steroid dose is gradually reduced over 4–6 months guided by clinical response and IgE. Relapse is common within 2–3 years of first episode, and often high doses of steroids are needed for a long time.

Pneumothorax

Spontaneous pneumothorax is uncommon in children with CF and mostly occurs in adults. The incidence also increases with underlying disease severity, with a lifetime risk of around 19% in the adult male CF population. Most patients have an FEV_1 < 40% at the time of first pneumothorax. The presence of a pneumothorax is a poor prognostic indicator and studies have quoted an average of 30 months survival after the first episode with a coexistent decline in lung function, although the occurrence reflects the severity of the underlying disease rather than being an independent risk factor. Most pneumothoraces in CF arise from rupture of apical pleural blebs, but bronchial cysts may also develop which, in the lung periphery, predispose to pneumothorax formation. Mucus plugging and inflammatory changes may also lead to air trapping within the alveoli; these may subsequently rupture and lead to a pneumothorax. There is a high rate of subsequent ipsilateral and contralateral pneumothoraces (40%). Because the lungs are usually stiff, complete collapse is unusual. Presentation is usually with acute chest pain, shortness of breath and unexpected deterioration. Small pneumothoraces may be asymptomatic and only detected on routine chest X-rays. A CT scan may sometimes be required to detect some pneumothoraces or to guide management.

The BTS guidelines suggest early and aggressive treatment of pneumothoraces in CF, and the treatment is similar to that for non-CF patients.[29] Oxygen saturations should be monitored and oxygen is provided. An intercostal chest drain should be inserted urgently in the emergency situation of a tension pneumothorax. A small pneumothorax without symptoms can be observed or aspirated but larger pneumothoraces require treatment with intercostal tube drainage. The collapsed lung can be stiff and take a long time to reexpand. All patients should receive antibiotic cover intravenously and adequate analgesia. Gentle physiotherapy should continue, but without positive expiratory pressure (PEP) masks or intermittent positive pressure breaths (IPPB). Further treatment options include pleurodesis, pleural abrasion, and pleurectomy, which all have markedly lower reported recurrence rates than observation or tube thoracostomy alone, which has an unacceptably high recurrence rate of 50%. Partial pleurectomy has a success rate of 95% with little reduction in pulmonary function associated with surgery, and it is generally felt to be the treatment of choice in CF patients with recurrent pneumothoraces who are fit to undergo surgery.[29] In those patients who are too ill to undergo surgery, it can take 2–3 weeks for the lung to reexpand with intubation and suction. In this group, talc instillation or repeated instillation of the patient's own blood are effective alternatives.

Pleural procedures were thought previously to make subsequent lung transplantation more difficult due to adhesions and transfusion requirements. More recent studies have shown that the outcome is not affected by previous pleural procedures (although sclerosants can make transplantation more difficult) and that these should not be a contraindication to lung transplantation.[30] Certainly, surgical intervention should be considered after the first episode, provided the patient is fit for the procedure.

Hemoptysis

Minor streaky hemoptysis is common with chronic infection due to chronic airway inflammation, but may be a manifestation of an acute infective exacerbation. Sputum should therefore be sent for microbiological analysis, and antibiotic cover should be provided as appropriate. It usually settles within a few days but can be frightening for the child the first time it occurs.

Rarely, massive hemoptysis may occur due to vessel rupture, particularly of collateral blood vessels formed secondary to bronchiectasis.[31] Massive hemoptysis is defined as >250 mL in a 24-h period. It is more common in older patients and those with severe lung disease and can be recurrent. It is important to remember that hemoptysis, particularly if associated with chest pain and breathlessness in a child with a totally implantable venous access device, may be a manifestation of underlying pulmonary embolus, although this is rare.

The bleeding may be significant enough to require resuscitative measures due to airway obstruction or hypotension, although this is unusual. Oxygen should be provided and the child should be positioned with the presumed side of bleeding down (the child can almost always locate the side due to a gurgling sensation). Blood should be sent to assess hemoglobin and platelet levels, as well as a coagulation profile and blood should be cross-matched. Chest radiographs are rarely helpful. Conventional resuscitative measures are paramount, with volume replacement and coagulopathy correction, using appropriate colloids, packed cells, or fresh frozen plasma.

Further management options may be required if bleeding is severe or persistent (daily for 7 days with >100 mL on 3 out of 7 days). Vasoconstrictor administration in the form of intravenous vasopressin infusion or terlipressin boluses may be given after a loading dose; they can lead to water intoxication and can cause bronchoconstriction, although terlipressin is said to have fewer side effects. Bronchoscopy may enable identification of a bleeding site or may facilitate clot removal (beware precipitating further bleeding), but rigid rather than flexible bronchoscopy is necessary if bleeding is severe. Tamponade with a Fogarty catheter may then be possible. Hemostasis may also be achieved with agents such as thrombin glue or lavage with iced saline or a vasoconstrictor agent. Oral tranexamic acid has been used long term in patients with recurrent bleeding with some success.

Selective bronchial angiography and embolisation is occasionally required. Numerous dilated tortuous bronchial arteries are often identified some of which may take origin from aberrant sources. The actual source of bleeding is difficult to discern but generally a number of large vessels (>2.5 mm) are embolised using variable sized gel foam pledgets. Great care must be taken to avoid the spinal artery (with consequent paraplegia). Postembolisation pain requiring narcotic analgesia and transient dysphagia are common. This is not a cure and many patients develop new vessels within months or years that may bleed and so require further embolisation.[32]

Pulmonary Resection

Occasionally the question of a lobectomy is considered in a child with CF. Generally, it is only an issue if there is very severe bronchiectasis confined to one area of the lung, while the rest of that side and the other lung are in good condition (confirmed on high resolution CT imaging). The rationale then is that the severely affected lobe is nonfunctioning but acting as a sump of infection for the rest of the lungs. Experience, however, is that although there may be short term advantages, the long term prognosis is unlikely to be altered.[33,34]

Gastrointestinal Disease

Pancreatic Insufficiency and Nutrition

Approximately 90% of CF patients are pancreatic insufficient. In some infants, pancreatic insufficiency can develop over time – at 6 weeks of age, 60% of infants are likely to be pancreatic insufficient but 90% of children within the same cohort are likely to exhibit pancreatic insufficiency by 12 months of age. Pancreatic insufficiency leads to malabsorption (particularly for fat), which is treated with pancreatic enzyme replacement (enteric-coated microspheres of pancreatin).[35] The dose should be titrated to provide normal stool formation, absence of abdominal symptoms, and satisfactory growth; the maximum dose should be 10–15 units lipase/kg/day. An apparent need for higher doses should prompt investigation for other causes of malabsorption e.g., coeliac disease, food intolerance/allergy, or an enteropathy. Stomach acid reduces the absorption of pancreatic enzymes so antacid therapy (e.g., ranitidine) may reduce the requirement. The most common preparations used in the UK contain 10,000 units of lipase per capsule as well as amylase and protease. The starting dose for an infant is usually ½ capsule per feed (6–8 g fat), whereas a toddler will typically require 2 capsules per meal and 1 for a snack. In babies, the capsule contents should be mixed with milk or apple puree and not placed directly in the child's mouth. The dose is generally titrated to clinical response and the enzyme requirement quite variable (usually 8–15 per meal in an older child/adult). High dose pancreatic enzyme capsules containing 25,000 units lipase are generally avoided due to an association with gut stricture formation and fibrosing colonopathy. There is not much a child can eat without first taking enzymes e.g., fruit, vegetables (except potatoes, beans, and peas), fruit juice, boiled sweets, etc. If the child is on special feeds such as neocate, enzymes are required, while if on pregestimil or emsogen, enzymes are not usually needed or given in smaller doses. Fat malabsorption means patients require supplementation with the fat-soluble vitamins A, D, and E, and sometimes K. Diets with a high fat and calorie content are encouraged.

Despite all this, a poor nutritional state is not uncommon. There are many factors that affect nutritional status, including reduced appetite, higher energy expenditure, and behavioral/psychological issues. Unfortunately, it is associated with a worse prognosis and those with poor nutritional status are more prone to chest infections.[36] Poor growth and nutrition are therefore treated aggressively and a dietitian is an integral part of the CF team. It is important to establish that the child has not developed CF-related diabetes or other concomitant diagnoses as discussed earlier. Correct enzyme dosage can be checked by assessing fat absorption, initially by looking for fat globules within the stool, and if necessary by a three-day fecal fat measurement with a fat intake diary. Extra nutritional supplementation may then be necessary. Initially, oral calorie supplements are used but if this fails, overnight enteral feeds are given via a gastrostomy. Percutaneous endoscopic gastrostomies (PEGs) are usually inserted by a surgeon and/or gastroenterologist. Traditionally a two-step procedure is performed, with a PEG inserted followed by a button type gastrostomy 6 weeks later; more recently buttons have been inserted in a single procedure (Fig. 35.4).

Distal Intestinal Obstruction Syndrome

Distal intestinal obstruction syndrome (DIOS), formerly known as meconium ileus equivalent, is caused by a number of factors including pancreatic insufficiency (it does not occur in pancreatic sufficient patients), thickened intestinal secretions, dehydration, and poor gastrointestinal motility. Viscid mucofeculent material obstructs the terminal ileum and/or right sided colon. It occurs in 7–15% CF patients and is more common in patients with a preceding history of meconium ileus. It may be exacerbated by inadequate enzyme therapy and there are often preceding issues with nonadherence to taking enzymes. It causes abdominal pain usually in the right lower quadrant and partial intestinal obstruction. There is usually abdominal fullness and there may be a palpable mass in the right iliac fossa. It quite often has an insidious onset with intermittent grumbling abdominal colic. Parents often report that the child is having diarrhoea (which is due to overflow of liquid stools); in this situation a plain abdominal radiograph should lead to the correct diagnosis showing a colon loaded with feces (Fig. 35.2a). The differential diagnosis of abdominal pain is shown in Table 35.2.

Management involves disimpaction by a water-soluble contrast preparation such as gastrografin given orally (or via a nasogastric tube if the child will not drink it). One or two doses are usually enough, and it is important the child is well hydrated (intravenous fluids may be necessary). Occasionally gastrografin is given rectally. If this fails, then use of alternative bowel cleansing solutions such as Klean-Prep can be used. Again care must be taken to prevent hypovolaemia, and it must not be used if there is evidence of peritonitis. Occasionally, a colonoscopy is required to clear the obstruction and rarely a laparotomy. Once the acute situation is resolved, underlying causes must be corrected and the pancreatic enzyme dosage may need to be adjusted (or taken in the first place!); fiber is encouraged in the diet. Children are sometimes discharged on regular lactulose or oral acetylcysteine.

Constipation is not uncommon in CF and may precede DIOS. It is treated aggressively to prevent progression, with laxatives and attention to enzyme intake and diet.

Gastro-Esophageal Reflux

Gastro-esophageal reflux (GER) is common in children and more so in the presence of underlying lung disease. It is estimated to

FIG. 35.4. (a) Child giving herself a feed through a percutaneous endoscopic gastrostomy (PEG). (b) Button gastrostomy with scar from Nissen's fundoplication.

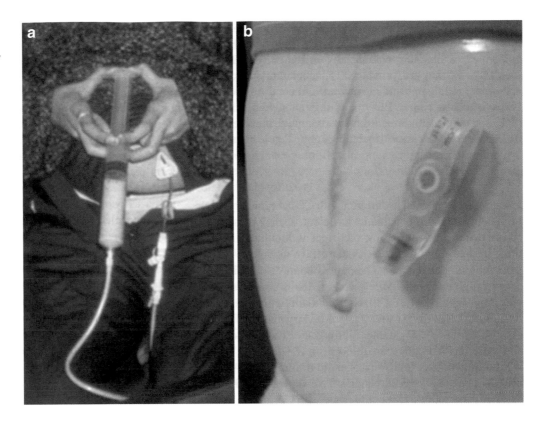

TABLE 35.2. The differential diagnosis of abdominal pain in cystic fibrosis.

Gastroesophageal reflux
Malabsorbtion
Constipation
Intestinal obstruction:
    Distal intestinal obstruction syndrome
    Volvulus
    Adhesions after previous surgery for meconium ileus
    Fibrosing colonopathy
    Intussusception
Appendicitis
Gallstones
Pancreatitis
Recurrent non-specific abdominal pain

occur in 1 in 4 children with CF under 5 years of age.[37] Proposed mechanisms include elevated abdominal pressure from chronic cough, hyperinflation with diaphragm depression, and medications which lower the lower oesophageal sphincter pressure (e.g., bronchodilators). The downwards head tilt position sometimes employed for chest physiotherapy may exacerbate GER. It is well established that GER impacts negatively on lung disease, particularly if there is associated aspiration. Symptoms that suggest GER are recurrent vomiting, epigastric pain, persistent wheezing, and recurrent dry cough. It should also be considered in any child with CF who has deteriorating lung function with frequent chest exacerbations.

Occasionally, a therapeutic trial of anti-reflux medication is carried out, but usually diagnostic proof is required before the child is given yet more drugs. A 24-h pH study is usually performed, with the probe placed just above the lower esophageal sphincter. In infants who are mainly milk fed, it is more useful to perform a dual probe pH study, whereby a second probe is the stomach. This allows recalculation of the reflux index to take into account the time the stomach is acidic to reduce the number of false-negative studies. For the study to be successful, children need to be on bolus rather than continuous feeds. If there is a naso-gastric tube in-situ, it is important to bear in mind that this will affect the integrity of the lower oesophageal sphincter and may worsen GER.

Treatment is with H_2-antagonists (e.g., ranitidine) or proton pump inhibitors (e.g., omeprazole) as well as a prokinetic agent (e.g., domperidone). Occasionally this fails and a Nissen's fundoplication is needed whereby the fundus of the stomach is wrapped around the distal esophagus. Gastric distension following a feed increases pressure around the wrap, thus preventing reflux of gastric contents. The parents must be warned that the child will no longer be able to vomit.

Fibrosing Colonopathy

Fibrosing colonopathy results in a thickened or narrowed segment of colon. Clinical features are similar to DIOS – usually insidious onset of abdominal pain, distension, vomiting and constipation, eventually resulting in intestinal obstruction. Occasionally onset is quicker, just a few days. It can also present with a colitic picture – bloody diarrhoea, pain, distension. Fibrosing colonopathy is associated with the use of high doses of pancreatic enzymes and perhaps with high-strength prepara-

36
Pulmonary Hemorrhage and Hemoptysis

Samantha J. Moss and David A. Spencer

Introduction

The lungs have a rich and complex vascular supply and so it is not surprising that episodes of pulmonary hemorrhage are not uncommon in pediatric respiratory medicine. The appearance of even a small amount of blood can be very alarming and often results in significant distress to both patient and carer. Assessment of this problem is rendered difficult because of the large number of potential sources, multiple possible pathologies, the inability of many children to expectorate, and the frequently intermittent nature of symptoms. True pulmonary hemorrhage, which we will define as bleeding into the lungs and conductive airways, is uncommon but potentially life-threatening. This group of problems needs to be differentiated from bleeding from the nose and nasopharynx, which is much more common and usually benign, and also from other rare causes, including factitious illness.

History

In the majority of cases, pulmonary hemorrhage occurs intermittently. It is important to document the nature and frequency of the episodes along with associated symptoms such as cough, pain, and possible localizing factors. The nature of the expectorate should be recorded, and whether this is apparently pure blood or mixed with sputum, vomitus, or other substances. A history of epistaxis should be sought, and whether the patient picks their nose, although it should be assumed that all children do so! A careful general medical history should be taken concentrating specifically on previous respiratory illnesses, bleeding diatheses, and renal disease.

Pathophysiology

Following an acute bleed, fresh red blood cells blood can be detected within the alveolar spaces and interstitium. Hemoglobin is then transformed into hemosiderin, which is ingested by macrophages. The presence of hemosiderin laden macrophages (HLM) in bronchoalveolar lavage fluid is usually considered to be diagnostic of pulmonary hemorrhage in the absence of conditions associated with transfusion-related iron overload such as thalassemia (Fig. 36.1). It takes several days before HLM appear, but they can then be detected for several weeks.[1] Macrophages produce proinflammatory cytokines resulting in inflammation and fibrosis with thickening of the alveolar epithelium and hyperplasia of type II pneumocytes if there is chronic or repeated hemorrhage.[2] Chronic bleeding causes an irritant bronchitis resulting in goblet cell hyperplasia and the production of large amounts of airway mucus.

Diffuse alveolar hemorrhage may be associated with a small vessel vasculitis. In these cases, infiltration of activated neutrophils results in necrosis of arteriolar walls, venules, and capillaries within the interstitial compartment. The accumulation of edema, fibrin, and neutrophilic infiltrate thickens the interstitial space resulting in fibrinoid necrosis. This decreases the integrity of the interstitial capillaries allowing red blood cells to enter the interstitial compartment and fill the alveolar spaces.[3] Small thrombi may be visible in capillaries and venules.

The lungs have two major sources of blood supply, the low pressure pulmonary arterial circulation and the smaller higher pressure bronchial circulation. There are natural links between the two circulations in the form of collateral vessels.[4] In lung, diseases associated with bronchiectasis chronic infection results in loss of connective tissue, proliferation of vessels, and bronchial artery enlargement. The formation of fragile bronchial-artery pulmonary artery fistulas and exposure to systemic pressures can then result in rupture of these vessels.[4,5]

Clinical Presentation and Physical Examination

Pulmonary hemorrhage does not necessarily result in frank hemoptysis. Presentations vary according to the total volume,

D.H. Parikh et al. (eds.), *Pediatric Thoracic Surgery*,
DOI: 10.1007/b136543_36, © Springer-Verlag London Limited 2009

a 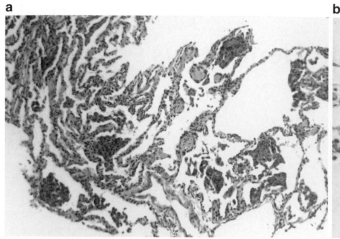 **b**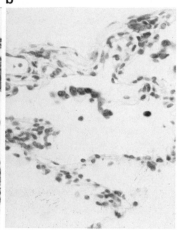

FIG. 36.1. Lung biopsy specimens demonstrating hemosiderrin laden macrophages within the alveoli **a** Hematoxylin stain (×4 magnification) and **b** Perls stain (×20 magnification)

rate of bleeding, and age of the child. These range from acute life threatening hemorrhage to chronic low grade hemorrhage presenting with features of iron deficiency anemia. Respiratory symptoms may include dyspnea, cough, and wheeze. On rare occasions massive blood loss results in cardiovascular instability and collapse. In some cases, patients with focal pulmonary hemorrhage may localize the site of bleeding as a "gurgling" on that side with associated focal chest pain.

Initial assessment should ensure that there are no features of cardiovascular compromise such as tachycardia, weak thready pulse, hypotension, or the high output state found in patients with arteriovenous malformations. Particular attention should be paid to examination of the nose and nasopharynx for evidence of hemorrhage and potential sites of bleeding including trauma to Little's area, the presence of nasal polyps, and active infection of the palatine tonsils. Examination of the skin may reveal evidence of a bleeding diathesis with bruising, signs of iron deficiency anemia, or other clues such as purpura or telangiectasia. General examination of the respiratory system may be normal, but evidence of clubbing, central cyanosis, and the presence of focal signs such as crackles and bronchial breathing should be sought. Careful general physical examination should always be performed for other signs including hepatosplenomegaly.

Specific Causes of Pulmonary Hemorrhage

Causes of pulmonary hemorrhage are summarized in Table 36.1 and the most common causes of pulmonary hemorrhage in children are discussed below.

Cystic Fibrosis (CF)

The management of CF lung disease has improved significantly in recent years. Significant pulmonary hemorrhage is now uncommon in pediatric practice compared with figures from previously reported series.[6] Although the production of blood streaked sputum is still relatively common, true pulmonary hemorrhage is now very unusual under ten years of age.

TABLE 36.1. Causes of pulmonary hemorrhage.

Localized hemorrhage		
	Infection	Abscess
		Pneumonia
		Bronchiectasis
		Herpes simplex
		Parasite
	Foreign body	
	Congenital defects	A-V malformations
		Sequestration
		Bronchogenic cysts
	Trauma	Contusion
		Fracture trachea/bronchus
		Gunshot wound
	Iatrogenic	Post surgical
		Post biopsy
	Tumors	Benign
		Malignant
Diffuse hemorrhage		
	Inflammatory	Henoch Schonein purpura
		Goodpasture's syndrome
		Wegener's granulomatosis
		Systemic lupus erythematosis
		Sarcoidosis
	Idiopathic pulmonary hemosiderosis	
	Congenital defects	Cardiac defects
	toxic	Penicillamine
		Cocaine
		Propylthiouracil
		Azothioprine

Presentation tends to be at an older age in boys than girls,[6] reflecting the relationship between sex and the severity of lung disease.

Acute pulmonary hemorrhage is frequently associated with exacerbations of respiratory infection. Most cases can be treated effectively with a conservative regime of intensive antibiotic therapy. Patients still require physiotherapy, but this must be administered gently to avoid precipitating a further acute bleed. It is important to exclude vitamin K deficiency and liver disease, which may exacerbate the bleeding tendency in this patient group.

Pulmonary Renal Syndromes

In all cases, patients should be examined for any systemic involvement such as sinusitis, glomerulonephritis, or synovitis that would indicate a systemic vasculitis or renal syndrome.

Henoch-Schönlein Purpura (HSP) is the most common vasculitis seen in children. Renal involvement is a common manifestation of the disease, which is characterized by purpura of the lower extremities. The presence of glomerular IgA distinguishes HSP from other vasculitic syndromes. Although pulmonary involvement is a rare complication of the disorder, it does significantly increase mortality.[7] If a biopsy is performed immunofluorescence may reveal IgA immune complexes.

Goodpasture's syndrome is characterized by the presence of anti-basement membrane antibodies that maybe detected in serum or as continuous linear deposits seen along the basement membrane in either pulmonary and/or renal tissue. In the majority of cases, lung and renal disease appear at the same time, although only one organ may be affected. Renal involvement manifests as hematuria, proteinuria, and progressive renal failure. Pulmonary hemorrhage is more common in patients who smoke tobacco.[8]

Systemic lupus erythematosus (SLE) is an auto-immune disease, which affects many organs including the lungs. Serum antinuclear antibodies and antidouble stranded DNA antibodies may be detected along with decreased complement levels. Immune complexes may be visible along alveolar walls, around small vessels and within glomerular capillaries.[3] Pulmonary hemorrhage is more common in adult patients, but is a recognized complication in children.[9] Hemoptysis is often severe and life-threatening.

Wegener's Granulomatosis is more likely to result in localized bleeding from a cavitating lesion than a diffuse bleed. The cytoplasmic staining anti-nuclear cytoplasmic antibody (cANCA) is usually detected in patient sera, while the perinuclear staining antibody (pANCA) is not. This condition is rare in children. The disease presents as a pulmonary granulomatous disease with frequent cavitation associated with midline upper airway lesions. There may also be vasculitic skin lesions and renal involvement. The prognosis is variable with some children dying from sepsis or multiorgan failure and others surviving into adulthood.[10]

Microscopic polyangitis shares many features with Wegener's Granulomatosis including necrotizing glomerulonephritis. However, circulating ANCA is generally of the "p" form and pulmonary capillaritis occurs in the absence of granulomatous disease of the respiratory tract.[11] Prognosis appears to be similar to that of Wegener's Granulomatosis.

Lymphoid granulomatosis is an angiocentric and angiodestrcutive lymphoproliferative disorder, which is very rare in childhood.[12] Skin, central nervous system, and renal involvement are common, and involvement of other systems including the upper airways, eyes, and gastrointestinal tract has been reported. Widespread destruction of lung parenchyma resulting in respiratory compromise with or without pulmonary hemorrhage is a major cause of death.[12] The prognosis is very variable with spontaneous resolution in some patients and progression to lymphoma on others.

Pulmonary hemorrhage has been reported in association with crescentic glomerulonephritis when no antibodies are present.[13] The prognosis from the renal disease is generally poor. ANCA-negative vasculitis is associated with restrictive lung disease, which in some cases is secondary to pulmonary hemorrhage.[14]

Pulmonary hemorrhage secondary to small vessel vasculitis can also be associated with drugs including Hydralazine and Propylthiouracil.

Idiopathic Pulmonary Hemosiderosis

Idiopathic pulmonary hemosiderosis (IPH) was first described as "brown lung induration" by Virchow in 1874. It is a condition of unknown etiology primarily affecting children under 10 years of age and should be considered as a diagnosis of exclusion after discounting all other known causes of pulmonary hemorrhage. A retrospective review of cases of IPH in Greece postulated that exposure to toxic insecticides may have been causal in some cases,[15] but this has not been reported elsewhere.

Symptoms are usually episodic although ongoing subclinical bleeding can be detected in some patients. Histology demonstrates the presence of HLM along with pulmonary fibrosis in some chronic cases, but there is no evidence of any inflammatory process. The estimated incidence is 0.24–1.23 cases per million[16,17] with males and females equally affected. There may be a genetic component to the condition as a high frequency of consanguinity is reported in some series.[18] Autoimmunity may be a factor in some cases as evidenced by the anecdotal response to immunosuppressive therapies in some patients.[18] Paradoxically, findings at lung biopsy are consistent with recurrent hemorrhage, *without* evidence of vasculitis.[19] IPH has an extremely variable course with some children dying within a few years of diagnosis and others surviving for decades. Spontaneous resolution has been reported in some patients who have not responded to treatment.[19] Of the patients that do go on to survive a proportion will have impaired respiratory function. A mean survival of only 2.5 years is frequently cited,[20] although this appears to have improved with more aggressive medical therapy in recent years and some series now quote a 5-year survival of 86%.[19,20]

Heiner's Syndrome

In 1962, Heiner described a cohort of seven infants and young children with chronic respiratory disease with high titres of serum precipitins to cow's milk proteins.[21] The cohort was selected after screening over 2,000 patients with respiratory symptoms.[22] Not all of the children displaying symptoms of IPH had hemoptysis, several had anemia and HLM were found in either gastric or bronchial aspirates.[4,5] Over a decade later, Boat described a similar cohort of six infants detected following screening of 160 infants with idiopathic chronic lung disease. All six infants demonstrated recurrent pulmonary infiltrates, but only five had HLM and four were anemic. As with Heiner's cohort, all six infants improved on a cow's milk free diet. The majority of infants subsequently became tolerant of milk in both series. The release of histamine, tryptase, and eosinophil cationic protein have been demonstrated in BAL following milk challenge along with bleeding into the alveolar spaces.[23] Despite this, the true existence of this condition is now questioned and many authorities are sceptical as to whether cow's milk allergy is a true cause of pulmonary hemorrhage.

The Cleveland "Epidemic"

An apparent epidemic of IPH was described in Cleveland, Ohio between 1993 and 2000. Presentation of these cases differed from that of typical IPH with patients presenting at a much younger age and having a worse prognosis. It has been suggested that the presence of the mould *Stachybotrys atra* in the home may have been relevant. However, a significant proportion of patients had other medical problems including developmental delay and seizures.[24] The true cause of this episode remains an enigma.

Pulmonary Hemorrhage Secondary to Cardiovascular Abnormalities

Alveolar hemorrhage secondary to cardiac failure results from high pulmonary capillary pressure causing mechanical injury to the epithelium.[25] Hemoptysis in congenital cardiac disease may be associated with pulmonary vascular obstruction. As the majority of patients with congenital cardiac disease undergo repair at an early age, the acquisition of aorto-pulmonary collateral arteries in conditions such as Tetralogy of Fallot is now rare.

Some patients with pulmonary atresia have congenital collateral vessels arising from the aorta. These patients are at risk of pulmonary hemorrhage, which is often precipitated by infection and may be fatal.

Infection

Infection is a common cause of hemoptysis in children, especially in the developing world where the majority of hemoptysis is secondary to tuberculosis.[26] The presence of an infectious process such as necrotising pneumonia, tuberculosis, lung abscess, or bronchiectasis leads to localized destruction of the lung parenchyma and erosion of blood vessels. Patients with pneumococcal pneumonia classically present with fever, chest pain, and a cough productive of rusty brown sputum. Pulmonary hemorrhage can also be caused by more unusual infections such as histoplasmosis.[27] Invasive aspergillus infection can cause pulmonary hemorrhage, usually in immune compromised patients. Hemorrhage can also occur when preexisting cavitatory disease is complicated by aspergilloma formation, or rarely in association with allergic bronchopulmonary aspergillosis.

The majority of cases of pulmonary hemorrhage following bone marrow transplantation are secondary to infection.

Foreign Body Aspiration

Pulmonary hemorrhage is an unusual presentation of foreign body aspiration. Hemorrhage is most likely to occur as a consequence of endobronchial infection in relation to the delayed diagnosis of retained organic objects.[22]

Pulmonary Hemorrhage in Newborn Infants

Neonatal pulmonary hemorrhage is most common in preterm infants. The immature vascular system and endothelial barrier make diffuse pulmonary hemorrhage relatively common. The reduced hematocrit of fluid aspirated during acute pulmonary hemorrhage suggests that there is often associated pulmonary edema.[28] Patent ductus arteriosus, surfactant deficient lung disease, infection, intracranial hemorrhage, and hypothermia are also more common in this group of patients, but the relative contributions and associations of these conditions to the causation of hemorrhage are not clearly defined. Antenatal corticosteroids protect against pulmonary hemorrhage.[29] Treatment primarily focuses on mechanical ventilation, in particular the increase of positive end-expiratory pressure, and the correction of any coagulopathy as well as treatment of any associated conditions. Mortality is related to coexistent pathologies, principally the degree of prematurity and severity of pulmonary insufficiency, and in some case series this approaches 40%.[29]

Pulmonary hemorrhage occurs rarely in term infants, usually within a few hours of birth. Many of these infants have intrauterine growth retardation, but the condition is also associated with meconium aspiration, delivery room resuscitation, and hypotension. Mortality is high, and often associated with the underlying risk factors.[29]

Trauma

Direct trauma to the chest can cause pulmonary contusions and occasionally overt pulmonary hemorrhage. Tracheo-bronchial rupture resulting from nonpenetrating trauma, or traumatic endobronchial intubation, can rarely result in fatal uncontrollable pulmonary hemorrhage.[30]

Pulmonary hemorrhage secondary to a tracheostomy is relatively common with some series reporting bleeding in approximately 10% of long-term patients.[31] Hemorrhage is generally secondary to abrasions and the formation of granulation tissue. Rarely, a tracheo-inominate artery fistula can cause life threatening hemorrhage. Symptoms usually resolve with minor changes to tracheostomy care such as the use of softer suction catheters and increased use of humidification.

Accidental or intentional smothering can cause intra-alveolar hemorrhage. A review of cases of sudden infant death syndrome found significant intra-alveolar hemorrhage in 47% of cases at autopsy[32] In some cases, mothers have subsequently confessed to having smothered their infants.[33]

Congenital Lung Abnormalities

Several congenital lung abnormalities may occasionally produce pulmonary hemorrhage, usually secondary to infection. Bronchogenic cysts result from abnormal budding of the primitive foregut during fetal growth. Pulmonary hemorrhage occurs either via the connecting bronchus, or rupture into a bronchus resulting in profuse bleeding. Pulmonary sequestration is pulmonary tissue that is isolated from normal functioning lung, receiving its blood supply from systemic arteries. The majority of patients with pulmonary sequestration do not present until adolescence, and hemoptysis is relatively common in older patients. Hemorrhage may also occasionally occur in children with congenital cystic adenomatous malformation (CCAM). Most of these problems are managed by surgical excision.

Neoplasm

Primary carcinoma of the lung is extremely rare in childhood with metastatic lesions including Wilm's tumour, osteogenic sarcoma, hepatoblastoma, and carcinoid being less uncommon. Hemoptysis is a relatively common presenting symptom of benign endo-bronchial tumours, of which the most common form is adenoma.

Pulmonary hemorrhage has been reported as a result of juvenile recurrent respiratory papillomatosis.[34] This is a relatively common benign neoplastic condition of the larynx in children caused by the human papilloma virus, which is acquired from mother in the birth canal. Wart like neoplasms may spread through the respiratory and digestive tracts, and in some cases can cause upper airway obstruction. Treatment is usually by excision. Surgical excision by microlaryngoscopy was common, although now many surgeons choose CO_2 laser or microdebrider excision as there is better control of hemostasis. There are reports that microdebrider excision is a less painful procedure that results in a quicker improvement in voice quality.[35] Spontaneous resolution occurs, but recurrence is also common. In these cases, adjuvant therapy including α interferon, indole-3-carbinol, and cidofovir has been used to slow the growth of the lesions. There have been reports of malignant transformation later in life.[35]

Pulmonary hemorrhage is also seen in acute lymphoblastic leukemia, both as an autopsy finding and as a finding at bronchoscopy. Bleeding may cause acute airway obstruction in these patients.[36]

Vascular Malformations

Pulmonary arterio-venous malformations can be isolated congenital abnormalities, be associated with hereditary hemorrhagic telangiectasia (Osler-Weber-Rendu disease), or be acquired as a result of chronic liver or cardiac disease. Pulmonary hemorrhage with or without hemothorax can result from rupture of these vascular malformations. Treatment depends on the nature of the underlying condition, but may include transvenous transcatheter embolotherapy using metal coils, detachable balloons, or gelfoam.

Diagnosis

Laboratory Investigations

The investigation of pulmonary hemorrhage depends upon the mode of presentation and nature of any underlying condition. A full blood count and film may show hypochromic, microcytic anemia with a reticulocytosis and low ferritin levels, if there has been chronic hemorrhage. Hemoglobin level will be normal during the initial phase of acute bleeding. It is unusual for disorders of coagulation to present as pulmonary hemorrhage, but clotting studies should be considered especially in cases where vitamin K, deficiency is likely such as such as in CF or liver disease. Fecal occult blood may be positive and HLM maybe present in gastric aspirates where blood has been swallowed. If possible sputum should be sent for microbial examination including acid fast bacilli. If tuberculosis is suspected a Mantoux test should be performed.

If the cause of pulmonary hemorrhage is not known, an auto-antibody screen may be useful in diagnosing a vasculitis or autoimmune problem. Urinalysis may detect signs of nephritis and hemoglobinuria may be present in diffuse brisk lung hemorrhage.[37]

Pulmonary Function Tests

Pulmonary function tests are not usually helpful, but may occasionally be useful in diagnosis and monitoring for disease progression. Single-breath carbon monoxide uptake may be elevated acutely as a result of the binding of carbon monoxide to the hemoglobin in intra-alveolar blood.[38] However, decreased uptake of carbon monoxide occurs if there is thickening of the alveolar septae as a result of repeated episodes of pulmonary hemorrhage. Fibrosis secondary to chronic hemorrhage may result in a restrictive defect.

Bronchoscopy

Bronchoscopy may reveal focal hemorrhage from localized endobronchial lesions such as hemangioma or adenoma. Bronchoalveolar lavage may be used to look for HML and for evidence of infection. Although flexible fibreoptic bronchoscopy is generally a safe and appropriate investigation, it is not an appropriate technique to use in the presence of massive pulmonary hemorrhage, for biopsy of a potentially hemorrhagic tissue mass or for removal of foreign bodies. Under these circumstances, it is necessary to use rigid bronchoscopy to control potential bleeding as rapid aspiration of large volumes of blood cannot be achieved using the suction channel of a flexible bronchoscope. Focal bleeding may also be controlled with the use of iced saline lavage, epinephrine, or balloon tamponade.[39]

Radiological Diagnosis

X-Ray

Plain chest radiograph may distinguish between localized and diffuse disease. In focal hemorrhage, a localized area of coalescent acinar nodules, dense consolidation, discrete mass, or atelectasis maybe seen.[5] Diffuse alveolar hemorrhage classically causes symmetrical ground glass alveolar opacity, more marked in the peri-hilar regions and lower zones and with sparing of the apices and costophrenic angles.[5] This may be difficult to differentiate from interstitial pneumonia or pulmonary oedema. Focal hemorrhage with secondary aspiration of blood in to the contralateral lung may give a similar picture to diffuse disease. In isolated hemorrhage, the radiographic signs resolve rapidly over 2–3 days. The chest radiograph may also demonstrate signs of the underlying disease such as collapse, bronchiectasis, or evidence of an inhaled foreign body. In chronic cases, decreased lung aeration and nodular lesions may be present. Hyperinflation of the lung fields and thickening of lung fissures is not uncommon during exacerbations. The chest radiograph is normal in approximately one third of cases.

Computed Tomography (CT)

CT may demonstrate underlying pathology as well as the extent, site, and severity of hemorrhage. The ground glass appearance of diffuse alveolar hemorrhage seen on the plain chest radiograph correlates with that on CT, with changes usually more marked in the lower lobes.

High resolution CT (HRCT) may demonstrate diffuse nodular opacities with no zonal predominance.[40] These nodules are thought to represent hemosiderrin laden macrophages. Findings suggestive of vasculitis such as centri-lobular perivascular densities both centrally and peripherally can be detected by both CT and HRCT.[5] In Wegener's Granulomatosis, CT may demonstrate diffuse centrilobular perivascular opacities.[41]

MRI

The ferrous component of hemosiderin causes T2 shortening. Therefore, an increased signal in T1 images and decreased signal in T2 images confirms the presence of hemosiderin within the lungs.

Radionulide Imaging

The use of 99m technetium labeled red blood cells can be used to localize the site of bleeding shortly after the initial bleed. 99m technetium colloid may also be used, but is less useful as it has a shorter half life.

Lung Biopsy

Open lung biopsy may be required where an underlying pathology has not been proven by other investigations. For example, in Goodpasture's syndrome, electron microscopy and immunofluorescence studies may demonstrate immune deposits with abnormalities of the basement membrane, even though all other investigations have proven normal.

Management

In acute life threatening pulmonary hemorrhage, initial management should focus upon resuscitation with adequate volume replacement, oxygen and cardiovascular support. It may be necessary to stabilize the airway by endotracheal intubation with mechanical ventilation to optimize oxygenation and very occasionally support with extracorporeal membrane oxygenation is required. Placing the patient with the affected lung in the dependent position may minimize bleeding into the unaffected lung. Occasionally, severe localized pulmonary hemorrhage has been managed by tamponade of the affected lung with selective intubation and ventilation of the unaffected lung. Case reports document the benefit of exogenous surfactant in infants with pulmonary hemorrhage requiring mechanical ventilation, although any benefit has not been proven by randomized controlled trial.[42]

It is clearly important to optimize the treatment of any known underlying conditions such as CF, bleeding disorders, and respiratory tract infections.

Conservative Management

Many cases of pulmonary hemorrhage may resolve spontaneously with conservative management of bed rest and treatment of the underlying condition.

Medical

Infection should be treated vigorously with the appropriate antimicrobial agents. This alone may resolve the problem in conditions such as primary bacterial pneumonia or infectious exacerbations exacerbations of CF.

If hemorrhage is due to a diffuse vasculitis then immunosuppression with corticosteroids and other antiinflammatory agents is usually indicated according to the precise nature of the condition. These cases should be managed in collaboration with pediatric immunologists or rheumatologists experienced in these problems.

The pulmonary vasculature is frequently abnormal in conditions characterized by chronic infection such as CF. There may be pulmonary hypertension with abnormally tortuous and thickened bronchial arteries. These vessels contract in response to vasoactive agents such as vasopressin, resulting in temporary slowing or cessation of bleeding.[43] Antifibrinolytic agents such as tranexamic acid have also been used with some success in both acute and chronic hemorrhage.[44,45]

Bronchial Artery Embolisation (BAE)

BAE was first reported by Remy et al. in 1974.[46] It is used to thrombose abnormal dilated arteries responsible for localized pulmonary hemorrhage in conditions such as CF to control the acute bleed and delay recurrence. The presence of enlarged and/or abnormally tortuous vessels emanating from the descending aorta and intercostal arteries is initially assessed by femoral artery catheterisation. Embolisation is then performed using a coil or embolic materials such as polyvinyl alcohol or gelfoam (Fig. 36.2). Although the technique is reasonably effective, it is less successful if there are multiple abnormal vessels and further bleeding may occur either from unembolized arteries or from recannulisation,[47] so that the procedure may need to be repeated on several occasions. Immediate success is reported as being as high as 75–98%,[6,47] but with reembolisation rates in children with CF ranging from 42–26%.

Complications of BAE are uncommon, but include chest pain, dysphagia, bronchial necrosis, bowel ischemia, and pyrexia. Paraplegia may occur as a consequence of interruption of spinal arteries arising from bronchial arteries, which are present in up to 55% of patients,[48] and the presence of these vessels is considered to be relative contraindication to this procedure. Pain following BAE can be sufficiently severe to require administration of intravenous analgesics, but usually resolves within a few days.[48]

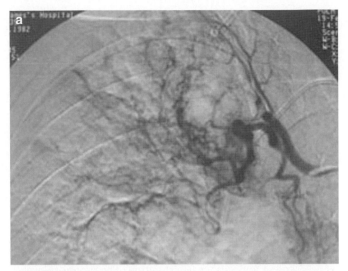

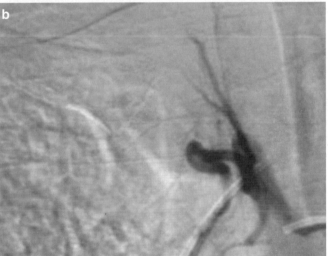

FIG. 36.2. Thoracic angiogram showing enlarged tortuous vessels before (**a**) and after (**b**) bronchial artery embolisation

Lobectomy

Successful conservative medical management and BAE have greatly reduced the need for acute lobectomy to control massive pulmonary hemorrhage, and this is now rarely required. Elective lobectomy may be indicated if hemorrhage is associated with significant localized pathology such as bronchiectasis, and favorable results have been reported in this situation.[49]

Complications

Pulmonary hemorrhage can be fatal. Risk of death is closely related to the etiology and is more common in cavitating TB, anaerobic lung abscesses, or endobronchial tumours. Predictors of mortality include age, volume of hemoptysis, receipt of blood products, pyrexia, and intermittent positive pressure ventilation. The acute mortality is reported as up to 13%.[50]

Chronic pulmonary hemorrhage results in a progressive fall in lung function secondary to pulmonary fibrosis. This has occasionally been managed with lung transplantation.

Conclusions

Pulmonary hemorrhage is a rare but potentially life threatening condition in children. Bleeding can either be localized or diffuse and occurs at a very variable rate. Clinicians need to be aware of both the acute and chronic management of such cases. Although many milder cases may be managed conservatively, all cases of significant hemorrhage require specialist assessment and further investigation. The prognosis varies greatly according to etiology of the condition.

Acknowledgments The authors thank Dr. Fiona Black, Dr. Catherine Owens, and Dr. David Kessel for their assistance with the photographs for this chapter.

References

1. Epstein CE, Elidemir O, Colasurdo GN, et al. Time course of hemosiderin production by alveolar macrophages in a murine model. Chest 2001;120(6):2013–20.
2. Malhotra P, Aggarwal R, Aggarwal AN, et al. Coeliac disease as a cause of unusually severe anaemia in a young man with idiopathic pulmonary haemosiderosis. Respir Med 2005;99(4):451–3.
3. Schwarz MI, Brown KK. Small vessel vasculitis of the lung. Thorax 2000;55(6):502–10.
4. Avital A, Springer C, Godfrey S. Pulmonary haemorrhagic syndromes in children. Paediatr Respir Rev 2000;1(3):266–73.
5. States LJ, Fields JM. Pulmonary hemorrhage in children. Semin Roentgenol 1998;33(2):174–86.
6. Barben JU, Ditchfield M, Carlin JB, et al. Major haemoptysis in children with cystic fibrosis: a 20-year retrospective study. J Cyst Fibros 2003;2(3):105–11.
7. Olson JC, Kelly KJ, Pan CG, et al. Pulmonary disease with hemorrhage in Henoch-Schoenlein purpura. Pediatrics 1992;89(6 Pt 2):1177–81.
8. Donaghy M, Rees AJ. Cigarette smoking and lung haemorrhage in glomerulonephritis caused by autoantibodies to glomerular basement membrane. Lancet 1983;2(8364):1390–3.
9. Beresford MW, Cleary AG, Sills JA, et al. Cardio-pulmonary involvement in juvenile systemic lupus erythematosus. Lupus 2005;14(2):152–8.
10. Belostotsky VM, Shah V, Dillon MJ. Clinical features in 17 paediatric patients with Wegener granulomatosis. Pediatr Nephrol 2002;17(9):754–61.
11. Ozen S, Ruperto N, Dillon MJ, et al. EULAR/PReS endorsed consensus criteria for the classification of childhood vasculitides. Annals of the rheumatic diseases 2006;65(7):936–41.
12. Ozaltin F, Aypar E, Besbas N, et al. Sino-Pulmonary-Renal disese in a child. Ped Rheum Online J 2004;2(1):51–62.
13. Seki Y, Maruyama K, Tomizawa S, et al. Fatal pulmonary haemorrhage and crescentic glomerulonephritis without autoantibodies: a paediatric case report. Pediatr Nephrol 1993;7(1):65–6.
14. Al Riyami BM, Al Kaabi JK, Elagib EM, et al. Subclinical pulmonary haemorrhage causing a restrictive lung defect in three siblings with a unique urticarial vasculitis syndrome. Clin Rheumatol 2003;22(4–5):309–13.
15. Cassimos CD, Chryssanthopoulos C, Panagiotidou C. Epidemiologic observations in idiopathic pulmonary hemosiderosis. J Pediatr 1983;102(5):698–702.
16. Kjellman B, Elinder G, Garwicz S, et al. Idiopathic pulmonary haemosiderosis in Swedish children. Acta Paediatr Scand 1984;73(5):584–8.
17. Ohga S, Takahashi K, Miyazaki S, et al. Idiopathic pulmonary haemosiderosis in Japan: 39 possible cases from a survey questionnaire. Eur J Pediatr 1995;154(12):994–5.
18. Kiper N, Gocmen A, Ozcelik U, et al. Long-term clinical course of patients with idiopathic pulmonary hemosiderosis (1979–1994): prolonged survival with low-dose corticosteroid therapy. Pediatr Pulmonol 1999;27(3):180–4.
19. Saeed MM, Woo MS, MacLaughlin EF, et al. Prognosis in pediatric idiopathic pulmonary hemosiderosis. Chest 1999;116(3):721–5.
20. Le Clainche L, Le Bourgeois M, Fauroux B, et al. Long-term outcome of idiopathic pulmonary hemosiderosis in children. Medicine 2000;79(5):318–26.
21. Heiner DC, Sears JW, Kniker WT. Multiple precipitins to cow's milk in chronic respiratory disease. A syndrome including poor growth, gastrointestinal symptoms, evidence of allergy, iron deficiency anemia, and pulmonary hemosiderosis. Am J Dis Child 1962;103:634–54.
22. Godfrey S. Pulmonary hemorrhage/hemoptysis in children. Pediatr Pulmonol 2004;37(6):476–84.
23. Torres MJ, Giron MD, Corzo JL, et al. Release of inflammatory mediators after cow's milk intake in a newborn with idiopathic pulmonary hemosiderosis. J Allergy Clin Immunol 1996;98(6 Pt 1):1120–3.
24. Dearborn DG, Smith PG, Dahms BB, et al. Clinical profile of 30 infants with acute pulmonary hemorrhage in Cleveland. Pediatrics 2002;110(3):627–37.
25. Boat T. Pulmonary Hemorrhage and Hemoptysis. In: Chernick, Boat, eds. Kendig's Disorders of the Respiratory Tract in Children. Sixth Editition ed. Philadelphia: WB Saunders; 1998:623–33.
26. Wong KS, Lien R, Hsia SH. Major hemoptysis in adolescents. Indian J Pediatr 2005;72(6):537–8.
27. Shaffer JP, Barson W, Luquette M, et al. Massive hemoptysis as the presenting manifestation in a child with histoplasmosis. Pediatr Pulmonol 1997;24(1):57–60.
28. Cole VA, Normand IC, Reynolds EO, et al. Pathogenesis of hemorrhagic pulmonary edema and massive pulmonary hemorrhage in the newborn. Pediatrics 1973;51(2):175–87.
29. Berger TM, Allred EN, Van Marter LJ. Antecedents of clinically significant pulmonary hemorrhage among newborn infants. J Perinatol 2000;20(5):295–300.
30. Roxburgh JC. Rupture of the tracheobronchial tree. Thorax 1987;42(9):681–8.
31. Wetmore RF, Handler SD, Potsic WP. Pediatric tracheostomy. Experience during the past decade. Ann Otol Rhinol Laryngol 1982;91(6 Pt 1):628–32.

32. Becroft DM, Thompson JM, Mitchell EA. Nasal and intrapulmonary haemorrhage in sudden infant death syndrome. Arch Dis Child 2001;85(2):116–20.

33. Bohnert M, Grosse Perdekamp M, Pollak S. Three subsequent infanticides covered up as SIDS. Int J Legal Med 2005;119(1):31–4.

34. Thompson JW, Nguyen CD, Lazar RH, et al. Evaluation and management of hemoptysis in infants and children. A report of nine cases. Ann Otol Rhinol Laryngol 1996;105(7):516–20.

35. Stamataki S, Nikolopoulos TP, Korres S, et al. Juvenile recurrent respiratory papillomatosis: Still a mystery disease with difficult management. Head Neck 2007;29(2):155–62.

36. Sanderson PM, Hartsilver E. Acute airway obstruction in a child with acute lymphoblastic leukaemia during central venous catheterization. Paediatr Anaesth 1998;8(6):516–9.

37. Boat T. Pulmonary Hemorrhage and Hemoptysis. In: Chernick, Boat, eds. Kendig's Disorders of the Respiratory Tract in Children. Sixth Editition ed. Philadelphia: WB Saunders; 2006:676–85.

38. Ewan PW, Jones HA, Rhodes CG, et al. Detection of intrapulmonary hemorrhage with carbon monoxide uptake. Application in goodpasture's syndrome. N Engl J Med 1976;295(25):1391–6.

39. Thompson JW, Nguyen CD, Lazar RH, et al. Evaluation and management of hemoptysis in infants and children. A report of nine cases. Ann Otol Rhinol Laryngol 1996;105(7):516–20.

40. Cheah FK, Sheppard MN, Hansell DM. Computed tomography of diffuse pulmonary haemorrhage with pathological correlation. Clin Radiol 1993;48(2):89–93.

41. Connolly B, Manson D, Eberhard A, et al. CT appearance of pulmonary vasculitis in children. AJR Am J Roentgenol 1996;167(4):901–4.

42. Mikawa K, Maekawa N, Nishina K, et al. Improvement of gas exchange following endobronchial instillation of an exogenous surfactant in an infant with respiratory failure by postoperative pulmonary haemorrhage. Intensive Care Med 1994;20(1):58–60.

43. Jougon J, Ballester M, Delcambre F, et al. Massive hemoptysis: what place for medical and surgical treatment. Eur J Cardiothorac Surg 2002;22(3):345–51.

44. Graff GR. Treatment of recurrent severe hemoptysis in cystic fibrosis with tranexamic acid. Respiration 2001;68(1):91–4.

45. Wong LT, Lillquist YP, Culham G, et al. Treatment of recurrent hemoptysis in a child with cystic fibrosis by repeated bronchial artery embolizations and long-term tranexamic acid. Pediatr Pulmonol 1996;22(4):275–9.

46. Remy J, Voisin C, Dupuis C, et al. Treatment of hemoptysis by embolization of the systemic circulation. Ann Radiol (Paris) 1974;17(1):5–16.

47. Brinson GM, Noone PG, Mauro MA, et al. Bronchial artery embolization for the treatment of hemoptysis in patients with cystic fibrosis. Am J Respir Crit Care Med 1998;157(6 Pt 1):1951–8.

48. Cohen AM, Doershuk CF, Stern RC. Bronchial artery embolization to control hemoptysis in cystic fibrosis. Radiology 1990;175(2):401–5.

49. Blyth DF, Buckcls NJ, Sewsunker R, et al. Pneumonectomy in children. Eur J Cardiothorac Surg 2002;22(4):587–94.

50. Coss-Bu JA, Sachdeva RC, Bricker JT, et al. Hemoptysis: a 10-year retrospective study. Pediatrics 1997;100(3):E7.

37
Interstitial Diseases of the Lung

Maya Desai

Introduction

Interstitial lung disease (ILD) in children comprises a heterogeneous group of rare conditions defined by diffuse infiltrates on chest X-ray and impairment of gas exchange. Interstitial infiltrates may cause inflammatory response, fibrosis, and damage to the lung parenchyma. Restrictive lung function abnormalities may be demonstrated. There are a large number of etiological agents and diseases described under this umbrella, many of them are exceedingly uncommon. ILD is a misleading term as pathology in many may show involvement of the interstitium, alveolar wall, vasculature, and airspaces. In clinical practice, the diagnosis is invariably made by histopathological evaluation of tissue samples. Therefore, the clinical presentation of tachypnoea, crackles on auscultation, and hypoxaemia associated with the diffuse interstitial changes on chest X-ray triggers a number of investigations to identify a more specific cause.

The etiology is varied and in many cases no cause is found. In addition to primary pulmonary ILDs, for example hypersensitivity and infectious pneumonitis, and systemic conditions with pulmonary involvement, for example connective tissue disease, there is a group of rare interstitial disorders, which have been thought to be idiopathic. These can be grouped together using the term pediatric interstitial lung disease (PILD). The classification of these cases is confusing, and there is some debate about which conditions should be included in the classification.

The natural history of ILD in children differs from that in the adult population, and depends on the underlying etiology. Outcome varies between complete resolution and death. Approaches to investigation and management also differ, although there is some overlap in conditions occurring in adolescence. Treatment modalities for PILD have been based on anecdotal evidence and have had variable benefit. Recent advances including the identification of genetic abnormalities in surfactant protein production are improving our understanding of the etiology and may lead to the development of novel approaches to treatment.

Historical Perspective

Acute ILD in adults was first described in the 1940s.[1] Further descriptions of more chronic conditions were made in subsequent years.[2,3] The presence of ILD was described in children in the late 1950s and early 1960s.[1,6] As more cases were described classifications were developed based on histological appearances.[7] Because of a lack of consensus of classification, a standardized classification of the interstitial pneumonias was formulated by the American Thoracic Society and European Respiratory Society.[8] The advantage of this scheme over previous ones is the correlation between histological and clinical/radiological/pathological diagnosis. This classification can be applied to a certain extent to pediatric ILD. However, even some of the more common diagnostic categories, for example UIP (usual interstitial pneumonia) has a different appearance in children. In addition, more recently some unique entities have been described in the pediatric age group, for example, neuro-endocrine hyperplasia of infancy (NEHI), which will be discussed later in the chapter. This raises the question of how applicable this classification is to all cases of pediatric ILD.

In an attempt to clarify the diagnostic categories in children less than 2 years of age, a collaborative research group in North America has drafted a new system of lung tissue classification in this age group.[9] This includes disorders specific to infancy, disorders of the previously abnormal host, disorders of the abnormal host, and disorders associated with systemic disease. It remains to be seen whether this reclassification will be of benefit in the clinical management of these patients and will be applicable to the older pediatric age group.

Epidemiology

Although known to be rare in children, the prevalence of ILD in children in unclear. In 2002, a national survey of pediatricians in UK and Ireland with an interest in respiratory disease revealed 46 cases of ILD proven on lung biopsy.[10] This gives an estimated prevalence of only 0.36/100,000. However, as already stated there is still controversy about the definition

D.H. Parikh et al. (eds.), *Pediatric Thoracic Surgery*,
DOI: 10.1007/b136543_37, © Springer-Verlag London Limited 2009

of ILD and establishing the diagnosis of ILD is difficult. This figure is, therefore, likely to be an underestimate.

Pathogenesis and Basic Science

There is a significant controversy on the definition of the "interstitium" of the lung. In the parenchyma of the lung, it is the spaces between pulmonary alveolar endothelium and capillary vasculature and tissues within the septa including peribronchiolar and perilymphatic tissues. There is usually a very close interrelationship between the exudates occurring in the alveolar walls, interstitium, and within the alveoli of the lung related to thin single basement layer pulmonary vascular and alveolar endothelium. ILD primarily involves the peripheral parts and is generally diffuse. Definition of ILD is nonspecific where the infiltrate including cells and extracellular matrix deposited within the interstitium of the lung, causing derangement of the lung architecture and parenchymal destruction depending on the inflammatory response.

The pathological processes that result in ILD are likely to vary depending on the cause and are not well understood. Recent research on the pathological processes that occur in the lung has led to new concepts about the etiology of ILD.[11] It is recognized that the essential feature of ILD is the derangement or disruption of the alveolar walls. It was previously accepted that an inflammatory process ensued and fibrotic changes resulted from the chronic inflammatory response.[12] Recent theories, however, emphasize the importance of the healing process following alveolar injury by the agents responsible for the disease, e.g., environmental inhalant or infectious pathogen. Part of an abnormal healing process includes failure of reepithelialization, migration and proliferation of fibroblasts, and deposition of extracellular matrix.[13] This leads to impaired gas exchange as seen in ILD. Although inflammation may not play the central role as previously thought, it still plays a role in the process. Lung development and growth is also likely to influence the remodeling process and may explain the some of the differences between pediatric and adult ILD.

Etiology

The term ILD can be applied to a number of different conditions with the same clinical pattern of presentation. The etiology is not always known or fully understood. In the past, the classification of conditions by histological characteristics has led to confusion and does not always reflect etiology. A comprehensive classification system would enable a logical diagnostic pathway to be followed and known causes to be identified. However, such a classification system does not exist.

One system of classification divides chronic pediatric ILD into primary and secondary causes and subdivides the primary causes onto known and unknown causes (Table 37.1).

This may be helpful when considering clinical features involving other systems, in particular, cardiovascular, skin and joints, and in identifying associated conditions that can give rise to ILD.

Primary ILD remains very difficult to classify. There are many known causes of primary ILD including infective agents, environmental inhalants, and drugs. However, many clinical presentations of ILD have no known etiology. As our understanding of lung physiology improves, this situation is likely to change. In recent years, greater understanding has been gained about the role of surfactant proteins in ILD; surfactant protein deficiencies have been identified in cases of familial ILD.[15] In due course, this may help in understanding some of the histological findings previously described. However, surfactant protein-C (SP-C) deficiency has been found in a variety of histological subtypes (UIP, DIP, NSIP)[15,16] and further work is still required before the etiology is fully understood.

Many causes of ILD occur across the age spectrum but may have a different clinical course in children compared with adults. Some conditions are described only in infants and young children.[9] These include chronic pneumonitis of infancy,[17] cellular interstitial pneumonitis,[18] neuro-endocrine cell hyperplasia of infancy (NEHI),[19] pulmonary interstitial glycogenosis (PIG),[20] and lymphangiectasia.[21] These conditions can be grouped into diffuse developmental abnormalities, surfactant dysfunction disorders, pre and postnatal growth abnormalities and undefined, possibly, reactive disorders. Further research will refine this classification.

The improved understanding we have about the etiology of complex pathological processes that occur in pediatric ILD are likely to lead to the development of new therapeutic approaches.

Clinical Features

Symptoms occur as a result of reduced lung compliance and abnormal gas exchange. Clinical presentation is very variable, ranging from asymptomatic to the development of hypoxaemia, respiratory failure, and pulmonary hypertension. Breathlessness is the commonest clinical symptom, sometimes occurring only with exertion. In infants and younger children, breathlessness is associated with difficulty in feeding and failure to thrive. Nonspecific symptoms such as failure to participate in sports, excessive tiredness or fatigue are common. In older children, hemoptysis, chest pain, and dry cough may occasionally be encountered.

In most instances, vital signs are normal but can show tachypnoea and tachycardia. Chest retractions can be present in younger children. Clinical examination showing deformity of the chest wall (for example, Harrison's sulci) and finger clubbing would suggest chronic and progressive disease. The presence of generalized inspiratory crackles on auscultation is much more common in generalized fibrosing disease and

TABLE 37.1. Classification of chronic interstitial lung disease in children (modified from Hilman and Amaro-Galvez, 2004).[14]

Primary causes	Secondary causes
Unknown causes	*Systemic diseases*
Usual interstitial pneumonitis (UIP)[a]	Collagen vascular diseases
Desquamative interstitial pneumonitis (DIP)	Juvenile idiopathic arthritis (JIA)
Non-specific interstitial pneumonitis (NSIP)	Dermatomyositis/polymyositis
Idiopathic pulmonary fibrosis (IPF)	Systemic lupus erythematosis (SLE)
Fibrosing alveolitis (FA)	Progressive systemic sclerosis (scleroderma)
Primary (idiopathic) pulmonary haemosiderosis	Ankylosing spondylitis
Pulmonary infiltrates with eosinophilia	Mixed connective tissue disease
Pulmonary alveolar proteinosis	Immunological disorders
Bronchiolitis obliterans (BO)	Sjogren's syndrome
Cryptogenic organising pneumonia (COP)[b]	Goodpasture's syndrome
Chronic pneumonitis of infancy (CPI)	Sarcoidosis
Cellular interstitial pneumonitis	Langerhans cell histiocytosis (Histiocytosis X)
Pulmonary microlithiasis	
	Associated with pulmonary vasculitides
	Polyarteritis
Known causes	Wegener's granulomatosis
Infectious or post-infectious	Churg-Strauss syndrome
(e.g. Adenovirus, Legionella, Pneumocystis, Mycoplasma)	Pulmonary vascular disorders
Lymphocytic interstitial pneumonitis (LIP)	Obstructive pulmonary venous disease (e.g. pulmonary vein atresia/stenosis,
(secondary to HIV)	anomalous pulmonary venous drainage)
Environmental inhalants (e.g. silica, asbestos, sulphuric acid, chlorine,	Veno-occlusive disease
ammonia, organic dusts[c], avian allergens†)	Diffuse arterio-venous malformations (e.g. hereditary haemorrhagic
Radiation – induced	telangiectasia)
Drug-induced (e.g. cyclophosphamide, methotrexate, azathioprine,cytosine	
arabinoside, vinblastine,	*Pulmonary lymphatic disorders*
bleomycin, nitrofurantoin)	
Surfactant protein B (SP-B) deficiency	*Aspiration syndromes*
Surfactant protein C (SP-C) deficiency	
	Miscellaneous
	Malignancies
	Metabolic disorders e.g. lipid storage disease
	Disorders associated with gastro-intestinal tract e.g. Crohn's disease,
	primary biliary cirrhosis
	Neurocutaneous syndromes e.g. neurofibromatosis

[a] may not occur in children
[b] previously known as bronchiolitis obliterans organising pneumonia
[c] can cause hypersensitivity pneumonitis

exudates. The general examination in children in systemic disorders such as systemic lupus erythematosus and dermatomyositis may give a clue to the diagnosis.

It is vital to establish the duration of symptoms and the speed with which they have developed as this gives a clue to the progression of the disease. Slowly progressive disease may only become apparent after attendance in Outpatient clinics and several visits to the Emergency Department with intermittent respiratory symptoms. The development of consistent symptoms only occurs when there is significant respiratory compromise. Reexamination of previously reported normal chest X-rays may reveal subtle changes. A positive family history may suggest systemic conditions or some primary disorders like desquamative interstitial pneumonitis or idiopathic pulmonary fibrosis.

The variable clinical presentation of children with ILD is mirrored by a varied outcome. The severity of symptoms, degree of hypoxia, and presence of pulmonary hypertension at presentation may reflect the likely survival as shown by Fan and Kozinetz.[22]

The problem faced by the clinician in this situation is that the spectrum of pathology is wide. The prudent approach for a clinician is to establish the nature of the disease process in terms of its acuteness from a careful history and clinical examination of the child as a whole. This clinical appraisal and the findings in the plain chest X-ray invariably leads to further investigations that may result in a diagnosis. The skill is to select the most appropriate investigations to produce a diagnostic yield.

Diagnosis

Laboratory Studies

The full blood count with differential count is not specific except in cases of raised eosinophil count would suggest allergic or eosinophilic lung disease. The erythrocyte sedimentation rate can be elevated in ILD but is nonspecific. Blood tests of hepatic and renal function are necessary to rule out involvement of these organs in a systemic disease. Cultures, skin tests, and serologic titers for infectious diseases may be useful.

Genetic studies can now be performed for surfactant B and C dysfunction. Angiotensin converting enzyme (ACE) can be raised in sarcoidosis.

Immunological Tests

The detection of serum antibodies to various allergens (in particular avian allergens in children, e.g., pigeon) would suggest extrinsic allergic alveolitis. High titers of nonspecific autoantibodies (antinuclear antibody, rheumatoid factors) are associated with systemic conditions like systemic lupus erythematosus, scleroderma and juvenile idiopathic arthritis (JIA). Anti-glomerular basement membrane (GBM) antibody would support the diagnosis of Goodpasture's syndrome. Other useful blood tests could include anti-cytoplasmic nuclear antibody (ANCA), which is usually raised in Wegener's granulomatosis.

Radiology

Chest Radiograph

Chest X-ray (CXR) is valuable in initial assessment and should be considered along with clinical features. CXR guides further investigation and help monitor the clinical progress of the disease. Invariably the plain CXR in most cases of ILD is normal unless fibrosis or oedema is present when the attenuation of the interstitium increases and becomes detectable on plain radiograph (Fig. 37.1). The infiltrate seen on X-ray becomes coarse as the disease advances until eventually honeycomb and cyst formation appears in late cases. Occasionally, it may give clue to the diagnosis depending on the distribution of the infiltrate and the nature of the opacification. Small round nodules may suggest either silicosis or sarcoidosis (rare in children), while small irregular nodules may suggest pneumoconiosis (rare in children), acute hemosiderosis, eosinophilic granuloma, extrinsic allergic alveolitis, or fibrosing alveolitis. In contrast very small nodules would suggest miliary tuberculosis or early pneumoconiosis, pneumocystis carinii or idiopathic chronic hemosiderosis.

Computed Tomography (CT Scan)

High resolution CT scan in these cases is particularly useful[23,24] (Fig. 37.2). CT scan gives the distribution and more accurate mapping of the disease process than plain chest

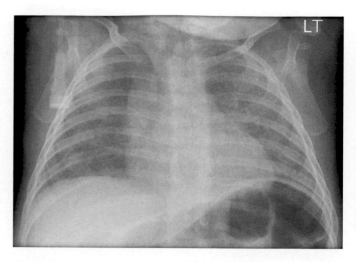

FIG. 37.1. Chest X-ray showing interstitial changes

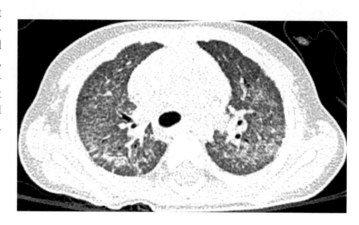

FIG. 37.2. HRCT section showing the typical "ground glass" appearance of the interstitium

X-ray. Mediastinal nodal disease, areas of emphysema, and the distribution of the nodular infiltrate is more accurately defined. The underlying lung disease is identified so that if biopsy is planned it can be directed to the specific areas to achieve a diagnostic sample. Therefore, CT scan is mandatory prior to consideration of obtaining a tissue sample.

Other Radiological Investigations

Ventilation Perfusion isotope scans invariably show abnormalities and defects depending on the clinical circumstances. These scans do not have any diagnostic value.

Barium swallow test may be useful as part of the assessment of possible chronic aspiration syndromes, excluding H-type fistulas, and sometimes identifying gastro-oesophageal reflux.

Lung Function Tests

The lung function tests typically show a restrictive pattern i.e., reduced functional residual capacity (FVC) and forced expiratory volume in 1 s (FEV_1). A mixed restrictive/obstructive pattern may also be seen. Although there results support a diagnosis of ILD, they are not diagnostic tests. They are usually performed for the assessment of the child's functional respiratory capacity and help in monitoring treatment. The restrictive lung disease in these cases tends to improve with a successful management.

Lung function is usually performed in children older than 5–6 years of age but infant lung function testing, which is available in some specialized centers can provide information regarding diagnosis and response to treatment in younger cases.

Oxygen saturation monitoring may reveal hypoxia at rest but in many cases of ILD, hypoxia is only apparent during sleep or exercise. Overnight oxygen saturation monitoring or a 6-min walk test may be necessary to identify moderately severe problems with gas exchange.

Other Noninvasive Investigations

If cardiac disease is suspected, ECG and echocardiography is essential. A pH study will provide more specific information about the presence of gastro-oesophageal reflux than a barium contrast study.

Bronchoalveolar Lavage (BAL)

BAL is very useful if appropriate investigations are carried out and may have high yield in diagnosis of ILD,[25] particularly in diagnosing infection in the immunocompromized host. Electron microscopic examinations of BAL showing lipo-proteinaceous material indicate alveolar proteinosis, intracellular X bodies indicate eosinophilic granuloma, while hemosiderin laden macrophages are seen in idiopathic pulmonary hemosiderosis. The presence of lipid laden macrophages may occur in chronic aspiration syndromes but are not specific to this. Bacteriological examination may show organisms especially pneumocystis carinii. Inorganic material in BAL can confirm specific exposure.

A differential count in BAL is helpful as high lymphocyte count favors the diagnosis of extrinsic allergic alveolitis, sarcoidosis, and chronic infections such as tuberculosis and fungal infections. Neutrophilia and raised eosinophilic count in BAL may suggest the diagnosis of idiopathic pulmonary fibrosis and exposure to inorganic dust. The cell counts are only indicative but not diagnostic of the diseases as superadded bacterial infections and chronicity of the disease may affect results.

Lung Biopsy

In most cases of ILD, a biopsy is required to obtain or confirm a diagnosis. The biopsy will provide information on the degree and type of inflammation and infiltrate as well as presence and extent of fibrosis. Widespread and extensive fibrosis and parenchymal destruction is unlikely produce a good response to medical therapy.

Two types of biopsy can be performed, namely transbronchial biopsy or via a transthoracic approach. Percutaneous needle biopsy has been described but may be associated with higher complication rates and lower yield. The decision about which technique to use depends to a certain extent on local expertise. The transbronchial biopsy is useful particularly if the disease distribution is central, but the yield may be lower than the transthoracic approach which remains the "gold standard." Generalized parenchymal disease is best diagnosed with open lung biopsy either with thoracotomy or with the help of video-assisted thoracoscopic (VAT) techniques.

In addition to routine light microscopy, the lung tissue should be subjected additionally to culture (fresh samples), immunoflorescent staining (using frozen samples), and electron microscopy (samples preserved in glutaraldehyde). Biopsy material should also be frozen in case further material is needed for more staining and other procedures.

Acute Interstitial Disease

Children with polytrauma may develop respiratory distress syndrome and a total "white out" is seen on the plain X-ray; or localized and confluent lesions due to hemorrhage and contusions are seen. Smoke and toxic fume inhalation results in delayed infiltrative changes on the chest X-ray. Acute infections related to viral pneumonia are common in epidemics and with family history as well in imunocompromized children. In children with HIV and hematological malignancies, sudden development of lung infiltration in presence of fever is more likely to be of infective origin. The diagnosis of pneumocystis carinii infection is important to achieve early especially as it responds well to treatment. Acute pulmonary eosinophilia in tropics due to parasitic infestation is suggested by high blood eosinophilic counts and IgE levels. A wide range of medications can also present with acute eosinophilia. Cytotoxic drugs used in chemotherapy can also give rise to acute infiltrative disease but care must be taken to differentiate this obvious diagnosis from infiltration caused by the opportunistic infections. More than usually empirical random use of antibiotics results in delayed diagnosis.

Once the known causes mentioned above are eliminated as the cause of acute infiltrative disease, other unknown causes and syndromes must be considered for the differential diagnosis. Further investigations such as HRCT, bronchoscopy, BAL, and lung biopsy should be considered to establish the diagnosis. In case of eosinophilic infiltrates and raised blood eosinophil counts, moderate doses of corticosteroids are usually given to treat cryptogenic pulmonary eosinophilia. A non-eosinophilic infiltrate creates diagnostic dilemma as lung histology is nonspecific but helpful in eliminating the infective cause. Pulmonary hemorrhage may be a presenting symptom with wide spread pulmonary infiltrative changes on X-rays and may be associated with anemia. There may be an underlying systemic condition for example, systemic lupus erythematosus, Wegener's granulomatosis, and Behcet's syndrome. Many causes of pulmonary hemorrhage such as Goodpasture's syndrome are immunologically mediated. Idiopathic pulmonary hemosiderosis is a diagnosis of exclusion, made when there is no cardiovascular abnormality and there is no identified systemic or immunological process.[26,27]

Chronic Interstitial Diseases

A careful clinical appraisal of history of breathlessness and progression of the symptoms in association with careful review of the radiology is essential in achieving the diagnosis. Recurrent history of viral pneumonia, heart disease, renal failure, and a specific history of oil inhalation are all important clues toward the diagnosis. Cytotoxic drugs for chemotherapy generally result in insidious onset interstitial disease and can be easily overlooked. In longstanding cases withdrawal of drug may not result in reversal of symptoms and pathology. A physician should keep in mind that secondary spread of tumours in the lung can simulate ILD. Generally, good detective work by the respiratory physician result in a diagnosis without the need for lung biopsy.

In children, however, the underlying cause can remain unknown in many chronic ILD cases. Histology becomes an essential part in these cases to classify and to get some prognostic clues. In most cases, a large amount of tissue would be required to assess the histological appearance in detail. A small sample may be sufficient for the diagnosis in certain types of chronic ILD such as sarcoidosis, alveolar proteinosis, and hemosiderosis.

Certain types of cell dysplasias in children such as lipoidosis can only be defined by lung biopsy. However, stigmata in systems suggesting syndromes such as tuberous sclerosis and neurofibromatosis may aid diagnosis, and would avoid lung biopsy.

The commonest chronic interstitial disease showing persisting pulmonary lesions and where BAL may show moderately raised lymphocyte count and mucosal biopsy may give a positive result showing chronic granulomata of sarcoidosis.[19] BAL may be useful is establishing the diagnosis in some conditions for example sarcoidosis and hypersensitivity pneumonitis.[28] BAL examined under electron microscope may show the Langerhans cells and a typical tubular structure within the cytoplasm suggestive of eosinophilic granulomata in Langerhans cell histiocytosis. Invariably the chest ray showing parenchymal lesions with bilateral hilar lymphadenopathy suggestive of tuberculosis, but in sarcoidosis the tuberculin test is negative and clinically otherwise relatively healthy patient. The lung shadows spares the bases and show bullae in the upper lobe. On many occasions sarcoidosis can be diagnosed with indirect evidence.

Wegener's chronic granulomata is diagnosed at open lung biopsy in absence of the systemic extrapulmonary features of lymphomatoid granulomatosis.

Widespread ILD with pulmonary architectural changes and fibrosis is commonly seen in connective tissue disorders. Clinically cryptogenic fibrosing alveolitis associated with widespread crepitations and breathlessness on exercise. BAL in this case is nonspecific with neutrophil predominance and occasionally eosinophilia within the aspirate. Histology on the open lung biopsy is the most reliable method of diagnosis but the changes within the lung parenchyma is dependent upon the stage of the disease. Histology helps to grade the disease in this disease which is associated with poor outcome. Importantly open biopsy rules out rare diseases and infection.

Management

Supportive Care

Supplementary oxygen for hypoxia is essential. Adequate nutrition with added calories is required as most of these children will have growth failure and vomiting related to secondary gastro-oesophageal reflux. Antibiotics for secondary and intercurrent infections are necessary. Some children may respond to bronchodilators. Avoiding environment containing irritants such as smoke within the house helps these children significantly.

Antiinflammatory Treatment

Corticosteroids mainly oral prednisolone and intravenous (iv) methylprednisolone are extremely useful in many of these conditions with dose reduction subsequently depending on the clinical response. There is no consensus as to the most effective regime. A high dose regime that aims to minimize potential side-effects gives a dose of iv methylprednisolone at 30 mg/kg per dose (up to a maximum of 1 g) on a monthly basis for six months (pulsed regime).[29]

Alternatively hydroxychloroquine, azathioprine, cyclophosphamide, ciclosporin, methotrexate, and intravenous gammaglobulin are given, although evidence to use cytotoxic agents in the management of ILD has not been evaluated. Hydroxychloroquine has been shown to be effective in some cases of desquamative pneumonitis. It is primarily anti-fibrotic.[30]

Lung transplantation can be considered for the progressive and end-stage ILD.

Specific Conditions

Disorders Specific to Infancy and Childhood

Some cases of ILD are particular to infancy presenting in neonates and children less than 2-years of age. The numbers of cases is small and their etiology is poorly understood.

To improve understanding of these cases, the children's ILD collaborative research group (CHILD) has developed a system of classification, which identifies four groups of patients.[9] These include diffuse developmental abnormalities, surfactant dysfunction disorders, pre and postnatal growth abnormalities and undefined, possibly, reactive disorders such as NEHI and PIG.

Developmental Abnormalities

Our understanding of this area is increasing rapidly. It is apparent that there is a complex interplay of genetics and processes, which can result in abnormal lung morphogenesis and function if defects occur. It is likely that in the future we will understand current idiopathic causes of ILD in this way.[31,32]

Surfactant Protein Disorders

Surfactant protein disorders are increasingly recognized as a cause of ILD in neonates and infants, particularly where there is a positive family history. Mutations in the surfactant protein-B (SP-B), surfactant protein-C (SP-C) gene, or ABCA3 gene (one of the ATP-binding cassette family) may be involved. The mode of presentation and clinical course is variable depending on the mutation. Autosomal recessive disorders of SP-B are fatal in the neonatal period. Pulmonary alveolar proteinosis occurring in neonates has been shown to be due to SP-B deficiency (see below). Recessive mutations in the *ABCA3* gene can lead to ILD of variable severity from fatal in the neonatal period to ILD in older children. Autosomal dominant mutations in the surfactant protein C results in ILD in older infants and children.

Treatment options are limited.[33] Administration of exogenous surfactant has not been beneficial. Lung transplantation may be an option in severe cases who survive beyond the neonatal period.

Other Rare Disorders of Infancy

NEHI (Neuroendocrine Hyperplasia of Infancy)

Neuroendocrine hyperplasia associated with persistent tachypnoea in infancy has been described in a small group of children less than 2 years of age.[19] These children have tachypnoea, hypoxia, crackles on auscultation and nondiagnostic findings on lung biopsy. The diagnosis is suggested by identification of increased amounts of bombesin (a neuroendocrine cell product) on immuno-histochemical staining of the biopsy. Although treatment with oxygen may be required initially, the outcome is good with reduction in symptoms with time.

PIG (Pulmonary Interstitial Glycogenosis)

This has been described in neonates presenting in the first month of life with ILD.[20] Lung biopsies show excessive amounts of glycogen storage in primitive interstitial mesenchymal cells. Treatment with steroids and hydroxychloroquine has been used with good outcome.

Desquamative Interstitial Pneumonitis (DIP)

Along with fibrosing alveolitis (FA), DIP represents part of the spectrum of conditions of unknown etiology described in terms of histological characteristics. They have different features compared with the same conditions presenting in adulthood.[34] The features seen on biopsy range between desquamation of cells of the alveolar lining and predominant fibrosis. The age of presentation is variable and is often during infancy or early childhood. The mainstay of treatment has been the use of steroids but chloroquine has been used as an adjunct to or instead of steroids. Other immunosuppressive agents such as methotrexate, cyclophosphamide, and ciclosporin have been used. There is a variable response to treatment, ranging from resolution through ongoing symptoms to decline and death. Some may be left with some functional impairment and be able to lead relatively normal lives and others will have significant morbidity.

It is likely that with increasing knowledge of the pathophysiology of surfactant disorders and other genetically determined processes occurring within the lung this heterogeneous group of patients will be more clearly defined.[15,16] Targeted treatment modalities can be expected.

Idiopathic Pulmonary Hemosiderosis (IPH)

Pulmonary hemosiderosis in children can be primary (idiopathic) or secondary to an autoimmune small vessel vasculitis, coagulation disorder, or diseases with increased venous pressure. IPH is a rare but serious and potentially life-threatening condition, which often presents late with anemia, diffuse interstitial changes on CXR and rarely with a history of hemoptysis. A lung biopsy may not be required if the BAL shows hemosiderin laden macrophages, and other diagnoses have been excluded. Lung function shows a falsely-elevated carbon monoxide diffusion (D_{CO}) during episodes of bleeding. Crises that can be life-threatening occur with acute episodes of hemorrhage. If the process is untreated progressive fibrosis can occur (Fig. 37.3). Most cases are treated with steroids, using higher doses to control symptoms and during crises with a background low dose to maintain control. Other agents such as cyclophosphamide and azothiaprine (as a steroid-sparing agent) have been used.[35] The prognosis has improved with early diagnosis and aggressive treatment.

Pulmonary Alveolar Proteinosis

This rare condition is characterized by accumulation of surfactant phospholipids and proteins within the lung alveoli. There are acquired and congenital forms.[36] Congenital forms may be due to SP-B deficiency (see above) or mutations of the genes encoding granulocyte-macrophage colony-stimulating factor (GM-CSF receptor) subunits. The clearance of surfactant by alveolar macrophages may be the key in acquired forms. Lung

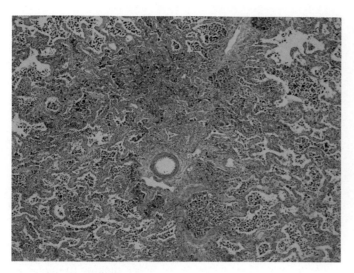

FIG. 37.3. Lung biopsy appearance in idiopathic pulmonary haemosiderosis showing debris in the alveoli with large haemosiderin deposits

lavage and administration of GM-CSF has been beneficial in some acquired forms but not in congenital alveolar proteinosis. The clinical course is variable but may result in early death.

Extrinsic Allergic Alveolitis (EAA)

The most common extrinsic allergens that cause EAA in children are from birds. This is an immune-mediated response, which results in susceptible individuals after repeated exposure.[37] A careful history can usually establish the diagnosis. Allergen avoidance usually results in the resolution of symptoms but steroids may be required in severe cases. The prognosis is generally good.

Primary Pulmonary Lymphangiectasia

Pulmonary lymphangiectasia results from abnormal drainage of the lymphatics in the interstitial and subpleural spaces. It can be secondary to obstruction of the pulmonary lymphatics or vein. Primary pulmonary lymphangiectasia presents in the neonatal period with respiratory distress. Although associated with early neonatal deaths, if survival occurs beyond the neonatal period with supportive therapy, the long-term outcome can be good.[21]

Systemic Diseases

ILD has been described in a wide variety of systemic conditions including SLE, scleroderma, dermatomyositis, Wegener's granulomatosis, and sarcoidosis.[38] SLE in particular has a range of potentially serious pulmonary complications. Although presentation in adulthood is the norm, cases have been described in adolescence and even earlier in childhood. Steroids are used in most cases, although D-penicillamine may be used in scleroderma and cyclophosphamide is often used in Wegener's granulomatosis with steroids.

Conclusion

The term ILD covers a wide range of conditions with overlap with other conditions, which are not strictly speaking interstitial. The type of investigation will be determined by age of presentation and associated presenting features. Tissue diagnosis is the "gold standard." The nature of the rare conditions presenting in the neonatal period and early infancy is being elucidated along with greater understanding of the physiological processes occurring during early lung growth and development. There is potential for more rapid diagnosis and therapeutic options in the future.

References

1. Hamman L, Rich A. Acute interstitial fibrosis of the lungs. Bulletin of Johns Hopkins Hospital 1944;74:177–212.
2. Liebow A, Steer A, Billingsley J. Desquamative interstitial pneumonia. American Journal of Medicine 1965;39:369–404.
3. Scadding J, Hinson K. Diffuse fibrosing alveolitis (diffuse interstitial fibrosis of the lungs): Correlation of histology at biopsy with prognosis. Thorax 1967;22:291–304.
4. Bradley C. Diffuse interstitial fibrosis of the lungs in children. Journal of Pediatrics 1956;48:442–450.
5. Hilton H, Rendle-Short J. Diffuse progressive interstitial fibrosis of the lungs in childhood (Hamman-Rich syndrome). Archives of Diseases in Childhood 1961;36:102–106.
6. Hewitt C, Hull D, Keeling J. Fibrosing alveolitis in infancy and childhood. Archives of Diseases in Childhood 1977;52:22–37.
7. Liebow A. New concepts and entities in pulmonary disease. In: Liebow A, Smith D, editors. The lung. Baltimore: Williams and Wilkins; 1968. pp. 332–365.
8. ATS, ERS. American Thoracic Society/European Respiratory Society International multidisciplinary consensus classification of the idiopathic interstitial pneumonias. American Journal of Respiratory and Critical Care Medicine 2002;165:277–304.
9. Dishop M, Deutsch G, Deterding R, Fan L, Young L, Cutz E, et al. A Working Histologic Classification of the Pediatric Interstitial Lung Disease Cooperative Group. Proceedings of the American Thoracic Society 2005;2:A474.
10. Dinwiddie R, Sharief N, Crawford O. Idiopathic interstitial pneumonitis in children: a survey in the United Kingdom and Ireland. Pediatric Pulmonology 2002;34:23–29.
11. Clement A, Henrion-Caude A, Faroux B. The pathogenesis of interstitial lung diseases in children. Paediatric Respiratory Reviews 2004;5:94–97.
12. Selman M, King T, Pardo A. Idiopathic pulmonary fibrosis: prevailing and evolving hypotheses about its pathogenesis and implications for therapy. Annals of Internal Medicine 2001;134:136–151.
13. Selman M, Pardo A. The epithelial/fibroblastic pathway in the pathogenesis of idiopathic pulmonary fibrosis: tying up loose ends. American Journal of Respiratory Cellular and Molecular Biology 2003;29:S93–S98.
14. Hilman B, Amaro-Galvez R. Diagnosis of interstitial lung disease in children. Paediatric Respiratory Reviews 2004;5(2):101–107.
15. Amin R, Wert S, Baughman R, Tomashefski J, Nogee L, A B, et al. Surfactant protein deficiency in familial interstitial lung disease? Journal of Pediatrics 2001;139(1):85–92.

16. Thomas A, Lane K, Phillips J, Prince M, Markin C, Speer M, et al. Heterozygosity for a surfactant protein C gene mutation associated with usual interstitial pneumonitis and cellular interstitial pneumonitis in one kindred. American Journal of Respiratory and Critical care Medicine 2002;165:1322–1328.

17. Katzenstein A, Gordon L, Oliphant M, Swender P. Chronic pneumonitis of infancy – a unique form of interstitial lung disease occurring in childhood. American Journal of Surgical Pathology 1995;19:439–447.

18. Schroeder S, Shannon D, Mark E. Cellular interstitial pneumonitis in infants – a clinicopathological study. Chest 1992;101:1065–1069.

19. Deterding R, Pye C, Fan L, Langston C. Persistent tachypnea of infancy is associated with neuroendocrine cell hyperplasia. Pediatric Pulmonology 2005;40(2):157–165.

20. Canakis A, Cutz E, Manson D, O'Brodovich H. Pulmonary interstitial glycogenosis: a new variant of neonatal interstitial lung disease. American Journal of Respiratory and Critical Care Medicine 2002;165(11):1466–1467.

21. Barker P, Esther C, Fordham L, Maygarden S, Funkhouser W. Primary pulmonary lymphangiectasia in infancy and childhood. European Respiratory Journal 2004;24:413–419.

22. Fan L, Kozinetz C. Factors influencing survival in children with chronic interstitial lung disease. American Journal of Respiratory and Critical Care Medicine 1997;156:939–942.

23. Copley S, Bush A. HRCT of paediatric lung disease. Paediatric Respiratory Reviews 2000;1(2):141–147.

24. Zompatori M, Bna C, Poletti V, Spaggiari E, Ormitti F, Calabro E, et al. Diagnostic imaging of diffuse infiltrative disease of the lung. Respiration 2004;71(1):4–19.

25. Fan L, Lung M, Wagener J. The diagnostic value of bronchoalveolar lavage in immunocompetent children with chronic diffuse pulmonary infiltrates [see comments]. Pediatric Pulmonology 1997;23:8–13.

26. Avital A, Springer C, Godfrey S. Pulmonary haemorrhagic syndromes. Paediatric Respiratory Reviews 2000;1(3):266–273.

27. Susarla S, Fan L. Diffuse alveolar hemorrhage syndromes in children. Current Opinion in Pediatrics 2007;19(3):314–320.

28. Costabel U, Guzman J. Bronchoalveolar lavage in interstitial lung disease. Current Opinion in Pulmonary Medicine 2001;7(5):255–261.

29. Fan L, RR D, C L. Pediatric interstitial lung disease revisited. Pediatric Pulmonology 2004;38:369–378.

30. Dinwiddie R. Treatment of interstitial lung disease in children. Paediatric Respiratory Reviews 2004;5:108–115.

31. Groenman F, Unger S, Post M. The molecular basis for abnormal human lung development. Biology of the neonate 2005;87(3):164–177.

32. Whitsett J, Wert S, Trapnell B. Genetic disorders influencing lung formation and function at birth. Human Molecular Genetics 2004;13:R207–R215.

33. Hamvas A. Inherited surfactant protein-B deficiency and surfactant protein-C associated disease: clinical features and evaluation. Seminars in Perinatology 2006;30(6):316–326.

34. Sharief N, Crawford O, Dinwiddie R. Fibrosing alveolitis and desquamative interstitial pneumonitis. Pediatric Pulmonology 1994;17:359–365.

35. Nuesslein T, Teig N, Rieger C. Pulmonary haemosiderosis in infants and children. Paediatric Respiratory Reviews 2006;7(1):45–48.

36. Ioachimescu O, Kavuru M. Pulmonary alveolar proteinosis. Chronic respiratory disease 2006;3(3):149–159.

37. Fan L. Hypersensitivity pneumonitis in children. Current Opinion in Pediatrics 2002;14(3):323–326.

38. Singsen B, Stilwell P, Platzker A. Pulmonary involvement in the rheumatic disorders of childhood. In: Chernick V, Boat T, editors. Kendig's disorders of the respiratory tract. Philadelphia: WB Saunders; 1998. pp. 1071–1102.

38
Pneumothorax

Timothy J. Bradnock and David C.G. Crabbe

Introduction

A pneumothorax is present when air accumulates in the pleural space. A pneumothorax may develop spontaneously or it may follow trauma, which may be iatrogenic.[1] Pneumothoraces can be classified as *primary* when the lung is otherwise normal and *secondary* when there is underlying lung pathology.[2] A spontaneous pneumothorax (SP) occurs when air enters the pleural space without an external cause. Primary spontaneous pneumothorax (PSP) is idiopathic and occurs in otherwise healthy individuals without preexisting lung disease. Secondary spontaneous pneumothorax (SSP) arises as a complication of underlying lung disease. Most pneumothoraces in children occur as the result of trauma, mechanical ventilation, or other iatrogenic causes.[2] Pneumothoraces in the newborn period usually occur in premature babies associated with meconium or blood aspiration. This chapter focuses chiefly on spontaneous pneumothoraces. Pneumothoraces arising in neonates or as a result of trauma are covered elsewhere in this book.

The incidence of PSP in children is unclear but is almost certainly considerably lower than the figure of approximately 10 per 100,000 reported in adults.[3,4] In a small retrospective study from the USA, SP accounted for one admission per 10,000 hospitalized children and 3.4 admissions per 10,000 hospitalized infants.[5] A review of hospital admissions to a tertiary pediatric hospital in Australia identified only 12 cases of SP over a 25-year period.[6] These findings are supported by another study from the USA, which recorded only 17 patients with SP under the age of 16-years over a 12-year period.[7]

In adults, there is a bimodal age distribution for pneumothorax with the first peak between the ages of 15–34 and the second after 55 years.[4] The first peak is due to PSP, which tends to occur in tall, thin young men who smoke and is rare after the age of 40.[1] The second peak in incidence is due to SSP. In adults between 70 and 80% of these cases are due to chronic obstructive pulmonary disease (COPD). Pediatric studies show similar findings: the incidence of PSP rises sharply in adolescence[6,8] and is higher in boys than girls,[3] particularly those with a tall, thin body habitus (ectomorphs).[9] In the western world, the most common cause of SSP in children is cystic fibrosis.[10] SP in infants and young children is almost always secondary to underlying lung disease.[5,7,8]

The literature concerning pneumothorax in children is scarce and consists primarily of small retrospective studies with variable, but generally limited, follow-up.[3,5,6] This has created an unhealthy but necessary dependence on adult guidelines for the management of children with pneumothoraces.[11,12] Unfortunately, the two most commonly used adult guidelines (British Thoracic Society and the American Academy of Chest Physicians) are divergent and poorly adhered to in practice.[13–16] It is questionable whether these recommendations should be applied to children because of clear differences in etiology,[17,18] higher recurrence rates,[3,19] and longer life expectancy.

Historic Perspective

Hippocrates described the use of incision, cautery, and metal tubes to drain empyemas 2,400 years ago, laying the foundations for the technique of thoracocentesis. In the sixteenth century, Vesalius noted the requirement for positive pressure ventilation to keep the lungs expanded once the pleural space had been opened. Itard, a student of Laennec, was the first to use the term pneumothorax in 1803. However, it was the development of the stethoscope by Laennec himself that allowed a detailed description of the condition.[11] Although predominantly seen as a complication of pulmonary tuberculosis, Laennec noted that pneumothorax could occur in otherwise healthy lungs. Despite his observations, tuberculosis was considered to be the primary cause of SP until 1932, when Kjaergaard discovered that the majority of cases occurred in adults with otherwise healthy lungs.[20]

The treatment of pneumothoraces was improved by the introduction of underwater seal drainage and chest tubes in 1875. Kenyon was the first to describe intercostal tube drainage in its modern form, when he published his "siphon" method for draining traumatic hemothoraces in 1916.[21] Closed tube drainage was popularized the following year during the influenza epidemic of 1917.[22]

The earliest attempts at pleurodesis stemmed from a need to create adhesions to facilitate lobectomy.[23,24] Intrapleural talc was first used in 1935[24] but its application to prevent recurrent pneumothorax was only realized in the late 1940s.[25] Despite initial concerns regarding asbestos contamination, talc quickly

D.H. Parikh et al. (eds.), *Pediatric Thoracic Surgery*,
DOI: 10.1007/b136543_38, © Springer-Verlag London Limited 2009

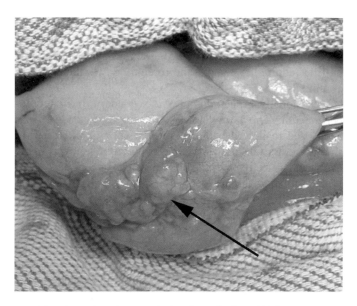

FIG. 38.1. Operative photograph showing sub-pleural blebs (*arrow*)

The colocalization of bullae, blebs, and air leaks to the apical regions of the lungs is likely to be related to the greater distending pressures that act across the alveoli in these regions.[48] Since the pressure expanding an area of lung is closely related to the intrapleural pressure in the adjacent pleural space, it follows that the apical alveoli are subjected to greater mechanical stress than those at the base. This theory is supported by observations that apical alveoli are more expanded than those in the lower zones. The most likely explanation for this is the effect of gravity compressing the lower regions of the lung. West used a lung-shaped elastic structure and an engineering technique called finite-element analysis to confirm that the apex of the upright lung is exposed to expanding stresses several times those at the base.[49] As West concludes, "it [the apex]… will be more vulnerable to mechanical failure in the event of randomly occurring weaknesses in the tissues or generalized parenchymal disease." Clinical studies confirming an association between PSP and an ectomorphic body habitus support this theory.[9] Ectomorphs are taller than average with a flat thorax in the antero-posterior plane. These changes in body habitus occur most rapidly between the ages of 11 and 14 years. It is possible that the disproportionate increase in negative intrathoracic pressure at the apex of the lung accompanying this period of rapid growth induces apical cyst formation predisposing to subsequent PSP.

The evidence for a causative link between ELCs and PSP remains circumstantial and is based on the high frequency with which these changes are found in patients with PSP. Even in nonsmokers, the incidence of ELCs in patients undergoing surgery or high resolution CT for PSP is between 75 and 100%.[49–51] In patients undergoing thoracotomy for PSP, the reported incidence of ELCs consistently approaches 100%. Baronofsky, for example, noted blebs in 25 of 26 young men undergoing thoracotomy for SP.[52] By contrast, in control patients without PSP matched by age, smoking, and gender, the incidence of ELCs is nearer 20%.[50,53]

It remains unclear whether ELCs are the site of air leakage. In the largest series of 1,199 patients with SP, including 218 patients with PSP, only 28% of patients undergoing surgery found to have visibly leaking ELCs.[54]

Although contralateral ELCs are found in 96% of patients with PSP,[52] contralateral recurrence is uncommon with estimates ranging between 2 and 26.7%.[55] In addition, the number and size of blebs does not correlate with the risk of PSP. Ohata and Suzuki examined blebs removed at thoracotomy in 126 patients with PSP.[56] In no case could a defect in the visceral pleura overlying the bleb be found. The external surface of the blebs appeared thinned with an absence of mesothelial cells resulting in exposure of the underlying collagen. In the absence of rupture, pores in the collagen 10–20 $\propto$m in diameter were observed and seen to correlate with the site of air leakage during surgery. These changes were not seen in giant bullae without pneumothorax and were less marked in bullae associated with pneumothorax. Such observations may in part explain the rarity with which leaking bullae are found at thoracoscopy and the fact that 25% of patients undergoing surgery for pneumothorax have no visible ELC's.[57] In nonrandomized studies comparing bullectomy alone with bullectomy and pleurodesis, significantly more recurrences were noted after isolated bullectomy.[58] Whether this observed difference reflects a failure of the surgeon to locate and resect all ELCs or is indicative of an alternative site of air leak is unclear.

Malignancy

A number of mechanisms have been suggested for malignancy-associated pneumothorax. Direct invasion of bronchioles by the metastasis may cause a ball-valve obstruction resulting in air-trapping and eventual rupture. Bronchopleural fistulae may develop from direct tumor invasion or as a consequence of tumor necrosis after chemotherapy. These mechanisms do not explain the well-recognized phenomenon of preclinical pulmonary metastases presenting with SP.[41] An alternative explanation is that small secondary deposits rupture into the lung itself causing free-air to track along vascular bundles to the mediastinum. Mediastinal air eventually ruptures through the mediastinal pleura resulting in pneumothorax.

It remains unclear why bone tumors are so frequently associated with SP. At diagnosis approximately 10% children will have pulmonary metastases, which are usually bilateral and multiple. Pneumothorax characteristically occurs approximately one week after starting chemotherapy and presumably this relates to tumor necrosis.

Cystic Fibrosis

SP in patients with cystic fibrosis is usually seen with advanced lung disease.[39] Most authors agree that pneumothorax in CF is the result of rupture of a subpleural bleb or bullus, which occurs after prolonged air entrapment. Recurrent small airway obstruction with mucus and infected viscous secretions creates a check-valve mechanism leading to atelectasis, air trapping, interstitial emphysema, bullus formation, bronchiectasis with cavitation and abscess formation. *Pseudomonas aeruginosa* infection causes pronounced inflammation in the lungs of CF patients and accelerates the cycle of airway obstruction, alveolar hyperinflation and lung destruction.[60] Postmortem studies have identified three types of pulmonary air cysts in CF patients – bronchiectatic cysts, interstitial cysts, and emphysematous bullae – all of which appear most commonly in the upper lobes.[61] Pneumonia, bronchiectasis, and mucous plugging invariably accompany these changes. SP occasionally occurs in CF patients without subpleural cysts. In this group interstitial air cyst rupture with air dissection along vascular sheaths appears to be the most likely mechanism.

Clinical Features

The typical patient with a PSP is a tall, thin boy with a below average body mass index,[3] a finding that is consistent with the adult literature. Most series suggest a male to female ratio of 2:1,[3,7] although this has not been a universal finding[6] and there may be a female preponderance below the age of 8.[17] SP usually presents with sudden onset pleuritic chest pain, shortness of breath and occasionally a dry cough. The onset is usually at rest and there is no association with exercise. Older children may describe the initial chest pain as "sharp" and later as a "steady ache." In SSP, other symptoms may occur related to the underlying disease process, e.g., pyogenic lung infection. In most cases symptoms resolve within 24 h, even in the absence of treatment. In the case of asthmatics, shortness of breath, without chest pain, appears to be the most common presentation. Rarely there may be a family history of pneumothorax.[62]

Clinical findings range from normal to acute respiratory distress. A simple pneumothorax occupying less than 15% of the thoracic cavity is difficult to detect on clinical examination.[1] The size of pneumothorax, however, correlates poorly with clinical manifestations. Chest wall movement may be reduced. Percussion of the affected thorax may be hyper-resonant. Auscultation may demonstrate decreased breath and heart sounds. Surgical emphysema is a rare finding. The presence of marked tachycardia, hypotension, cyanosis, neck vein engorgement, contralateral tracheal deviation, or a cardiac arrest with electromechanical dissociation suggests a pneumothorax under tension.

The severity of respiratory distress in a child with a pneumothorax depends on their age, pulmonary reserve, the etiology of the pneumothorax, and whether the pleural gas is under tension. As a general rule, signs and symptoms are more marked in SSP where pulmonary reserve is lower.[63] Typically, infants present respiratory distress with marked subcostal recession, intercostal indrawing and widespread accessory muscle use, particularly in the neck. A high proportion of infant pneumothoraces present under tension. In child receiving positive pressure ventilation, the onset of a pneumothorax will be heralded by an abrupt deterioration in gas exchange and hypotension.

Diagnosis

Radiological Diagnosis

A pneumothorax can usually be diagnosed with a plain postero-anterior (PA) chest radiograph (Fig. 38.2). This is best performed with the patient in the upright position.[3] The presence of a thin visceral pleural line without distal lung markings is diagnostic of a pneumothorax. When a pneumothorax is suspected clinically, but not confirmed on the upright PA chest radiograph, a lateral radiograph provides useful information in 14% of cases.[64] Lateral or decubitus chest radiographs with the affected hemithorax positioned superiorly are particularly useful in neonates or ventilated patients and in cases where the patient cannot be positioned upright.[65] In this projection, the visceral pleural line is seen in a retrosternal position or overlying the vertebrae parallel to the chest wall. The lateral decubitus radiograph is as sensitive as CT scanning in the diagnosis of pneumothorax and is a useful adjunct to a standard PA chest radiograph in children with chronic lung disease in whom a small undiagnosed pneumothorax is likely to have significant consequences.[66] Expiratory chest radiographs are not helpful.[67] In the supine patient air in the pleural space is most easily seen in the cardiophrenic recess where it enlarges the costophrenic

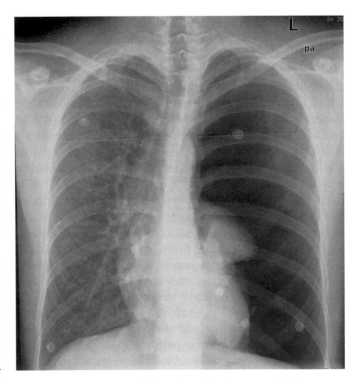

FIG. 38.2. Chest radiograph showing a simple pneumothorax

The British Thoracic Society currently recommends early and aggressive treatment of AIDS-related SP with early tube drainage and talc pleurodesis, early VATS-assisted talc poudrage or unilateral/bilateral pleurectomy.[11]

Cystic Fibrosis

Improvements in pulmonary and neonatal intensive care, earlier diagnosis through the introduction of a national newborn screening programme and advances in postural drainage techniques, antibiotics, and aggressive physiotherapy have improved the longevity of patients with cystic fibrosis (CF).[10] The mean survival of patients with CF was 4 years in 1950, 19 years in 1976, and over 30 years in 2006. One consequence of improved survival in these patients has been a rise in the overall incidence of SP, which now tends to occur in older adolescents and young adults.[108,109] The largest study to date of SP in CF patients reports an annual incidence of 0.64% with as many as 40% presenting under tension.[108]

The onset of SP reflects the severity of the underlying lung disease and usually heralds a grave prognosis. The incidence of SP in CF rises sharply once FEV_1 falls below 50% of the predicted value. 75% of CF patients suffering SP have an FEV_1 of less than 40% predicted.[108] In one large series, the median survival from the date of first pneumothorax was 29.9 months.[39] Around one third of patients will die in the first year following SP.[108] Most die of end-stage cardiorespiratory failure secondary to CF,[110] although a risk of mortality between 6.3% and 14.3% directly attributable to the pneumothorax itself has been described.[108]

Conservative management of CF with tube drainage has an unacceptably high recurrence rate, which has been reported between 64 and 83%.[111] The initial size and presenting symptoms of the pneumothorax do not predict the risk of recurrence. As many as 60% of small, asymptomatic pneumothoraces recur with observation alone. For this reason, current guidelines recommend surgical intervention after a first SP.[60] Several studies have confirmed the efficacy and safety of thoracotomy and pleurectomy or pleural abrasion in selected patients. Thoracotomy and partial pleurectomy has a success rate of 95% and is considered the treatment of choice in CF patients with recurrent pneumothoraces.[39] Chemical pleurodesis with talc or instillation of the patient's own blood may be acceptable alternatives for patients who cannot tolerate thoracotomy.[11] However, sclerosants should only be used after consultation with the regional lung transplant team as they make transplantation considerably more difficult. Specifically, it takes longer to remove the lungs, prolonging the ischaemic time for the donor lungs, and results in heavy bleeding.

These complex patients should be managed in a tertiary centre. Since SP in CF may be preceded or precipitated by an acute exacerbation of an underlying pulmonary infection, management should include aggressive intravenous antibiotic therapy. This reduces the risk of sputum retention, which may delay reexpansion of the collapsed lung. SP in CF is associated with pathogens such as *Pseudomonas aeruginosa* and *Aspergillus spp.*[108] The importance of postoperative chest physiotherapy and analgesia cannot be underestimated.[109]

Malignancy

The association of pulmonary metastases with SP in children is well described. The most frequently implicated primary tumor is a bone sarcoma,[41] although associations with other tumors have been described including primary pulmonary rhabdomyosarcoma,[112] metastatic Wilm's tumor,[113] and pleuropulmonary blastoma.[114] Some authors have suggested that the occurrence of a SP in a child with a bone sarcoma but no known pulmonary metastases is highly suggestive that occult pulmonary metastases are present.[41] Cytotoxic agents and radiotherapy have also been implicated in causing spontaneous pneumothoraces. The occurrence of a pneumothorax in a patient with pulmonary metastases does not appear to adversely affect the overall prognosis, with survival being dependent on the underlying tumor. Management of these patients should be in close cooperation with the oncologists. Nonoperative treatment with tube drainage has been used with good success.

Alveolar-Pleural Fistula

Air leaks, or alveolar-pleural fistulas, are the most common complication of elective pulmonary resections and video-assisted procedures.[115] Although air leaks are often described as "bronchopleural fistulas" (BPF), this is not technically correct. An alveolar-pleural fistula represents a communication between the pulmonary parenchyma distal to a segmental bronchus and the pleural space. In contrast, a BPF is a communications between the pleural space and the bronchial tree at the mainstem, lobar, or segmental level. Bronchopleural fistulae are uncommon, have a high morbidity and mortality, and almost always require reoperation. Air leaks occur in around 33% of patients after elective pulmonary resection and will usually cease spontaneously. They are more likely to follow bi-lobectomy and upper lobectomy as postoperative apposition of the parietal to visceral pleural occurs less rapidly than following lower lobectomy. As an air leak diminishes it will change from being continuous throughout the respiratory cycle to being present during expiration only and then only on forced expiration (i.e., coughing). Spontaneous closure of an air leak will generally only occur when there is no longer a pneumothorax – in other words apposition of the parietal and visceral pleura. For this reason low pressure high volume suction (10–20 cm water) will aid closure of an air leak if there is a persistent pneumothorax.

Persistent large air leaks may require further surgery or pleurodesis. A randomized controlled study comparing instillation of autologous blood with continued tube thoracostomy alone in patients with prolonged air leak after lobectomy, found a reduction in length of drainage and hospitalisation in the instillation group.[116] They concluded that the instillation of 50 mL autologous blood is effective in sealing postoperative air leaks.

Tension Pneumothorax

Tension pneumothorax is an emergency, which requires decisive and prompt intervention to avoid an adverse outcome. In a child with a pneumothorax, the presence of marked tachycardia, hypotension, cyanosis, neck vein engorgement, contralateral tracheal deviation suggest the diagnosis of pleural air under tension. In the intensive care setting, unexplained deterioration or a cardiac arrest with electromechanical dissociation in a mechanically ventilated patient may herald the onset of tension pneumothorax. Tension pneumothorax occurs when the intrapleural pressure exceeds atmospheric pressure throughout inspiration as well as expiration. This situation arises as a result of a one-way valve system which admits air to enter the pleural space during inspiration but prevents its escape during expiration.

The management of tension pneumothorax is based on Advanced Pediatric Life Support guidelines. High concentration oxygen should be administered and a large-bore cannula introduced into the pleural space via the second anterior intercostal space in the mid-clavicular line. A rush of air is heard as the cannula breaches the parietal pleura, which confirms the diagnosis of tension pneumothorax. Following cannulation of the pleural space air should be aspirated until the patient has stabilized at which point a formal tube thoracostomy is performed. The cannula should remain in-situ until bubbling from the underwater seal system confirms the chest drain to be functioning correctly.

Prognosis/Long-Term Outcome

The recurrence rates for PSP and SSP have been discussed elsewhere in this chapter. There is little accurate data regarding the mortality rate for pneumothorax in children. In adults the mortality rate in the UK is 1.26 per million per year in men and 0.62 per million per year in women.[4] The case-fatality rate in the UK is 0.09% and 1.8% in men and 0.06% and 3.3% in women for the ages 15–34 and 55+, respectively.[4] PSP can be considered an essentially benign but troublesome condition with a significant recurrence rate in children.

In SSP, the long-term prognosis is related to the underlying condition of the lungs. In cystic fibrosis, the onset of SP, reflecting advanced pulmonary disease, is associated with a dramatic increase in mortality, with mean survival times of 30 months reported in some series.[39] In patients with AIDS, SP has an in-patient mortality rate of 34%.[63]

Advice on Air Travel

The traditional advice that travels in pressurized aircraft should be deferred for 6 weeks following thoracic surgery or a pneumothorax has been revised recently.

Current BTS guidelines advise a minimum delay of 1 week after full radiographic resolution on chest X-ray before air travel and 2 weeks delay in the case of a traumatic pneumotho-

rax or thoracic surgery.[117] The Aerospace Medical Association guidelines suggest that air travel can be undertaken safely 2–3 weeks after drainage of a pneumothorax or uncomplicated thoracic surgery.[118] The presence of an untreated pneumothorax is, of course, an absolute contraindication to flight in a pressurized aircraft because of the risk of expansion or development of a tension pneumothorax.

Following thoracotomy with surgical pleurodesis or talc insufflation (at thoracotomy), the risk of recurrent pneumothorax is so low that no subsequent travel restrictions are necessary.[92] For children who have not undergone a definitive surgical procedure, there remains a significant risk of recurrence, which is maximal within the first year. These children may be advised to consider alternative forms of transport for at least one year after a first PSP.

Conclusion/Future Perspective

There is little direct evidence to underpin the management of pneumothorax in children. Recent guidelines concerning the management of pneumothorax in adults are contradictory and their recommendations not readily applicable to children. Pneumothorax remains an uncommon clinical entity before late adolescence. In this younger age-group, the majority of pneumothoraces are secondary to overt or occult lung disease and a thorough search for the precipitating condition must be undertaken. Adolescents with a PSP can be managed according to adult guidelines. In younger patients, particularly those with an SSP, management is empirical out of necessity. Recurrence rates are higher in children than adults. Surgical treatment is highly effective and generally preferable to chemical pleurodesis.

As with most areas of pediatric surgery, there is a desperate need for good-quality evidence upon which to establish guidelines specifically for children. The relative infrequency of pneumothoraces in children suggests this will only be possible through multicentre collaboration. Small-bore pigtail catheters are gaining popularity and may prove a valuable tool for aspiration of pneumothoraces in children. The optimum surgical approach for children with recurrent pneumothoraces remains unclear.

References

1. Sahn SH, Heffner JE. Spontaneous pneumothorax. N Eng J Med 2000; 342: 868–875.
2. Karnik, A., Management of pneumothorax and barotrauma: current concepts. Comp Ther 2001; 27: 311–321.
3. Poenaru D, Yazbeck S, Murphy S. Primary spontaneous pneumothorax in children. J Pediatr Surg 1994; 29: 1183–1185.
4. Gupta D, Hansell A, Nichols T, et al. Epidemiology of pneumothorax in England. Thorax 2000; 55: 666–671.
5. Alter S. Spontaneous pneumothorax in infants: A 10-year review. Pediatr Emerg Care 1997; 13: 401–403.
6. Davis AM, Wensley DF, Phelan PD. Spontaneous pneumothorax in paediatric patients. Respir Med 1993; 87: 531–534.

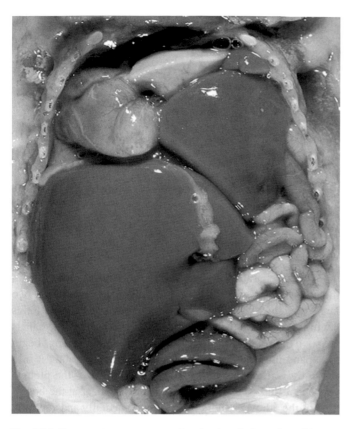

FIG. 39.1. Postmortem appearance showing herniation of small bowel through a left CDH with shift of the thoracic organs to the right and a hypoplastic left lung

week 5 the lung buds enlarge to form the right and left bronchi and then branch further. There is continuing growth both caudally and laterally as the developing lungs begin to fill the pericardioperitoneal canals, which, in turn, become the pleural cavities. By the end of the embryonic period the lungs can be identified as two separate organs within the thoracic cavity.

During the pseudoglandular stage repeated divisions of the tracheal diverticulum create the bronchial tree. This period of extensive epithelial branching is regulated by a complex network of signaling molecules. In the cannalicular stage the bronchioles continue to divide into smaller and more abundant canals. As the saccular stage is entered the number of respiratory bronchioles and terminal sacs (alveoli) increases further, a process which continues during postnatal life.

Pulmonary Vascular Development

To understand the consequences of lung hypoplasia in CDH it is necessary to understand development of the pulmonary vasculature. The pulmonary vascular bed evolves in parallel with airway development. The prime role of the lung is gas exchange, and the arrangement of the pulmonary vasculature to allow sufficient blood flow to the alveolar bed is crucial for this to occur efficiently. Some argue that vessel growth is driven, in part, by development of the airways.[14-16] It has also been suggested that the pulmonary vasculature is the driving force behind lung branching morphogenesis and that abnormal vascular development may be one of the key causes of abnormal lung development.[17] Either way, a complex network

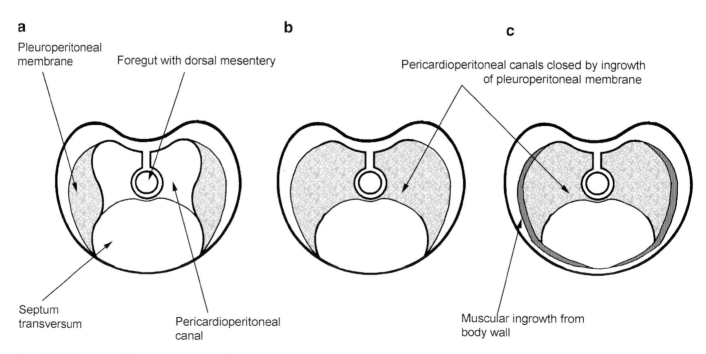

FIG. 39.2. Transverse illustrations showing the embryology of the normal human diaphragm. A: Pleuroperitoneal folds appear at the beginning of the 5th week, B: Pleuroperitoneal folds fuse with the septum transversum and mesentery of the esophagus in the 7th week, C: A rim of muscle derived from the body wall forms the peripheral part of the diaphragm

of vessels must develop from the mesenchyme surrounding the lung bud and form a circuit between the right and left sides of the heart.[16]

Blood vessel development is the result of two complimentary mechanisms, vasculogenesis, and angiogenesis. Vasculogenesis is the process whereby vessels form de novo through recruitment of multipotential mesenchymal progenitors coalescing to create endothelial tubes.[18,19] Angiogenesis is the formation of new vessels by capillary outgrowth from existing vessels. Subsequently, periendothelial support cells are recruited from the mesenchyme to become pericytes and vascular smooth muscle cells. The initial establishment, and subsequent maturation of vessels, is controlled by an intricate network of biochemical signals.

Blood vessel formation occurs at all stages of lung development mostly by vasculogenesis.[14,15] As early as 34 days of gestation the new lung bud has an accompanying pulmonary vessel extending from the outflow tract of the heart, a capillary plexus, and a vein returning to the primitive heart.[13,15] This primary vascular plexus develops from endothelial precursors or angioblasts that form within the mesenchyme around the terminal buds of the airways.[20] Growth factors produced by the airway epithelium are thought to influence organization of these early vessels.[21] Alongside the larger airway branches capillaries coalesce into larger vessels, which, in turn, become continuous with vessels adjacent to the main airway branches. Rather than being concentrated in a specific period of lung development there is continuous development of the vasculature corresponding with lung morphogenesis.[14] The pulmonary veins also develop throughout this stage from the same mesenchyme although independently from the pulmonary arteries. Some of the primitive arteries remodel and increase in size with time gaining an investment of smooth muscle as they become mature pulmonary arteries. This muscle layer is essential to control vascular tone and pulmonary blood flow.[22]

Prevalence of Congenital Diaphragmatic Hernia

The estimated prevalence of CDH is 1 in 2,500 with CDH representing 8% of all major congenital anomalies.[23–25] The estimated prevalence in live births is nearer to 1 in 5,000.[25,26] The reported ratio of male to female infants affected with CDH varies widely, from 0.6 to 1.58.[1]

Accurate determination of the prevalence of CDH is difficult. Individual reports should be scrutinized for the source and type of data used to arrive at the figures presented as studies may be based on antenatal detection rates, hospital admissions, or population-based registries. The latter, which attempt to identify all CDH cases in a given population, probably offer the most accurate estimated prevalence.[26,27]

Six percent of affected pregnancies end in spontaneous abortion or stillbirth.[26–28] In addition, a number of infants succumb to severe respiratory distress within the first few hours of life. Consequently, a significant number of cases of CDH are never recognized.[28]

Pathophysiology

The pathology of CDH comprises three elements: the diaphragmatic hernia, pulmonary hypoplasia, and herniation of the abdominal organs into the thorax. A patent ductus arteriosus and patent foramen ovale are also frequently seen, as well as nonrotation of the intestines.[29] The hernia is located on the left side in 84%, the right in 13%, and in 2% of cases there are bilateral herniae.[1] The defect is usually complete but in approximately 10%, there is a sac of peritoneum/pleura separating the thoracic and abdominal organs.[5]

The lung on the side of the diaphragmatic defect is invariably hypoplastic but the contralateral lung is also affected to a lesser degree.[30–32] The hypoplastic lung has fewer airway generations and fewer, smaller, alveoli with a delay in differentiation of pulmonary epithelial cells. Lung hypoplasia precedes formation of the diaphragm in the teratogenic nitrofen model of CDH.[33,34] As outlined earlier, lung growth is intricately linked to pulmonary vascular development such that a deficiency in one will contributes to a deficiency in the other.[35] The vascular bed is hypoplastic with a reduced number of arterial branches. Further, these vessels are abnormally small with thickened media and adventitia. The excess smooth muscle of the media extends peripherally into the normally nonmuscularized intra-acinar arteries. These changes are most exaggerated in the ipsilateral lung but the contralateral lung is also affected. These findings contribute to the increase in pulmonary vascular resistance seen in CDH.[31,32,36–39]

The precise sequence of events that results in the posterolateral defect of a Bochdalek hernia remain incompletely understood. However, based on rodent models, normal diaphragmatic development has been studied extensively and a number of pathological mechanisms have been suggested. These include the following:

1. A primary lung abnormality
2. Defective innervation of the diaphragm by the phrenic nerve
3. Improper myotubule formation
4. Failure of the pleuroperitoneal canal(s) to close
5. Defective embryogenesis of the pleuroperitoneal fold(s)[40]

Which elements of these theories are correct is unclear although current data from animal models of CDH point to a defect in the developing pleuroperitoneal folds as the cause of the diaphragmatic defect.[41–43] Nevertheless, this model may not be directly applicable to human CDH.[44] What is widely accepted, however, is the presence of a mesenchymal lesion that results in the diaphragmatic defect.[45] Subsequent linking of the diaphragmatic defect and lung hypoplasia, and the timing of these two pathologies, again evokes a number of theories.

One hypothesis, supported by observation that abnormal lung morphogenesis precedes development of CDH in the teratogenic nitrofen model, implicates development of a diaphragmatic hernia as a consequence of primary lung hypoplasia.[33] However, the murine $fgf10$ null mutant mouse model raises doubts about this since these mice have no lungs yet a normal diaphragm.[46] A second hypothesis, based on generation of lung hypoplasia following surgical creation of CDH, suggests that the lung lesion follows development of CDH and may be caused by it.[45,47] A further hypothesis, in keeping with the evidence both for and against the previous hypotheses, merges the two lines of thought, postulating that the lungs are affected both prior to and after the development of the diaphragmatic defect, i.e., there is a "dual-hit."[48]

A final hypothesis focuses on the mesenchyme as the site of faults that result in both diaphragmatic and lung lesions, as well as many of the other anomalies associated with CDH.[45] Indeed, a mesenchymal lesion affecting normal development of the vascular smooth muscle (VSM) conveniently accounts for the pulmonary vascular aberrations and pulmonary hypertension seen in CDH.

Pulmonary Hypertension in CDH

A key factor in mortality associated with CDH is development of persistent pulmonary hypertension of the newborn (PPHN). This is usually evident through poor oxygenation with, in particular, a difference between pre- and postductal arterial oxygen saturation. Echocardiography reveals raised pulmonary vascular resistance and high right ventricular pressures.[49] In a number of cases, adaptation from fetal to newborn circulation is impaired and the pressure in the pulmonary vascular bed remains high or becomes abnormally high after birth. Blood flow through the lungs is hampered and blood flows preferentially into the systemic circulation via the ductus arteriosus and foramen ovale – right-to-left shunting.[22]

The etiology of PPHN is varied but can be divided conveniently into lung hypoplasia and underdevelopment of the pulmonary vascular bed, such as that seen in CDH, or failure of adaptation of the vascular bed due to a number of perinatal or early postnatal insults including acidosis and hypoxia, factors which may also occur in CDH.[50] The pathophysiology of PPHN is complex, involving endothelial and smooth muscle dysfunction. In addition, there is imbalance of circulating vasodilator and vasoconstrictive factors, each with a differing contribution at various stages of the disease.[51] Nitric oxide (NO), made chiefly in the endothelial cells, is one critical factor that causes smooth muscle relaxation. A lack of NO may be caused by stimuli such as hypoxia. Inhaled NO (iNO) therapy has greatly improved outcome for babies with PPHN from many causes although sadly this does not include CDH.[50,52]

Pulmonary hypertension in CDH has two components. There is an exaggerated, but reversible, pulmonary vasoconstriction and secondly there is a fixed resistance from the hypoplastic vascular bed associated with hypoplasia of the lung.[53]

In approximately 50% of infants with CDH pulmonary hypertension is transitory and resolves over the first few weeks of life.[11,54] Other infants have intractable pulmonary hypertension with persistently raised pulmonary vascular pressures, despite therapeutic interventions. Historically, infants with refractory pulmonary hypertension rarely survived. In recent years survival of these severely affected infants is improving largely due to the acceptance of hypercarbia, which allows "gentle ventilation" of the lungs and avoids iatrogenic lung damage.[11] There remains a cohort of babies who die or are left with long-term pulmonary hypertension.[53] Persistent pulmonary hypertension has been recorded in up to 35% of CDH survivors and, not surprisingly, is associated with increased overall morbidity.[53,55]

Etiology and Genetics

Most cases of CDH are sporadic and the cause is unknown. The etiology of CDH is considered to be multifactorial with environmental, genetic, gene/gene, and gene/environmental factors each contributing.[2] Genetic factors are increasingly thought to play a key role.[56,57] Familial cases account for less than 2% and the recurrence risk within the same family is equally low.[23,58] In some kindreds, familial patterns emerge with autosomal recessive, autosomal dominant, and X-linked – all reported.[2]

Overall CDH is considered to be genetically heterogeneous but there are a number of rare syndromes that include CDH.[1] The commonest is Fryns syndrome. This is a heterogeneous autosomal recessive syndrome with a large number of potential features but CDH is almost always present.[59] CDH is also a cardinal feature of the Donnai-Barrow syndrome.[57] In most syndromes where CDH may feature, no consistent genetic defect has been confirmed. These include Beckwith-Wiedemann syndrome, Coffin-Siris, Brachman-de-Lange, and Perlman syndromes. CDH has, however, been reported as part of syndromes with identified genetic aberrations, including, Denys Drash (gene $wilms\ tumour\ 1,\ wt1$), Simpson-Golabi-Behmel ($glipican-3$), Marfan ($fibrillin1$), and craniofrontonasal syndrome ($ephrin-B1$).[2,60]

The gene most prominently associated with CDH is $wt1$. Syndromes with $wt1$ mutations associated with CDH include Denys-Drash[61] and Meacham syndrome[62] while in Beckwith-Wiedemann syndrome abnormal imprinting has been found in a gene that is repressed by $wt1$. The WAGR syndrome (Wilms tumour, aniridia, genitourinary anomalies, and mental retardation) is a contiguous gene deletion syndrome involving $wt1$ and has been associated with CDH in two cases (although in one case the hernia was a Morgagni type).[63] It is interesting to note that a proportion of $wt1$ null-mutant mice also have Bochdalek-type diaphragmatic hernia.[43,64] However, screening of a CDH population failed to identify any defects in $wt1$, so it is unlikely that this gene plays a major role in the pathogenesis of CDH.

Sex reversal syndromes such as Meacham syndrome have also been reported with CDH.[62] There is large variation in the male to female ratio for CDH reported in the literature. This figure ranges from 0.6 to 1.58, suggesting no definitive sex linkage.[1] Interestingly, in a large study in teratogen-induced CDH the male to female ratio was equal and there was no discordance of internal and external genitalia to suggest sex reversal or other intersex states.[65]

Finally, CDH has also been described in various chromosomal numerical abnormalities including trisomies 13, 18, 21, and Turner's syndrome.[2] CDH has been associated with a number of recurrent chromosome deletions including 1q42, 8p, 15q26, and distal Xp. Complex "high-resolution" genome studies are currently underway, which may, in turn, reveal more of the etiology of CDH.[56]

Experimental Models

A number of experimental models for CDH have been described. None of the models is ideal, which is not surprising given the variable environmental factors and changeable genetic background associated with CDH.[66] Established CDH models include teratogenic (nitrofen-induced), dietary (vitamin A deficiency), genetic modification (murine knockouts), and surgically created defects (CDH lamb).

Teratogen-Induced CDH Models

Several teratogens result in CDH, including 4-biphenyl carboxylic acid, SB-210661, and bis-diamine. The best recognized teratogen model is based on administration of nitrofen to pregnant rodents.[34,67–71] A number of reports confirm the similarity of the embryopathy created by nitrofen exposure in both rats and mice to human CDH. Not only is there a diaphragmatic defect and lung hypoplasia, but the pulmonary vasculature is comparable to that in human PHT.[67,72] Other malformations such as cardiac defects and intestinal malrotation are present in nitrofen-induced CDH, in keeping with the incidence of these anomalies in human disease.[73–77] These similarities suggest that the embryological "hit" caused by nitrofen exposure may be comparable to the developmental insult(s) that result in human CDH. These considerations together with the fact that the model is reproducible and comparatively inexpensive make it popular for studies of CDH pathophysiology, including evaluation of new therapies.[5,68,78]

Vitamin A-Deficient Rodents

The association between maternal vitamin A deficiency and diaphragmatic defects was first reported in 1941.[79] Vitamin A has three active forms, two of which – retinol and retinoic acid – act as signaling molecules controlling the expression of genes important for growth and differentiation. With this in mind it is not surprising that vitamin A deficiency and excess

can both result in birth defects.[79,80] In a study of human CDH newborns with diaphragmatic hernia and their mothers were found to have abnormal retinol levels.[81] A "retinoid hypothesis" for the etiology of CDH has been proposed.[82]

A number of factors implicate a problem with the retinoid signaling pathway in CDH although much of the evidence has come from animal models making direct comparison with the human condition difficult. Nonetheless, links between CDH and the pathway surrounding vitamin A and its retinoid derivatives are numerous:

1. Vitamin A deficiency prior to and during pregnancy in rodents leads to predominantly right-sided CDH in 67% of the offsprings.[43,79,83]
2. Administration of vitamin A during vitamin A-deficient pregnancies reduces the incidence of CDH.[83]
3. The incidence of nitrofen-induced CDH is reduced by giving vitamin A or retinoic acid.[84]
4. Posterolateral diaphragmatic defects are seen in a proportion of offsprings in a compound (dual) retinoic acid receptor (RAR) knockout model.[85]
5. Infants with CDH have lower retinol and retinol binding protein levels than control newborns, while retinol levels are elevated in mothers of CDH-affected infants.[81]
6. Nitrofen inhibits a retinoic acid response element in mice embryos and this effect is reversed by retinoic acid supplements.[86]
7. Retinal dehydrogenase-2 is inhibited by four teratogens that all cause CDH.[70]
8. CDH is associated with gene defects in chromosome 15q, a region that encodes cellular retinoic acid-binding protein-1.[2,70,87]
9. Disruption of retinoic acid signaling inhibits lung bud formation in embryonic cultures and retinoic acid deficiency results in lung agenesis.[88]

These data support a role for the retinoid signaling pathway in experimental CDH at least. However, there has been only a single report in humans of abnormal retinol levels in a small cohort of infants with CDH,[81] and the association with the genetic defect in chromosome 15q is by no means universal in CDH patients.[2] A role for the pathway in normal lung and diaphragmatic development is likely but it is crucial to note that a severe embryopathy due to excess use of retinoids in pregnancy has also been described.[80,87] Over 20% of affected pregnancies end in miscarriage or stillbirth while 11% of liveborn infants have malformations, which precludes attempting to reduce the incidence of CDH through maternal vitamin A supplementation.[80]

Genetic Models

Recent sequencing of the human genome has paved the way for studies of the role of individual genes in normal development and disease. A wide variety of methodologies have been described that allow gene expression to be reduced or eliminated either from the beginning of development or at a predetermined time point. Such genetic models have been applied to the problem of CDH but lack of a single genetic defect has hindered identification of an ideal model. While diaphragmatic defects have been described in several gene-knockout mouse models in a number of these the diaphragm is either complete but abnormally muscularized (e.g., the Fog2 mutant mouse) or there is a central ventral defect, as seen in Slit3- and Gata4-deficient mice.[89–91] However, posterior defects more comparable to the Bochdalek-type hernia have also been reported. This type of hernia is found in MyoR and Capsulin double mutants, Wilms' tumour 1 (wt1) null mutant mice, retinoic acid receptor (RAR) α, and RARβ2 double mutants and in conditional COUP-TFII null mutant animals.[64,85,92,93] Of particular interest are the wt1 knockout model, because of the link with Denys-Drash syndrome and its link with vitamin A metabolism. It should be noted that in many of these genetic modes a wide range of other defects are present, which are not found in human CDH. In wt1 knockout mice the lungs grow down through the diaphragmatic defect and heterozygote mice do not show the predisposition to Wilms' tumor that is seen in humans with a wt1 mutation.[64] Equally, a diaphragmatic defect is not seen in all mutant fetuses, and the classic pulmonary vasculopathy has not been described in these models.[43] The genetic contributions from these elegant studies may unravel molecular clues to further our understanding of the etiology and treatment of CDH.[56]

Lamb CDH Model

First described in 1967, this was the earliest model for CDH.[94] A diaphragmatic defect is created in mid-late gestational surgical creation based on the theory that lung hypoplasia is caused by compression of the lung by herniated abdominal organs in the chest.[94–97] This model has permitted detailed studies of CDH pathophysiology. Indeed, the surgical model has proven to be invaluable for studying the effects of antenatal tracheal occlusion and its role in management of antenatally diagnosed human CDH.[98–101]

Associated Anomalies/Malformations

CDH may be isolated or occur in association with a wide range of other congenital malformations and genetic aberrations. The rate of associated anomalies is reported to be between 40 and 60%.[102,103] Combining data from various reports suggests that 50–60% of fetuses have isolated CDH while 40–50% have major associated malformations, mostly independent of recognized syndromes.[1,27,29] In some cases the associated anomaly may be detected prenatally and may alert the sonographer to the presence of other anomalies although CDH may remain undetected until after birth.[87,104]

The majority of associated anomalies are congenital cardiac defects, most commonly ventricular septal defects, tetralogy

of Fallot and aortic coarctation.[29,104–106] Less serious cardiac conditions such as patent ductus arteriosus and patent foramen ovale are also common in babies with CDH. Anomalies are also found in other systems including the genitourinary system (23%), gastrointestinal tract (14–17%), central nervous system (14%), skeletal system (10%), and other pulmonary anomalies in 5%, while 10% have chromosomal defects.[29,105] Associated anomalies are significantly more frequent in fetuses with bilateral CDH but the incidence of almost all anomalies does not appear to correlate with the side of the defect.[26,107] However, a recent report based on the California Birth Defects Monitoring Program found differing frequencies of a number of anomalies according to the side of the diaphragmatic defect.[108] The significance of this finding is unknown.

Diagnosis and Management

Antenatal Diagnosis

Up to 56% of CDHs are now diagnosed antenatally, usually on a 20-week routine fetal anomaly ultrasound (US) scan (Fig. 39.3).[26–28,109] The stomach or bowel is seen within the chest and the mediastinum is displaced from the side of the lesion.[110] The rate of antenatal detection is increasing and is likely to rise further with advances in USS technology making first trimester diagnosis possible.[26] Antenatal diagnosis has a significant impact on the outcome for an infant with CDH. This is not only through planning of perinatal care but also because many parents will opt for termination of pregnancy. Fetuses with an antenatally diagnosed CDH are more likely to have other anomalies, which have a significant adverse effect on the prognosis. Survival is lower in the antenatally detected group due largely to associated anomalies rather than CDH per se, i.e., antenatal diagnosis on its own is not a poor prognostic factor.[26,105,111] Nonetheless, the rate of elective termination of pregnancy is rising following antenatal

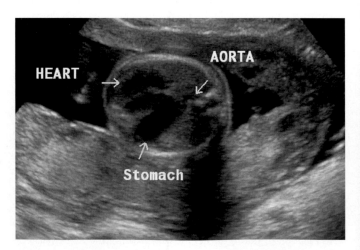

FIG. 39.3. Antenatal ultrasound image showing the fetal heart and stomach in the chest

diagnosis of a CDH with recent studies reporting termination rates of 19–24%.[26–28]

For babies detected in utero antenatal counseling, ideally from a multidisciplinary team, should be offered. Termination of pregnancy may be considered. Karyotyping by amniocentesis or chorionic villus sampling should be offered. Parents should be informed of the unpredictable postnatal course for these babies. Delivery should be planned in a tertiary obstetric center with access to specialist neonatal and surgical care. There is debate over the merits of centralizing CDH care and delivery of affected babies in "high-volume" specialized centers.[103,112]

The first question that many parents will ask when a congenital anomaly is detected is the likely outcome for the pregnancy. Unfortunately, there is no consensus regarding the ideal method by which to predict prognosis due to CDH, particularly in infants with isolated CDH.[110] A number of features appear to have some predictive value including bilateral hernia, the position of the liver, and fetal lung–head ratio. Other factors such as polyhydramnios and mediastinal shift previously considered important now seem to be poor predictors of outcome.[113,114]

Measurement of fetal lung to head ratio (LHR) has gained popularity in recent years as a method of determining prognosis. Two-dimensional US is used to calculate the ratio of the area of the contralateral fetal lung at the level of the four chamber view of the heart to the fetal head circumference at the level of the lateral ventricles (Fig. 39.4).[115] There results of antenatal prognostication by LHR are unfortunately not consistent. This is probably due to inconsistencies in measurement of lung as well as the variable gestational age at which the measurements are taken.[116–118] Moreover, a recent systematic review and meta-analysis found that calculation of prognosis from LHR is not supported by current evidence.[119] More recently, Cannie et al. reported the use of magnetic resonance imaging (MRI) as a new method for predicting outcome in antenatally diagnosed CDH.[120] They correlated total fetal lung volume with total fetal body volume to generate a lung volume observed–expected ratio. A ratio below 35% predicted a poor prognosis although thus far the patient numbers are small, and the technique requires validation before being used for antenatal counseling.

Antenatal Surgery

With the concept that mortality in isolated CDH is related to pulmonary hypoplasia much interest has centered on fetal intervention to improve lung growth. The first strategy involved in-utero repair of the diaphragm. While this was technically possible outcome was no better following antenatal repair than with conventional postnatal treatment.[121] An alternative strategy arose from the observation that congenital laryngeal atresia results in lung *hyperplasia*.[122] From this came the concept of tracheal occlusion (TO) to promote lung growth in CDH – the so-called *plug the lung until it grows* strategies.[123] Subsequent experimental studies in both surgically created and teratogen-induced CDH confirmed lung enlargement following TO.[78,100,101,123] Improvement in pulmonary vascular morphology and physiology was also demonstrated in animal models although the timing and duration of TO were critical.[23,78,101,124,125]

When these experiments were first translated into humans, the procedure involved TO via a hysterotomy with reversal at the time of delivery by an ex-utero intrapartum procedure (EXIT). Mortality from premature delivery and respiratory insufficiency was unacceptably high.[126] The technique of fetal TO evolved to less invasive endoscopic tracheal clipping followed by an EXIT procedure. The latest methods for TO involve percutaneous "fetoscopic" endoluminal tracheal occlusion (FETO) with a detachable balloon at 26–28-weeks gestation and prenatal balloon retrieval

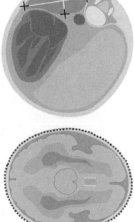

FIG. 39.4. Measurement of the lung-to-head ratio in a section through the four-chamber view, both schematically (*right*) and on an ultrasound image (*left*). The contralateral lung is proportionated over the head circumference (bottom right). With permission from Deprest et al.[115]

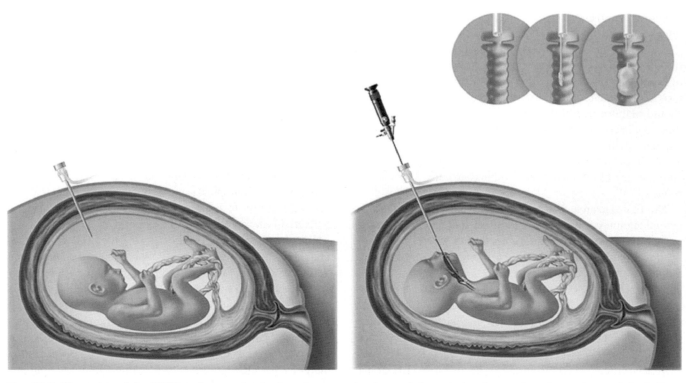

FIG. 39.5. Illustration of the FETO technique: the fetal tracheoscope is advanced through the pharynx into the trachea and the balloon deployed (insert). With permission from Deprest et al.[25]

at around 34-weeks gestation (Fig. 39.5).[25,127] Morbidity includes premature prelabor rupture of membranes and subsequent premature delivery in more than 15% of patients although this is a marked improvement from the more invasive techniques.[115,128] Maternal issues include an increase in the cesarean section rate.

Given that open fetal surgery did not improve survival Harrison and coworkers led a trial of FETO with EXIT to seek improved survival in severe CDH.[128] As already outlined, predicting outcome in antenatally diagnosed CDH is difficult. This study used LHR <1.4 and liver herniation in an attempt to select severe cases but survival was not significantly different between the FETO (73%) and conventional (77%) treatment groups. Preterm delivery was, however, significantly greater in the FETO group. FETO is now reserved for fetuses that fulfill stricter criteria of severity in an attempt to select babies with the poorest chance of postnatal survival.[117] A recent nonrandomized nonblinded report found survival of 50% in the FETO-treated group compared with 9% survival of infants who did not undergo surgery.[127]

Antenatal surgery for CDH is still in evolution with patient selection proving to be a bigger hurdle than the procedure itself. These interventions should be offered in specialized fetal treatment centers as part of clinical trials.[11] In Europe the "FETO" groups are working to refine trial criteria (J. Deprest, personal communication). Outcomes from these European studies are awaited with interest.

Antenatal Steroid Therapy

For normal infants at risk of premature delivery antenatal steroids (dexamethasone) improve lung maturity and reduce the incidence of surfactant-deficient lung disease.[129] Data from animal models of CDH support the administration of antenatal glucocorticoids for the fetus with CDH. Studies show improved pulmonary morphology, compliance, biochemistry, and fetal survival.[68,69,130–132] However, a recent multicenter randomized trial was inadequately powered and failed to show a survival benefit in human CDH.[133] With such compelling animal data, an adequately powered randomised trial is required to answer the question although large patient numbers will be necessary to detect a significant advantage.

Delivery

For those infants with an in-utero diagnosis of CDH delivery should be planned to optimize postnatal care. In most cases obstetric care will be given in a tertiary unit with surgical services on site. The delivery itself, unless indicated for obstetric reasons, is usually vaginal although some centers elect to deliver these infants by cesarean section.[134] There is no evidence to support cesarean delivery.[135] Bag-valve-mask ventilation should be avoided and the infant intubated as soon as possible to minimize gaseous distension of the stomach. For this purpose a nasogastric tube should be inserted, and this may help confirm the diagnosis if the tube is seen within the chest on X-ray.

Exogenous surfactant therapy has been offered to newborns with CDH due to improved pulmonary hemodynamics reported in the lamb model.[136] However, while both human and animal studies suggest a deficiency of surfactant in CDH, use is only recommended in premature infants. No benefit has been identified in term neonates and surfactant may even be harmful in this group.[109,137]

Postnatal Diagnosis

Around 50% of babies with a CDH remain undiagnosed until birth. The classical presentation in these babies is of a term infant with acute respiratory distress shortly after, or within, 12 h of birth. These infants may have clinically apparent mediastinal shift, a scaphoid abdomen and, instead of breath sounds, bowel sounds may be heard within the chest. An X-ray then reveals the characteristic combination of bowel loops within the chest, lung hypoplasia, and mediastinal shift away from the side of the hernia (Fig. 39.6). A proportion of infants presenting in this way will succumb soon after birth from lung hypoplasia. At the other end of the spectrum a small number of cases are asymptomatic and the CDH goes undetected for months or years. This subset has normal lungs and the transition to extrauterine life is unremarkable. Such patients are not usually included in studies of management and outcome for CDH as their pre- and postoperative course cannot be compared with that of infants who present with acute respiratory distress.

Postnatal Management

Since the realization that CDH is a physiological insult as well as a surgical one there has been a move away from emergency surgery. It has become apparent that the method of ventilation in these infants is crucial, not least because they are very susceptible to PPHN. In the 1980s hyperventilation and alkalinization were the mainstay of treatment for pulmonary hypertension because experimental data showed reversal of ductal blood flow and shunting with aggressive ventilation.[138,139] Unfortunately this strategy resulted in significant barotrauma and it is now accepted that mortality actually increases. "Gentle ventilation" is emerging as the standard of care.[109,112] If adequate oxygenation cannot be achieved using conventional ventilation high-frequency oscillating ventilation (HFOV), extracorporeal membrane oxygenation (ECMO), and inhaled nitric oxide (iNO) are used as adjunctive treatments.[140–142]

Gentle Ventilation and Permissive Hypercapnia

One important recent advance in management of infants with CDH began with the report by Wung et al. describing "gentle ventilation" for respiratory failure and PPHN.[143] The infant is intubated but allowed to breath spontaneously and hypercapnia is tolerated (permissive hypercapnia). Crucially, high

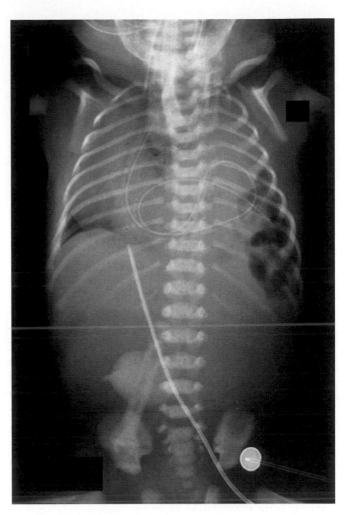

FIG. 39.6. Radiograph of a newborn with a left-sided CDH showing herniation of bowel into the thoracic cavity and mediastinal shift away from the lesion

ventilator pressures are avoided with the aim of minimizing iatrogenic/ventilator-induced lung injury.[112] Although individual centers have differing ventilation protocols, typical settings are shown in Table 39.1.[112,144] This ventilatory strategy was not universally embraced at first but when others began to employ the technique survival rates for CDH improved considerably. Permissive hypercarbia is associated with fewer complications notably a reduced incidence of pneumothorax. Survival in infants treated by gentle ventilation reaches 76% and if infants with lethal associated anomalies are excluded, survival approaches 100% in some centers.[142]

High-Frequency Oscillating Ventilation

High-frequency oscillating ventilation (HFOV) is a method of ventilation that aims to reduce the barotra-uma associated with high airway pressures. The rate of ventilation is very high with a mean airway pressure of 18–20 cmH$_2$O. Gas exchange takes place through diffusion rather than bulk gas flow. The chief benefit

TABLE 39.1. "Gentle" ventilation strategy in CDH.[144]

PIP (peak inspiratory pressure)	20–25 cmH$_2$O
PEEP (positive end expiratory pressure)	5 cmH$_2$O
Preductal O$_2$ saturation	>90%
PaCO$_2$ (arterial partial pressure of CO$_2$)	<60 mmHg

of HFOV is recruitment of lung with minimal barotrauma. The advantages of HFOV have been reported in many centers caring for infants with CDH.[134,145–147]

Inhaled Nitric Oxide

Native NO is produced by the vascular endothelium and acts as a vasorelaxant. Inhaled NO (iNO) is an established therapy for PPHN. Inhaled NO has been shown to lower pulmonary artery pressure in infants with CDH although the effect is transient.[54] This transient physiological benefit does not, unfortunately, translate into improved clinical outcome.[112] Indeed, a Cochrane Database Systematic Review also found that iNO therapy does not benefit infants with CDH and may increase requirement for ECMO.[52] However, many units continue to use this therapy although the effect of treatment should be monitored using echocardiography.[54]

Extracorporeal Membrane Oxygenation (ECMO)

Extracorporeal membrane oxygenation (ECMO) is a treatment for potentially reversible hypoxemic respiratory failure. It is identical to cardiopulmonary bypass but rather than being used for the duration of an operation it may be used for days or weeks to support cardiac and pulmonary function.[148] ECMO has been used for selected CDH infants since the late 1980s.[149] Initially it was used as rescue therapy postsurgical repair of CDH but it is now also employed during the preoperative stabilization phase.[150] ECMO is associated with a significant morbidity, so the eligibility criteria for ECMO therapy are strict.

The evidence surrounding the use of ECMO in infants with CDH is conflicting. In their parallel publications, the "tale of two cities," Azarow et al. and Wilson et al. reported equivalent survival either with and without ECMO.[140,145] A Cochrane Database of Systematic Reviews report found only a short-term benefit with ECMO, and the overall effect of ECMO use in CDH was unclear.[151] Indeed, many long-term survivors have significant disability.[152]

Liquid Ventilation

Liquid ventilation was first investigated in the 1950s for use by astronauts. The technique has evolved considerably since that time and now utilizes perfluorocarbons, which are inert liquids capable of carrying considerable amounts of O$_2$ and CO$_2$. The perfluorocarbon liquid fills and ventilates the lung.

Barotrauma is minimized and liquid ventilation promotes lung growth through mechanical stretching.[153] Experimental animal studies and initial human studies have confirmed that the technique is feasible but trials in a range of children with respiratory failure are currently halted due to an excess mortality in the liquid ventilation group.[154,155]

Surgery

The necessity for surgical repair of the diaphragmatic defect to reduce the intestines from the thoracic cavity and repair the diaphragmatic defect is undisputed. However, the timing of surgery remains a question for debate. Current practice favors delayed over immediate surgery.[156] However, a recent Cochrane Database Systematic Review concluded that there is no clear evidence to favor delayed over immediate repair although an advantage could not be ruled out.[157] Most centers continue to allow a period of stabilization prior to surgery.[112,142,157] Surgery is scheduled when the newborn has stabilized. Criteria vary between centers – surgery may be undertaken within days or 1–2 weeks following birth. Ideally operative repair should take place during normal working hours as a semielective case.

Repair of the diaphragmatic hernia is usually performed through the abdomen through a subcostal or transverse muscle cutting incision on the side of the diaphragmatic defect. The abdominal viscera are gently returned to the abdomen and the defect visualized (Fig. 39.7). Where a hernial sac is found this is excised. Following mobilization of the posterior rim of the diaphragmatic defect primary repair will be possible in the majority of infants using interrupted nonabsorbable sutures. Care should be taken to ensure that significant chest wall deformity is not created by aggressive attempts to close the defect primarily. Where there is inadequate native diaphragm the defect can be closed with a patch of prosthetic material or native tissue. Most surgeons use a prosthetic sheet such as Gore-tex (W.L. Gore & Associates, USA) or a bioprosthetic material such as Surgisis Gold (Cooke Surgical, USA), although some prefer to rotate native tissue such as the latissimus dorsi or abdominal wall muscles.[158–160] Once the viscera are returned to the abdomen it is sometimes difficult to close the abdominal wound without causing an abdominal compartment syndrome. In such cases, the abdominal wall may also be closed with a prosthetic patch. A chest drain is best avoided to prevent overdistension of the ipsilateral lung and pneumothorax.[144,161]

Alternatives to the traditional surgical technique described earlier include laparoscopic and thoracoscopic repair of the diaphragmatic hernia.[162–164] Most reported series are based around late presenting CDH in adults and older children although a number of them include infants of less than 1 week of age.[162,164] Although there is still some question over the best approach to CDH repair, Yang et al. have, using strict selection criteria, undertaken successful thoracoscopic repair in a series of newborns.[164]

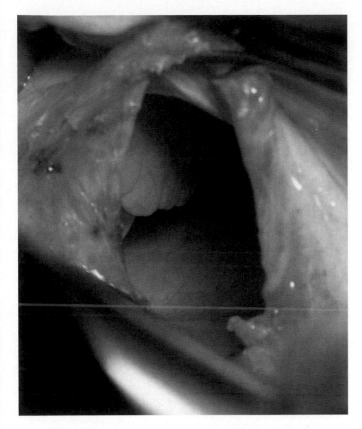

Fig. 39.7. Operative photograph showing margins of the diaphragmatic defect and the underlying lung

Complications related directly to repair of the diaphragmatic hernia include recurrent herniation, small bowel obstruction, pleural effusion, chylothorax, and patch-associated problems such as infection. Chest wall deformity may also be seen in the long term. Recurrence of CDH is seen in up to 7% of children who have undergone a primary repair, occurring most commonly in the first year of life.[165,166] Recurrent herniation (44–46%) and small bowel obstruction (7%) both occur more frequently in the first year of life following patch repair. Recurrence of CDH in patch repairs is likely to relate to the inability of the patch to expand with the children as they grow. Pleural effusions are more common following patch repair and may require drainage. Chylous effusions have been treated successfully with octreotide.[167,168]

Postnatal Prognosis

A number of prognostic factors have been identified for infants with CDH after birth. Birth weight, Apgar score, best postductal partial pressure of oxygen (pO_2), age at presentation, side of the hernia, and the need for and duration of extracorporeal membrane oxygenation (ECMO) have all been associated with prognosis.[140,169,170] Unfortunately none is universally accepted.[134] An alternate predictor is pulmonary to systemic artery pressure ratio, by serial echocardiograms.[54]

Overall Survival

Survival rates for babies with CDH vary considerably from 50 to 80%.[26–28,114,115] There are a number of explanations for the variation in survival. These include the following:

(1) Patient population
(2) True differences in pathology severity, e.g., CDH associated with another lethal malformation
(3) Other CDH-specific factors, e.g., bilateral herniae
(4) Postnatal management

Case selection bias is crucial. The sickest infants may never reach a tertiary pediatric surgery center and, thus, may not be included in outcome figures. A substantial fetal and early neonatal loss rate is well recognized for CDH and the diagnosis is not made for many, if not the majority, of these cases. Reports citing impressive survival figures must always be viewed with scepticism about ascertainment bias, even though this is rarely mentioned.

The presence of another major anomaly or chromosomal defect reduces the survival chances for newborns with CDH significantly.[105,171] In a recent population-based study, the overall survival was 47% rising to 63% for isolated CDH.[26] These authors reported a survival of only 19% in babies with major associated anomalies. Cardiac anomalies account for the bulk of the increased mortality.

The pathophysiology of CDH also affects outcome. Postnatal mortality is, by and large, the result of respiratory failure due to a combination of pulmonary hypoplasia and pulmonary hypertension.[53] The degree of pulmonary hypoplasia is variable with some infants succumbing very soon after birth while others have apparently normal lungs.[172] The position of the fetal liver has also been related to survival although its predictive value is not universally accepted.[118] Two recent publications suggest that liver position alone is the best prognostic indicator for isolated left-sided CDH.[117,173] Herniation of the liver into the thoracic cavity on antenatal USS ("liver up") is associated with greater postnatal mortality than when the liver is confined to the abdomen ("liver down"). Historically the side of the hernia was thought to predict outcome, with right-sided hernias carrying a worse prognosis than left.[27] However, emerging data show no difference in survival although newborns with bilateral herniae do have greater mortality.[26,28,140]

The fourth factor that may influence survival rates in CDH is postnatal care. The Canadian Neonatal Research Network recently reported better than expected outcome in centers caring for greater numbers of infants with CDH.[174] A recent systematic review included reports from centers treating >20 infants/year and with survival of >75% in isolated CDH in order to seek a benchmark of care.[109] The overall survival in the combined studies was 79% (range 69–93%) with survival of 85% (78–96%) in isolated CDH. Management strategies based on gentle ventilation were cited consistently.

Improved postnatal survival correlates with the termination rate following antenatal diagnosis.[28] The effect of termination is to "replace" some of the neonatal deaths with aborted fetuses. Case selection bias of this type has a profound effect on survival.[26,28,115]

Long-Term Sequelae

A large number of babies with CDH survive with apparently normal lung function although up to 25% will have some CDH-related symptoms in later life.[175,176] This subset of children mostly suffer from respiratory and gastrointestinal symptoms with a proportion also having neurodevelopmental sequelae including hearing loss.[175,177–179] Gastrointestinal morbidity is largely due to gastroesophageal reflux although there is a small incidence of adhesional obstruction.[180] Failure to thrive may require nutritional support via a gastrostomy in up to one-third of patients with up to 20% requiring fundoplication for intractable reflux.[178,181,182] Other long-term problems in CDH patients include spine and chest wall deformities including pectus excavatum and scoliosis.[175,181]

Respiratory symptoms are related to primary lung hypoplasia, the sequelae of neonatal ventilation, and the effects of gastroesophageal reflux. A proportion of children develop chronic lung disease, similar to that seen in premature infants, and require prolonged oxygen therapy.[180] Even some seemingly well children are found to have reduced inspiratory muscle strength and a degree of small airways obstruction.[181] A recent report documenting postnatal lung growth, measured by serial ventilation–perfusion (V/Q) scintigraphy, showed persisting abnormalities, especially in children with a patch repair.[183] Whether the need for a patch is a marker of worse lung hypoplasia or the patch impairs stretch-induced lung growth is unknown. Lastly, a small subset of patients have residual chronic pulmonary hypertension requiring long-term pulmonary vasodilator therapy.[184] The implications of increased survival rates in babies with severe CDH for long-term lung function remain to be seen.[175,181,185]

Future Directions

Work continues in many areas related to CDH care and research. At the time of writing these include the following:

- Accurate case selection of the "high risk" fetus for tracheal occlusion (FETO)
- Improving survival raises debate on centralizing CDH care to high-volume centers
- Pharmacological therapies – can we find better selective treatment of pulmonary hypertension (e.g., PDE5 inhibitors – Sildenafil)
- Novel agents to stimulate lung growth prenatally (e.g., growth factors)
- International registries to define "best practice" and link the contributions of the CDH study group and its parent organization CHERUBS.

References

1. Enns GM, Cox VA, Goldstein RB, et al. Congenital diaphragmatic defects and associated syndromes, malformations, and chromosome anomalies: a retrospective study of 60 patients and literature review. Am J Med Genet 1998; 79: 215–25.
2. Slavotinek AM. The genetics of congenital diaphragmatic hernia. Semin Perinatol 2005; 29: 77–85.
3. Bochdalek VA. Einige Betrachtungen uber die entstehung des angeborenen zwench fellbrunches als bietrag zur patholoischen anatomie der ilernien. Viertefjahrschrift fur die praktische. Heilkunde 1848; 19: 89–97.
4. Irish MS, Holm BA, Glick PL. Congenital diaphragmatic hernia. A historical review. Clin Perinatol 1996; 23: 625–53.
5. Chinoy MR. Pulmonary hypoplasia and congenital diaphragmatic hernia: advances in the pathogenetics and regulation of lung development. J Surg Res 2002; 106: 209–23.
6. Hedblom CA. Diaphragmatic hernia: a study of three hundred and seventy-eight cases in which operation was performed. JAMA 1925; 85: 947–53.
7. Rickham PP. Some congenital malformations necessitating emergency operations in the newborn period. Br Med J 1971; 4: 286–90.
8. Ladd WE, Gross RE. Congenital diaphragmatic hernia. N Engl J Med 1940; 223: 917–23.
9. Potter EL. Pathology of the Fetus and of the Newborn, 1st Edition. Chicago: Year Book Publishers, 1952.
10. Campanale RP, Rowland RH. Hypoplasia of the lung associated with congenital diaphragmatic hernia. Ann Surg 1955; 142: 176–89.
11. Muratore CS, Wilson JM. Congenital diaphragmatic hernia: where are we and where do we go from here? Semin Perinatol 2000; 24: 418–28.
12. Sadler TW. Langman's Medical Embryology, 8th Edition. Philadelphia, PA: Lippincott Williams & Wilkins, 2000.
13. Hislop AA. Airway and blood vessel interaction during lung development. J Anat 2002; 201: 325–34.
14. Schachtner SK, Wang Y, Scott BH. Qualitative and quantitative analysis of embryonic pulmonary vessel formation. Am J Respir Cell Mol Biol 2000; 22: 157–65.
15. Hall SM, Hislop AA, Pierce CM, Haworth SG. Prenatal origins of human intrapulmonary arteries: formation and smooth muscle maturation. Am J Respir Cell Mol Biol 2000; 23: 194–203.
16. Hislop AA, Pierce CM. Growth of the vascular tree. Paediatr Respir Rev 2000; 1: 321–7.
17. Chinoy MR, Miller SA. Relevance of tenascin-C and matrix metalloproteinases in vascular abnormalities in murine hypoplastic lungs. Biol Neonate 2006; 90: 185–96.
18. Risau W, Lemmon V. Changes in the vascular extracellular matrix during embryonic vasculogenesis and angiogenesis. Dev Biol 1988; 125: 441–50.
19. Hanahan D. Signalling vascular morphogenesis and maintenance. Science 1997; 277: 48–50.
20. Stenmark KR, Mecham RP. Cellular and molecular mechanisms of pulmonary vascular remodeling. Annu Rev Physiol 1997; 59: 89–144.
21. Shifren JL, Doldi N, Ferrara N, et al. In the human fetus, vascular endothelial growth factor is expressed in epithelial cells and myocytes, but not vascular endothelium: implications for mode of action. J Clin Endocrinol Metab 1994; 79: 316–22.

22. Lakshminrusimha S, Steinhorn RH. Pulmonary vascular biology during neonatal transition. Clin Perinatol 1999; 26: 601–19.

23. Narayan H, De Chazal R, Barrow M, et al. Familial congenital diaphragmatic hernia: prenatal diagnosis, management, and outcome. Prenat Diagn 1993; 13: 893–901.

24. Tonks A, Wyldes M, Somerset DA, et al. Congenital malformations of the diaphragm: findings of the West Midlands Congenital Anomaly Register 1995 to 2000. Prenat Diagn 2004; 24: 596–604.

25. Deprest J, Jani J, Van Schoubroeck D, et al. Current consequences of prenatal diagnosis of congenital diaphragmatic hernia. J Pediatr Surg 2006; 41: 423–30.

26. Gallot D, Boda C, Ughetto S, et al. Prenatal detection and outcome of congenital diaphragmatic hernia: a French registry-based study. Ultrasound Obstet Gynecol 2007; 29: 276–83.

27. Skari H, Bjornland K, Haugen G, et al. Congenital diaphragmatic hernia: a meta-analysis of mortality factors. J Pediatr Surg 2000; 35: 1187–97.

28. Stege G, Fenton A, Jaffray B. Nihilism in the 1990s: the true mortality of congenital diaphragmatic hernia. Pediatrics 2003; 112: 532–5.

29. Skarsgard ED, Harrison MR. Congenital diaphragmatic hernia: the surgeon's perspective. Pediatr Rev 1999; 20: e71–e78.

30. Areechon W, Reid L. Hypoplasia of lung with congenital diaphragmatic hernia. Br Med J 1963; 1: 230–3.

31. Kitagawa M, Hislop A, Boyden EA, et al. Lung hypoplasia in congenital diaphragmatic hernia. A quantitative study of airway, artery, and alveolar development. Br J Surg 1971; 58: 342–6.

32. Geggel RL, Murphy JD, Langleben D, et al. Congenital diaphragmatic hernia: arterial structural changes and persistent pulmonary hypertension after surgical repair. J Pediatr 1985; 107: 457–64.

33. Iritani I. Experimental study on embryogenesis of congenital diaphragmatic hernia. Anat Embryol 1984; 169: 133–9.

34. Jesudason EC, Connell MG, Fernig DG, et al. Early lung malformations in congenital diaphragmatic hernia. J Pediatr Surg 2000; 35: 124–7.

35. Grover TR, Parker TA, Balasubramaniam V, et al. Pulmonary hypertension impairs alveolarization and reduces lung growth in the ovine fetus. Am J Physiol Lung Cell Mol Physiol 2005; 288: L648–L654.

36. Levin DL. Morphologic analysis of the pulmonary vascular bed in congenital left-sided diaphragmatic hernia. J Pediatr 1978; 92: 805–9.

37. Tenbrinck R, Gaillard JL, Tibboel D, et al. Pulmonary vascular abnormalities in experimentally induced congenital diaphragmatic hernia in rats. J Pediatr Surg 1992; 27: 862–5.

38. Yamataka T, Puri P. Pulmonary artery structural changes in pulmonary hypertension complicating congenital diaphragmatic hernia. J Pediatr Surg 1997; 32: 387–90.

39. Taira Y, Yamataka T, Miyazaki E, Puri P. Adventitial changes in pulmonary vasculature in congenital diaphragmatic hernia complicated by pulmonary hypertension. J Pediatr Surg 1998; 33: 382–7.

40. Greer JJ, Cote D, Allan DW, et al. Structure of the primordial diaphragm and defects associated with nitrofen-induced CDH. J Appl Physiol 2000; 89: 2123–9.

41. Kluth D, Tenbrinck R, Vonekesparre M, et al. The natural history of congenital diaphragmatic hernia and pulmonary hypoplasia in the embryo. J Pediatr Surg 1993; 28: 456–63.

42. Allan DW, Greer JJ. Pathogenesis of nitrofen-induced congenital diaphragmatic hernia in fetal rats. J Appl Physiol 1997; 83: 338–47.

43. Clugston RD, Klattig J, Englert C, et al. Teratogen-induced, dietary and genetic models of congenital diaphragmatic hernia share a common mechanism of pathogenesis. Am J Pathol 2006; 169: 1541–9.

44. Fisher JC, Bodenstein L. Computer simulation analysis of normal and abnormal development of the mammalian diaphragm. Theor Biol Med Model 2006; 3: 9.

45. Jesudason EC. Small lungs and suspect smooth muscle: congenital diaphragmatic hernia and the smooth muscle hypothesis. J Pediatr Surg 2006; 41: 431–5.

46. Min H, Danilenko DM, Scully SA, et al. Fgf-10 is required for both limb and lung development and exhibits striking functional similarity to Drosophila branchless. Genes Dev 1998; 12: 3156–61.

47. Starrett RW, de Lorimier AA. Congenital diaphragmatic hernia in lambs: hemodynamic and ventilatory changes with breathing. J Pediatr Surg 1975; 10: 575–82.

48. Keijzer R, Liu J, Deimling J, et al. Dual-hit hypothesis explains pulmonary hypoplasia in the nitrofen model of congenital diaphragmatic hernia. Am J Pathol 2000; 156: 1299–306.

49. Mohseni-Bod H, Bohn D. Pulmonary hypertension in congenital diaphragmatic hernia. Semin Pediatr Surg 2007; 16: 126–33.

50. Perreault T. Persistent pulmonary hypertension of the newborn. Paediatr Respir Rev 2006; 7S: S175–S176.

51. Dakshinamurti S. Pathophysiologic mechanisms of persistent pulmonary hypertension of the newborn. Pediatr Pulmonol 2005; 39: 492–503.

52. Finer NN, Barrington KJ. Nitric oxide for respiratory failure in infants born at or near term. Cochrane Database Syst Rev 2006; CD000399.

53. Iocono JA, Cilley RE, Mauger DT, et al. Postnatal pulmonary hypertension after repair of congenital diaphragmatic hernia: predicting risk and outcome. J Pediatr Surg 1999; 34: 349–53.

54. Dillon PW, Cilley RE, Mauger D, et al. The relationship of pulmonary artery pressure and survival in congenital diaphragmatic hernia. J Pediatr Surg 2004; 39: 307–12.

55. Keller RL, Moore P, Teitel D, et al. Abnormal vascular tone in infants and children with lung hypoplasia: findings from cardiac catheterization and the response to chronic therapy. Pediatr Crit Care Med 2006; 7: 589–94.

56. Kantarci S, Donahoe PK. Congenital diaphragmatic hernia (CDH) etiology as revealed by pathway genetics. Am J Med Genet C Semin Med Genet 2007; 145: 217–26.

57. Scott DA. Genetics of congenital diaphragmatic hernia. Semin Pediatr Surg 2007; 16: 88–93.

58. Norio R, Kaariainen H, Rapola J, et al. Familial congenital diaphragmatic defects: aspects of etiology, prenatal diagnosis, and treatment. Am J Med Genet 1984; 17: 471–83.

59. Slavotinek AM. Fryns syndrome: a review of the phenotype and diagnostic guidelines. Am J Med Genet A 2004; 124: 427–33.

60. Klaassens M, van Dooren M, Eussen HJ, et al. Congenital diaphragmatic hernia and chromosome 15q26: determination of a candidate region by use of fluorescent in situ hybridization and array-based comparative genomic hybridization. Am J Hum Genet 2005; 76: 877–82.

61. Devriendt K, Deloof E, Moerman P, et al. Diaphragmatic hernia in Denys-Drash syndrome. Am J Med Genet 1995; 57: 97–101.

62. Suri M, Kelehan P, O'Neill D, et al. WT1 mutations in Meacham syndrome suggest a coelomic mesothelial origin of the cardiac and diaphragmatic malformations. Am J Med Genet A 2007; 143: 2312–20.

63. Scott DA, Cooper ML, Stankiewicz P, et al. Congenital diaphragmatic hernia in WAGR syndrome. Am J Med Genet A 2005; 134: 430–3.

64. Kreidberg JA, Sariola H, Loring JM, et al. WT-1 is required for early kidney development. Cell 1993; 74: 679–91.

65. Connell MG, Corbett HJ, Purvis A, et al. Sex and congenital diaphragmatic hernia. Pediatr Surg Int 2006; 22: 95–8.

66. Hösgor M, Tibboel D. Congenital diaphragmatic hernia; many questions, few answers. Paediatr Respir Rev 2004; 5 (Suppl A): S277–S282.

67. Kluth D, Kangah R, Reich P, et al. Nitrofen-induced diaphragmatic hernias in rats: an animal model. J Pediatr Surg 1990; 25: 850–4.

68. Losty PD, Suen HC, Manganaro TF, et al. Prenatal hormonal therapy improves pulmonary compliance in the nitrofen-induced CDH rat model. J Pediatr Surg 1995; 30: 420–6.

69. Okoye BO, Losty PD, Lloyd DA, Gosney JR. Effect of prenatal glucocorticoids on pulmonary vascular muscularisation in nitrofen-induced congenital diaphragmatic hernia. J Pediatr Surg 1998; 33: 76–80.

70. Mey J, Babiuk RP, Clugston R, et al. Retinal dehydrogenase-2 is inhibited by compounds that induce congenital diaphragmatic hernias in rodents. Am J Pathol 2003; 162: 673–9.

71. Fujino H, Nakagawa M, Nishijima S, et al. Morphological differences in cardiovascular anomalies induced by bis-diamine between Sprague-Dawley and Wistar rats. Congenit Anom (Kyoto) 2005; 45: 52–8.

72. Tenbrinck R, Tibboel D, Gaillard JLJ, et al. Experimentally induced congenital diaphragmatic-hernia in rats. J Pediatr Surg 1990; 25: 426–9.

73. Losty PD, Connell MG, Freese R, et al. Cardiovascular malformations in experimental congenital diaphragmatic hernia. J Pediatr Surg 1999; 34: 1203–7.

74. Kim WG, Suh JW, Chi JG. Nitrofen-induced congenital malformations of the heart and great vessels in rats: an animal model. J Pediatr Surg 1999; 34: 1782–6.

75. Baoquan Q, Diez-Pardo JA, Tovar JA. Intestinal rotation in experimental congenital diaphragmatic hernia. J Pediatr Surg 1995; 30: 1457–62.

76. Migliazza L, Otten C, Xia H, et al. Cardiovascular malformations in congenital diaphragmatic hernia: human and experimental studies. J Pediatr Surg 1999; 34: 1352–8.

77. Migliazza L, Xia H, Diez-Pardo JA, Tovar JA. Skeletal malformations associated with congenital diaphragmatic hernia: experimental and human studies. J Pediatr.Surg 1999; 34: 1624–9.

78. Kanai M, Kitano Y, von Allmen D, et al. Fetal tracheal occlusion in the rat model of nitrofen-induced congenital diaphragmatic hernia: tracheal occlusion reverses the arterial structural abnormality. J Pediatr Surg 2001; 36: 839–45.

79. Andersen DH. Incidence of congenital diaphragmatic hernia in the young of rats bred on a diet deficient in vitamin A. Am J Dis Child 1941; 62: 888–889.

80. Lammer EJ, Chen DT, Hoar RM, et al. Retinoic acid embryopathy. N Engl J Med 1985; 313: 837–41.

81. Major D, Cadenas M, Fournier L, et al. Retinol status of newborn infants with congenital diaphragmatic hernia. Pediatr Surg Int 1998; 13: 547–9.

82. Greer JJ, Babiuk RP, Thebaud B. Etiology of congenital diaphragmatic hernia: the retinoid hypothesis. Pediatr Res 2003; 53: 726–30.

83. Wilson JG, Roth CB, Warkarny J. An analysis of the syndrome of malformations induced by maternal vitamin A deficiency. Effects of restoration of vitamin A at various times during gestation. Am J Anat 1953; 92: 189–217.

84. Babiuk RP, Thebaud B, Greer JJ. Reductions in the incidence of nitrofen-induced diaphragmatic hernia by vitamin A and retinoic acid. Am J Physiol Lung Cell Mol Physiol 2004; 286: L970–L973.

85. Mendelsohn C, Lohnes D, Decimo D, et al. Function of the retinoic acid receptors (RARs) during development (II). Multiple abnormalities at various stages of organogenesis in RAR double mutants. Development 1994; 120: 2749–71.

86. Chen MH, MacGowan A, Ward S, et al. The activation of the retinoic acid response element is inhibited in an animal model of congenital diaphragmatic hernia. Biol Neonate 2003; 83: 157–61.

87. Gallot D, Marceau G, Coste K, et al. Congenital diaphragmatic hernia: a retinoid-signaling pathway disruption during lung development? Birth Defects Res A Clin Mol Teratol 2005; 73: 523–31.

88. Desai TJ, Malpel S, Flentke GR, et al. Retinoic acid selectively regulates Fgf10 expression and maintains cell identity in the prospective lung field of the developing foregut. Dev Biol 2004; 273: 402–15.

89. Ackerman KG, Herron BJ, Vargas SO, et al. Fog2 is required for normal diaphragm and lung development in mice and humans. PloS Genet 2005; 1: 58–65.

90. Liu J, Zhang L, Wang D, et al. Congenital diaphragmatic hernia, kidney agenesis and cardiac defects associated with Slit3-deficiency in mice. Mech Dev 2003; 120: 1059–70.

91. Jay PY, Bielinska M, Erlich JM, et al. Impaired mesenchymal cell function in Gata4 mutant mice leads to diaphragmatic hernias and primary lung defects. Dev Biol 2007; 301: 602–14.

92. Lu JR, Bassel-Duby R, Hawkins A, et al. Control of facial muscle development by MyoR and capsulin. Science 2002; 298: 2378–81.

93. You LR, Takamoto N, Yu CT, et al. Mouse lacking COUP-TFII as an animal model of Bochdalek-type congenital diaphragmatic hernia. Proc Natl Acad Sci USA 2005; 102: 16351–6.

94. de Lorimer A, Tierney D, Parker H. Hypoplastic lungs in fetal lambs with surgically produced congenital diaphragmatic hernia. Surgery 1967; 62: 12–17.

95. Ohi R, Suzuki H, Kato T, Kasai M. Development of the lung in fetal rabbits with experimental diaphragmatic hernia. J Pediatr Surg 1976; 11: 955–9.

96. Harrison MR, Jester JA, Ross NA. Correction of congenital diaphragmatic hernia in utero. I. The model: intrathoracic balloon produces fatal pulmonary hypoplasia. Surgery 1980; 88: 174–82.

97. Harrison MR, Bressack MA, Churg AM, de Lorimier AA. Correction of congenital diaphragmatic hernia in utero. II. Simulated correction permits fetal lung growth with survival at birth. Surgery 1980; 88: 260–8.

98. Bratu I, Flageole H, Laberge JM, et al. Pulmonary structural maturation and pulmonary artery remodeling after reversible fetal ovine tracheal occlusion in diaphragmatic hernia. J Pediatr Surg 2001; 36: 739–44.

99. Lipsett J, Cool JC, Runciman SI, et al. Effect of antenatal tracheal occlusion on lung development in the sheep model of congenital diaphragmatic hernia: a morphometric analysis of pulmonary structure and maturity. Pediatr Pulmonol 1998; 25: 257–69.

100. Bealer JF, Skarsgard ED, Hedrick MH, et al. The 'PLUG' odyssey: adventures in experimental fetal tracheal occlusion. J Pediatr Surg 1995; 30: 361–4.

101. Roubliova XI, Verbeken EK, Wu J, et al. Effect of tracheal occlusion on peripheric pulmonary vessel muscularization in a fetal rabbit model for congenital diaphragmatic hernia. Am J Obstet Gynecol 2004; 191: 830–6.

102. Sweed Y, Puri P. Congenital diaphragmatic hernia: influence of associated malformations on survival. Arch Dis Child 1993; 69: 68–70.

103. Colvin J, Bower C, Dickinson JE, Sokol J. Outcomes of congenital diaphragmatic hernia: a population-based study in Western Australia. Pediatrics 2005; 116: e356–e363.

104. Harmath A, Hajdu J, Csaba A, et al. Associated malformations in congenital diaphragmatic hernia cases in the last 15 years in a tertiary referral institute. Am J Med Genet A 2006; 140: 2298–304.

105. Fauza DO, Wilson JM. Congenital diaphragmatic hernia and associated anomalies: their incidence, identification, and impact on prognosis. J Pediatr Surg 1994; 29: 1113–17.

106. Graziano JN. Cardiac anomalies in patients with congenital diaphragmatic hernia and their prognosis: a report from the Congenital Diaphragmatic Hernia Study Group. J Pediatr Surg 2005; 40: 1045–9.

107. Losty PD, Vanamo K, Rintala RJ, et al. Congenital diaphragmatic hernia – does the side of the defect influence the incidence of associated malformations? J Pediatr Surg 1998; 33: 507–10.

108. Slavotinek AM, Warmerdam B, Lin AE, Shaw GM. Population-based analysis of left- and right-sided diaphragmatic hernias demonstrates different frequencies of selected additional anomalies. Am J Med Genet A 2007; 143: 3127–36.

109. Logan JW, Cotten CM, Goldberg RN, Clark RH. Mechanical ventilation strategies in the management of congenital diaphragmatic hernia. Semin Pediatr Surg 2007; 16: 115–25.

110. Kitano Y. Prenatal intervention for congenital diaphragmatic hernia. Semin Pediatr Surg 2007; 16: 101–8.

111. Cohen MS, Rychik J, Bush DM, et al. Influence of congenital heart disease on survival in children with congenital diaphragmatic hernia. J Pediatr 2002; 141: 25–30.

112. Logan JW, Rice HE, Goldberg RN, Cotten CM. Congenital diaphragmatic hernia: a systematic review and summary of best-evidence practice strategies. J Perinatol 2007; 27: 535–49.

113. Laudy JA, Van Gucht M, Van Dooren MF, et al. Congenital diaphragmatic hernia: an evaluation of the prognostic value of the lung-to-head ratio and other prenatal parameters. Prenat Diagn 2003; 23: 634–9.

114. Bedoyan JK, Blackwell SC, Treadwell MC, et al. Congenital diaphragmatic hernia: associated anomalies and antenatal diagnosis. Outcome-related variables at two Detroit hospitals. Pediatr Surg Int 2004; 20: 170–6.

115. Deprest J, Jani J, Cannie M, et al. Prenatal intervention for isolated congenital diaphragmatic hernia. Curr Opin Obstet Gynecol 2006; 18: 355–67.

116. Heling KS, Wauer RR, Hammer H, et al. Reliability of the lung-to-head ratio in predicting outcome and neonatal ventilation parameters in fetuses with congenital diaphragmatic hernia. Ultrasound Obstet Gynecol 2005; 25: 112–18.

117. Jani J, Keller RL, Benachi A, et al. Prenatal prediction of survival in isolated left-sided diaphragmatic hernia. Ultrasound Obstet Gynecol 2006; 27: 18–22.

118. Arkovitz MS, Russo M, Devine P, et al. Fetal lung-head ratio is not related to outcome for antenatal diagnosed congenital diaphragmatic hernia. J Pediatr Surg 2007; 42: 107–10.

119. Ba'ath ME, Jesudason EC, Losty PD. How useful is the lung-to-head ratio in predicting outcome in the fetus with congenital diaphragmatic hernia? A systematic review and meta-analysis. Ultrasound Obstet Gynecol 2007; 30: 897–906.

120. Cannie M, Jani JC, De Keyzer F, et al. Fetal body volume: use at MR imaging to quantify relative lung volume in fetuses suspected of having pulmonary hypoplasia. Radiology 2006; 241: 847–53.

121. Harrison MR, Adzick NS, Bullard KM, et al. Correction of congenital diaphragmatic hernia in utero VII: a prospective trial. J Pediatr Surg 1997; 32: 1637–42.

122. Silver MM, Thurston WA, Patrick JE. Perinatal pulmonary hyperplasia due to laryngeal atresia. Hum Pathol 1988; 19: 110–13.

123. Hedrick MH, Estes JM, Sullivan KM, et al. Plug the lung until it grows (PLUG): a new method to treat congenital diaphragmatic hernia in utero. J Pediatr Surg 1994; 29: 612–17.

124. Sylvester KG, Rasanen J, Kitano Y, et al. Tracheal occlusion reverses the high impedance to flow in the fetal pulmonary circulation and normalizes its physiological response to oxygen at full term. J Pediatr Surg 1998; 33: 1071–4.

125. Luks FI, Wild YK, Piasecki GJ, De Paepe ME. Short-term tracheal occlusion corrects pulmonary vascular anomalies in the fetal lamb with diaphragmatic hernia. Surgery 2000; 128: 266–72.

126. Flake AW, Crombleholme TM, Johnson MP, et al. Treatment of severe congenital diaphragmatic hernia by fetal tracheal occlusion: clinical experience with fifteen cases. Am J Obstet Gynecol 2000; 183: 1059–66.

127. Jani J, Gratacos E, Greenough A, et al. Percutaneous fetal endoscopic tracheal occlusion (FETO) for severe left-sided congenital diaphragmatic hernia. Clin Obstet Gynecol 2005; 48: 910–22.

128. Harrison MR, Keller RL, Hawgood SB, et al. A randomized trial of fetal endoscopic tracheal occlusion for severe fetal congenital diaphragmatic hernia. N Engl J Med 2003; 349: 1916–24.

129. Roberts D, Dalziel S. Antenatal corticosteroids for accelerating fetal lung maturation for women at risk of preterm birth. Cochrane Database Syst Rev 2006; 3: CD004454.

130. Losty PD, Pacheco BA, Manganaro TF, et al. Prenatal hormonal therapy improves pulmonary morphology in rats with congenital diaphragmatic hernia. J Surg Res 1996; 65: 42–52.

131. Schnitzer JJ, Hedrick HL, Pacheco BA, et al. Prenatal glucocorticoid therapy reverses pulmonary immaturity in congenital diaphragmatic hernia in fetal sheep. Ann Surg 1996; 224: 430–7.

132. Hedrick HL, Kaban JM, Pacheco BA, et al. Prenatal glucocorticoids improve pulmonary morphometrics in fetal sheep with congenital diaphragmatic hernia. J Pediatr Surg 1997; 32: 217–21.

133. Lally KP, Bagolan P, Hosie S, et al. Corticosteroids for fetuses with congenital diaphragmatic hernia: can we show benefit? J Pediatr Surg 2006; 41: 668–74.

134. Bagolan P, Casaccia G, Crescenzi F, et al. Impact of a current treatment protocol on outcome of high-risk congenital diaphragmatic hernia. J Pediatr Surg 2004; 39: 313–18.

135. Frenckner BP, Lally PA, Hintz SR, Lally KP. Prenatal diagnosis of congenital diaphragmatic hernia: how should the babies be delivered? J Pediatr Surg 2007; 42: 1533–8.

136. O'Toole SJ, Karamanoukian HL, Sharma A, et al. Surfactant rescue in the fetal lamb model of congenital diaphragmatic hernia. J Pediatr Surg 1996; 31: 1105–8.

137. Van Meurs K. Is surfactant therapy beneficial in the treatment of the term newborn infant with congenital diaphragmatic hernia? J Pediatr 2004; 145: 312–16.

138. Rudolph AM, Yuan S. Response of the pulmonary vasculature to hypoxia and H^+ ion concentration changes. J Clin Invest 1966; 45: 399–411.

139. Drummond WH, Gregory GA, Heymann MA, Phibbs RA. The independent effects of hyperventilation, tolazoline, and dopamine on infants with persistent pulmonary hypertension. J Pediatr 1981; 98: 603–11.

140. Wilson JM, Lund DP, Lillehei CW, Vacanti JP. Congenital diaphragmatic hernia – a tale of two cities: the Boston experience. J Pediatr Surg 1997; 32: 401–5.

141. Kays DW, Langham MR, Ledbetter DJ, Talbert JL. Detrimental effects of standard medical therapy in congenital diaphragmatic hernia. Ann Surg 1999; 230: 340–8.

142. Boloker J, Bateman DA, Wung JT, Stolar CJ. Congenital diaphragmatic hernia in 120 infants treated consecutively with permissive hypercapnea/spontaneous respiration/elective repair. J Pediatr Surg 2002; 37: 357–66.

143. Wung JT, James LS, Kilchevsky E, James E. Management of infants with severe respiratory failure and persistence of the fetal circulation, without hyperventilation. Pediatrics 1985; 76: 488–94.

144. Wung JT, Sahni R, Moffitt ST, et al. Congenital diaphragmatic hernia: survival treated with very delayed surgery, spontaneous respiration and no chest tube. J Pediatr Surg 1995; 30: 406–9.

145. Azarow K, Messineo A, Pearl R, et al. Congenital diaphragmatic hernia – a tale of two cities: the Toronto experience. J Pediatr Surg 1997; 32: 395–400.

146. Kinsella JP, Truog WE, Walsh WF, et al. Randomized, multicenter trial of inhaled nitric oxide and high-frequency oscillatory ventilation in severe, persistent pulmonary hypertension of the newborn. J Pediatr 1997; 131: 55–62.

147. Cacciari A, Ruggeri G, Mordenti M, et al. High-frequency oscillatory ventilation versus conventional mechanical ventilation in congenital diaphragmatic hernia. Eur J Pediatr Surg 2001; 11: 3–7.

148. Khan AM, Lally KP. The role of extracorporeal membrane oxygenation in the management of infants with congenital diaphragmatic hernia. Semin Perinatol 2005; 29: 118–22.

149. Wilson JM, Bower LK, Lund DP. Evolution of the technique of congenital diaphragmatic hernia repair on ECMO. J Pediatr Surg 1994; 29: 1109–12.

150. Kunisaki SM, Barnewolt CE, Estroff JA, et al. Ex utero intrapartum treatment with extracorporeal membrane oxygenation for severe congenital diaphragmatic hernia. J Pediatr Surg 2007; 42: 98–104.

151. Elbourne D, Field D, Mugford M. Extracorporeal membrane oxygenation for severe respiratory failure in newborn infants. Cochrane Database Syst Rev 2002; CD001340.

152. Davis PJ, Firmin RK, Manktelow B, et al. Long-term outcome following extracorporeal membrane oxygenation for congenital diaphragmatic hernia: the UK experience. J Pediatr 2004; 144: 309–15.

153. Hirschl RB. Current experience with liquid ventilation. Paediatr Respir Rev 2004; 5 (Suppl A): S339–S345.

154. Wilcox DT, Glick PL, Karamanoukian HL, et al. Partial liquid ventilation and nitric oxide in congenital diaphragmatic hernia. J Pediatr Surg 1997; 32: 1211–15.

155. Hirschl RB, Philip WF, Glick L, et al. A prospective, randomized pilot trial of perfluorocarbon-induced lung growth in newborns with congenital diaphragmatic hernia. J Pediatr Surg 2003; 38: 283–9.

156. Harting MT, Lally KP. Surgical management of neonates with congenital diaphragmatic hernia. Semin Pediatr Surg 2007; 16: 109–14.

157. Moyer V, Moya F, Tibboel R, et al. Late versus early surgical correction for congenital diaphragmatic hernia in newborn infants. Cochrane Database Syst Rev 2002; CD001695.

158. Bianchi A, Doig CM, Cohen SJ. The reverse latissimus dorsi flap for congenital diaphragmatic hernia repair. J Pediatr Surg 1983; 18: 560–3.

159. Scaife ER, Johnson DG, Meyers RL, et al. The split abdominal wall muscle flap – a simple, mesh-free approach to repair large diaphragmatic hernia. J Pediatr Surg 2003; 38: 1748–51.

160. Joshi SB, Sen S, Chacko J, et al. Abdominal muscle flap repair for large defects of the diaphragm. Pediatr Surg Int 2005; 21: 677–80.

161. Cloutier R, Allard V, Fournier L, et al. Estimation of lungs' hypoplasia on postoperative chest x-rays in congenital diaphragmatic hernia. J Pediatr Surg 1993; 28: 1086–9.

162. Becmeur F, Reinberg O, Dimitriu C, et al. Thoracoscopic repair of congenital diaphragmatic hernia in children. Semin Pediatr Surg 2007; 16: 238–44.

163. Schaarschmidt K, Strauss J, Kolberg-Schwerdt A, et al. Thoracoscopic repair of congenital diaphragmatic hernia by inflation-assisted bowel reduction, in a resuscitated neonate: a better access? Pediatr Surg Int 2005; 21: 806–8.

164. Yang EY, Allmendinger N, Johnson SM, et al. Neonatal thoracoscopic repair of congenital diaphragmatic hernia: selection criteria for successful outcome. J Pediatr Surg 2005; 40: 1369–75.

165. Hajer GF, vd Staak FH, de Haan AF, Festen C. Recurrent congenital diaphragmatic hernia; which factors are involved? Eur J Pediatr Surg 1998; 8: 329–33.

166. Grethel EJ, Cortes RA, Wagner AJ, et al. Prosthetic patches for congenital diaphragmatic hernia repair: surgisis vs Gore-Tex. J Pediatr Surg 2006; 41: 29–33.

167. Goyal A, Smith NP, Jesudason EC, et al. Octreotide for treatment of chylothorax after repair of congenital diaphragmatic hernia. J Pediatr Surg 2003; 38: E19–E20.

168. Casaccia G, Crescenzi F, Palamides S, et al. Pleural effusion requiring drainage in congenital diaphragmatic hernia: incidence, aetiology and treatment. Pediatr Surg Int 2006; 22: 585–8.

169. The Congenital Diaphragmatic Hernia Study Group. Estimating disease severity of congenital diaphragmatic hernia in the first 5 minutes of life. J Pediatr Surg 2001; 36: 141–5.

170. Rygl M, Pycha K, Stranak Z, et al. Congenital diaphragmatic hernia: onset of respiratory distress and size of the defect: analysis of the outcome in 104 neonates. Pediatr Surg Int 2007; 23: 27–31.

171. Witters I, Legius E, Moerman P, et al. Associated malformations and chromosomal anomalies in 42 cases of prenatally diagnosed diaphragmatic hernia. Am J Med Genet 2001; 103: 278–82.

172. Miniati D. Pulmonary vascular remodeling. Semin Pediatr Surg 2007; 16: 80–7.

173. Hedrick HL, Danzer E, Merchant A, et al. Liver position and lung-to-head ratio for prediction of extracorporeal membrane oxygenation and survival in isolated left congenital diaphragmatic hernia. Am J Obstet Gynecol 2007; 197: 422–4.

174. Javid PJ, Jaksic T, Skarsgard ED, Lee S. Survival rate in congenital diaphragmatic hernia: the experience of the Canadian Neonatal Network. J Pediatr Surg 2004; 39: 657–60.

175. Bagolan P, Morini F. Long-term follow up of infants with congenital diaphragmatic hernia. Semin Pediatr Surg 2007; 16: 134–44.

176. Koivusalo A, Pakarinen M, Vanamo K, et al. Health-related quality of life in adults after repair of congenital diaphragmatic defects – a questionnaire study. J Pediatr Surg 2005; 40: 1376–81.

177. Nobuhara KK, Lund DP, Mitchell J, et al. Long-term outlook for survivors of congenital diaphragmatic hernia. Clin Perinatol 1996; 23: 873–87.

178. Muratore CS, Utter S, Jaksic T, et al. Nutritional morbidity in survivors of congenital diaphragmatic hernia. J Pediatr Surg 2001; 36: 1171–6.

179. Muratore CS, Kharasch V, Lund DP, et al. Pulmonary morbidity in 100 survivors of congenital diaphragmatic hernia monitored in a multidisciplinary clinic. J Pediatr Surg 2001; 36: 133–40.

180. Jaillard SM, Pierrat V, Dubois A, et al. Outcome at 2 years of infants with congenital diaphragmatic hernia: a population-based study. Ann Thorac Surg 2003; 75: 250–6.

181. Trachsel D, Selvadurai H, Bohn D, et al. Long-term pulmonary morbidity in survivors of congenital diaphragmatic hernia. Pediatr Pulmonol 2005; 39: 433–9.

182. Su W, Berry M, Puligandla PS, et al. Predictors of gastro-esophageal reflux in neonates with congenital diaphragmatic hernia. J Pediatr Surg 2007; 42: 1639–43.

183. Hayward MJ, Kharasch V, Sheils C, et al. Predicting inadequate long-term lung development in children with congenital diaphragmatic hernia: an analysis of longitudinal changes in ventilation and perfusion. J Pediatr Surg 2007; 42: 112–16.

184. Keller RL, Hamrick SE, Kitterman JA, et al. Treatment of rebound and chronic pulmonary hypertension with oral sildenafil in an infant with congenital diaphragmatic hernia. Pediatr Crit Care Med 2004; 5: 184–7.

185. Downard CD, Jaksic T, Garza JJ, et al. Analysis of an improved survival rate for congenital diaphragmatic hernia. J Pediatr Surg 2003; 38: 729–32.

40
Diaphragmatic Eventration and Phrenic Palsy

David C.G. Crabbe

Introduction

The term eventration is used to describe an abnormal elevation of the diaphragm. This may be congenital or acquired and one cause for the latter is phrenic nerve palsy. The distinction between a congenital diaphragmatic hernia with a sac and a congenital eventration is often confused. Margins of normal diaphragm should be apparent in a diaphragmatic hernia with a sac whereas an eventration will have a uniform contour. Congenital eventration may present in the newborn period with respiratory symptoms or they may be detected coincidentally in later life. Phrenic nerve palsies will usually present with respiratory failure.

Historical Perspective

The term eventration was used first by Becklard in 1829 although Petit probably described the condition in 1790.[1] Bingham described plication of the diaphragm in 1954.[2]

Basic Science, Embryology, and Pathogenesis

The muscular part of the diaphragm functions most efficiently if stretched to an optimal length. This length correlates with the functional residual capacity of the lungs and, in this position, the diaphragm adopts the typical dome shape. If the diaphragm is paralyzed or the muscle component is deficient the diaphragm will bulge upward, or *eventrate*, into the thorax. This is usually associated with paradoxical movement – the normal hemidiaphragm descends during inspiration and the abnormal hemidiaphragm rises.[3] The respiratory consequences of a diaphragmatic eventration are more severe in infants than in older children and adults. The physiological basis for this involves three factors[4,5]:

1. The minimal contribution intercostal muscles make to ventilation in infancy.
2. The extreme mobility of the mediastinum in infancy.
3. The decrease in chest wall compliance with age.
4. Infants are habitually supine and their abdominal viscera press on the diaphragm from below.

These factors are cumulative and reduce the functional residual capacity (FRC) of the lungs to the critical closing volume at which point atelectasis occurs. The work of breathing then increases substantially, leading to a vicious cycle of fatigue and hypoxia.

The diaphragm is innervated by the phrenic nerves. The phrenic nerves arise chiefly from the fourth cervical nerve root, receiving branches from C3 and C5. The phrenic nerves descend to the root of the neck beneath the prevertebral fascia on the anterior surface of the scalenus anterior muscles. The fibers from C5 may arise separately from the superior trunk of the brachial plexus lateral to the anterior scalene as an accessory phrenic nerve, which joins the main phrenic nerve a variable distance into the thorax. The phrenic nerves usually enter the chest sandwiched between the subclavian vein and artery, medial to the internal mammary artery, although occasionally they may descend anterior to the subclavian vein or, rarely, penetrate the vein.[6] The nerves descend under the mediastinal pleura in front of the hila of the lungs to the diaphragms. At this point the nerves divide into two terminal branches, which enter the diaphragm, and then each branch subdivides into two rami, which innervate the muscle. The course of the terminal rami of the phrenic nerves over the diaphragms is fairly constant,[7] a matter of some relevance when planning incisions in the diaphragm (Fig. 40.1). The phrenic nerves are liable to injury at any point along their course.

Congenital eventration of the diaphragm affects the left side more commonly than the right.[8,9] The embryology of diaphragmatic eventration is incompletely understood but pulmonary hypoplasia is uncommon, in contradistinction to congenital diaphragmatic hernia. As a consequence the condition may go

D.H. Parikh et al. (eds.), *Pediatric Thoracic Surgery*,
DOI: 10.1007/b136543_40, © Springer-Verlag London Limited 2009

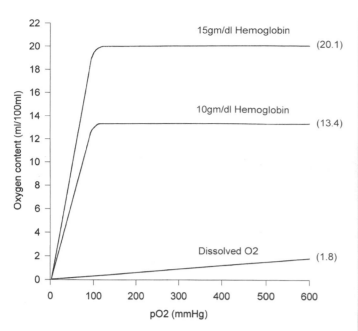

FIG. 41.2. Oxygen delivery graph

addition to respiratory support and is the method of choice for patients with isolated cardiac failure or combined cardiac and respiratory failure. The blood draining into the ECLS circuit is "true venous" blood and, if some cardiac output is maintained, the reduced proportion of deoxygenated blood not drained through the circuit continues to flow through the pulmonary circulation. Blood ejected from the left ventricle into the aortic arch will mix with the richly oxygenated blood from the ECLS circuit. In pulmonary hypertension, the pulmonary arterial pressures will markedly drop due to drainage of blood from the right atrium into the ECLS circuit. Excellent oxygenation is achieved with this modality. Potential disadvantages reflect the method of cannulation and the direct return of blood into the aorta and, in turn, the cerebral circulation. There are concerns, particularly in the neonate, about delivery of supersaturated blood to the cerebral circulation.[9] Additionally, any particulate matter or entrapped air from the circuit will be returned directly into the systemic circulation leading to the possibility of cerebral emboli.[10] Despite excellent tissue oxygenation, there is some evidence that blood returning from the ECMO circuit does not adequately perfuse the coronary arteries limiting myocardial perfusion to the relatively poorly saturated blood that is ejected from the left ventricle.[11,12] Most ECLS circuits in current use are nonpulsatile, and so, although circulatory support is offered, alterations in pulsatility are seen. A phenomenon peculiar to VA ECLS is the development of "cardiac stun," where myocardial contractility diminishes leading to a barely perceptible pulse pressure after the initiation of ECLS.[13] This may be due to the previously hypoxic myocardium being exposed to "hyperoxic" blood and it tends to be a transient phenomenon. The diagnosis must be confirmed with echocardiography as loss of pulse pressure may be due to cardiac tamponade or incorrect arterial cannula placement.

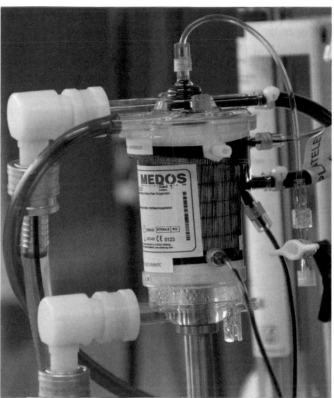

FIG. 41.3. The membrane oxygenator

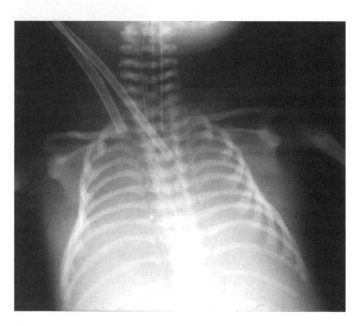

FIG. 41.4. Chest X-ray showing VA ECMO cannulae

Methods of Cannulation for VA ECLS

The commonest vessels for cannulation in VA ECLS are the RIJV and the RCCA. The patient is positioned over a shoulder roll to extend the neck and the head is turned to the left.

Paralysis and analgesia/sedation are recommended. An open cut down technique is usually employed where the vessels are exposed through either a transverse or oblique incision with sternocleidomastoid split with blunt dissection. When the carotid sheath is opened and the RCCA exposed, a loading dose of intravenous heparin is administered (usually 50 units/kg). The RCCA is controlled with two 2/0 silk ties (Fig. 41.5a) and, at least 90 s following the heparin injection, the cranially placed ligature is tied. The artery is occluded caudally and opened with a size 11 blade. The arteriotomy is dilated with dilators (e.g., Garrett), and a lubricated, clamped, arterial cannula is advanced through the arteriotomy after release of the caudal occlusion clamp (Fig. 41.5b). The tip of the arterial cannula should be sited one-third of the distance between the sternal notch and the xiphoid. The clamp is released to fill the cannula with blood and secured with the two silk ties over a plastic "sloop." The RIJV is controlled in an identical fashion and a lubricated, clamped venous cannula is advanced through the venotomy so that the tip is located halfway between the sternal notch and the xiphoid. Pressure on the liver is often required before release of the clamp to fill the cannula with blood and prevent entrainment of air. Once the cannulae are secured (Fig. 41.5c) they are connected to the ECLS circuit, taking care to ensure that the arterial cannula is connected to the postoxygenator tubing.

Utilizing the neck vessels for cannulation involves occlusion of the RCCA for the duration of the ECLS run. This raises theoretical concerns regarding perfusion of the right cerebral hemisphere although there is a lack of consensus regarding this risk in the literature. Reports utilizing EEG monitoring,[14,15] near infrared spectroscopy,[16] and Doppler imaging[17] yield conflicting results.

Following successful weaning from ECLS (see later) both RCCA and RIJV are usually permanently ligated though some authors advocate repair of the RCCA with variable success.[18,19] In our center we have recently developed a method of percutaneous insertion of both RIJV and RCCA cannulae using Seldinger technique in infants and children that does not require ligation of either vessel. Doppler studies at 12–36 months following ECLS showed normal flow in each vessel with no evidence of stenosis.

In patients requiring support for a low cardiac output state following cardiac surgery, VA ECLS cannulation can also be undertaken through the sternotomy wound. The venous cannula is placed directly into the right atrium (through the appendage) and the arterial cannula in the ascending aorta. Follow-up studies in pediatric cardiac surgery patients show no difference in outcome between chest cannulation and neck cannulation,[20] although the open chest wound can lead to increased bleeding complications.[21] We prefer neck cannulation where possible with sternotomy wound closure to reduce blood loss and facilitate chest physiotherapy.

In adults, particularly when ECLS is instituted during cardiopulmonary arrest, VA ECLS can be carried out through cannulae inserted into the femoral artery and vein.[22,23] Case reports of femoral arterial cannula placement also described this technique in the child[24] and neonate.[25]

Venovenous ECLS

In venovenous ECLS (VV ECLS) the oxygenated blood from the circuit is returned into the venous circulation, either directly into the right atrium (Fig. 41.6) or via the femoral vein. Adequate native cardiac output is mandatory for this method of support although, in patients where myocardial contractility is reduced secondary to hypoxia, the improved oxygenation resulting from VV ECLS can result in improved cardiac function and a reduction in inotrope requirements.[26] As the oxygenated blood reenters the venous circulation, all blood is directed through the pulmonary circulation and the pulmonary arterial system is exposed to fully saturated blood resulting in pulmonary arterial vasodilatation facilitating resolution of pulmonary hypertension. Venous blood drained into the ECLS circuit will inevitably be mixed with some returned oxygenated blood, leading to a degree of "recirculation" of oxygenated blood in the venous cannula. The in-line SvO_2 is, therefore, not a true indication of venous oxygenation, so it is less useful in determining the efficacy of tissue oxygenation. Venovenous ECMO avoids the need for arterial cannulation and, in the absence of a large ASD or VSD, should not be associated with cerebral embolic phenomena. In adults, if

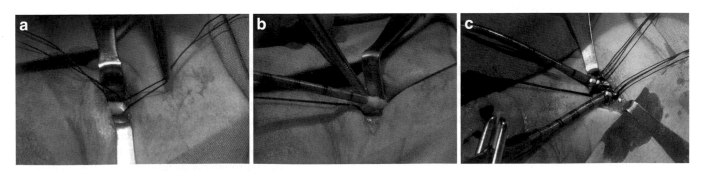

FIG. 41.5. Cannulation for VA ECMO. (a) Control of the RCCA between silk slings, (b) Insertion of the arterial cannula, (c) Arterial and venous cannulae in place

coagulation, drug therapy, and surgical treatment.[37] Optimization of coagulation is achieved with acceptance of lower ACTs by maintaining circuit blood flows at a high level and platelet transfusion to achieve a platelet level above 150,000/μl. Drug therapy includes vitamin K administration, antifibrinolytics, and recombinant activated factor VII.

Commonly used antifibrinolytics are epsilon-aminocaproic acid (Amicar) and Aprotinin. Amicar works by displacing plasminogen from fibrin, thereby preventing fibrinolysis. The most widespread indication for Amicar use is to control bleeding from surgical sites during an ECLS run.[38] One group described the prophylactic use of Amicar on ECLS in high-risk patients, demonstrating a reduced incidence of bleeding complications compared with historical controls,[39] although another multicenter randomized controlled study did not support this practice.[40] Standard ACT parameters should be set during Amicar infusion.

In the United Kingdom, Aprotinin is the most commonly used antifibrinolytic that acts through inhibition of plasmin and both plasma and tissue kallikrein. There is good evidence to support its use to prevent and treat bleeding after cardiac surgery,[41,42] and its use during ECLS has also been described.[43] The main concern with antifibrinolytic use is clot formation in the circuit and that accurate ACT monitoring is essential. In our experience, the administration of Aprotinin leads to inaccurate results when using celite-based ACT tubes, and we have changed our practice to use kaolin-based ACT tubes for more reliable monitoring. Some centers continue to use celite-based tubes but increase the ACT parameters by 20 s.[43]

Administration of recombinant factor VII (rFVIIa) enhances the rate of thrombin formation, leading to a more stable fibrin plug. This is a novel therapy for bleeding complications during ECLS and reports are limited, so far, to small case series.[44,45] There does appear to be evidence for the cautious use in refractory bleeding. We currently ensure that there is a spare circuit primed to crystalloid in the event of oxygenator failure due to thrombus.

Sedation/Paralysis

Neonates, children, and adults are routinely sedated during ECLS, predominantly to decrease pain and anxiety, reduce oxygen consumption and CO_2 production, and prevent cannula displacement. The most commonly used drugs for sedation are benzodiazepines (e.g., midazolam), morphine, and fentanyl.[46] The pharmacokinetics of these drugs are altered from the larger volume of distribution, changes in intra- and extracellular volumes, nonpulsatile flow, and reduced plasma protein concentration.[47] There has been a reduction in the use of paralyzing agents during ECLS and lower levels of sedation, resulting in increased awareness of the patient.[48]

Nutritional Support During ECLS

Patients on ECLS are catabolic and nutritional support is essential to preserve lean body mass.[49] Historically, due to con-

cerns regarding gut mucosal integrity in previously hypoxemic patients, the parenteral route was preferred during ECLS. However, recent reports demonstrate the feasibility in using enteral feeds in neonates,[50] children,[51] and adults[52] with no evidence of increased septic complications secondary to translocation of gut organisms.[53]

Weaning and Decannulation

When native cardiopulmonary function shows signs of recovery, the level of extracorporeal support is gradually reduced (or *weaned*). In VV ECLS two modes of weaning are commonly employed – reducing ECLS blood flow or reducing the oxygen fraction in the gas flow through the oxygenator. At low blood flows, an increased level of heparinization is required to avoid the risk of thrombus, so in high-risk patients a higher flow with weaning the blender is preferable. When a low level of support is reached (typically ~10–15% cardiac output) a "trial off ECLS" is undertaken. In VV ECLS this can be achieved by "capping off" the oxygenator, disconnecting the gas flow, thereby stopping oxygen and CO_2 diffusion. Unaltered venous blood circulates through the ECLS circuit and with continued cardiopulmonary stability, the cannula(e) can be removed.

In VA ECLS reducing the ECLS blood flow reduces the level of extracorporeal oxygenation. Reducing the oxygen fraction in the blender gas through the oxygenator has a similar effect although at low oxygen levels this introduces a large right-to-left shunt of poorly oxygenated blood. The patient needs to be excluded from the ECLS circuit to "trial-off" before removing the cannulae. During this trial blood recirculates through the oxygenator circuit through the bridge. Clamping and unclamping of the bridge ("flashing") is advisable every 15 min to avoid blood clotting in the cannulae.

Decannulation from ECLS when cannulae have been placed percutaneously (or with an open-assisted technique) does not require surgical involvement. In an appropriately sedated patient (we prefer paralysis to avoid entrainment of air), the cannulae are removed and direct pressure is applied over the site. Bleeding usually ceases after 10–15 min and the skin can be closed with sutures or adhesive dressings. Open decannulation requires a surgical team. The RCCA and RIJV are usually ligated although some advocate repair of the RCCA, especially after a short ECLS run.

Complications

ECLS specialists carry out regular monitoring of circuit and patient to allow prompt recognition of potential complications. Fortunately, serious complications are rare but a rigorous critical incident reporting system coupled with regular multidisciplinary meetings to discuss "near-misses" in a non-judgmental environment is essential to the smooth running of an ECLS service. All ECLS specialists undergo formal training and then keep a record of "pump-hours" to demonstrate adequate exposure. In our unit we use an ECLS clinical simulator and scenario-based training to augment our practice of regular water drills.

Oxygenator Failure

Impending oxygenator failure can be recognized by reduced efficacy of gaseous exchange (rising pCO_2 or falling pO_2), or from increased preoxygenator pressures, which are monitored continuously. Occasionally, the membrane can become saturated with condensation ("wet lung") leading to poor gaseous exchange. This is resolved by increasing the blender gas flow rate to "sigh" the membrane, resulting in improvement in the blood gases. If this step does not rectify the problem, thrombus formation should be suspected and the membrane changed. In cases where the circuit is relatively new and there is little evidence of clot elsewhere, the membrane can be changed in isolation, although in a circuit over 1-week old or with other sites of thrombus, changing the whole circuit is advisable. During circuit or membrane changes, the patient will be off extracorporeal support, so a full team is required to support the patient throughout.

Tubing or Raceway Rupture

Since the introduction of Super Tygon raceway tubing (Norton Performance Plastics, Akron, OH), this complication has become rare. The raceway is put under repeated occlusive stress from the occlusive roller-head pump and in prolonged ECLS runs it should be "walked" to avoid excessive exposure to an individual segment. In neonates, where smaller tubing is used, we usually walk the raceway every 7 days but in older patients this is carried out more frequently.

Air Embolism

A bolus of air in the ECLS circuit can circulate quickly and be delivered to the patient with potentially catastrophic consequences. In VA ECLS air embolus can result in cerebral infarction and in VV ECLS it will be delivered to the pulmonary circulation. Possible sources of air include bubbles in infusions (imperative to avoid), entrainment of air from cracked tubing or connections, and supersaturation with oxygen at low blood flow rates. When air is recognized in the circuit the patient should be taken off support by opening the circuit bridge. By manipulation of the tubing bubbles can be positioned close to a pigtail where they can be aspirated safely. If an air embolus is inadvertently delivered to the patient the head should be lowered to encourage any emboli away from the cerebral circulation. Inotropic support may be required if air enters the coronary arteries leading to myocardial dysfunction. Close vigilance by the ECLS team is essential to recognize and prevent this complication.

Bleeding

Bleeding is the most common complication of ECLS. Bleeding from cannulae sites can be controlled by direct pressure, application of hemostatic dressings, or placement of a purse-string suture. Bleeding from other surgical sites such as the chest and abdomen may require repeated exploration for hemostasis. Intracranial hemorrhage (ICH) is a devastating complication that occurs in 6% of neonates and 5% of pediatric patients.[54] The appearance of a new ICH or enlargement of a preexisting bleed is an indication to discontinue ECLS. Measures to prevent bleeding have been described previously. Ensuring optimal platelet count, fibrinogen levels, and close control of heparinization are incorporated into the daily routine. Rarely, heparin-induced thrombocytopenia is encountered, and hematological advice should be sought before changing to an alternative anticoagulant.

Infection

Many patients who receive ECLS have severe infections and are colonized with a multitude of potentially pathogenic organisms. They are usually already on broad-spectrum antibiotics. The incidence of septic complications in neonates, children, and adult ECLS patients ranges from 10 to 22%.[54] Regular surveillance cultures should be performed with a low threshold for commencing or changing antibiotic regimes. We recommend routine antifungal prophylaxis for all patients on broad-spectrum antibiotics.

Renal Failure

Many patients requiring ECLS have significant fluid overload and have some degree of renal compromise. Acute renal failure is often attributed to the pre-ECLS hypoxemia and poor renal perfusion. Oliguria is common during ECLS. An aggressive diuretic policy is warranted to remove excess fluid, and it is not unusual to require slow continuous ultrafiltration (SCUF) due to refractory oliguria. Continuous hemofiltration (CVVH) or hemodialysis/diafiltration (CVVHD/CVVHDF) is easily achieved by attaching a hollow fiber hemodialysis filter or dialysis machine to the ECLS circuit.[55] Careful management of fluid balance is essential as there can be large fluid shifts, especially in smaller patients. Renal ultrasonography is recommended to exclude structural anomalies.

Common Conditions Requiring ECLS and Outcome

Neonatal Respiratory Failure

Refractory respiratory failure in the neonate represents the most common indication for ECLS and comprises over 60% of all reported patients (nearly 21,000 patients) in the most

5. Greenough A, Emery E. ECMO and outcome of mechanical ventilation in infants of birthweight over 2 kg. Lancet 1990: 336; 760.

6. Anonymous. UK collaborative randomised trial of neonatal extracorporeal membrane oxygenation. UK Collaborative ECMO Trail Group. Lancet 1996: 348; 75–82.

7. Roberts TE. Economic evaluation and randomised controlled trial of extracorporeal membrane oxygenation: UK collaborative trial. The Extracorporeal Membrane Oxygenation Economics Working Group. BMJ 1998: 317; 911–915.

8. Bennett CC, Johnson A, Field DJ, Elbourne D. UK collaborative randomised trial of neonatal extracorporeal membrane oxygenation: follow-up to age 4 years. Lancet 2001: 357; 1094–1096.

9. Short BL. The effect of extracorporeal life support on the brain: a focus on ECMO. Semin Perinatol 2005: 29; 45–50.

10. Fink SM, Bockman DE, Howell CG, et al. Bypass circuits as the source of thromboemboli during extracorporeal membrane oxygenation. J Pediatr 1989: 115; 621–624.

11. Kato J, Seo T, Ando H, Takagi H, Ito T. Coronary arterial perfusion during venoarterial extracorporeal membrane oxygenation. J Thorac Cardiovasc Surg 1996: 111: 630–636.

12. Secker-Walker JS, Edmonds JF, Spratt EH, Conn AW. The source of coronary perfusion during partial bypass for extracorporeal membrane oxygenation (ECMO). Ann Thorac Surg 1976: 21; 138–143.

13. Martin GR, Short BL, Abbott C, O'Brien AM. Cardiac stun in infants undergoing extracorporeal membrane oxygenation. J Thorac Cardiovasc Surg 1991: 101; 607–611.

14. Streletz LJ, Bej MD, Graziani LJ, et al. Utility of serial EEGs in neonates during extracorporeal membrane oxygenation. Pediatr Neurol 1992: 8; 190–196.

15. Hahn JS, Vaucher Y, Bejar R, Coen RW. Electroencephalographic and neuroimaging findings in neonates undergoing extracorporeal membrane oxygenation. Neuropediatrics 1993: 24; 19–24.

16. Ejike JC, Schenkman KA, Seidel K, et al. Cerebral oxygenation in neonatal and pediatric patients during veno-arterial extracorporeal life support. Pediatr Crit Care Med 2006: 7; 154–158.

17. Weber TR, and Kountzman B. The effects of venous occlusion on cerebral blood flow characteristics during ECMO. J Pediatr Surg 1996: 31; 1124–1127.

18. Cheung PY, Vickar DB, Hallgren RA, et al. Carotid artery reconstruction in neonates receiving extracorporeal membrane oxygenation: a 4-year follow-up study. Western Canadian ECMO Follow-Up Group. J Pediatr Surg 1997: 32; 560–564.

19. Desai SA, Stanley C, Gringlas M, et al. Five-year follow-up of neonates with reconstructed right common carotid arteries after extracorporeal membrane oxygenation. J Pediatr 1999: 134; 428–433.

20. Kolovos NS, Bratton SL, Moler FW, et al. Outcome of pediatric patients treated with extracorporeal life support after cardiac surgery. Ann Thorac Surg 2003: 76; 1435–1441.

21. Weinhaus L, Canter C, Noetzel M, et al. Extracorporeal membrane oxygenation for circulatory support after repair of congenital heart defects. Ann Thorac Surg 1989: 48; 206–212.

22. Sasako Y, Nakatani T, Nonogi H, et al. Clinical experience of percutaneous cardiopulmonary support. Artif Organs 1996: 20; 733–736.

23. Sung K, Lee YT, Park PW, et al. Improved survival after cardiac arrest using emergent autopriming percutaneous cardiopulmonary support. Ann Thorac Surg 2006: 82; 651–656.

24. Inoue Y, Kaneko H, Yoshizawa Y, Morikawa A. Rescue of a child with fulminant myocarditis using percutaneous cardiopulmonary support. Pediatr Cardiol 2000: 21; 158–160.

25. Booth KL, Guleserian KJ, Mayer JE, Laussen PC. Extracorporeal membrane oxygenation support of a neonate with percutaneous femoral arterial cannulation. Ann Thorac Surg 2006: 81; 1514–1516.

26. Roberts N, Westrope C, Pooboni SK, et al. Venovenous extracorporeal membrane oxygenation for respiratory failure in inotrope dependent neonates. ASAIO J 2003: 49; 568–571.

27. Osiovich HC, Peliowski A, Ainsworth W, Etches PC. The Edmonton experience with venovenous extracorporeal membrane oxygenation. J Pediatr Surg 1998: 33; 1749–1752.

28. Skarsgard ED, Salt DR, Lee SK. Venovenous extracorporeal membrane oxygenation in neonatal respiratory failure: does routine, cephalad jugular drainage improve outcome? J Pediatr Surg 2004: 39; 672–676.

29. Reickert CA, Schreiner RJ, Bartlett RH, Hirschl RB. Percutaneous access for venovenous extracorporeal life support in neonates. J Pediatr Surg 1998: 33; 365–369.

30. Foley DS, Swaniker F, Pranikoff T, et al. Percutaneous cannulation for pediatric venovenous extracorporeal life support. J Pediatr Surg 2000: 35; 943–947.

31. Pranikoff T, Hirschl RB, Remenapp R, et al. Venovenous extracorporeal life support via percutaneous cannulation in 94 patients. Chest 1999: 115; 818–822.

32. Moront MG, Katz NM, Keszler M, et al. Extracorporeal membrane oxygenation for neonatal respiratory failure. A report of 50 cases. J Thorac Cardiovasc Surg 1989: 97; 706–714.

33. Fortenberry J, Pettignano R, Dykes F. Principles and practice of venovenous ECMO. In: Extracorporeal Cardiopulmonary Support in Critical Care, Van Meurs KP, Lally KP, Peek G, Zwischenberger JB, eds. Extracorporeal Life Support Organisation, Ann Arbor, MI, 2005.

34. Tourner S, Roth SJ. Venoarterial perfusion for resuscitation and cardiac procedures. In: Extracorporeal Cardiopulmonary Support in Critical Care, Van Meurs KP, Lally KP, Peek G, Zwischenberger JB, eds. Extracorporeal Life Support Organisation, Ann Arbor, MI, 2005.

35. Bartlett R. 2005. Physiology of ECLS. In: Extracorporeal Cardiopulmonary Support in Critical Care, Van Meurs KP, Lally KP, Peek G, Zwischenberger JB, eds. Extracorporeal Life Support Organisation, Ann Arbor, MI, 2005.

36. Aiyagari RM, Rocchini AP, Remenapp RT, Graziano JN. Decompression of the left atrium during extracorporeal membrane oxygenation using a transseptal cannula incorporated into the circuit. Crit Care Med 2006: 34; 2603–2606.

37. Peek G, Wittenstein B, Harvey C, Machin D. Management of bleeding during ECLS. In: Extracorporeal Cardiopulmonary Support in Critical Care, Van Meurs KP, Lally KP, Peek G, Zwischenberger JB, eds. Extracorporeal Life Support Organisation, Ann Arbor, MI, 2005.

38. Downard CD, Betit P, Chang RW, et al. Impact of AMICAR on hemorrhagic complications of ECMO: a ten-year review. J Pediatr Surg 2003: 38; 1212–1216.

39. Wilson JM, Bower LK, Fackler JC, et al. Aminocaproic acid decreases the incidence of intracranial hemorrhage and other hemorrhagic complications of ECMO. J Pediatr Surg 1993: 28; 536–540.

40. Horwitz JR, Cofer BR, Warner BW, et al. A multicenter trial of 6-aminocaproic acid (Amicar) in the prevention of bleeding in infants on ECMO. J Pediatr Surg 1998: 33; 1610–1613.

41. Jamieson WR, Dryden PJ, O'Connor JP, et al. Beneficial effect of both tranexamic acid and aprotinin on blood loss reduction in reoperative valve replacement surgery. Circulation 1997: 96; 96–100.

42. Codispoti M, Mankad PS. Management of anticoagulation and its reversal during paediatric cardiopulmonary bypass: a review of current UK practice. Perfusion 2000: 15; 191–201.

43. Peek GJ, Firmin RK. The inflammatory and coagulative response to prolonged extracorporeal membrane oxygenation. ASAIO J 1999: 45; 250–263.

44. Wittenstein B, Ng C, Ravn H, Goldman A. Recombinant factor VII for severe bleeding during extracorporeal membrane oxygenation following open heart surgery. Pediatr Crit Care Med 2005: 6; 473–476.

45. Dominguez TE, Mitchell M, Friess SH, et al. Use of recombinant factor VIIa for refractory hemorrhage during extracorporeal membrane oxygenation. Pediatr Crit Care Med 2005: 6; 348–351.

46. DeBerry BB, Lynch JE, Chernin JM, et al. A survey for pain and sedation medications in pediatric patients during extracorporeal membrane oxygenation. Perfusion 2005: 20; 139–143.

47. Buck ML. Pharmacokinetic changes during extracorporeal membrane oxygenation: implications for drug therapy of neonates. Clin Pharmacokinet 2003: 42; 403–417.

48. Frenckner B, Tibboel D. Sedation and management of pain on ECLS. In: Extracorporeal Cardiopulmonary Support in Critical Care, Van Meurs KP, Lally KP, Peek G, Zwischenberger JB, eds. Extracorporeal Life Support Organisation, Ann Arbor, MI, 2005.

49. Jaksic T. Nutritional support of the ECMO Patient. In: Extracorporeal Cardiopulmonary Support in Critical Care, Van Meurs KP, Lally KP, Peek G, Zwischenberger JB, eds. Extracorporeal Life Support Organisation, Ann Arbor, MI, 2005.

50. Hanekamp MN, Spoel M, Sharman-Koendjbiharie I, et al. Routine enteral nutrition in neonates on extracorporeal membrane oxygenation. Pediatr Crit Care Med 2005: 6; 275–279.

51. Pettignano R, Heard M, Davis R, et al. Total enteral nutrition versus total parenteral nutrition during pediatric extracorporeal membrane oxygenation. Crit Care Med 1998: 26; 358–363.

52. Scott LK, Boudreaux K, Thaljeh F, et al. Early enteral feedings in adults receiving venovenous extracorporeal membrane oxygenation. J Parenter Enteral Nutr 2004: 28; 295–300.

53. Wertheim HF, Albers MJ, Piena-Spoel M, Tibboel D. The incidence of septic complications in newborns on extracorporeal membrane oxygenation is not affected by feeding route. J Pediatr Surg 2001: 36; 1485–1489.

54. Deberry B, Lynch JE, Chung D, Zwischenberger JB. Emergencies during ECLS and their management. In: Extracorporeal Cardiopulmonary Support in Critical Care, Van Meurs KP, Lally KP, Peek G, Zwischenberger JB, eds. Extracorporeal Life Support Organisation, Ann Arbor, MI, 2005.

55. Sell LL, Cullen ML, Whittlesey GC, et al. Experience with renal failure during extracorporeal membrane oxygenation: treatment with continuous hemofiltration. J Pediatr Surg 1987: 22; 600–602.

56. Roy BJ, Rycus P, Conrad SA, Clark RH. The changing demographics of neonatal extracorporeal membrane oxygenation patients reported to the Extracorporeal Life Support Organization (ELSO) Registry. Pediatrics 2000: 106; 1334–1338.

57. Walker GM, Coutts JA, Skeoch C, Davis CF. Paediatricians' perception of the use of extracorporeal membrane oxygenation to treat meconium aspiration syndrome. Arch Dis Child Fetal Neonatal Ed 2003: 88; F70–F71.

58. Anonymous. Does extracorporeal membrane oxygenation improve survival in neonates with congenital diaphragmatic hernia? The Congenital Diaphragmatic Hernia Study Group. J Pediatr Surg 1999: 34; 720–724.

59. Davis PJ, Firmin RK, Manktelow B, et al. Long-term outcome following extracorporeal membrane oxygenation for congenital diaphragmatic hernia: the UK experience. J Pediatr 2004: 144; 309–315.

60. Green TP, Timmons OD, Fackler JC, et al. The impact of extracorporeal membrane oxygenation on survival in pediatric patients with acute respiratory failure. Pediatric Critical Care Study Group. Crit Care Med 1996: 24; 323–329.

61. Peek G, Tirouvopaiti R, Firmin R. ECLS for adult respiratory failure: etiology and indications. In: Extracorporeal Cardiopulmonary Support in Critical Care, Van Meurs KP, KP Lally, G Peek and JB Zwischenberger, Eds:. Extracorporeal Life Support Organisation, Ann Arbor, MI, 2005.

62. Kolla S, Awad SS, Rich PB, et al. Extracorporeal life support for 100 adult patients with severe respiratory failure. Ann Surg 1997: 226; 544–564.

63. Boehmer JP, Popjes E. Cardiac failure: mechanical support strategies. Crit Care Med 2006: 34; S268–S277.

64. Delius RE, Bove EL, Meliones JN, et al. Use of extracorporeal life support in patients with congenital heart disease. Crit Care Med 1992: 20; 1216–1222.

65. Ziomek S, Harrell JE, Jr., Fasules JW, et al. Extracorporeal membrane oxygenation for cardiac failure after congenital heart operation. Ann Thorac Surg 1992: 54; 861–867.

66. Duncan BW, Hraska V, Jonas RA, et al. Mechanical circulatory support in children with cardiac disease. J Thorac Cardiovasc Surg 1999: 117; 529–542.

67. Asaumi Y, Yasuda S, Morii I, et al. Favourable clinical outcome in patients with cardiogenic shock due to fulminant myocarditis supported by percutaneous extracorporeal membrane oxygenation. Eur Heart J 2005: 26; 2185–2192.

68. Reddy SL, Hasan A, Hamilton LR, et al. Mechanical versus medical bridge to transplantation in children. What is the best timing for mechanical bridge? Eur J Cardiothorac Surg 2004: 25: 605–609.

69. Morris MC, Wernovsky G, Nadkarni VM. Survival outcomes after extracorporeal cardiopulmonary resuscitation instituted during active chest compressions following refractory in-hospital pediatric cardiac arrest. Pediatr Crit Care Med 2004: 5; 440–446.

70. Megarbane B, Leprince P, Deye N, et al. Emergency feasibility in medical intensive care unit of extracorporeal life support for refractory cardiac arrest. Intens Care Med 2007: 33; 758–764.

71. Younger JG, Schreiner RJ, Swaniker F, et al. Extracorporeal resuscitation of cardiac arrest. Acad Emerg Med 1999: 6; 700–707.

72. Horan M, Ichiba S, Firmin RK, et al. A pilot investigation of mild hypothermia in neonates receiving extracorporeal membrane oxygenation (ECMO). J Pediatr 2004: 144; 301–308.

73. Nobuhara KK, Fauza DO, DiFiore JW, et al. Continuous intrapulmonary distension with perfluorocarbon accelerates neonatal (but not adult) lung growth. J Pediatr Surg 1998: 33; 292–298.

74. Fauza DO, Hirschl RB, Wilson JM. Continuous intrapulmonary distension with perfluorocarbon accelerates lung growth in infants with congenital diaphragmatic hernia: initial experience. J Pediatr Surg 2001: 36; 1237–1240.

75. Hirschl RB, Philip WF, Glick L, et al. A prospective, randomized pilot trial of perfluorocarbon-induced lung growth in newborns

with congenital diaphragmatic hernia. J Pediatr Surg 2003: 38; 283–289.

76. Walker GM, Kasem KF, O'Toole SJ, et al. Early perfluorodecalin lung distension in infants with congenital diaphragmatic hernia. J Pediatr Surg 2003: 38; 17–20.

77. Boedy RF, Howell CG, Kanto WP, Jr. Hidden mortality rate associated with extracorporeal membrane oxygenation. J Pediatr 1990: 117; 462–464.

78. Wilson BJ, Jr., Heiman HS, Butler TJ, et al. A 16-year neonatal/ pediatric extracorporeal membrane oxygenation transport experience. Pediatrics 2002: 109; 189–193.

79. Heulitt MJ, Taylor BJ, Faulkner SC, et al. Inter-hospital transport of neonatal patients on extracorporeal membrane oxygenation: mobile-ECMO. Pediatrics 1995: 95; 562–566.

80. Foley DS, Pranikoff T, Younger JG, et al. A review of 100 patients transported on extracorporeal life support. ASAIO J 2002: 48; 612–619.

81. Linden V, Palmer K, Reinhard J, et al. Inter-hospital transportation of patients with severe acute respiratory failure on extracorporeal membrane oxygenation – national and international experience. Intensive Care Med 2001: 27; 1643–1648.

82. Rossaint R, Pappert D, Gerlach H, et al. Extracorporeal membrane oxygenation for transport of hypoxaemic patients with severe ARDS. Brit J Anaesth 1997: 78; 241–246.

83. Westrope C, Roberts N, Nichani S, et al. Experience with mobile inhaled nitric oxide during transport of neonates and children with respiratory insufficiency to an extracorporeal membrane oxygenation center. Pediatr Crit Care Med 2004: 5; 542–546.

42
Diaphragmatic Pacing in Children

Hélène Flageole and Michael G. Davis

Introduction

Diaphragmatic pacing was first reported in 1966 by Dr. William Glenn, a pioneer of cardiac pacemaker technology, to help adults with central hypoventilation secondary to quadriplegia.[1] The use of phrenic nerve pacing to treat infants and children with primary Congenital Central Alveolar Hypoventilation Syndrome (CCAHS) was reported by Hunt et al. in 1978.[2] The focus of this chapter will be the indications for diaphragmatic pacing in children, a detailed description of the surgical aspects of diaphragmatic pacers, and the long-term follow-up information available for this group of patients.

Historical Background: Ondine's Curse

Ondine (Undine in some texts) was a mythological figure of European tradition. She was a water nymph destined to become human when she fell in love with a mortal. The mortal was doomed to die if he was unfaithful to her. In the medical literature, Ondine's curse is synonymous with disorders of central hypoventilation, sleep apnea, and loss of autonomic ventilation.[3–6] In these writings, Ondine is regarded as having "cursed" her husband with loss of automatic breathing as a result of his infidelity.[7,8] How did disorders of respiration become associated with this legend?

In the early 1950s abnormalities of respiratory control resulting in hypoventilation were observed in patients afflicted with bulbar poliomyelitis.[9] The term Ondine's curse was first used by Severinghaus and Mitchell in 1962. The authors reported postoperative respiratory problems in a group of patients who had undergone high bilateral spinothalamic cordotomies for relief of chronic pain. They observed prolonged periods of apnea in these patients who were, nonetheless, able to breathe on command.[10] The authors considered their observations to match the description of the German legend of Undine. In 1973, Mellins et al. applied the term "Ondine's curse" to infants with congenital alveolar hypoventilation in whom there was a failure of automatic control of ventilation by the central nervous system.[11]

There is, however, one small problem attributing these abnormalities of respiratory control to Ondine. In none of the classic writings does Ondine ever curse her husband! Although less prosaic, the term congenital central alveolar hypoventilation syndrome is, therefore, factually more accurate.

Pathophysiology

Congenital central hypoventilation syndrome (CCAHS) is defined as a congenital defect of automatic breathing control. Acquired abnormalities of respiratory control have been reported in association with viral encephalitis, asphyxia, trauma, brain tumors, brainstem infarction, and some rare inborn errors of metabolism (Leigh's disease, pyruvate dehydrogenase deficiency, and carnitine deficiency).

In children with CCAHS ventilation is most severely affected during quiet sleep, a state during which automatic neural control is predominant. Ventilatory patterns may also be abnormal during active sleep and during wakefulness, depending upon the severity of the disorder. The severity of respiratory dysfunction in CCAHS ranges from mild hypoventilation during quiet sleep, with relatively good ventilation and oxygenation during wakefulness, to complete apnea during sleep and severe hypoventilation during wakefulness. Other symptoms indicative of brainstem or autonomic dysfunction may be present, but these are not essential components of CCAHS. While there is some evidence for deterioration of respiratory control with age, the usual reason for decline in respiratory function is incremental lung damage from recurrent infection. It is important to realize that children with CCAHS are unable to respond automatically to stress, such as intercurrent illness, with the result that rapid accumulation of CO_2 is liable to occur.

The pathophysiology of CCAHS has been the subject of intense speculation and research. It has been postulated that the condition arises from prenatal genetic damage to respiratory center in the brainstem, or from a more widespread involvement of the central nervous system.[4] Replication of

D.H. Parikh et al. (eds.), *Pediatric Thoracic Surgery*,
DOI: 10.1007/b136543_42, © Springer-Verlag London Limited 2009

the abnormalities of ventilatory control typical of CCAHS has been reproduced in cats by localized destruction of the intermediate area of the ventral surface of the medulla oblongata in the brainstem. Other investigators have suggested hypoplasia of the arcuate nucleus in the ventral surface of the medulla as the probable cause of CCAHS.[12] Although this experimental data seem compelling careful radiological surveys of the brainstem in patients with CCAHS have failed to identify any recognizable lesion.[13]

Physiologic Abnormalities in Ventilatory Control

CCAHS was initially thought to be a disorder of central chemoreceptors rendering them insensitive to carbon dioxide. The ventilatory response to both low oxygen and high carbon dioxide was essentially random, without any evidence of progressive ventilatory stimulation, suggesting that children with CCAHS have absent chemoreceptor responses to both hypercapnea (central) and hypoxia (peripheral) while awake.[14] There has also been speculation that the defect in CCAHS lies in the central integration of chemoreceptor signals.[15]

Ventilatory and arousal responses to respiratory stimulation apparently involve separate pathways. Consequently, if children with CCAHS have a disorder of chemoreceptor input integration they should still respond to other respiratory stimuli. Marcus and coworkers, however, concluded that most children with CCAHS do respond to hypercapnea, indicating some central chemoreceptor sensitivity.[16] They speculated that because these children are able to respond to hypercapnea, the most probable mechanism for CCAHS is a brainstem lesion in the region responsible for integration of chemoreceptor information.

Despite absent rebreathing ventilatory responses to both hypercapnea and hypoxia, most patients with CCAHS are able to maintain adequate ventilation during wakefulness. Gozal et al. hypothesized that the ability of children with CCAHS to maintain waking ventilation was due to intact peripheral chemoreceptor (chemoreceptors in the great vessels responding to changes in oxygen and carbon dioxide levels) function.[17] Tidal breathing of 100% oxygen results in patients with CCAHS and normal controls result in a similar decreases in ventilation, suggesting that peripheral chemoreceptors are indeed intact. Acute hypoxia produces similar increases in minute ventilation in the two groups although children with CCAHS increased their minute ventilation by a preferential increase in respiratory rate as opposed to tidal volume. Vital capacity breaths of each of 5 and 15% CO_2-containing gas mixtures induced similar increases in minute ventilation in CCAHS and controls. Gozal et al. concluded that peripheral chemoreceptor function, when assessed by acute hypoxia, hyperoxia, or hypercapnea, is preserved in children with CCAHS who are able to sustain adequate ventilation during wakefulness.[17] They speculated that the apparent large variability in CCAHS results from defective brainstem integration of chemoreceptor information.

Chemoreceptors play an important role in respiratory control during exercise. During maximal exercise, oxygen consumption and minute ventilation appear lower in CCAHS. The increase in minute volume is the result of increasing respiratory rate rather than tidal volume. Furthermore, respiratory rate and ventilation increase proportionately to exercise intensity in CCAHS, suggesting that exercise-induced increases in ventilation can occur in the absence of chemoreceptor function. Paton et al. also speculated that, in the absence of ventilatory response to progressive chemoreceptor stimulation from rising carbon dioxide or reduction in oxygen levels in blood, motion has a direct effect on respiratory rate, and consequently minute ventilation, during exercise.[15] They demonstrated this by strapping the legs of subjects with CCAHS to the pedals of a motorized bicycle to produce passive leg motion. Motion at pedal frequency above 40 cycles per minute results in an increase in minute ventilation in both CCAHS subjects and normal controls. Proprioceptive stimuli from joint and muscle receptors are probably responsible for this increase.

In controls, the increase in ventilation is tightly coupled to the increase in metabolic requirements. However, in CCAHS, passive leg motion is associated with ventilation in excess of metabolic requirements, resulting in normalization of carbon dioxide levels. Normalization of CO_2 levels with motion in subjects with CCAHS lends support to the theory that there is a basic defect affecting integration of sensor inputs to the brain center responsible for matching breathing with the metabolic requirements of the body.

CCAHS is characterized by abnormal ventilatory control in the absence of a recognized anatomic lesion resulting in disturbances of autonomic nervous system (ANS) function. Another symptom of malfunction of the ANS is a reduction in heart rate variability.[18,19] Patients with CCAHS show disturbed moment-to-moment heart rate variability. A prospective Holter study by Silvestri et al. demonstrated baseline bradycardia, coupled with atrial and ventricular premature beats.[20] These changes are found with increasing frequency with advancing age. The long-term significance of these findings is unclear, but it certainly justifies close monitoring as these aberrant cardiac rhythms occur more frequently under general anesthesia although they usually resolve spontaneously. However, Kolb et al. recently reported a patient with CCAHS who received a diaphragmatic pacing system in early childhood who, at the age of 17 years, also required a cardiac pacemaker.[21] It is noteworthy that this could be done without significant interaction between the devices.

Genetics of CCAHS

The first few years of the twenty-first century saw a breakthrough in the understanding of CCAHS. Mutations in the *PHOX2B* gene have been identified in subjects with CCAHS.[22] Pursuing a genetic explanation for CCAHS was supported by data from familial occurrences and genetic segregation analyses. Instead of being considered a disorder restricted to abnormalities of breathing control, CCAHS has come to be regarded as a more generalized ANS dysfunction. Using the candidate approach to search for CCAHS-susceptibility genes, Amiel et al. reported their findings in 2003.[23] They identified mutations in the homeobox gene *PHOX2B* in patients with CCAHS that were not found in normal controls. These mutations consisted mostly of polyalanine repeat expansions although they also identified frameshift mutations in some patients. These initial findings were subsequently corroborated even more convincingly by Weese-Mayer et al., adding weight to the theory that *PHOX2B* is the disease-defining gene in CCAHS.[24,25]

PHOX2B is a gene located on chromosome 4p12, which encodes a highly conserved transcription factor known to play a key role in the development of ANS reflex circuits in mice. *PHOX2B* normally encodes a protein that contains two poly-alanine repeat sequences of 9 and 20 residues in length. In CCAHS, expansions of 25–33 repeats have been identified in these polyalanine sequences.

PHOX2B encodes a transcriptional activator involved in promoting pan-neuronal differentiation in early embryologic development of the nervous system.[26] Through a separate pathway, it represses expression of neurogenesis inhibitors. In addition, *PHOX2B* is required to express tyrosine hydroxylase, dopamine beta-hydroxylase, and receptor tyrosine kinase, thereby confirming its regulatory role in the noradrenergic phenotype in vertebrate neural cells.[27] Pattyn et al. studied *PHOX2B* extensively and were able to demonstrate an early expression pattern in the rhombencephalon, suggesting a link between early patterning events and later neurogenesis in the hindbrain.[28] The original references are included for the avid reader. For the purpose of this text, it will suffice that there is now solid data to establish *PHOX2B* as a key transcription factor in development of autonomic reflex pathways. In children with CCAHS there seems to be an imbalance in the sympathetic and parasympathetic nervous systems as well as relative dysfunction in the enteric nervous system.

These recent discoveries have not only advanced our understanding of the basic science of this rare disease. They also have critical clinical implications. There is now a reliable molecular genetic test to diagnose CCAHS. The disease is inherited in an autosomal dominant fashion and it is, therefore, recommended that parents and siblings of affected children are screened.

Associated Anomalies

Hirschsprung's disease has been associated with CCAHS. In 1978, Haddad et al. described three patients with CCAHS and Hirschsprung's disease, including two siblings with total colonic aganglionosis.[29] Several further reports have appeared since then.[30–35] There would appear to be a female preponderance of around 2:1 in patients with Hirschsprung's disease and CCAHS, in contrast to the 4:1 male predominance seen in isolated Hirschsprung's disease. The majority of patients with Hirschsprung's disease and CCAHS have total colonic aganglionosis.

Neuroblastoma, ganglioneuroblastoma, and neurofibromatosis have also been seen in children with CCAHS.[36–39] These associations hint at a primary defect of neural crest cell migration. In 1974, Bolande coined the term "neurocristopathy" to describe lesions resulting from maldevelopment of the neural crest tissues.[40] Twenty years later, the same author published a review describing the advances in neural crest ontogeny as well as the increase in number and variety of neurocristopathies.[41] Advances in the molecular genetics offer the tantalizing prospect of unifying the neurocristopathy concept with the phenotypic abnormalities seen in CCAHS, Hirschsprung's disease, and other malformations of the ANS.

Clinical Features of CCAHS

The clinical presentation of CCAHS is variable, dependent on the severity of the disorder.[42] Although most infants are vigorous at birth, with normal Apgar scores, the severely affected become apneic as soon as they fall asleep and will require assisted ventilation in the newborn nursery. Some spontaneous improvement is observed in infancy but this apparent improvement results from normal maturation of the respiratory system and alteration of the normal wake/sleep cycle rather than a real change in the underlying disorder. Apnea or hypoventilation will persist during sleep.

Some individuals with CCAHS will present with cyanosis, edema, and signs of right-sided heart failure during later childhood. Almost invariably these children are thought initially to have a cyanotic congenital heart anomaly, only to be found to have severe pulmonary hypertension at the time of cardiac catheterization.

Patients with milder forms of CCAHS may present with tachycardia, diaphoresis, and/or cyanosis during sleep. Fortunately, these children generally come to medical attention before they develop intractable right heart failure. Finally, some children present with unexplained apnea, or an apparent life-threatening event.

Diagnosis of CCAHS

Diagnostic criteria for CCAHS are shown in Table 42.1.[43] Confirmation of the diagnosis of CCAHS clinically requires continuous noninvasive monitoring of ventilation during sleep. This is best accomplished using transcutaneous oxygen and carbon dioxide measurements, pulse oximetry, and end-tidal capnography. Intermittent blood gas sampling by arterial puncture or arterialized capillary sampling is not helpful because it will invariably result in arousal of the patient and therefore not represent gas exchange during sleep. Typically, infants with CCAHS have a decreased or

TABLE 42.1. Diagnostic criteria for congenital central hypoventilation syndrome.

Hypoventilation (hypopnea) during quiet sleep leading to progressive hypercarbia ($pCO_2 > 60$ torr) and hypoxemia
Absent or negligible ventilatory and arousal sensitivity to hypercarbia during sleep
Variable deficiency in hypoxic ventilatory responsiveness, with absent or negligible hypoxic arousal responsiveness during sleep
Lack of response to respiratory stimulants
Absence of autoresuscitation
Onset of symptoms during the first year of life
Absence of primary pulmonary disease or neuromuscular dysfunction to explain the hypoventilation

TABLE 42.2. Selection criteria for diaphragmatic pacing quadriplegic patients.

Stable cervical spinal cord injuries at C3 level or above
At least 3 months postinjury to allow time for spontaneous recovery
Intact phrenic nerves, assessed by transcutaneous stimulation of the phrenic nerves in the neck
Normal lung function
Low-pressure urinary drainage, controlled urinary tract infections
No significant musculoskeletal deformities
Age > 10 years
Supportive family network, including domestic stability and financial security
Normal cognitive function and motivation to pursue independence

absent ventilatory response to hypercapnea and/or hypoxia, although these abnormalities may not be seen in all patients depending on the methodology used.[14] Genetic mutation analysis should be performed in suspected cases.

Respiratory Failure Associated with Spinal Cord Trauma

Some degree of respiratory insufficiency is present in all persons with cervical spinal cord injuries and tetraplegia because of loss of intercostal muscle innervation. However, injuries at or above C4 level will also damage the phrenic nerve. Although spontaneous recovery of diaphragmatic function occurs in some patients during the first year after injury, patients with cervical cord injuries above the level of C3 invariably require long-term respiratory support.[44]

Conventional treatment consists of mechanical ventilation through a tracheostomy. Provided suitable financial and domestic support is available it may be possible to rehabilitate children to home on long-term mechanical ventilation.

Diaphragmatic pacing following cervical cord trauma was first described by Glenn in 1972.[45] Considerable advances in microelectronics since then have made diaphragmatic pacing for respiratory support in tetraplegic patients a viable proposition.[46] Elefteriades et al. have proposed a series of selection criteria for pacing quadriplegic patients (Table 42.2).[47]

Management

Pharmacologic Management

Over the years all known (and some only suspected) respiratory stimulants have been used to treat CCAHS without sustained benefit. Theophylline and caffeine may have limited use in the mildest forms of CCAHS. Progesterone may be of use although feminizing side effects limit its utility. Methylphenidate has some effect but excessive doses results in sleep deprivation. Doxapram is a respiratory stimulant occasionally given to babies with apnea of prematurity when caffeine fails, or for respiratory depression following anesthesia. It has been of some use in CCAHS but long-term treatment is limited by the nonspecific adrenergic stimulation.

Mechanical Ventilation

Positive pressure ventilation through a tracheotomy is the most commonly used method of support for children with CCAHS and now considered the standard treatment.[48] However, there are many inherent problems associated with long-term tracheotomy in children, including a significant mortality.[49] Speech and language development is hindered, and lower respiratory tract infections are frequent.[50,51]

Noninvasive positive pressure ventilation (NPPV) avoids the need for tracheotomy. Positive pressure ventilation can be applied using a nasal mask. The first use of this method of ventilation to treat a 6-year old with CCAHS appeared in 1987.[52] Subsequently this technique has been used to treat a 9-month-old infant.[53] Noninvasive ventilation in the home setting requires a considerable degree of patient cooperation and an even greater degree of parental supervision, rendering it impractical for many families. Prolonged use of nasal mask ventilation may lead to pressure-induced distortion of maxillary growth from the tight-fitting mask. Growth of the maxilla fails to follow growth of the mandible creating a *pseudoprognathis* deformity of the mid-face.[54] Gas exchange is apt to become inadequate during respiratory tract infections because of either nasal obstruction or excessive secretions with the result that ICU admission and endotracheal intubation become necessary.

Negative pressure ventilation using a chest shell (cuirass) provides another alternative for noninvasive ventilation. Negative pressure ventilation has the additional advantages of augmenting normal breathing patterns and avoiding a tracheotomy. However, this technique is of limited value in the presence of lung disease, especially as lung compliance declines. Moreover, frequent refitting becomes necessary because of growth, and the equipment is cumbersome.

Diaphragmatic Pacing

Diaphragmatic pacing was first described in 1966 for patients with respiratory failure secondary to quadriplegia.[1] Subsequently, Hunt et al. developed a modified method of diaphragmatic pacing for infants and children.[2] Diaphragmatic pacing allows ventilation of the lungs by diaphragmatic excursion (i.e., negative pressure). For patients with normal waking ventilation the real benefit of diaphragmatic pacing at night is freedom from positive-pressure ventilation. In children who also require ventilatory support while awake, pacing can improve their quality of life substantially. This is accomplished mainly as a result of increased mobility, which brings considerable benefits for general physical and mental development through independent living.[55] Normal breathing patterns can be simulated. The need for a face mask or cuirass and equipment for mechanical ventilation is avoided. Feeding and speech are not compromised. From a financial point of view, although the initial cost of diaphragmatic pacing is expensive, the savings incurred in ventilator-related expenses are such that, on average, the pacemaker will pay for itself within 4–5 years. Thereafter, diaphragmatic pacing is approximately $20,000 per annum, which is less expensive than mechanical ventilation at home.

Diaphragmatic pacing becomes feasible in children over the age of 1 year. Below this age the chest wall is too compliant to allow effective pacing. In addition to age, there are several general criteria that must be met before considering diaphragmatic pacing (Table 42.3).[55] Traditionally phrenic nerve and diaphragm function is evaluated by documenting the contractile response of each hemidiaphragm to electrical stimulation of each phrenic nerve by surface electrodes.[56] More recently, the relationship between cerebral and diaphragmatic function has been evaluated using cortical and cervical magnetic stimulation.[57] The principle of magnetic stimulation is to create a brief and intense magnetic field that, unlike electrical current, is only mildly attenuated by natural barriers such as skin and bone. This enables magnetic fields to reach deeply seated structures. Furthermore, magnetic stimulation is less painful and therefore better tolerated than electrical stimulation, particularly in children.

There are two diaphragmatic pacing systems available commercially in the USA.[58] The Avery breathing pacemaker system (Avery Laboratories, Commack, NY) is FDA approved and has been in clinical use for many years.[59] The Atrostim phrenic nerve stimulator (Atrotech, Tampere, Finland) is FDA approved for investigational use only although this system is widely used outside the USA.[60] A third system is manufactured

by MedImplant Biotechnisches Labor, Vienna, Austria but this is not available in the USA.

The main differences between the three pacing systems lie in the electrodes. The Avery system uses monopolar or bipolar nerve cuff electrodes. The Atrostim system uses a four-pole sequential stimulation. Each electrode comprises four contacts evenly spaced around the phrenic nerve, which are stimulated sequentially activating different parts of the nerve with the aim of delaying diaphragmatic muscle fatigue. The MedImplant system features a similar system with four electrodes sutured to each phrenic nerve.

Diaphragmatic pacing systems used in clinical practice consist of four components (Fig. 42.1).

Nerve electrode. A titanium or platinum noncircumferential electrode is attached to the phrenic nerve. This connects to the receiver via a high-flexibility stainless steel cable insulated by a silicone sheath (Fig. 42.2).

Receiver. The receiver is a totally implanted device about the size of a Canadian dollar coin. This receives radiofrequency energy and converts it into electrical impulses, which in turn stimulate the phrenic nerve to elicit contraction of the diaphragm (Fig. 42.3).

TABLE 42.3. General criteria for diaphragmatic pacing in children.

Chronic respiratory failure requiring long-term respiratory support by mechanical ventilation via a permanent tracheotomy on either a temporary, intermittent, or continuous basis

A defined central neurologic cause such as alveolar hypoventilation or spinal cord trauma interrupting neuronal conduction at C3 level or above

Intact phrenic nerves, assessed by transcutaneous stimulation of the phrenic nerves in the neck

Normal, or near normal, lung function

Supportive family network, including domestic stability and financial security

Normal cognitive function and motivation to pursue independence

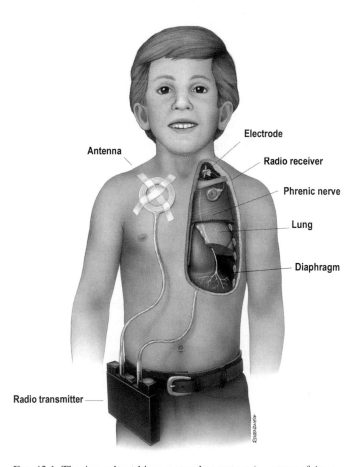

FIG. 42.1. The Avery breathing pacemaker system (courtesy of Avery Biomedical Devices, Commack, NY, USA)

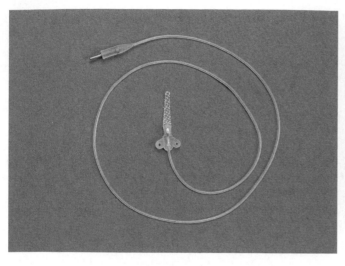

FIG. 42.2. The nerve-stimulating electrode

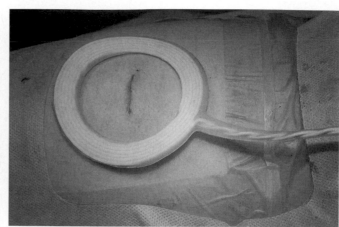

FIG. 42.4. The external antenna, worn over each implanted receiver coil

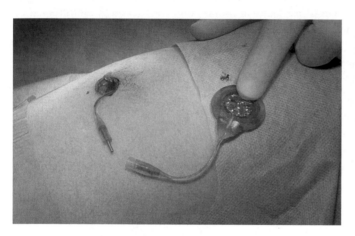

FIG. 42.3. The receiver coil, which is implanted subcutaneously

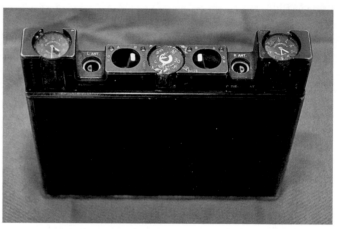

FIG 42.5. The external pulse generator. This is a dual-channel device for simultaneous control of both pacing electrodes

External antenna. An antenna is worn over each implanted receiver. The antennae send radio signals transcutaneously from the transmitter to the internal receiver (Fig. 42.4).

Pulse generator. The external generator provides the signals for phrenic nerve stimulation. The power and frequency of the signals can be adjusted (Fig. 42.5).

The phrenic nerves can be exposed for attachment of pacing electrodes through the neck or through the chest. The preferred site for electrode placement is the intrathoracic segment of the phrenic nerve, just above the reflection of the pericardium. The intrathoracic phrenic nerve can be approached using several routes. It can be reached by an anterior thoracotomy incision although the resulting scar is cosmetically unsatisfactory. When using an open technique, we prefer a transaxillary approach through the third intercostal space. A small incision is made in the inferior aspect of the axilla, extending between the latissimus dorsi muscle posteriorly and the pectoralis major anteriorly. The exposure provided by this approach

is satisfactory and, since no muscle is divided, postoperative discomfort is minimal. The cosmetic result is excellent.

The phrenic nerve is exposed approximately 5 cm above the pericardial reflection by incising the mediastinal pleura over a distance of 1.5 cm. Extreme care must be exercised to avoid damage to the nerve by overzealous dissection of the epineurium. The electrode is secured in position using fine nonabsorbable sutures placed in the pleura. We do not routinely leave a chest tube at the end of the procedure because of the potential risk of infection.

In recent years we have used thoracoscopy for electrode placement. The procedure takes us longer thoracoscopically than through an axillary thoracotomy, and the postoperative analgesia requirements are similar. This probably relates to the learning curve for an uncommon procedure and it seems likely that thoracoscopy will provide advantages for adult patients.

The phrenic nerve can also be exposed in the neck, where it lies on the anterior scalene muscle.[61] Unfortunately the phrenic nerve may comprise the C3/4 root only in the neck. The C5 component then forms an accessory phrenic nerve, which joins the C3/4 root only in the lower thorax.[62] Consequently, one might only capture 75% of the fibers in the neck. Moreover, cervical electrodes may inadvertently stimulate the brachial plexus giving rise to undesirable neck or arm twitches, particularly in small patients. For these reasons, we reserve the cervical approach for patients who have a hostile thoracic cavity, e.g., following previous thoracic surgery or an empyema.

Whether the thoracic or cervical approach is used to affix the electrodes to the phrenic nerves, the connecting wires are tunneled to a subcutaneous location on the lower lateral chest wall on each side. A subcutaneous pocket is created for the receiver (Fig. 42.3). At the end of the procedure all components are totally implanted and the wounds are closed in a standard fashion. Before leaving the operating room correct functioning of the pacing system must be verified. The surface antenna is placed over the receiver and the generator is activated (Fig. 42.6).

The pacing generator is left inactive for several days after surgery, to allow recovery and general convalescence. There then follows a period of diaphragmatic training, which usually lasts 3–4 months.[47,63] Diaphragmatic conditioning is a process whereby the fast-contracting muscle fibers that are anaerobic, highly glycolytic, and susceptible to fatigue, are progressively transformed into slow-contracting, fatigue-resistant fibers. This process makes long-term diaphragmatic pacing possible. Pacing is started at 1–2h per day, and increased by 30–60min each week. Once diaphragmatic conditioning is complete long-term pacing continues at a rate of about 7–10 breaths per minute. The long-term risk of diaphragmatic fatigue appears to be minimal when these pacing frequencies are used.

Most children requiring long-term respiratory support will have a tracheostomy. Diaphragmatic pacing offers a small chance of life without a permanent tracheostomy. In practice this is realized infrequently.[64] Although phrenic nerve stimulation

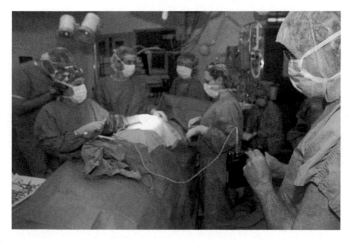

FIG. 42.6. Before leaving the operating room correct functioning of the pacing system is verified

causes contraction of the diaphragmatic muscle resulting in inhalation, exhalation is passive. Diaphragmatic pacing is, therefore, not capable of producing an effective cough in tetraplegic patients.

Pacing can produce upper airway obstruction as a result of vigorous diaphragm contraction, which is not coordinated with phasic muscle control of the upper airway. All infants and young children require tracheostomy to prevent upper airway obstruction during sleep. A small number of older children and adults (<10%) are eventually able to manage without a tracheostomy.[65]

Although patient numbers remain small there is some long-term follow-up data available for diaphragmatic pacing. This includes information on a limited number of children (Table 42.4). In a retrospective study of quadriplegic adults, Carter et al. suggested that there was a survival advantage in patients supported by phrenic pacing.[70] The patients reported in this study were paced for a mean duration of 13.7 years, which is impressive given the limited life expectancy that follows traumatic quadriplegia.

Complications

The perioperative morbidity associated with implantation of a diaphragmatic pacing system is low and the mortality approaches zero. Intraoperative complications include damage to the phrenic nerve, especially in redo situations. One of our patients developed an empyema postoperatively and, as a consequence, we chose to replace the electrode in his neck rather than returning to the hostile thoracic cavity.[71] Immediate postoperative complications include a pneumothorax and, as alluded to earlier, infections. We do not leave a chest tube routinely at the end of the procedure since the visceral pleura is usually not damaged and we feel that this may add an unnecessary risk of infection. One patient developed a pneumothorax shortly after returning to the intensive care unit post-op. A chest tube was placed, the lung reexpanded immediately, and the tube was removed the following day.

The most common long-term issue is equipment failure. The receiver requires replacement most frequently. The subcutaneous location of the receiver makes this a relatively simple procedure, which can be performed as an outpatient. In recent years the longevity of the pacing receivers has increased considerably. Pacing electrodes occasionally need replacement because of fracture of the silicone sheath surrounding the wire. The most feared complication for these patients with diaphragmatic pacing devices is entrapment of the phrenic nerve as a consequence of scar tissue formation around the electrode. We have experienced this in one patient. A segmental phrenic nerve resection with primary reanastomosis was performed with partial recovery. Two other groups have reported successful recovery after phrenic nerve damage.[72,73]

Intramuscular electrode placement has been proposed as a method of avoiding intrathoracic dissection of the phrenic

TABLE 42.4. Diaphragmatic pacing in children – outcome series.

Author	No. of patients	Age	Diagnoses	Duration of pacing	Outcome
Eleftriades et al.[47]	4	7–15 years	C1/2 trauma = 4	2.5–18 years	3 continue on long-term pacing, 1 institutionalized on long-term IPPV after 2.5 years
Shaul et al.[66]	9	5–15 years	Cervical cord trauma = 1 CCAHS = 8	15–49 months	Successful pacing in 8
Weese-Mayer[67]	35	1–18 yearrs	Quadriplegia = 19 CCAHS = 14 Other = 2	0.1–3.6 years	Successful pacing with no reported complications in 60% children
Girsch[68]	8	2–13 years	CCAHS = 1 High cervical cord lesions = 7		
Flageole et al.[55]	3	1–5 years	CCAHS = 3	0.5–10 years	
Cahill et al.[69]	4	7.5–19 years	Cervical cord trauma = 47	9–47 months	All paced successfully, 1 died myocarditis 32m

nerves.[74] The abdominal surface of the diaphragm is approached laparoscopically, and electrodes are placed at the sites where the phrenic nerves enter the diaphragm. This requires electrophysiologic mapping to determine the optimum site for electrode placement since the phrenic nerves are not visible on the inferior surface of the diaphragm. Preliminary results appear comparable to conventional electrode placement.

Summary

Infants with CCAHS whose parents choose to continue treatment should be offered diaphragmatic pacing after the age of 1 year. It has an acceptably low complication rate and leads to greatly enhanced quality of life for these unfortunate children. Children with less severe forms of CCAHS who can breathe spontaneously during the day benefit from overnight pacing and thereby become free from mechanical ventilation. Patients with a more severe disease require overnight mechanical ventilation but can be paced during the day and, again, this augments their freedom greatly.

We now have three patients with diaphragmatic pacing systems who have reached adulthood. One young man, now aged 21, is a computer technician, and we have a young lady who is a member of her school's basketball team. These patients attest to the long-term benefits of diaphragmatic pacing technology.

References

1. Glenn WW, Anagnastopoulos CE. Electronic pacemakers of the heart, gastrointestinal tract, phrenic nerve, bladder, and carotid sinus: current status. Surgery 1966: 60; 480–94.
2. Hunt CE, Matalon SV, Thompson TR, et al. Central hypoventilation syndrome: experience with bilateral phrenic nerve pacing in 3 neonates. Am Rev Respir Dis 1978: 118; 23–8.
3. Nannapeneni R, Behari S, Todd NV, et al. Retracing "Ondine's Curse". Neurosurgery 2005: 57; 354–63.
4. Deonna T, Arczynska W, Torrado A. Congenital failure of automatic ventilation (Ondine's curse): a case report. J Pediatr 1974: 84; 710–14.
5. Furukawa T: Ondine's curse. Brain Nerve 2002: 54; 385–8.
6. Kuhn M, Lutolf M, Reinhart WH. The eye catcher: Ondine's curse. Respiration 1999: 66; 265.
7. Comroe JH Jr. Frankenstein, Pickwick, and Ondine. Am Rev Respir Dis 1975: 111; 689–92.
8. Sugar O. In search of Ondine's curse. JAMA 1978: 240; 236–7.
9. Sarnoff FJ, Whittenberger JL, Affeldt JE. Hypoventilation syndrome in bulbar poliomyelitis. JAMA 1951: 147; 30–6.
10. Severinghaus JW, Mitchell RA. Ondine's curse: failure of respiratory center automaticity while awake. J Clin Res 1962: 10; 122.
11. Mellins RB, Balfour HH Jr, Turino GM, et al. Failure of automatic control of ventilation (Ondine's curse). Medicine 1973: 49; 487–504.
12. Shannon DC, Marsland DW, Gould JB, et al. Central hypoventilation during quiet sleep in two infants. Pediatrics 1976: 57; 342–6.
13. Weese-Mayer DE, Brouillette RT, Naidich TP, et al. Magnetic resonance imaging and computerized tomography in central hypoventilation. Am Rev Respir Dis 1988: 137; 379–87.
14. Paton JY, Swaminathan S, Sargent CW, et al. Hypoxic and hypercapneic ventilatory responses in awake children with congenital hypoventilation syndrome. Am Rev Respir Dis 1989: 140; 368–72.
15. Paton JY, Swaminthan CW, Sargent A, et al. Ventilatory response to exercise in children with congenital central hypoventilation syndrome. Am Rev Respir Dis 1993: 147; 1185–91.
16. Marcus CL, Batista DB, Amihyia A, et al. Hypercapneic arousal responses in children with congenital central hypoventilation syndrome. Pediatrics 1991: 88; 993–8.
17. Gozal D, Marcus CL, Shoseyov D, et al. Peripheral chemoreceptor function in children with congenital central hypoventilation syndrome. J Appl Physiol 1993: 74; 379–87.
18. Woo Ms, Woo MA, Gozal D, et al. Heart rate variability in congenital central hypoventilation syndrome. Pediatr Res 1992: 1; 291–6.
19. Ogawa T, Kojo M, Fukushima N, et al. Cardio-respiratory control in an infant with Ondine's curse: a multivariate autoregressive modeling approach. J Auton Nerv Syst 1993: 42; 41–52.

20. Silvestri JM, Hanna BD, Volgman AS, et al. Cardiac rhythm disturbances among children with idiopathic congenital central hypoventilation syndrome. Pediatr Pulmonol 2000: 29; 351–8.
21. Kolb C, Eicken A, Zrenner B, et al. Cardiac pacing in a patient with diaphragm pacing for congenital central hypoventilation syndrome (Ondine's curse). J Cardiovasc Electrophysiol 2006: 17; 789–91.
22. Weese-Mayer DE, Berry-Kravis EM, Marazita ML. In pursuit (and discovery) of a genetic basis for congenital central hypoventilation syndrome. Respir Physiol Neurobiol 2005: 149; 73–82.
23. Amiel J, Laudier B, Attie-Bitach T, et al. Polyalanine expansion and frameshift mutations of the paired-like homeobox gene PHOX2B in congenital central hypoventilation syndrome. Nat Genet 2003: 33; 459–61.
24. Weese-Mayer DE, Berry-Kravis EM, Zhou L, et al. Idiopathic congenital central hypoventilation syndrome: analysis of genes pertinent to early autonomic nervous system embryologic development and identification of mutations in PHOX2B. Am J Med Genet 2003: 123A; 267–78.
25. Trang H, Dehan M, Beaufils F, et al. The French CCHS working group: the French congenital central hypoventilation syndrome registry: general data, phenotype, and genotype. Chest 2003: 127; 72–9.
26. Dubreuil V, Hirsch MR, Jouve C, et al. The role of Phox2b in synchronizing pan-neuronal and type-specific aspects of neurogenesis. Development 2002: 129; 5241–53.
27. Lo L, Morin X, Brunet JF, et al. Specification of neurotransmitter identity by Phox2 proteins in neural crest stem cells. Neuron 1999: 22; 693–705.
28. Pattyn A, Morin X, Cremer H, et al. The homeobox gene Phox2b is essential for the development of autonomic neural crest derivatives. Nature 1999: 399; 366–70.
29. Haddad GG, Mazza NM, Defendini R, et al. Congenital failure of automatic control of ventilation, gastrointestinal motility and heart rate. Medicine 1978: 57; 517–26.
30. Minutillo C, Pemberton PJ, Goldblatt J. Hirschsprung's disease and Ondine's curse: further evidence for a distinct syndrome. Clin Genet 1989: 36; 200–3.
31. Stern M, Hellwage HH, Gravinghoff L, et al. Total aganglionosis of the colon (Hirschsprung's disease) and congenital failure automatic control of ventilation (Ondine's curse). Acta Pediatr Scand 1981: 70; 121–4.
32. O'Dell K, Staren E, Bassuk A. Total colonic aganglionosis (Zuelzer-Wilson syndrome) and congenital failure of automatic control of ventilation (Ondine's curse). J Pediatr Surg 1987: 22; 1019–20.
33. Roshkow JE, Haller JO, Berdon WE, et al. Hirschsprung's disease, Ondine's curse and neuroblastoma: manifestations of neurocristopathy. Pediatr Radiol 1988: 19; 45–9.
34. Fodstad H, Ljunggren B, Shawis R. Ondine's curse with Hirschsprung's disease. Br J Neurosurg 1990: 4; 87–93.
35. El-Halaby E, Coran A. Hirschsprung's disease associated with Ondine's curse: report of three cases and review of the literature. J Pediatr Surg 1994: 29; 530–5.
36. Gaisie G, Kook SO, Young LW. Coexistent neuroblastoma Hirschsprung's disease – another manifestation of the neurocristopathy. Pediatr Radiol 1979: 8; 161–3.
37. Hunt CE, Matalon SV, Thompson TR, et al. Central hypoventilation syndrome: experience with bilateral phrenic nerve pacing in 3 neonates. Am Rev Respir Dis 1978: 188; 23–8.
38. Garcia RD, Carillo A, Bartolome M, et al. Central hypoventilation syndrome associated with ganglioneuroblastoma. Eur J Pediatr Surg 1995: 5; 292–4.
39. Sforza E, Colomaria V, Lugaresi E. Neurofibromatosis associated with central hypoventilation syndrome during sleep. Acta Pediatr 1994: 83; 794–6.
40. Bolande RP. The neurocristopathies: a unifying concept of disease arising in neural crest maldevelopment. Human Pathol 1974: 5; 409–29.
41. Bolande RP. Neurocristopathy: its growth and development in 20 years. Pediatr Pathol Lab Med 1997: 17; 1–25.
42. Guilleminault C, McQuitty CJ, Ariagno RL, et al. Congenital central alveolar hypoventilation syndrome in six infants. Pediatrics 1982: 70; 684–94.
43. Keens T, Hoppenbrouwers T. Congenital central hypoventilation syndrome (770.81). In: Diagnostic Classification Steering Committee of the American Sleep Disorders Association. The International Classification of Sleep disorders: Diagnostic and Coding Manual. Allen Press Inc., Lawrence, KS, 1990, pp. 205–9.
44. Wick AB, Menter RR. Long-term outlook in quadriplegic patients with initial ventilator dependency. Chest 1986: 90; 406–10.
45. Glenn WW, Holcomb WG, McLaughlin AJ, et al. Total ventilatory support in a quadriplegic patient with radiofrequency electrophrenic respiration. N Engl J Med 1972: 286; 513–16.
46. Ragnarsson KT. Functional electrical stimulation after spinal cord injury: current use, therapeutic effects and future directions. Spinal Cord 2008: 46; 255–74.
47. Elefteriades JA, Quin JA, Hogan JF et al. Long-term follow-up of pacing of the conditioned diaphragm in quadriplegia. J Pacing Clin Electrophysiol 2002: 25; 897–906.
48. Tibbals J, Henning RD. Noninvasive strategies in the management of a newborn infant and three children with congenital central hypoventilation syndrome. Pediatr Pulmonol 2003: 36; 544–8.
49. Midwinter KI, Carrie S, Bull PD. Pediatric tracheostomy: Sheffield experience. J Laryngol Otol 2002: 116; 532–5.
50. Hill BP, Singer LT. Speech and language development after infant tracheostomy. J Speech Hear Disord 1990: 55; 15–20.
51. Morar P, Singh V, Makura Z, et al. Orophrayngeal carriage and lower airway colonization/infection in 45 tracheostomised children. Thorax 2002: 57; 1015–20.
52. Ellis ER, McCauley VB, Mellis C, et al. Treatment of alveolar hypoventilation in a six-year-old girl with intermittent positive pressure ventilation through a nose mask. Am Rev Respir Dis 1987: 136; 188–91.
53. Villa MP, Dotta A, Castello D, et al. Bi-level positive airway pressure (BiPAP) ventilation in an infant with central hypoventilation syndrome. Pediatr Pulmonol 1990: 9; 44–5.
54. Tibballs J, Henning RD. Noninvasive ventilatory strategies in the management of a newborn infant and three children with congenital central hypoventilation syndrome. Pediatr Pulmonol 2003: 36; 544–8.
55. Flageole H. Central hypoventilation and diaphragmatic eventration: diagnosis and management. Semin Pediatr Surg 2003: 12; 38–45.
56. Moxham J, Shneerson JM. Diaphragmatic pacing – clinical commentary. Am Rev Respir Dis 1993: 148; 533–6.
57. Similowski T, Straus C, Attali V, et al. Assessment of the motor pathway to the diaphragm using cortical and cervical magnetic stimulation in the decision-making process of phrenic pacing. Chest 2006: 110; 1551–7.

58. Creasey G, Elefteriades J, DiMarco A, et al. Electrical stimulation to restore respiration. J Rehab Res Dev 1996: 33; 123–32.
59. Avery Biomedical Devices, Inc. Commack, NY, USA. www.averylabs.com.
60. Atrotech Ltd, Tampere, Finland. http://www.atrotech.com.
61. Glenn WWL, Phelps ML. Diaphragm pacing by electrical stimulation of the phrenic nerve. Neurosurgery 1985: 17; 974–84.
62. Loukas M, Kinsella CR, Louis RG, et al. Surgical anatomy of the accessory phrenic nerve. Ann Thorac Surg 2006: 82; 1870–5.
63. Garrido-Garcia H, Alvarez JM, Escribano PM, et al. Treatment of chronic ventilatory failure using a diaphragmatic pacemaker. Spinal Cord 1998: 36; 310–14.
64. Weese-Mayer DE, Hunt CE, Brouillette RT, et al. Diaphragm pacing in infants and children. J Pediatr 1992: 120; 1–8.
65. Chervin RD, Guilleminault C. Diaphragm pacing: review and reassessment. Sleep 1994: 17; 76–87.
66. Shaul DB, Danielson PD, McComb JG, et al. Thoracoscopic placement of phrenic nerve electrodes for diaphragmatic pacing in children. J Pediatr Surg 2002; 37: 974–8.
67. Weese-Mayer DE, Silvestri JM, Kenny AS, et al. Diaphragm pacing with a quadripolar phrenic nerve electrode: an international study. Pacing Clin Electrophysiol 1996; 19: 1311–19.
68. Girsch W, Koller R, Holle J, et al. Vienna phrenic pacemaker – experience with diaphragm pacing in children. Eur J Pediatr Surg 1996; 6: 140–3.
69. Cahill JL, Okamoto GA, Higgins T, et al. Experiences with phrenic nerve pacing in children. J Pediatr Surg 1983; 18: 851–4.
70. Carter RE, Donovan WH, Halstead L, et al. Comparative study of electrophrenic nerve stimulation and mechanical ventilatory support in traumatic spinal cord injury. Paraplegia 1987; 25: 86–91.
71. Flageole H, Adolph VR, Davis GM, et al. Diaphragmatic pacing in children with congenital central hypoventilation syndrome. Surgery 1995: 118; 25–8.
72. Shoemaker M, Palmer G, Brown JM, et al. Aggressive treatment of acquired phrenic nerve paralysis in infants and small children. Ann Thorac Surg 1981: 32; 258–9.
73. Brouillette RT, Hahn YS, Noah ZL, et al. Successful reinnervation of the diaphragm after phrenic nerve transection. J Pediatr Surg 1986: 21; 63–5.
74. DiMarco AF, Onders RP, Ignagni A, et al. Phrenic nerve pacing via intramuscular diaphragm electrodes in tetraplegic subjects. Chest 2005: 127; 671–8.

Section 9
Chest Wall Abnormalities

43
Pectus Excavatum

Robert E. Kelly and Donald Nuss

Introduction

Pectus excavatum (Latin: excavated chest) is a depression of the anterior chest wall and is the most frequent chest wall deformity, occurring in 1 in 400 to 1 in 1,000 children.[1] It constitutes about 90% of childhood chest wall deformities. It is to be distinguished from pectus carinatum, in which the sternum and costal cartilages protrude too far anteriorly, producing what has been called a "pouter pigeon chest" or "keel" chest. Although often present at birth, the depression may arise from a normal chest or progress in a congenital case at the time of puberty. Although the physiologic and psychologic consequences vary for a large number of patients, the lesion is troublesome enough that they welcome corrective surgery.

Historical Perspective

Pectus excavatum was recognized and described at least as early as the sixteenth century. Johan Schenck (1531–1590) collected literature on the subject, as cited in Ebstein.[2] Symptoms of dyspnea and paroxysmal cough were attributed to severe pectus excavatum by Bauhinus in 1594.[3] It was not until the twentieth century that general anesthesia permitted surgical treatment for the condition.

In 1911 in Germany, Meyer made a failed attempt at treatment by resection of the second and third costal cartilages.[4] Two years later Sauerbruch succesfully treated a watch maker with a pectus excavatum incapacitated by dyspnea and palpitations.[5] Surgical treatment involved excision of a section of the anterior chest wall, including the left fifth to ninth costal cartilages, and a segment of the adjacent sternum. After recovery the patient was able to resume work without dyspnea in his father's watch factory, despite visible cardiac pulsations beneath a muscle flap. He was married three years later. By the 1920s, Sauerbruch performed the first pectus repair utilizing bilateral costal cartilage resection and sternal osteotomy,[6] a technique popularized by Ravitch's reports more than 20

years later. Sauerbruch advocated external traction for six weeks after operation.

Oschsner and Debakey published a review in 1939 of all the published cases and surgical approaches for pectus repair up to that time.[7] Simple line drawings depicted the varied resections utilized. That same year, Lincoln Brown proposed that shortened diaphragmatic ligaments attached to the undersurface of the sternum caused the condition.[8] Though clearly disproven by thoracoscopy, some physicians still mistakenly adhere to this theory today.

In 1948, Ravitch had success with an extensive operation at Johns Hopkins which mobilized the sternum completely, divided all sternal attachments including the intercostal bundles, rectus muscles, diaphragmatic attachments, and excised the xiphisternum.[9] By 1958, Welch at Boston Children's Hospital advocated a less radical approach, preserving the intercostal bundles.[10]

Internal support was suggested in 1950 by Dorner, who utilized homologous rib.[11] Metal support was described first in 1956 by Wallgren and Sulamaa, who pushed a slightly curved stainless steel bar through the caudal end of the sternum from side to side and bridged the newly created gap between the sternum and ribs.[12] In 1961, Adkins and Blades suggested passing the bar behind the sternum rather than through it.[13] A variety of other techniques have been reported to be effective: Titanium miniplates,[14] Dacron vascular graft strut,[15] seagull wing self retaining prosthesis,[16] bioabsorbable weave,[17] and substernal mesh bands.[18] Plastic surgeons have treated pectus excavatum by implantation of silicone bags in the depression, which restores the external contour of the chest, but does not address the shape of the chest wall.[19,20] Sternal turnover was a totally new concept introduced in 1954 by Judet.[21] In 1968, Wada of Japan reported a large series.[22] He removed the whole deformed sternum, turned it over, and sutured it back in place. This procedure was not widely adopted outside Japan, because of major complications in the event of infection.

Concern regarding the growth of the chest after resection of the entire length of the costal cartilages was voiced by Pena and associates in a 1990 report describing failure of growth of

D.H. Parikh et al. (eds.), *Pediatric Thoracic Surgery*,
DOI: 10.1007/b136543_43, © Springer-Verlag London Limited 2009

the thoracic cage following costochondral cartilage resection in baby rabbits.[23] The human counterpart of this phenomenon was described in 1996 by Haller and associates, who reported chest wall constriction after too extensive and too early operations.[24]

In 1997, Nuss presented a 10-year experience with a minimally invasive technique requiring no cartilage incision or resection, no sternal osteotomy, relying instead on placement of an internal brace with a stainless steel bar.[25] This technique was made possible by the flexibility of costal cartilage. The rationale for this technique was based on the malleability of the pediatric chest.[26,27] Chest reconfiguration occurs in adults who develop a barrel-shaped chest in response to the stiff lungs of chronic obstructive pulmonary disease.[28] The technique has been adopted world wide with positive results.

Pathogenesis and Basic Science

The etiology of pectus excavatum is unknown. Epidemiological hints its cause may lie in the animal kingdom and geographic distribution and heritability. Animals occasionally affected include dogs and cats.[29] The incidence of pectus excavatum in man varies from 38 per 10,000 births among white infants to 7 per 10,000 births among African-American infants in a 1975 Collaborative Perinatal Project in the United States. This study represented a collaborative endeavor by 12 major medical centers and the National Institute of Neurological and Communicative Disorders and Stroke of the National Institutes of Health.[1] Reports of large numbers of cases treated surgically have appeared from the Far East and in the Indian subcontinent.[22,30] A report of congenital chest wall malformations in Nigerians surveying 2,195 autopsies from the University of Ilorin reported one patient with Poland's syndrome, one with Cantrell's syndrome, and none with pectus excavatum, suggesting it is an uncommon occurrence among black Africans.[31] However, it may be that the condition was simply not recorded, as was the case in autopsies at Johns Hopkins until 1947.

Pectus excavatum has a strong familial tendency. A family with three affected brothers was reported by Coulson in 1820.[32] Fifty years later, a 17-year-old patient born with pectus excavatum was reported by Williams, who noted that his father and brother were also affected.[33] In our series of patients, about 45% of patients with pectus excavatum have a family history.[34] The mode of inheritance was sought in 34 families with more than one affected individual. Of the 34 families, 14 families suggested autosomal dominant inheritance, 4 families suggested autosomal recessive inheritance, 6 families suggested X-linked recessive inheritance, and 10 families had complex inheritance patterns.[35]

The effects on longevity and health after childhood attributable to untreated pectus excavatum remain unclear. To examine this, a study of all patients noted to have pectus excavatum at autopsy at a major medical center with a longstanding interest in the condition over a 112-year period was made. Pectus excavatum was identified in 62 of 50,496 cases at Johns Hopkins between 1889 and 2001. Of those 62 patients, 17 were 65 years or older and appeared to have died of causes unrelated to pectus excavatum, the oldest being 91 years. The severity of the deformity could not be determined from the autopsy data. Survival analysis indicated that pectus excavatum patients had a different survival than controls. Pectus excavatum patients tended to die earlier; but pectus excavatum patients who survived past the age of 56 years tended to survive longer than their matched controls. There were no reported cases of pectus excavatum before 1947, roughly coincident with Ravitch's reports from the same institution.[28]

No consistent histological abnormalities have been identified in the cartilage of patients with pectus excavatum but associations with several connective tissue abnormalities were identified in the autopsy series report.[28] These associations include Marfan syndrome, in about 25% of patients, and Ehlers Danlos syndrome in 5% of patients.[34]

Pulmonary function tests in affected patients have shown that preoperative forced vital capacity (FVC) and forced expiratory volume (FEV_1) medians lower than normal by 13%. Forced expiratory flow (FEF_{25-75}) medians are lower than normal by 20%. Postoperative patients show statistically significant improvement after surgery by the Nuss procedure for all parameters. Patients older than 11 years at the time of surgery had lower preoperative values and larger mean postbar removal improvement than younger patients. An older patient with a preoperative FEF_{25-75} score of 80% of normal would be predicted by our data to have a postoperative FEF_{25-75} of 97%, indicating almost complete normalization for this function. FVC and FEV_1 also improved by clinically significant amounts. These results are consistent with patient reports of clinical improvement.

Since patients with pectus excavatum seldom complain of shortness of breath at rest, but rather during heavy exertion like running or swimming, exercise pulmonary function tests should be expected to show more profound differences. A comprehensive search of the literature identified eight studies that met all inclusion criteria. Those studies of 169 pectus excavatum patients indicated that surgical repair of pectus excavatum significantly improves cardiovascular function. Malek reported a metaanalysis of cardiovascular function following surgical repair of pectus excavatum in 2006.[36] Previously, Malek et al. had reported on 21 patients with severe pectus excavatum who underwent exercise pulmonary functions testing. Maximum oxygen uptake (VO_2max) and oxygen pulse (VO_2max/cardiac frequency) – both indices of maximum aerobic exercise capacity – were significantly lower than the reference values. Patients exhibited cardiovascular limitation, but not ventilatory limitation. The metabolic threshold for lactate accumulation was abnormally low (41% of the reference value), and was consistent with cardiovascular impairment rather than physical deconditioning.[37]

Clinical Features

Pectus excavatum is a depression of the anterior chest wall and is almost always worst in the region of the inferior sternum. The depth and shape of the depression are variable. Often asymmetric, the depression of the chest can be localized and deep (cup-shaped Fig. 43.1), diffused and shallow (saucer-shaped Fig. 43.2), or may extend cephalad to the clavicles (furrow-shaped). A depression on one side of the sternum may be associated with a protrusion on the other side (a mixed carinatum/excavatum deformity).[38] Many but not all patients are tall and thin suggesting a connective tissue disorder. About 20% patients show physical signs of Marfan syndrome, and 2% of Ehlers-Danlos syndrome.[34] Mild scoliosis is present in about 20% of patients and severe scoliosis in another 10%. The depression may be noted at birth or appear during childhood. It tends to progress as the child grows and is especially prone to progress during puberty. Whether patients "outgrow" pectus excavatum remains dubious. Patients tend to stand with a posture characterized by thoracic kyphosis, rounded shoulders, and a protuberant abdomen (Fig. 43.3). In severe cases, symptoms are frequent (Table 43.1) and are dominated by complaints of easy fatigability, shortness of breath on exertion, and short-duration chest pain, often over the mid or lower sternum of just to one side of the sternum. Ravitch noted 50 years ago that while some patients have no limitation of activity, "it is more common to hear of a boy who can 'fool around' shooting basketball but not play a game, or play a game of tennis but not a set."[9]

Self consciousness about the appearance of the chest arises in many. Usually children develop this concern around school age, since classmates often point out their previously unrecognized "flaw" using unflattering words. Many school-age patients become unwilling to go swimming or play sports they might otherwise play to avoid ridicule.[39] Just as one would not leave cleft lip untreated, surgical correction of such a disruptive problem should be undertaken when practical.

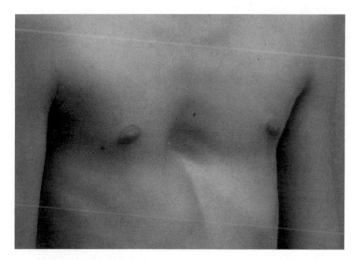

FIG. 43.1. Cup-shaped excavatum deformity

Diagnosis

Diagnosis of pectus excavatum is made by physical examination. On visual examination, the patients not only have an obvious depression of the anterior chest wall but also have the classic pectus posture, consisting of rounded shoulders and protuberant abdomen (Fig. 43.3). It is important to examine the patient in different positions, since seated or standing positions can exaggerate the defect by flexion of the thoracic spine. The supine position gives the most reproducible result. Palpation is helpful to determine cardiac displacement and sternal torsion. Determining the location of the deepest part of the depression is helpful in planning surgical correction. Usually the deepest point is at the xiphoid or inferior of the sternum. If the deepest point is not in the midline, the depression is asymmetric (Fig. 43.4). The costal cartilages inferior to the sternum are sometimes "flared" that is they protrude anteriorly in the upper abdomen inferior to the depression.

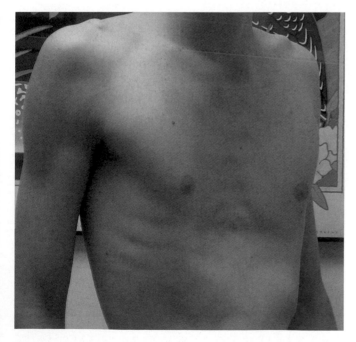

FIG. 43.2. Saucer-shaped excavatum deformity

Investigations

Since many patients with pectus excavatum complain of exercise intolerance, easy fatigability, or chest pain, we obtain pulmonary function studies and echocardiography on all patients. Static pulmonary function tests (PFT's) do not generally show profound deficits but in a large series of patients (more than 600) we have found that the mean forced vital capacity

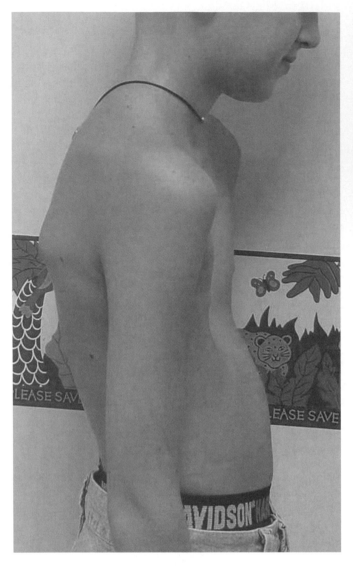

Fig. 43.3. Posture characterized by thoracic kyphosis, rounded shoulders, and a protuberant abdomen

Table 43.1. Preoperative symptoms in patients undergoing repair of pectus excavatum ($N = 900$).

Exercise intolerance	739 (82%)
Chest pain (with or without exercise)	615 (68%)
Lack of endurance	603 (67%)
Shortness of breath	386 (43%)
Asthma or asthma-like symptoms	257 (29%)
Frequent URI	226 (25%)
Mild scoliosis	150 (17%)
Severe scoliosis	91 (10%)

(FVC), forced expiratory volume in one second (FEV_1), and the midportion of the forced expiratory flow (FEF_{25-75}) are in the low normal range of 80–89% of predicted values, whereas in the normal population, the majority are in the 90–110%

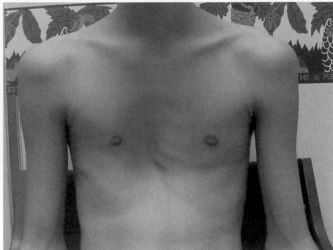

Fig. 43.4. Asymmetric excavatum deformity

range. It is frequently the case that static PFTs are 85% predicted while the VO_2 max in the same patient is in the 50–65% predicted range. It is important that the exercise PFTs be done by a protocol that seeks to measure gas exchange. Recent reports verify the sustained improvement in performance following repair.[40]

Cardiology

Common cardiology protocols such as the Bruce protocol will be reported as showing a normal response to exercise, since the patient will not have EKG findings of cardiac ischemia, and will increase heart rate in a normal way.

Cardiology evaluation is important since a significant fraction of patients will have findings of right ventricular compression or mitral valve prolapse.[41] It is also useful in patients with exertional chest pain for whom one contemplates a major thoracic operation to assure normal cardiac function. For example, we have uncovered an unrecognized AV canal defect requiring surgical repair during pre-operative testing for pectus repair. Some of the decreased ability to do work noted in the exercise studies may be explained by decreased cardiac output due to compression of the heart, which results in incomplete filling and decreased stroke volume. Compression can also interfere with normal valve function. Mitral valve prolapse was present in 17% of our patients, and in up to 65% of those in other series, compared with only 1% in the normal pediatric population.[41–43] Dysrhythmias, including first-degree heart block, right bundle branch block, and Wolff-Parkinson-White syndrome were present in 16% of our series.[28]

Radiological Diagnosis

Radiological evaluation of pectus excavatum can be carried out with plain lateral chest X-ray by measuring the distance

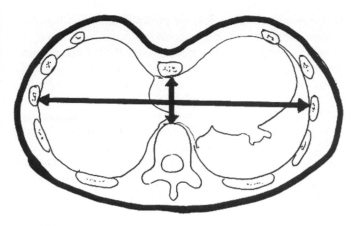

FIG. 43.5. Pectus index

from the posterior surface of the sternum to the anterior edge of the body of the spine. Computed tomographic (CT) scan provides much more information regarding the anatomy of the defect. Haller suggested dividing the transverse diameter by the AP diameter, which gives a useful indicator of severity (Fig. 43.5).[44] In normal patients, the ratio is 2.0 or less.[45] Haller and associates reported severe pectus corresponded to an index of 3.2 or greater. CT scans should by convention be obtained in quiet respiration, not at full inspiration, since the pectus index is markedly changed at full inspiration. In measuring the pectus index in a patient with a deep (barrel) chest that arithmetic will reduce the Haller index and under-represent the severity of the depression. CT scans also give much better assessment of cardiac compression and displacement: Asymmetry of the cartilaginous component of the chest wall, the three-dimensional nature of the depression is better seen by CT, and the vertical extent of the depression and the amount of sternal torsion associated with twisted costal cartilages are better seen and measured by CT. These factors may allow better determination of appropriate surgical treatment such as where to place the bars and whether two or more bars are needed. Most of the advantages of CT are accrued by MRI without radiation but most radiologists believe that bony structures like the chest wall are better evaluated by CT. Also, the CT images can be acquired in about a minute, without the concerns for sedation or claustrophobia, which often occurs during the 20 min or so in a dark noisy tunnel to get the MRI scan. Respiratory motion of the chest wall is insignificant on CT, but not on MRI.

Management

Antenatal/Perinatal Management

Pectus excavatum has been rarely noted antenatally.[46] In our perinatal center, which cares for 5,000 deliveries per year, we have encountered only one case in ten years (personal communication, Alfred Abuhamad MD, 2007), although pectus excavatum is common at birth. Shamberger states 33% of pectus deformities are present at birth.[41]

Medical

Prior to the twentieth century, treatment was confined to fresh air and exercise without success. Various exercises, efforts to improve posture and braces such as the "figure of eight" clavicular fracture splint have been employed. Critical studies of their effectiveness are lacking. Because compression braces have been very successful in correcting pectus carinatum,[47] novel approaches to treat pectus excavatum with external suction[48] and implanted magnets[49] have been attempted without success to date. The external suction approach has suffered from recurrence and skin injury. The implanted magnet approach is moving to phase I clinical trial.

Surgical

Conventional Operative Techniques: Description of Modified Ravitch Operation

Because of the occurrence of asphyxiating thoracic chondrodystrophy following extensive cartilage resection, most surgeons perform a less extensive resection than previously.[50] In the open technique, an anterior thoracic incision is made, which can be either infra-mammary or vertical. Skin flaps are elevated, and the pectoralis major and rectus abdominal muscles are reflected off the sternum. The third through sixth costal cartilages are exposed. The perichondrium is incised. The standard approach is to make a longitudinal incision through the perichondrium and then remove the entire deformed cartilage, preserving the perichondrium. An increase in number of surgeons now favor removing two short segments of the cartilage, each about a centimeter long, at either end of the cartilage, taking care to preserve the bone – cartilage junction as it is the epiphyseal growth plate. An osteotomy is performed through the anterior table of the sternum at the location of the angulation. The posterior table is fractured, and then the sternum is elevated and untwisted if necessary. The osteotomy is closed with nonabsorbable sutures. A strut may be inserted under the sternum to bridge the gap between the ribs and the sternum and prevent the sternum from sinking back into the chest. The perichondrial "sleeves" are resutured, drains are inserted, the muscle flaps sutured back into position and the incisions are closed. Postoperative management is similar to that of the closed technique, except that patients are required to refrain from contact sports for at least three months vs. six weeks for the closed technique.

Minimally Invasive Operative Techniques: Description of Nuss Operation

In the minimally invasive approach, a convex stainless steel or titanium bar (Biomet Microfixation, Jacksonville, Florida) (Fig. 43.6) is inserted under the sternum, elevating it anteriorly

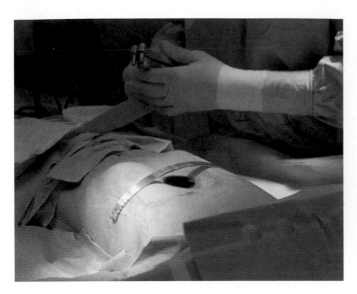

FIG. 43.6. Pectus bar bent to the contour of the chest

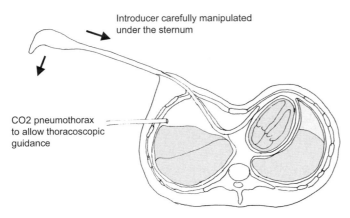

Introducer carefully manipulated under the sternum

CO2 pneumothorax to allow thoracoscopic guidance

FIG. 43.7. Bar introducer

and holding it in the desired position. Incisions on each side of the chest are used to create a subcutaneous tunnel from the lateral chest to the top of the pectus ridge on each side. The pectus ridge is the most anterior prominence lateral to the depression on each side. At the top of the ridge, bilateral thoracostomy incisions are made, and then a centimeter wide, flat, appropriately curved metal tunneler (an introducer Fig. 43.7) is inserted into the chest under thoracoscopic guidance.

Very carefully, with the thoracoscope in place and the introducer and vital structures under good vision, the pleura and pericardium are dissected off the undersurface of the sternum (Fig. 43.8). The introducer is slowly advanced across the mediastinum and then brought out through the thoracostomy incision on the contralateral side (Fig. 43.9). When the introducer has been passed across the mediastinum, it is lifted anteriorly, while at the same time applying pressure on the lower costal margin. Elevating the sternum with the introducer is repeated until the sternal depression has been corrected. An umbilical tape is attached to the introducer, and the introducer

is slowly pulled back across the mediastinum by withdrawing it from the chest. A pectus support bar is then attached to the umbilical tape and slowly guided through the substernal tunnel by applying traction on the umbilical tape under thoracoscopic scope control, with the convexity of the bar facing posteriorly until it emerges on the contralateral side (Fig. 43.10).

The length of the bar is determined by measuring the distance from the mid-axillary line to mid-axillary line and subtracting 2.5 cm (1 in.). The bar is bent to the desired configuration at the operating table. Once the bar is in position inside the chest with the convexity facing posteriorly, it is turned over by using specially designed bar flippers (Fig. 43.11). This gives instant correction of the pectus excavatum. The bar is stabilized by wiring a stabilizer to one end of the bar (Fig. 43.12) and by placing sutures around the bar and underlying ribs. The sutures are usually placed with thoracoscopic guidance by using an autosuture needle. It is essential that the bar be adequately stabilized or it will displace with activity after recovery. Once the bar is in position, the incisions are closed. The thoracoscope is removed, and the pneumothorax is evacuated by using a water-seal system. Postoperative analgesia is provided by a thoracic epidural for three postoperative days. Discharge from hospital is usually possible on the fourth or fifth day. Patients need to refrain from sporting activities for six weeks after surgery. All patients are started on an exercise and posture program to facilitate chest expansion and to maintain a good posture.

Severe scoliosis associated with pectus excavatum and acquired thoracic dystrophy may be managed by the vertically expandable prosthetic titanium rib (VEPTR). Expansion thoracoplasty with this device allows serial expansion of the chest wall to allow continued growth of the thorax and spine until skeletal maturity is achieved. More than 300 patients with various disorders have been treated with this technique, developed by Campbell and associates.[51] Anterior rib osteotomies adjacent to the costochondral junction and posterior osteotomies adjacent to the transverse process of the spine in ribs three to nine are performed in Jeune's asphyxiating thoracic dystrophy. The mobilized segment of thoracic wall is distracted, moved postero-laterally, and anchored to a curved metallic device that is attached to the second and tenth ribs. The mobilized section of chest is secured to the VEPTR with 2 mm titanium rings stabilizing the segment and allowing healing of the multiple osteotomies. A second stage is done three months later. The devices can be expanded every six months as necessary.[52]

Complications

Description and Incidence

Until now complications following the open operation have all been recorded retrospectively. Table 43.2 shows the prospectively obtained operative complication rates from a

FIG. 43.8. Transthoracic dissection under thoracoscopic guidance

Underside of sternum

Pericardium

Tip of introducer negotiated under sternum, avoiding the pericardium

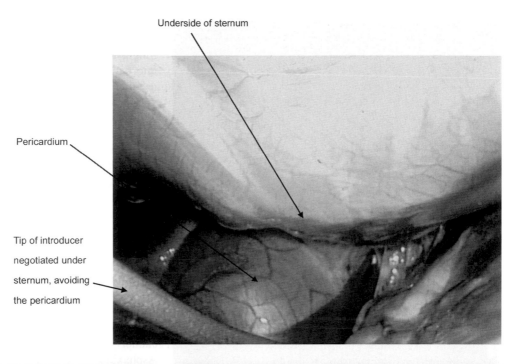

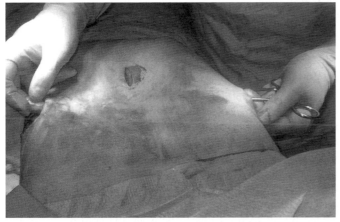

FIG. 43.9. Bar introducer emerging from the opposite side of the thorax. Instead of using thoracoscopy, a short incision has been made below the xiphisternum to allow the surgeon's finger to guide the introducer through the chest

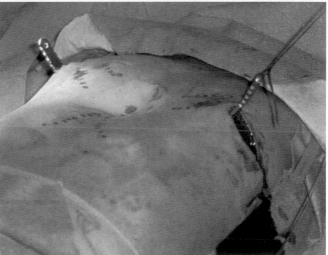

FIG. 43.10. Pectus bar drawn through the thorax

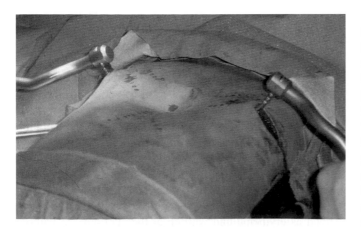

FIG. 43.11. Pectus bar "flippers" applied in preparation to rotate the bar

multicenter study of pectus excavatum in the US and Canada. Collected by study nurses, these data have been compiled by centers performing both Nuss and Ravitch-type operations. Overall, the initial postoperative complication rates are low and similar for the open and closed operations. With either type of operation rare bizarre complications have occurred: With open operation, cardiac perforation by the stabilizing bar,[53] migration of the stabilizing bar into the ventricle of the heart,[54–55] hemopericardium,[56] laceration of the phrenic artery,[57] and movement of the bar into the abdomen have been reported.[58] Nuss operation patients have suffered cardiac perforation,[59–60] erosion of the pectus bar into the great vessels following untreated displacement,[61] and pulmonary injury in published reports.

References

1. Chung CS, Myrianthopoulos NC. Factors affecting risks of congenital malformations. I. Analysis of epidemiologic factors in congenital malformations. Report from the Collaborative Perinatal Project. Birth Defects Orig Artic Ser 1975; 11(10):1–22.

2. Ebstein E. Die Trichterbrust in inhren Beziehungen zur Konstitution. Zeitschr. F. Konstitutionslehre 1921; 8:103.

3. Bauhinus J. Observationum Medicariam. Liber II, Observ. 264, Francfurti 1600; 507.

4. Meyer L. Zurchirurqishen Behandlung der augeborenen Trichterbrust. Verh Bel Med Gest 1911; 42:364.

5. Sauerbruch F. Die Chirurgie der Brustorgane, Vol 1. Berlin, Springer, 1920; 437.

6. Sauerbruch F. Operative Beseitigung der Angeborenen Trichterbrust. Deutsche Zeitschr f. Chir 1931; 234:760–4.

7. Ochsner A, DeBakey M. Chone-Chondrosternon: report of a case and review of the litterature. J Thorac Surg 1939; 8:469–511.

8. Brown AL. Pectus excavatum. J Thorac Surg 1939; 9:164–84.

9. Ravitch MM. The chest wall. Pediatric Surgery, 4th edition. Year Book Medical Publishers, 1986; 568.

10. Welch KJ. Satisfactory surgical correction of pectus excavatum deformity in childhood. J Thorac Surg 1958; 36:697–713.

11. Dorner RA, Keil PG, Schissel DJ. Pectus excavatum. J Thorac Surg 1950; 20:444.

12. Wallgren GR, Sulamaa M. Surgical treatment of funnel chest. Exhib. VIII, Internat. Cong Paediat 1956; 32.

13. Adkins PC, Blades BA. A stainless steel strut for correction of pectus excavatum. Surg Gynecol Obstet 1961; 113:111–3

14. De Agustin-Asensio JC, Banuelos C, Vazquez JJ. Titanium miniplates for the surgical correction of pectus excavatum. J Am Coll Surg 1999; 188:455–8.

15. Lane-Smith DM, Gillis DA, Roy PD. Repair of pectus excavatum using a Dacron vascular graft strut. J Pediatr Surg 1994; 29:1179–82.

16. Actis Dato GM, Cavaglia M. Ruffini E. The seagull wing self retaining prosthesis in the surgical treatment of pectus excavatum. J Cardiovasc Surg (Torino) 1999; 40:139–46.

17. Brooks JP, Tripp HF. Bioabsorbable weave technique for repair of pectus excavatum. J Thorac Cardiovasc Surg 2000; 119:176–8.

18. Karagounis VA, Wasnick J, Gold JP. An innovative signle-stage repair of severe asymmetric pectus excavatum defects using substernal mesh bands. Ann Thorac Surg 2004; 78:e19–21.

19. Marks MW, Argenta LC, Lee DC. Silicone implant correction of pectus excavatum: indications and refinement in technique. Plast Reconstr Surg 1984; 74:52–8.

20. Sorensen JL. Subcutaneous silicone implants in pectus excavatum. Scand J Plast Reconstr Surg Hand Surg 1988: 22; 173–6.

21. Judet J, Judet R. Thorax en entonnoir. Un Procede Operatoire. Rev Orthop 1954; 40:248–57.

22. Wada J, Ideda K, Ishida T. Results of 271 funnel chest operations. Ann Thorac Surg 1970; 10(6):526–32.

23. Martinez D, Juame J, Stein T, et al. The effect of costal cartilage resection on chest wall development. Ped Surg Int 1990; 5:170–3.

24. Haller JA, Columbani PR, Humphries C. Chest wall reconstruction after too extensive and too early operations for pectus excavatum. Ann Thorac Surg 1996; 61:1618–25.

25. Nuss D, Kelly RE, Croitoru DP. A 10-year review of a minimally invasive technique for the correction of pectus excavatum. J Pediatr Surg 1998; 33:545–52.

26. Kelley SW. Surgical diseases of children. Dislocations, congenital and acquired, Vol 1, 3rd edition. St. Louis, C.V. Mosby Co, 1929; 537.

27. Haller JA. Thoracic injuries. In Welch KJ, Randolph JG, Ravitch MM (eds.) Pediatric Surgery, Vol 1, 4th edition. Chicago, Year Book Medical Publishers, 1986; 147.

28. Nuss D, Croitoru DP, Kelly RE. Congenital chest wall deformities. In Ashcraft KW, Holcomb GW III, Murphy JP (eds.) Pediatric Surgery, 4th edition. Philadelphia, Elsevier Saunders, 2005; 245–63.

29. Fossum TW, Boudrieau RJ, Hobson HP, et al. Surgical correction of pectus excavatum, using external splintage in two dogs and a cat. J Am Vet Med Assoc 1989: 195: 91–97.

30. Park HJ, Lee SY, Lee CS. Complications associated with the Nuss procedure: Analysis of risk factors and suggested measure of prevention of complications. J Pediatr Surg 2004; 39:391–5.

31. Odelowo EO. Congenital chest wall malformations in Nigerians. Afr J Med Sci 1989; 18:263–8.

32. Coulson W. Deformities of the chest. London Med Gaz 1820; 4:69–73.

33. Williams CT. Congenital malformation of the thorax: Great depression of the sternum. Tr Path Soc London 1872; 24:50.

34. Croitoru DP, Kelly RE, Nuss D. Experience and modification update for the minimally invasive Nuss technique for pectus excavatum repair in 303 patients. J Pediatr Surg 2002; 37:437–45.

35. Creswick H, Stacey MW, Kelly RE. Family study of the inheritance of pectus excavatum. J Pediatr Surg 2006; 41:1699–703.

36. Malek MH, Berger DE, Housh TJ. Cardiovascular function following surgical repair of pectus excavatum: A metaanalysis. Chest 2006; 130:506–16.

37. Malek MH, Fonkalsrud EW, Cooper CB. Ventilatory and cardiovascular responses to exercise in patients with pectus excavatum. Chest 2003; 124:870–82.

38. Cartoski MJ, Nuss D, Goretsky MJ. Classification of the dysmorphology of pectus excavatum. J Pediatr Surg 2006; 41:1573–81.

39. Lawson M, Cash T, Akers R. A pilot study of the impact of surgical repair on disease-specific quality of life among patients with pectus excavatum. J Pediatr Surg 2003: 38; 916–8.

40. Sigalet DL, Montgomery M, Harder J. Long term cardiopulmonary effects of closed repair of pectus excavatum. Pediatr Surg Int 2007; 23:493–7.

41. Shamberger RC, Welch KJ, Sanders SP. Mitral valve prolapse associated with pectus excavatum. J Pediatr 1987; 111:404–7.

42. Saint-Mezard G, Duret JC, Chanudet X. Mitral valve prolapse and pectus excavatum. Presse Med 1986; 15:439.

43. Warth DC, King ME, Cohen JM. Prevalence of mitral valve prolapse in normal children. J Am Coll Cardiol 1985; 5:1173–7.

44. Haller JA, Kramer SS, Lietman SA. Use of CT scans in selection of patients for pectus excavatum surgery: a preliminary report. J Pediatr Surg 1987; 22:904–6.

45. Daunt SW, Cohen JH, Miller SF. Age-related normal ranges for the Haller index in children. Pediatr Radiol 2004; 34:326–30.

46. Salamanca A, Girona A, Padilla M, et al. Prenatal diagnosis of pectus excavatum and its relation to Down's syndrome. Ultrasound Obstet Gynecol 1992; 2:446–7.

47. Haje SA, Bowen JR. Preliminary results of orthotic treatment of pectus deformities in children and adolescents. J Pediatr Orthop 1992; 12:795–800.

48. Schier F. Vacuum treatment of pectus excavatum. Eur J Cardiothorac Surg 2006; 30:687.

49. Harrison MR, Estefan-Ventura D, Fechter R. Magnetic mini-mover procedure for pectus excavatum: development, deisgn and simulations for feasibility and safety. J Pediatr Surg 2007; 42:81–6.

50. Fonkalsrud EW, DeUgarte D. Choi E. Repair of pectus excavatum and carinatum deformities in 116 adults. Ann Surg 2002; 236:304–12.

51. Campbell RM, Smith M. Treatment of thoracic insufficiency syndrome associated with congenital scoliosis. J Bone Joint Surg 79B 1997; 1:82.

52. Waldhausen JHT, Redding GH, Song KM. Vertical expandable prosthetic titanium rib for thoracic insufficiency syndrome: a new method to treat an old problem. J Pediatr Surg 2007; 42:76–80

53. Pircova AA, Sekarski-Hunkeler N, Jeanrenaud X, et al. Cardiac perforation after surgical repair of pectus excavatum. J Pediatr Surg 1995; 30:1506–8.

54. Dalrymple-Hay MJ, Calver A, Lea RE, et al. Migration of pectus excavatum correction bar into the left ventricle. Eur J Cardiothorac Surg 1997; 12:507–9.

55. Onursal E, Toker A, Bostanci K. A complication of pectus excavatum operation: endomyocardial steel strut. Ann Thorac Surg 1999; 68:1082–3.

56. Elami A. Lieberman Y. Hemopericardium: a late complication after repair of pectus excavatum. J Cardiovasc Surg (Torino) 1991; 32:539–40.

57. Paret G, Taustein I, Vardi A. Laceration of the phrenic artery. A life-threatening complication after repair of pectus excavatum. J Cardiovasc Surg (Torino) 1996; 37:193–4.

58. Stefani A, Morandi U, Lodi R. Migration of pectus excavatum correction metal support into the abdomen. Eur J Cardiothorac Surg 1998; 14:434–6.

59. Nuss D, Kelly RE, Croitoru DP. Repair of pectus excavatum. Pediatric Surgery & Innovative Techniques 1998; 2:205–221.

60. Hebra A, Swoveland B, Egbert M, et al. Outcome analysis of minimally invasive repair of pectus excavatum: review of 251 cases. J Pediatr Surg 2000; 35:252–7; discussion 257–8.

61. Hoel TN, Rein KA, Svennevig JL. A life-threatening complication of the Nuss procedure for pectus excavatum. Ann Thorac Surg 2006; 81:370–2.

62. Ellis DG, Snyder CL, Mann CM. The 'redo' chest wall deformity correction. J Pediatr Surg 1997; 32:1267–71.

63. Lacquet LK, Morshuis WJ, Folgering HT. Long-term results after correction of anterior chest wall deformities. J Cardiovasc Surg (Torino) 1998; 39:683–8.

64. Pretorius ES, Haller JA, Fishman EK. Spiral CT with 3D reconstruction in children requiring reoperation for failure of chest wall growth after pectus excavatum surgery. Preliminary observations. Clin Imaging 1998; 22:108–16.

65. Weber TR, Kurkchubasche A. Operative management of asphyxiating thoracic dystrophy after pectus repair. J Pediatr Surg 1998; 33:262–5.

66. Shin S, Goretsky MJ, Morales M. When it's not an infection: Metal allergy after the Nuss procedure for repair of pectus excavatum. J Pediatr Surg 2007; 42:3–7.

67. Calkins CM, Shen SB, Sharp RJ. Management of postoperative infections after the minimally invasive pectus excavatum repair. J Pediatr Surg 2005; 40:1004–7. Discussion 1007–8.

68. Elves MRWJ, Scales JT, Kemp HBS. Incidence of metal sensitivity in patients with total hip replacement. Br Med J 1975; 4:376–8.

69. Jensen CS, Lisby S, Baadsgaard O. Decrease in nickel sensitization in a Danish schoolgirl population with ears pierced after implementation of a nickel-exposure regulation. Br J Dermatol 2002; 146:636–42.

70. Johansen J, Menne T, Christophersen J. Changes in the pattern of sensitization to common contact allergens in Denmark between 1985–86 and 1997–98, with a special view to the effect of preventive strategies. Br J Dermatol 2000; 142:490–5.

71. Hebra A, Jacobs JP, Feliz A. Minimally invasive repair of pectus cxcavatum in adult patients. Am Surg 2006; 72:837–42.

72. Mansour KA, Thourani VH, Odessey EA. Thirty-year experience with repair of pectus deformities in adults. Ann Thorac Surg 2003; 76:391–5.

73. Kim do H, Hwang JJ, Lee MK. Analysis of the Nuss procedure for pectus excavatum in different age groups. Ann Thorac Surg 2005; 80:1073–7.

74. Coln D, Gunning T, Ramsay M. Early experience with the Nuss minimally invasive correction of pectus excavatum in adults. World J Surg 2002; 26:1217–21.

75. Schalamon J, Pokall S. Windhaber J. Minimally invasive correction of pectus excavatum in adult patients. J Thorac Cardiovasc Surg 2006; 132:524–9.

76. Roberts J, Hayashi A, Anderson JO. Quality of life of patients who have undergone the Nuss procedure for pectus excavatum: preliminary findings. J Ped Surg 2003; 38:779–83.

77. Krasopoulos G, Dusmet M. Nuss procedure improves the quality of life in young male adults with pectus excavatum deformity. Eur J Cardiothorac Surg 2006; 29:1–5.

through the posterior aspect of the median scalene muscle to cross the postero-lateral border of the first rib on its way to supplying the scalenus anterior muscle. The posterior scalene muscle follows the posterior border of the median but inserts onto the second rib and does not form a part of the scalene triangle.

Note should be made of the scalene fat pad, which offers a protective covering to the vessels and nerves crossing the supraclavicular fossa, lying deep to the supraclavicular cutaneous nerves and the platysma muscle.

Causation and Pathological Anatomy

Cervical ribs are found in about 1% of the general population, in about 5% of all cases of thoracic outlet syndrome, and in over 80% of those cases presenting with arterial compression (Fig. 44.1). In a proportion of cases the cervical rib, which normally articulates with the C7 transverse process behind and the scalene tubercle of the first rib in front, is incomplete or vestigial, comprising little more than a prominent C7 transverse process. In such cases, a fibrous band may replace the anterior component of the rib and such structures are undoubtedly capable of producing TOCS.

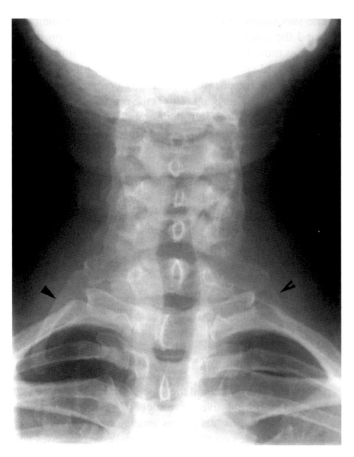

FIG. 44.1. Thoracic outlet X-ray demonstrating bilateral cervical ribs

Neurovascular compression in the scalene triangle can result from skeletal abnormality such as a congenital cervical rib, a prominent scalene tubercle, congenital pseudoarthrosis of the clavicle,[5] or from acquired bony encroachment in cases of traumatic callus, neoplasia, functional hypertrophy, or sepsis. The Klippel-Fiel syndrome has been implicated in neurogenic TOCS in children.[6]

Compression can also arise from encroachment by soft tissue structures discrete from cervical ribs such as fibro-muscular bands, as classified by Roos,[7] or from spasm or fibrosis of the scalene muscles, which may arise as a late consequence of "whiplash injury", producing characteristic histological appearances.[8]

Direct overstretching of the brachial plexus in cervical hyperextension–hyperflexion injury can result in entrapment in fibrous scar tissue, producing TOCS symptoms, which may be relieved by neurolysis.[9]

Cervical roots C5 and 6 are vulnerable to compression by the origins of the scalene muscles but the C8 and T1 roots, which contribute to the ulnar nerve, are most likely to be affected by cervical ribs inserting on the first rib or associated fibrous bands; most patients suffering nontraumatic TOCS experience pain in these dermatomes. Soft tissue tumors in the root of the neck and apex of the thorax may invade or distort the brachial plexus, producing TOCS symptoms.[10,11] One study recorded the anatomical abnormalities found in patients with clinical TOCS and found that similar abnormalities were detectable on bilateral neck dissection in 46% out of 250 cadavers.[12]

Violent or repetitive arm movements associated with sports or related occupations have been implicated in arterial[13,14] and neurological[14,15] injuries at the thoracic outlet.

Hypertrophy of the subclavius and scalene muscles may result from overuse arising from increased sporting or occupational activity. This may account for a proportion of cases of neurogenic TOCS and is implicated in the majority of cases of venous TOCS (Paget-Schroetter syndrome[4]).

When arterial compression is the predominant presenting feature, pathological manifestations may include focal stenosis, intimal injury, and post-stenotic aneurysm formation, all capable of producing thrombo-embolic complications in the ipsilateral arm or even stroke.[16]

Presentation and Management

Neurogenic TOCS

This syndrome characteristically presents in young adults (20 to 40-years old) and affects women twice as often as men. Patients complain of pain, dysaesthesia, numbness, and weakness in a variable distribution affecting the neck, shoulder, arm, hand, and back and as many as 50% of patients may have symptoms resembling Raynaud's phenomenon.[17] Sometimes there is associated occipital headache[18] and often symptoms are exacerbated by posture particularly that associated with work, or with sustained use of the arm in elevation. There may be a history of hyperextension injury ("whiplash") preceding the development of symptoms.[19] Physical signs may be minimal and it is rare to find identifiable weakness or wasting of muscles, probably because the neural compression at the thoracic outlet is usually intermittent. The detection of thenar wasting in the affected hand should raise the suspicion of carpal tunnel compression, and if this is excluded then the presence of this sign in TOCS points to the probability of a prominent cervical rib or band and of irreversible fibrotic changes in the brachial plexus. Tenderness or hypersensitivity of the brachial plexus elicited by gentle thumb compression in the supraclavicular fossa is a common finding but the most useful sign is a positive elevated arm stress test (EAST), where the patient is asked to raise both arms in the "surrender" position and repeatedly grip and release the hands. This exercise should provoke the onset of the patient's typical shoulder and arm pain within a minute. Other tests designed to provoke symptoms by placing the scalene muscles on the stretch are less useful.

It is important to exclude alternative causes of pain in the arm or neck through careful examination of the cervical spine and the shoulder, elbow and wrist joints, checking movement, sensation and strength in the hand.

Evidence of arterial involvement in neurogenic TOCS is rare and the finding of radial pulse diminution with full abduction of the arm has little discriminatory value, being observed in 10–20% of normal individuals. However, the C8/T1 root lies close to the subclavian artery as it crosses the first rib so that duplex ultrasound evidence of arterial flow disturbance when the arm is raised to a position where neural symptoms are provoked may be used as a surrogate maker of compression. It is necessary to undertake bilateral brachial blood pressure measurement in all cases.

Plain X-rays will detect significant cervical spondylosis, cervical ribs, and obvious deformity of the first rib, clavicle and gleno-humeral joint, while MRI scans are capable of detecting some fibrous cervical bands in expert hands. Neurophysiolgical tests commonly prove normal in neurogenic TOCS,[20] although reversible changes in motor-evoked potentials on elevation of the affected arm have been described.[21] The main value of neurophysiological testing is to exclude other disorders and to establish a baseline for medico-legal reasons.

Arterial TOCS

Although arterial involvement (Fig. 44.2) features in less than 5% of adult TOCS cases, its prompt recognition is important since thrombo-embolic complications can threaten the viability of the arm. Bony abnormality, usually a cervical rib, is present in over 80% of cases and surgical correction is usually required.[22]

Sometimes the condition will come to light when examination prompted by neurological symptoms reveals reduced pulsation or blood pressure in the affected arm or the patient gives a history of unilateral Raynaud's phenomenon or of coldness or claudication in the arm. Otherwise, presentation can be acute, with a range of thrombo-embolic symptoms ranging from digital micro-embolisation to acute ischemia of the arm. Usually the age of the patient will provide a clue but in patients at risk of atherosclerosis or cardiac disease the differential diagnosis may be confusing.

Compression of the subclavian artery at the thoracic outlet can produce local intimal injury resulting in the formation of intra-luminal thrombus, or else turbulent flow can lead to a post-stenotic dilatation or aneurysm. Either condition can generate local or distant thrombosis. If this is treated by peripheral embolectomy alone, overlooking the subclavian lesion, recurrence of the ischemia is inevitable and the viability of the arm will be compromised unnecessarily. It is, therefore, essential to undertake a careful history and examination to detect possible thoracic outlet problems and to request Duplex scanning of the subclavian artery if there is any suspicion of compromise. Cross-sectional imaging or arteriography (angiography) used selectively will resolve doubt.

The three essentials in treating arterial TOCS are to remove the source of subclavian compression, to repair any damaged section of artery and to restore distal patency. Adjunctive measures such as cervical sympathectomy and arm fasciotomy are rarely necessary, and the prognosis, providing the three essential objectives are met, is good. Endovascular therapy will seldom provide a better option in these cases.

Venous TOCS

Deep venous thrombosis (DVT) affects the lower limb about 30 times more frequently than the upper limb. In the modern era of intravenous monitoring, therapy and haemodialysis, 40% of upper limb DVTs is secondary to catheterization, another 35% are secondary to trauma, neoplasia, irradiation, or infection, and only about 25% represent primary subclavian vein thrombosis, of which the majority is associated with TOCS (Fig. 44.3).[23–27]

Catheter-related upper limb DVT produces pain and swelling in the affected arm. The diagnosis should be confirmed by duplex ultrasound scanning and treatment involves catheter removal and anticoagulation.

Non-thrombotic venous obstruction in the upper limb is uncommon and can be difficult to evaluate. The patient may give a history of intermittent heaviness, discoloration, and swelling of the arm, and in some cases suspicion of TOCS may be raised by associated pains and paraesthesia in the neck, shoulder and arm. There may be a history of positional or occupational exacerbation and obesity or mammary hyperplasia may be contributory. If the hand is not cyanotic or edematous and the veins on the dorsum collapse when the arm is elevated to the horizontal position, the problem is likely to be postural so that reassurance and general advice are all that is required. If signs of venous congestion are more severe and persistent, duplex insonation of the subclavian vein should

normal, venography should be repeated with a view to balloon venoplasty. A recent approach is to undertake on-table venography and venoplasty at the time of surgical decompression.[38]

Conservative Management in TOCS

As always, treatment is founded on a thorough diagnostic assessment. Conservative measures should constitute the first line of management in neurogenic TOCS, unless there is compelling evidence of progressive neurological injury (muscle wasting, intractable pain, deranged nerve conduction). Evidence of vascular compromise, whether arterial or venous, warrants decompressive surgery.

Conservative management of TOCS should be a holistic exercise. A sympathetic and supportive approach is essential since many patients are anxious and depressed about their condition after months or years of disability, diagnostic confusion, and ineffective interventions. An explanation of the mechanisms of the condition usually helps. Patients who have become confused by their own researches may require clarification and reassurance.

It is important to identify occupational stresses and poor posture so that factors that reinforce symptoms can be altered. Issues of inadequate sleep, obesity, poor diet and abuse of tobacco, drugs or alcohol abuse need to be identified and addressed. Psychosocial strains at work or at home may be a source of muscle tension and insomnia.

The object of physiotherapy is to alleviate irritation of the brachial plexus and related nerves by expanding the bony thoracic outlet and relaxing muscle spasm in the neck and shoulder girdle. Attention should focus on improved posture through elevation of the shoulder girdle on the thorax,[39] deep breathing and developing extension of the thorax, neck, and shoulders. Exercises of the thoracic, scalene, paravertebral, parascapular, and trapezius muscle groups are designed to relieve spasm and improve strength and flexibility. Active conservative management along these lines should demonstrate improvement within 1 month and at 6 months 70–80% of patients should report continued benefit. Patients showing a poor response are more likely to be seeking compensation for work-related strain, suffering from obesity or to be affected by concomitant carpal tunnel syndrome.[40]

A more recent approach in patients suffering pain and spasm in the scalene muscles is to employ intra-muscular injection of local anesthetic or botulinum toxin.[41] A temporary response may predict a more durable benefit following surgery.

Surgical Techniques for Thoracic Outlet Decompression

Selection of the optimal surgical approach is tailored to the individual and will depend on the perceived anatomical cause of compression, the need to deal with complications and secondary factors such as cosmesis, or the need for adjunctive procedures such as cervical sympathectomy. The informed consent process should include a clear explanation of the procedure and a realistic appraisal of its potential benefit. An account of possible complications should include injuries to nerves (cutaneous: supraclavicular or intercosto-brachial, phrenic, sympathetic or brachial plexus), vessels (subclavian artery and vein and their branches, thoracic duct) and intrathoracic structures. The possible need for transfusion, chest drains, and thoracotomy should be covered as should the likelihood of postoperative pain and stiffness. At least one member of the surgical team should be fully trained and experienced in thoracic outlet surgery.

The main decision concerns the choice of a supra-clavicular or a trans-axillary approach; opinion has shifted over the decades. When there is clear evidence of arterial compression attributable to a cervical rib or band, most surgeons would select a supraclavicular approach. Similarly most would regard a transaxillary approach to first rib resection as first choice for the relief of venous TOCS. Neither of these strategies is standardized, and the literature contains reports of satisfactory outcomes using either approach for arterial or venous TOCS cases.

The debate continues as to how best to manage the largest group of TOCS patients, those presenting with neurogenic symptoms refractory to conservative management. In this group, durable decompression of the brachial plexus may involve the removal of cervical ribs and bands, anterior scalenectomy and first rib resection. However, too radical an approach to thoracic outlet surgery may precipitate the development of peri-neural fibrosis leading to chronic pain and stiffness. Current opinion favors a supraclavicular approach combining scalenectomy with removal of bands to achieve brachial plexus decompression with the option of removing the first rib through the same incision if this appears to be necessary.[42] Occasionally, a separate anteromedial infraclavicular approach may facilitate removal of the inaccessible anterior section of the first rib, reducing the risk of damaging the subclavian vein.[43]

The Supraclavicular Approach

Endotracheal general anesthesia is advisable, and the patient is positioned supine with the table inclined 5° head up in order to reduce venous filling. The skin incision commences 1 cm above the clavicle, 2 cm lateral to the midline and extends postero-laterally, following the root of the neck for 6–8 cm (Fig. 44.4). The external jugular vein and the supra-clavicular nerves are encountered immediately beneath the platysma; the former can be divided but the latter should be mobilized carefully and preserved. The clavicular head of sterno-cleido-mastoid can be divided to improve exposure but the sternal head should always be preserved to maintain the contour of the neck. The scalene fat pad should then be divided inferiorly and reflected upwards, to reveal the omo-hyoid and anterior scalene muscles, the brachial plexus and the superior aspect of the subclavian artery. The omo-hyoid muscle can be retracted

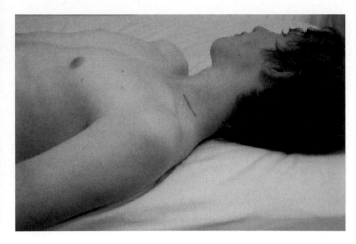

FIG. 44.4. Supraclavicular decompression of the thoracic outlet

but excision is easier and incurs no morbidity. The phrenic nerve should be dissected carefully off the front of the anterior scalene muscle and retracted with a soft elastic sling and the subclavian artery is mobilised and slung, dividing costo-cervical and thyro-cervical branches as required. At this point, the bony inferior border of the thoracic outlet should be assessed, noting the first rib, the scalene tubercle and any cervical rib or band, after which the anterior and median scalene muscles are inspected to detect fibrous thickening and tightness. Once the strategic compass of the operation has been decided, dissection of the brachial plexus and scalene muscles proceeds. The attachment of the anterior scalene muscle to the first rib is divided, and the muscle reflected superiorly to uncover the brachial plexus before being resected. Sibson's fascia can now be separated from the concavity of the first rib, protecting the pleura and lung, after which a cervical rib can be identified, freed from its attachment to the first rib anteriorly, then followed back to the cervical spine using a combination of sharp and blunt dissection (a Pennybacker dissector is useful here). If the first rib is to be resected, it should first be divided anteriorly then followed posteriorly, in the same way as the cervical rib is removed. To join the brachial plexus, the T1 root has to cross the necks of both the first rib and of any cervical rib so it must be retracted and protected before the posterior origins of these ribs are divided using bone shears and nibblers. Spikes of bone should be trimmed meticulously. When detaching the middle scalene muscle from the first rib, care must be taken to remain in the sub-periosteal plane to avoid damaging the long thoracic nerve (c 5–7), which innervates the serratus anterior muscle. Bone nibblers are used to trim back the anterior stump of the first rib but since this is covered by the subclavian vein, it occasionally requires removal through a separate anterior infraclavicular approach.

After confirming the removal of all constricting bones, bands and muscle, hemostasis is secured and the neurovascular structures are inspected. Stricture, aneurysm, or intimal injury of the subclavian artery should be detected and corrected at this stage, if necessary with the help of intraoperative ultrasonography. Decompression of the brachial plexus should seek to avoid disturbing the perineural connective tissue in order to minimize adhesions. For the same reason, the scalene fat pad should be sutured back in place before wound closure.

Providing there is no air leak from the lung, an underwater seal chest drain is not needed and closed suction drainage will deal with hemoserous exudates. A suction drain is adequate if the pleura is breached providing the lung is intact, to reduce the likelihood of postoperative pleuritic pain.

Providing pain control is adequate, and clinical examination or chest X ray confirm normal ventilation, patients can be discharged home on the second postoperative day.

The Transaxillary Approach

Under general anesthesia, the patient is positioned in 45° of lateral tilt with the arm wrapped and suspended in a sling above the axilla to permit a full range of movement. A horizontal skin incision is made 2–3 cm below the apex of the axilla, extending from the pectoralis major muscle anteriorly to the latissimus dorsi muscle posteriorly and this is then deepened through the axillary fat pad, taking care to preserve the intercosto-brachial and latissimus dorsi nerves. An assistant then elevates the arm in a cephalad direction, effectively lifting it off the chest, enabling the operating surgeon to palpate the first rib, and identify the neurovascular bundle at the thoracic outlet. The anterior scalene muscle should be palpated separating the subclavian artery and vein and the presence of abnormal cervical ribs or bands noted. To remove the first rib, an incision in the first intercostal space is developed in the sub-periosteal plane, so that the lateral aspect can be dissected anteriorly to the costo-clavicular ligament and posteriorly to the neck of the rib, again taking care to protect the long thoracic nerve as it pierces the middle scalene muscle.

The attachment of the anterior scalene muscle to the rib is divided well away from the phrenic nerve, the accessible muscle cut back, and any fibrous bands are excised similarly. Removal of the first rib is usually facilitated by dividing its mid part, then following the two stumps anteriorly and posteriorly. On completion of rib resection, the brachial plexus posteriorly and the subclavian vein anteriorly should be free of all bony impingement.

At this stage, in cases of venous TOCS, all peri-venous fibrous tissue should be removed until the vein is fully compressible and free to dilate. It should be possible to resect the anterior end of the first rib sufficiently to free the subclavian vein but if this remains inaccessible, it can be removed under the same anaesthetic through a separate medial infra-clavicular approach.

After hemostatic checks, the axillary wound is closed with suction drainage same as for the supraclavicular operation.

Endoscopic approaches to thoracic outlet decompression, with or without robotic assistance, have been developed in recent years.[44] They offer excellent visualization with a modest cosmetic benefit but are expensive in terms of equipment and increased operative time. As with other minimally-invasive innovations, technical advance will make them increasingly relevant in the future.

Outcomes After TOCS Surgery

There are numerous reports of the results of thoracic outlet decompression procedures in the world of literature, with general agreement that interventions for arterial complications are successful in relieving ischemia and providing durable symptom relief in over 90% of cases.

In venous TOCS, initial restoration of venous patency may be followed by late re-stenosis or thrombosis. However, because of the development of collateral venous drainage, many of these late failures are asymptomatic, overlooked, and unreported; significant long-term morbidity is confined largely to patients who elude adequate primary treatment.

The picture with respect to neurogenic TOCS is more diverse, presumably owing to the subjective nature of the symptomatology and the intractability of psycho-social factors. A number of scoring systems have been employed to provide an objective evaluation of outcome. Altobelli and colleagues[45] used a 10 point patient-scored scale to evaluate return to normality in 254 operations for neurogenic TOCS in 185 patients treated between 1994 and 2002. The transaxillary first rib resection with lower part scalenectomy was the primary intervention and supraclavicular residual scalenectomy was performed for patients with persistent or recurrent symptoms. Only 46% of the primary operations were judged successful, with most symptomatic recurrences developing in the second postoperative year. Eighty percent of the secondary procedures were performed for recurrent symptoms of which 56% showed sustained success. The authors concluded that symptomatic improvement was often transient and that patients should be followed for a minimum of 18 months to evaluate outcome.

Degeorges and colleagues[46] reported on 176 procedures in 155 patients between 1979 and 1999, utilizing a variety of operative approaches for all forms of presentation, 54.5% comprising mixed neurovascular symptoms. Follow-up was for a mean of 7.5 years, using Derkash's classification by means of a telephone survey. They recorded excellent to good outcomes in 84% of cases with the worst results occurring in patients suffering from poorly systematized neurological symptoms. The authors recommended caution in offering surgical treatment to this subset of patients.

The "DASH" questionnaire[47] (Gummeson 2003) may prove to be the most appropriate tool for the objective evaluation of outcome in TOCS surgery. One recent study[48] appears to confirm its potential. Between 1998 and 2005, 23 consecutive patients undergoing decompressive surgery for TOCS (14 venous and 9 neurogenic) completed the DASH questionnaire before and after the operation. The results showed a clear separation between the two clinical groups, with venous TOCS proving less incapacitating than neurogenic TOCS. Surgery produced a striking early improvement in the neurogenic group.

Providing surgery is offered selectively and providing operations are planned and performed with skill and care. Eighty percent of patients undergoing intervention should achieve sustained benefit with few complications. Particular caution is warranted in patients with diffuse neurological symptoms, who should be offered counseling and physiotherapy as first line treatment. Follow-up should be maintained for a minimum of two years and a proportion of patients will require more than one intervention.

TOCS in children is rare. Review of the literature, much of which comprises single case reports, suggests that recognizable skeletal abnormality with vascular involvement is responsible for a higher proportion of presentations than in the adult population. In general, management of TOCS-related complications in children should adhere to the same principles that apply in adults.[49] Children appear to be less likely than adults to present with neurological symptoms in the absence of recognizable skeletal abnormality. Because growth offers an opportunity of skeletal remodeling, it is logical that neurogenic cases should be offered physiotherapy and that surgery is reserved for persistent symptoms.[50]

Conclusion

Success in the treatment of TOCS is contingent on distinguishing the three main types of presentation, recognizing the need for prompt intervention to correct arterial and venous complications and for conservatism in the management of exclusively neurogenic symptoms.

References

1. Adson AW, Coffey JR: Cervical rib. Ann Surg 1927; 85:839.
2. Kieffer E: Arterial complications of thoracic outlet syndrome. In Bergan JJ, Yao JST (eds.): Evaluation and Treatment of Upper and Lower Extremity Circulatory Disorders. Orlando, Grune and Stratton, 1984; pp. 249–275
3. Coote H: Exostosis of the left transverse process in the 7th cervical vertebra surrounded by blood vessels and nerves: Successful removal. Lancet 1861; 1:360–361.
4. Kahn SN, Stansby G: Paget Schroetter Syndrome. Phlebology 2003; 18:2–11.
5. Sales de Gauzy J, Baunin C, Puget C, Fajadet P, Cahuzac JP: Congenital pseudarthrosis of the clavicle and thoracic outlet syndrome in adolescence. J Paediatr Orthop B 1999; 8:299–301.
6. Konstantinou DT, Chroni E, Constantoyiannis C, Dougenis D. Klippel-Feil syndrome presenting with bilateral thoracic outlet syndrome. Spine 2004; 29:E189–92.
7. Roos DB: Congenital anomalies associated with thoracic outlet syndrome. Am J Surg 1976; 132:771–8.
8. Sanders RJ, Jackson CG, Banchero N, Pearce WH: Scalene muscle abnormalities in traumatic thoracic outlet syndrome. Am J Surg 1990; 159:231–6.

9. Alexandre A, Coro L, Azuelos A, Pellone M: Thoracic outlet syndrome due to hyperextension-hyperflexion cervical injury. Acta Neurochir Suppl 2005; 92:21–4.

10. Gehman KE, Currie I, Ahmad D, Parrent A, Rizkalla K, Novick RJ. Desmoid tumour of the thoracic outlet: an unusual cause of thoracic outlet syndrome. Can J Surg 1998; 41:404–6.

11. Atasoy E. Thoracic outlet compression caused by a Schwannoma of the C7 nerve root. J Hand Surg (Br) 1997; 22:662–3.

12. Redenbach DM, Nelems B: A comparative study of structures comprising the thoracic outlet in 250 human cadavers and 72 cases of thoracic outlet syndrome. Eur J Cardiothoracic Surg 1998; 13:353–60.

13. Rohrer MJ, Cardullo PA, Pappas AM: Axillary artery compression and thrombosis in throwing athletes. J Vasc Surg 1990; 11:761–9.

14. Casbas L, Chauffour X, Bossavy JP, Midy D, Baste JC, Barret A. Post-traumatic thoracic outlet syndromes. Ann Vasc Surg 2005; 19:25–8.

15. Carmichael KD. Brachial plexus injury by non-violent means in an adolescent baton-twirler. Am J Orthop 2003; 32:306–8.

16. Lee TS, Hines GL. Cererbral embolic stroke and arm ischaemia in a teenager with arterial thoracic outlet syndrome: a case report. Vasc Endovasc Surg 2007; 41:254–7.

17. Pistorius MA, Planchon B. The incidence of Thoracic Outlet Syndrome on the epidemiology and clinical presentation of apparently primary Raynaud's phenomenon. A prospective study in 570 patients. Int Angiol 1995; 14:60–4.

18. Raskin NH, Howard MW, Ehrenfeld WK. Headache as the leading symptom of the thoracic outlet syndrome. Headache 1985; 25:208–10.

19. Capistrant TD. Thoracic outlet syndrome in whiplash injury. Ann Surg 1977; 185:175–8.

20. Komanetsky RM, Novak CB, Mackinnon SE et al. Somatosensory evoked potentials fail to diagnose thoracic outlet syndrome. J Hand Surg (Am) 1996; 21:662–6.

21. Haghigi SS, Baradarian S, Bagheri R. Sensory and motor evoked potentials findings in patients with thoracic outlet syndrome. Electromyogr Clin Neurophysiol 2005; 45:149–54.

22. Durham JR, Yao JST, Pearce WH, et al. Arterial injuries in the thoracic outlet syndrome. J Vasc Surg 1995; 21:57–70.

23. Adams JT, McEvoy RK, DeWeese JA. Primary deep venous thrombosis of upper extremity. Arch Surg 1965; 91:29–42.

24. Coon WW, Willis PW. Thrombosis of axillary and subclavian veins. Arch Surg 1967; 94:657–63.

25. Hill SL, Berry RE. Subclavian vein thrombosis: a continuing challenge. Surgery 1990; 108:1–9.

26. Horattas MC, Wright DJ, Fenton AH, et al. Changing concepts of deep venous thrombosis of the upper extremity: report of a series and review of the literature. Surgery 1988; 104:561–7.

27. Lindblad B, Tengborn L, Bergqvist D. Deep vein thrombosis of the axillary-subclavian veins. Eur J Vasc Surg 1988; 2:161–5.

28. Sanders RJ, Hammond SL. Subclavian vein obstruction without thrombosis. J Vasc Surg 2005; 41:285–90.

29. Sanders RJ, Rao NM. Pectoralis minor obstruction of the axillary vein: report of six patients. J Vasc Surg 2007; 45:1206–11.

30. Meier GH, Pollak JS, Rosenblatt M, et al. Initial experience with venous stents in exertional axillary-subclavian vein thrombosis. J Vasc Surg 1996; 24:974–83.

31. Cassada DC, Lipscomb AL, Stevens SL, Freeman MB, Grandas OH, Goldman MH. The importance of thrombophilia in the treatment of the Paget-Schroetter syndrome. Ann Vasc Surg 2006; 20:596–601.

32. Harley DP, White RA, Nelson RJ, et al. Pulmonary embolism secondary to venous thrombosis of the arm. Am J Surg 1984; 147:221–4.

33. Hingorani A, Ascher E, Lorenson E et al. Upper extremity deep venous thrombosis and its impact on morbidity and mortality rates in a hospital-based population. J Vasc Surg 1997; 26:853–60.

34. Monreal M, Lafoz E, Ruiz J et al. Upper-extremity deep venous thrombosis and pulmonary embolism. Chest 1991; 99:280–3.

35. Divi V, Proctor MC, Axelrod DA, Greenfield LJ. Thoracic outlet decompression for subclavian vein thrombosis: experience in 71 patients. Arch Surg 2005; 140:54–7.

36. Thompson JF. Transaxillary first rib resection. In: Vascular and endovascular techniques. Greenhalgh RM (ed.). New York, WB Saunders, 2001

37. Sanders RJ, Cooper MA. Surgical management of subclavian vein obstruction, including six cases of subclavian vein bypass. Surgery 1995; 118:856–63.

38. Schneider DB, Dimuzio PJ, Martin ND, et al. Combination treatment of venous thoracic outlet syndrome: open surgical decompression and intraoperative angioplasty. J Vasc Surg 2004; 40:599–603.

39. Kenny RA, Traynor GB, Withington D, Keegan DJ. Thoracic outlet syndrome: a useful exercise treatment option. Am J Surg 1993; 165:282–4.

40. Novak CB, Collins ED, MacKinnon SC. Outcome following conservative management of thoracic outlet syndrome. J Hand Surg (Am) 1995; 20:542–8.

41. Jordan SE, Ahn SS, Freischlag J, Gelabert HA, Machleder HI. Selective botulinum chemodenervation of the scalene muscles for treatment of neurogenic thoracic outlet syndrome. Ann Vasc Surg 2000; 14:365–9.

42. Sanders RJ, Pearce WH. The treatment of thoracic outlet syndrome: A comparison of different operations. J Vasc Surg 1989; 10:626–34.

43. Robicsek F, Eastman D. "Above under" exposure of the first rib: a modified approach for the treatment of thoracic outlet syndrome. Ann Vasc Surg 1997; 11:304–6.

44. Martinez BD, Wiegand CS, Evans P, Gerhardinger A, Mendez J. Computer-assisted instrumentation during endoscopic transaxillary first rib resection for thoracic outlet syndrome: a safe alternative approach. Vascular 2005; 13:327–35.

45. Altobelli GG, Kudo T, Haas BT, Chandra FA, Moy JL, Ahn SS. Thoracic outlet syndrome: pattern of clinical success after operative decompression. J Vasc Surg 2005; 42:122–8.

46. Degeorges R, Reynaud C, Becquemin JP. Thoracic outlet syndrome surgery: long term functional results. Ann Vasc Surg 2004; 18:558–65.

47. Gummeson C, Atroshi I, Ekdahl C. The disabilities of the arm, shoulder and hand (DASH) outcome questionnaire: longitudinal construct validity and measuring self-rated health change after surgery. BMC Musculoskeletal disorders 2003; 4:11.

48. Cordobes-Gual J, Lozano-Vilardell P, Torreguitart-Mirada N, Lara-Hernandez R, Riera-Vasquez R, Julia-Montoya J. Prospective study of the functional recovery after surgery for thoracic outlet syndrome. Eur J Vasc Endovasc Surg 2008; 35:79–83.

49. Vercellio G, Baraldini V, Gatti G, Coletti M, Cipolat L. Thoracic outlet syndrome in paediatrics: clinical presentation, surgical

treatment and outcome in a series of eight children. J Paediatr Surg 2003; 38:58–61.

50. Yang J, Letts M. Thoracic outlet syndrome in children. J Pediatr Orthop 1996; 16:514–7.

51. Thompson RW. Treatment of thoracic outlet syndromes and cervical sympathectomy. In: Springer Surgical Atlas Series - Vascular Surgery. London, Springer-Verlag, 2004.

45
Thoracopagus Conjoined Twins

Alastair J.W. Millar, Heinz Rode, Jenny Thomas, and John Hewitson

"A soul with two thoughts. Two hearts that beat as one."
McCoy sisters

Introduction

Conjoined twins represent rare and most challenging congenital malformations, the etiology of which remains obscure. The birth of conjoined twins has always fascinated mankind with the public's view of malformed children greatly influenced by the prevailing culture and religious beliefs. Surgeons over the years have attempted to separate these twins with variable success. Systematic preoperative surgical planning is essential. Knowledge of the anatomy and its variations including understanding of physiology of the conjoined twins, the use of newer imaging techniques along with a multidisciplinary team approach to the complex surgical problem has also improved outcome. The management of thoracopagus conjoined twins is not only surgically challenging, and poses moral and ethical dilemmas, but also has obstetric implications, anesthetic considerations, and demands significant and complex postoperative care (Fig. 45.1).

Conjoined twins are always joined at homologous sites, and the clinical classification is based on the most prominent site of union, combined with the suffix "pagus" meaning "that which is fixed."[1] Conjoined twins are individual and deformed but symmetrical and proportional, truly a "harmony in form." There are also asymmetrical forms. Eight symmetrical configurations are recognized, i.e., thoracopagus (chest), omphalopagus (umbilicus), ischiopagus (hip), pygopagus (rump), rachipagus (spine), craniopagus (cranium), cephalopagus (head), and parapagus (side). Asymmetrical or incomplete conjoined twins (heteropagus) result from the demise of one twin with remnant structures attached to the complete twin but the junction remains at or near one of the common sites of union.(Fig. 45.2) Fetus-in-feto are asymmetrical monozygotic di-amniotic intra-parasitic twins.[2] Conjoined triplets are exceptionally rare and their pathogenesis remains even more

obscure[3] (Fig. 45.3). Conjoined twins often have discordant anomalies occurring in one twin, especially reversal of cardiac situs (71%), congenital diaphragmatic hernia, and anomalous pulmonary and hepatic venous drainage.

"E pluribus unum – out of many, one
Ex uno plures – out of one, many"

Incidence

Although the worldwide incidence of monozygotic twinning is the same in all ethnic groups, the incidence of conjoined twins appears to be higher in Sub-Saharan Africa, ranging from 1:50,000 to 1:100,000 live births, or 1 in 400 monozygotic twin births.[4–6] The natural history that follows a prenatal diagnosis of conjoined twins confirms that a large number of infants die either in utero (28%) or immediately after birth (54%); in fact, only around 20% survive.[7]

Conjoined twins are monozygotic, mono-amniotic, and mono-chorionic and are always of the same gender with a 3:1 female preponderance. In human gestations, no factors have been consistently linked to the incidence of conjoined twins. Conjoined twins can also occur in association with triplet and quadruplet pregnancies. Two theories are proposed: The first is the fission theory in which the fertilized egg splits partially. Their formation occurs after the primitive streak begins to form and is the consequence of incomplete separation of the embryonic plate between 15 and 17 days gestation with two centers of embryonic growth arising. The second is the fusion theory, in which a fertilized egg completely separates, but stem cells (which search for similar cells) find like-stem cells on the other twin and fuse the twins together. This results in early reattachment of two separate embryonic discs at the dorsal neural tube or ventral yolk sac areas at 3–4 weeks gestation. Spencer's extensive embryological studies appear to favor the latter theory (as did Aristotle), but this remains controversial – a theory that was also held by Aristotle. Although genetically identical, one infant is almost always weaker or smaller than

D.H. Parikh et al. (eds.), *Pediatric Thoracic Surgery*,
DOI: 10.1007/b136543_45, © Springer-Verlag London Limited 2009

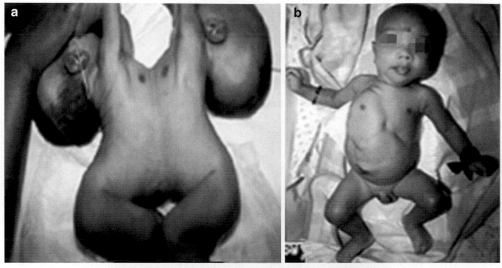

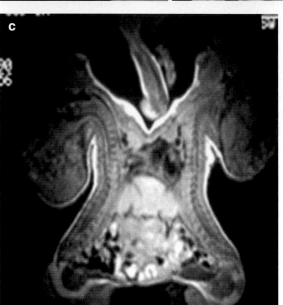

FIG. 45.1. (a) Thoraco-omphalopagus twins operated on with a view to attempting to save one with a more normal heart. The thoracotomy was made to incorporate much of the thoracic wall of the chest of the twin on the right. (b) Note the surviving twin with a mild chest deformity indicating successful thoracic wall and skin closure. (c) MRI showing the shared internal organs including fused liver

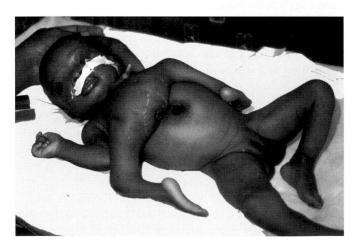

FIG. 45.2. A parasitic thoracopagus twin with heterotopic attachment of the parasite of pelvis, buttocks and legs to the chest of the autosite

the other and may have additional congenital defects. Despite their anatomical conjunction and same genetic and environmental factors, different personality traits can be distinguished from an early age.[8–10]

Historical Perspective

In prehistoric times, conjoined twins were depicted in cave drawings, on pottery or as figurines and often assumed the female form. In folklore, they were generally regarded as an omen of impending disaster; eliciting strong emotions ranging from wonder and admiration to rejection and hostility. Although malformed children were treated compassionately at times, historical records show that infanticide was frequently practiced, and the mother often held responsible for causing the malformation.[11,12] A 17-cm marble statue of a parapagus twin excavated

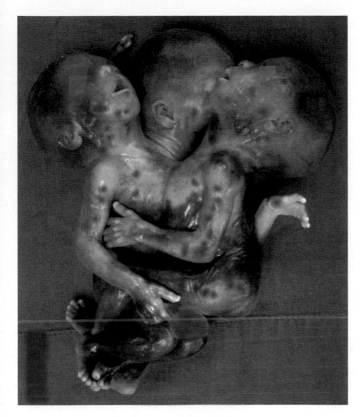

FIG. 45.3. Conjoined triplets – one set of thoracopagus twin with a parapagus twin attached to the one thoracopagus twin

from a Neolithic shrine in Anatolia is the earliest example of a pair of conjoined twins. Three thousand years later Australian Aborigines inscribed a memorial to a dicephalus conjoined twin on a rock, and 2,000 years later (700 BC) conjoined Molionides brothers appeared in Greek geometric art. Double-headed human figures have also been described in ancient South Pacific chalk drawings, pre-Columbian clay figures from Mexico, and in woodcuts from Middle Aged Europe.

Mary and Eliza Chalkhurst, the Biddenden pygopagus twins, were born in 1100 AD in Kent, England and lived together for 34 years. The statement filled with pathos "As we came together, we will also go together" is ascribed to the surviving twin on the death of her sister. She died 6 h later.

During the sixteenth century, conjoined twins were commonly described and radically different opinions developed between the concepts of deformity as divine design and deformity as an accident – this became known as the "quarrel of the monsters." Ambroise Pare, a distinguished surgeon from sixteenth century described in his book "Of Monsters and Prodigies" possible causes of conjoined twins (Pare A. Complete works (Translation) by Johnson T. 1678.). The most celebrated twins were Eng and Chang Bunker who were "discovered" in 1811 in Siam; and were responsible for the inappropriate term "Siamese" twins over the years. They were joined by a short anterior abdominal band containing fibrous tissue and liver. They were taken to America where they were first portrayed as human anomalies but later performed as acrobats in a circus.

Later on they became wealthy cotton plantation owners in North Carolina. They married sisters and between them had 22 children. They died within hours of each other at the ripe age of 63 years.

The first recorded unsuccessful attempt at separation was made in 907 AD in Armenia on male ischiopagus twins at the age of 30 years, and the first successful separation was performed by Johannes Fatio in 1689 in Basel, Switzerland on xypho-omphalopagus twins. Both children survived.[13,14] Since then more than 1,200 cases had been reported in the literature by 2000.

Clinical Features

Thoracopagus twins are joined predominantly at the sternum but this conjunction may extend to the umbilical region, thoraco-omphalopagus, which are the most frequently seen variety. Reportedly, 75% of these cases have various degrees of cardiac fusion. Prenatal ultrasonography can accurately diagnose significant cardiac fusion as well as cardiac anomalies, allowing a choice regarding termination of the pregnancy. Fetal MRI may be especially useful in defining detail of conjunction and associated anomalies. Clinical outcome of thoracopagus twins are related to their cardiac anomalies. The typical conjunction is along the whole length of the sternum from the suprasternal notch to the xiphisternum. The join frequently extends to the upper abdomen and may also be associated with an exomphalos. The twins face each other and of necessity the necks are extended in an almost opisthotonic posture. Each twin has a nipple in the appropriate position in relation to the fused but separated sternums. The ribs on each side join a sternum with a wide central oval shaped area of conjunction in which lie the two hearts most often in a single pericardial cavity. Lung hypoplasia, usually in one twin more than the other, along with rib abnormalities may occur. Although the sternal conjunction is variable, if there is any upper abdominal conjunction, this usually extends to the umbilicus and is always associated with extensive liver fusion. In this case, the foregut of each twin is separate with again a varying degree of join from the duodenum distally.

Thoracopagus conjoined twins may be classified according to the degree of cardiac conjunction (Leachman's Classification):

1. Type A completely separate hearts
2. Type B atrial connection only
3. Type C both atrial and ventricular connections

Diagnosis

Prenatal Diagnosis

The main objective of prenatal diagnosis is to define the extent of the abnormalities and to counsel the parents accordingly. Prenatal assessment of the extent of organ involvement is often difficult for technical reasons i.e., the position of the fetuses in utero, and the presence of oligo or polyhydramnios. A team approach for prenatal counseling and management is highly recommended combining the experience of the ultrasonographer, obstetricians, neonatologists, geneticists, pathologists and pediatric surgeons of all subspecialty disciplines. Recent advances in ultrasound technology, the usage of color Doppler flow studies, prenatal MRI and multi-slice CT scans have improved prenatal diagnosis[15] (Figs. 45.1c, 45.4a, b).

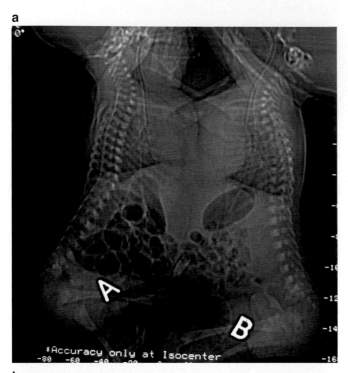

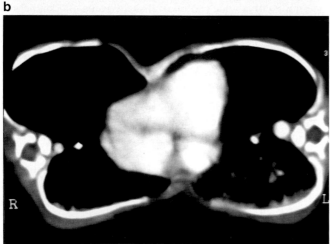

FIG. 45.4. (a) Scout coronal view prior to CT scan of a set of thoraco-omphalopagus twins with extensive abdominal conjunction and less marked cervical spine extension. In this case the hearts were separate, the liver was fused, and the gastrointestinal tracts were separate. Successful separation was achieved. (b) Axial CT of a set of thoracopagus twins. Note the central pericardium. Although the hearts look fused in fact they were separate and lay one on top of the other. The rib cage is slightly asymmetrical with each sternum receiving ribs from a mirror image of the other twin

In 1950, Gray proposed radiological criteria for diagnosing ventrally fused twins. Roentological findings are: both fetal heads are at the same level and in the same plane; an unusual opisthotonic position of the cervical spines, which becomes more pronounced with time; an extremely narrow space between the lower cervical and upper thoracic spines not allowing the development of a normal thoracic cage; no change in the relative positions after maternal movement or manual manipulation. Other features include persistent alignment of the two fetuses facing each with continuity of the skin and mirror image body parts with limbs close together.[16]

The wide prevalence of the use of prenatal ultrasound investigations has undoubtedly resulted in an increased detection of conjoined twins with the diagnosis having been made as early as 9 weeks gestation.[17,18] The bifid appearance of the first trimester fetal pole is an early sonographic feature. However, due to the complexity of conjunction prenatal diagnosis is more accurate from 20 weeks gestation. The presence of a single heart and fused liver would confirm the diagnosis. Additional findings include same sex twins, a single placenta, more than three umbilical cord vessels and shared organs. The diagnosis is seldom missed by those experienced in obstetrical ultrasound. Ultrasound is also important in evaluating the fetuses for other anomalies that may affect outcome. Serial scans in the second and third trimesters may be necessary to further define anatomy.

Fetal echocardiography is essential in establishing the presence and severity of cardiac anomalies. The ECG is generally unreliable as two separate ECGs do not rule out significant sharing of cardiac structures. Serial fetal echocardiography can be used as a prognostic indicator determining postnatal feasibility of successful separation. Termination of pregnancy is offered when fetal echocardiography shows a shared heart, if the anticipated deformities following separation are extensive and in the presence of cerebral conjunction. Fetal MRI is also useful in complex cases to define anatomy and may help in the decision making. Management of parents who opt to continue with the pregnancy is aimed at maximizing the potential for survival of the twins and minimizing maternal morbidity.

Obstetric Implications

In human gestations, no maternal factors have been consistently linked to the development of conjoined twins. In the majority, the prenatal course is uneventful. The birth of conjoined twins may be unexpected, particularly in rural communities, resulting in obstructive labor with difficult transvaginal delivery or emergency caesarean section (CS).[6,19] These complications can be avoided by planned CS at 36–38 weeks once the lungs have reached maturity because of the high rate of stillbirths and dystocia. Children weighing less than 3 kg, including thoracopagus and ischiopagus have been born vaginally, and this is made possible through prematurity and tissue pliability. Most children born vaginally do not sustain any damage to the connecting sites (bridges), except where there is an omphalocoele associated with thoraco-omphalopagus conjunction. Rupture of the exomphalos and evisceration of liver and bowel may occur.[20] Maternal mortality during labor has also been reported.

Ideally the immediate perinatal management of the babies is also planned, and in one case in which a twin with a normal heart perfused the co-twin with a rudimentary heart, the ex utero intrapartum treatment procedure (EXIT) was utilized because of concern that the normal twin would suffer immediate cardiac decompensation at birth.[7] This EXIT to separation strategy allowed prompt control of the airway and circulation before clamping the umbilical cord and optimized management of a potentially lethal situation with survival of the normal twin.

Postnatal Diagnosis and Management

Immediate postnatal management consists of resuscitation and stabilization of the twins. This is followed by a thorough physical examination with special investigations to define the anatomy of conjunction, feasibility of separation, and additional abnormalities. In general, it is better to wait until 6–9 months age before attempting separation as outcomes are better and greater preparation can be made in planning the operation. If emergency surgery is anticipated, all twins should undergo echo-cardiography and plain roentgenography, which provides limited but essential information. The site of conjunction will determine the type and order of special investigations. The information obtained will determine the surgical approach, the timing of separation, the allocation of organs and structures, and the eventual prognosis regarding survival and functional outcome.[21,22]

These imaging studies must include a thorough evaluation of the cardiovasular, diaphragmatic, hepatobiliary, pulmonary, upper gastro-intestinal tract, and vascular systems (Table 45.1). These investigations should provide excellent anatomical detail, demonstrating organ position, shared viscera and vascular anatomy. Contrast imaging evaluates the gastrointestinal tract. A routine search for other anomalies is made. Radioisotope scanning can assess regional perfusion fields. Multiplanar imaging techniques provide the best overall anatomical detail, but CT scan is more useful if bony detail is required. The use of diagrams, 3D organ models, and surgical rehearsal of the planned separation procedure if feasible will ensure the best possible outcome. Despite all these investigations and careful analysis of findings, preoperative interpretation may still be difficult with incorrect conclusions drawn.

Ethical and Moral Considerations

Ethical considerations, which need to reconcile the best options for the twins and their parents, are playing an increasing role in present day decision-making.[23–25] The sacrifice of one twin, because of inability to sustain life alone, is the

TABLE 45.1. Investigation of conjoined twins

System	Evaluation
Cardio respiratory	Electrocardiogram
	Echocardiography/Doppler ultrasound
	MRI/CT with contrast
	Cardiac catheterization and Angiography
Alimentary tract	Contrast meal and enema
	Ultrasound
	Radio-isotope scans (liver); technetium
	Tc99m-(Sn) colloid and excretion Tc99m
	mebrofenin
	Radio-isotope scintigraphy
Genito-urinary	Ultrasound
	Isotope renography
	Micturating cystourethrography
	Genitogram
Skeletal system	Radiography
	MRI (spinal cord)
	Ultrasound
Vascular	Doppler ultrasound
	Angiography
Cross-circulation	Radio-isotope scan Tc99m-DMSA

controversy that evokes the most anguish. The decision whether to operate or not is rendered more complex by those about surviving conjoined twins who consciously elected not to be separated and report that they have lived socially acceptable lives.[26] Equally, controversy surrounds those few conjoined twins who have survived to adulthood and then decide that separation should be attempted despite the operative risks and the potential for significant long-term morbidity as life in conjunction was considered unbearable.

Being conjoined does not necessarily negate individual development. Religious views may only support minimal surgical interference, especially when one twin will be sacrificed at surgery, "We cannot accept one baby must die so that the other one may live. It is not God's will," which differs from the legal opinion "Why I must order twin baby to die," or a twin's own opinion, "As we came together, we will also go together," Eliza Chulkhurst.[12]

From a practical point of view, the Great Ormond Street Ethical Guidelines for Conjoined Twin Separation have been generally accepted; where separation is feasible with a reasonable chance of success it should be carried out; when surgery is not possible, custodial care should be offered and nature allowed to take its course; where one twin is dead or has a lethal abnormality and cannot survive independently from its normal twin and if unoperated both twins could die, separation to save the healthy twin should be attempted.[24]

Anesthetic Considerations

Anesthesia for separation of conjoined twins is a complex, demanding procedure, which is facilitated by having two color-coded anesthetic teams representing each child.[27,28]

Preoperative planning and rehearsals are essential for elective separations. The extent of cross-circulation between the infants is unpredictable despite detailed and thorough preoperative work-up. The preoperative planning should include availability of additional team members in case of prolonged anesthesia and surgery, to provide rest. Thoracopagus conjunctions are associated with a significant risk of anesthetic complications; therefore, the anesthetic team should also be aware preoperatively of ethical issues and decisions made in favor of one twin to the detriment of the other in case where unfortunate and unavoidable sacrifice of one twin in favor of the other has to be made. It may only be possible to make this decision during the separation procedure when the true anatomy is exposed and defined.

Anesthetic Challenges

Although the neck and head are not often involved in the conjunction of twins where separation is considered, access to these structures for anesthesia and vascular access is a considerable challenge. The higher the conjunction, the greater is the degree of hyperextension of the babies' heads and necks, and the more difficult is airway access (Fig. 45.1).

Thoracopagus twins have the highest mortality of all the types of conjoined twins[29,27] as an isolated abnormality and may be further complicated by additional complex conjunctions at other levels – either cephalad (head and neck) or caudad (abdomen, pelvis, spine). In many series, early morbidity and the inability to separate the twins occurs in this group. The EXIT (ex utero intrapartum treatment) procedure has presented an unusual approach to this problem and may offer a realistic option in managing these infants prior to delivery.[7,30] The EXIT procedure is aimed at maintaining both oxygenation and cardiopulminary stability for the conjoined twins.[31] If one baby is not viable, surgery may be performed at this time using placental "cardiopulmonary bypass" while separation is achieved.

Preoperative Work-Up

All of the above factors will impact on many aspects of preoperative workup for separation, as well as those investigations that are necessary prior to separation. The two major factors that determine survival are the degree of conjunction of the hearts and their anatomical structures, and how feasible it is to provide enough cover for the deficit of skin and chest wall (i.e., ribs and sternum) to enable functional and stable chest dynamics for both babies after their separation. Therefore, a thorough evaluation of cardiac and lung function and their anatomy help the anesthetist plan and manage the surgery more effectively.

There has been very little emphasis placed on investigating the respiratory system of these babies. Lung abnormalities when assessed by bronchoscopy have been identified as tracheomalacia and the presence of aberrant bronchi. These findings raise the consideration that all thoracopagus twins should undergo bronchoscopy during the work-up to surgery.[32,33]

Cardiac and circulatory effects will depend on the complexity of the conjunction and the anatomical abnormalities

in either or both twins' hearts. Pericardium is usually shared but the variation in the rest of the heart structures is unpredictable, and each set of twins needs to be assessed in their own right. Angiography under general anesthetic may still be needed, but it remains a high risk procedure with an unpredictable response to anesthesia. In a set of twins with venous-pole sharing, induction of anesthesia resulted in asystole in the twin with a myopathic ventricle – resulting in brain death in that twin, an emergency separation with survival of the other.[4]

Vascular access: Venous access may become reduced during a prolonged hospital stay. Ultrasound scanning is useful in finding vessels as they are not always in the normal anatomical positions.

Airway management is usually difficult. These babies lie face to face in proximity to each other. The larynx is very anterior and endotracheal intubation with the aid of a fibreoptic bronchoscope has been used successfully but depends on operator ability and the availability of a small caliber bronchoscope for the neonatal age-group. The use of lignocaine local anesthesia to the vocal cords is advised. It is necessary to employ an anesthetist for each twin to manage the airways, and muscle relaxation should not be administered until the airway can be controlled. Awake intubation should not be attempted except in moribund patients. Emergency intubation in these babies should be avoided if possible. Their deterioration should be anticipated, and intubation performed in a controlled planned way.

Positioning for surgery and the changes required for the different disciplines needs to be discussed with each surgical team. Where cardiopulmonary bypass is required, space for the bypass machine needs to be identified and the placement of the cannulas in the patient(s) needs to be clarified. In general, the babies' heads are at the top end of a normal operating table with the anesthetic machines on either side. In older, bigger twins, it is important to ensure that the twins will fit onto the table in the space available, and it may be necessary to use a wider table or modify the one planned for use.

Equipment Preparation and/or Adaptation

Providing anesthesia for two babies simultaneously requires organization and preparation of the environment. Numerous options have been reported. A Carlens (Y) adaptor to fashion a connector to both babies' airways to allow for synchronous ventilation has been used successfully.[33] We have used a "splitter" for the gas pins at the main supply plug to enable the use of two machines from one gas outlet in the cardiac catheterization laboratory.

Anesthesia for Procedures Prior to Separation

Computerized tomography scanning (CT), magnetic resonance imaging (MRI), radioisotope studies, and cardiac catheterization may all be necessary for determining the anatomical structures and deciding whether surgery is possible or not. In complex conjunctions, transthoracic echocardiography may be limited and transesophageal echo, MRI angiography, and cardiac catheterization with angiography may be required.[33]

Surgical procedures prior to separation include examination under anesthesia for clarification of anatomical structures, bronchoscopy, systemic to pulmonary shunts where the anatomy of the heart is abnormal, laparotomy for necrotizing enterocolitis, decompression of intestinal obstruction where the conjunction has involved bowel, and placement of tissue expanders. Also these infants may require surgery that is common for any child, for example, adenoidectomy for upper airway obstruction.[27]

Surgical Management

Preoperative Preparation

Preoperative assessment should include all parameters prior to normal pediatric anesthesia. Documentation of all investigations is essential and any anticipated difficulties discussed with the surgical team. Features of cardiac failure and respiratory compromise should be identified and treated. In general, these babies are fairly similar in size so that the medication administered can be calculated by taking the combined weight and dividing this in half. Unless there is significant discrepancy between the sizes of the infants, each baby should have its own medication given on a dose/kg per individual, regardless of the cross-over between circulations. Color labeling for each twin's medication allows easier identification. In the period prior to planned surgery for separation, the upper limbs should not be used for phlebotomy or vascular access to spare these vessels for use intra-operatively.

Planning of the operating room environment is vital to successful peri-operative management.

Intraoperative Management

In thoracopagus infants, there is extensive cross circulation. With complex cardiopagus, inhalational anesthesia given to one twin may affect the twin not receiving the agent before the one receiving the anesthetic (personal experience). One has to be prepared for any eventuality.

During surgery difficulties with vascular access, hemodynamic stability, temperature control, and blood loss can be expected. Because of cross circulation, pharmacokinetics, and pharmacodynamics are inconsistent and altered drug responses must be expected. Prior to separation, the surgeon may still not know the exact nature of venous connections, coronary arterial anatomy, and the branching anatomy of the head and neck vessels and the true size of the atria and ventricles.

General Principles of Surgery

The surgical separation of conjoined twins presents a great challenge. Improved survival rates for conjoined twins are due to advances in perinatal and postnatal diagnostic techniques, meticulous interpretation of the special investigations, and correct anesthetic and surgical management carried out by an experienced multidisciplinary team.[26,29,34–39]

Many descriptions of surgical procedures to separate the various types of conjoined twins have been published.[26,29,35–38,40] Technical details are determined by the anatomy of conjunction, the allocation of sharing of organs and structures, and the planned reconstruction. Standard approaches are normally utilized but variations may demand a novel surgical approach or alternative techniques. Major factors that will govern successful separation include the order of separation, the distribution of organs between the twins, meticulous aseptic surgical techniques, the reconstruction of divided organs, and structures and wound closure. It is also necessary to distinguish between structures that are shared by both twins and those belonging only to one individual.[8] Unexpected anatomical variations are often encountered, including previously unrecognized cardiac, gastrointestinal, and hepatobiliary anomalies. Operation time is prolonged with the separation of the more complex thoracopagus twins in the order of 7–13 h.

Emergency surgery is indicated when there is damage to the connecting bridge or when correctable anomalies threaten the survival of one or both twins, and there is the possibility of saving at least one of the twins. Emergency separation has resulted in up to a 70% mortality rate compared with 20% for elective procedures, emphasizing the need to stabilize the infants initially and to postpone surgery until the basic investigations have been completed.[7] In our experience, emergency surgery was necessary to alleviate intestinal obstruction, to manage a ruptured exomphalos and for deteriorating cardiac-respiratory status, threatening survival of one or both twins.

Elective surgery is best scheduled for when the infants are thriving, and all investigations have been completed, providing a comprehensive and functional description of normal and fused anatomy. Delaying separation into early childhood may result in increased postnatal deformities and psychological problems. If separation is possible and desirable, it is proposed that surgery should be performed within the first 6–9 months before an awareness of their condition develops. Motor skills, sensory integration, and personality need to develop in a separate state.[41]

Skin Closure

Whenever there is extensive sharing of body surface areas, closure of the disconnected surfaces may pose major problems, especially when separation is undertaken as an emergency.[42–44] A wide variety of techniques have been described, including elevation of wide skin flaps, use of relaxation incisions, insertion of prosthetic material, delayed split skin grafts, and the use of prior tissue expanders to develop abundant native skin to allow for tension free closure without causing increase in intracompartmental pressure, local wound problems or restriction of respiratory excursion. Cardiovascular and respiratory failures are the most frequent causes of death in the immediate postoperative period. Subcutaneous tissue expansion is used to

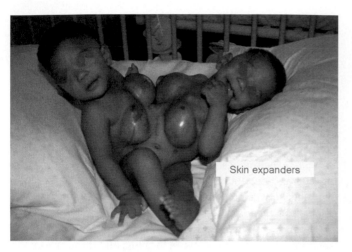

Skin expanders

FIG. 45.5. Skin expanders inserted over the chest wall of omphalo-ischiopagus twins illustrating the gain in skin cover that can be achieved

provide tissue for reconstruction or closure where insufficient natural tissue exists[44-46] (Fig. 45.5). Closure under tension is poorly tolerated, and it is preferred that both chest and abdomen cavities be left open if necessary for later staged closure with plastic reconstruction using skin and muscle flaps or split skin grafting onto granulation tissue. Vacuum dressings may assist a more rapid healing, earlier grafting, and wound closure. Unfortunately, tissue expansion is not always possible, and has a nearly 60% incidence of complications such as bleeding, wound sepsis, and skin necrosis. Skin expanders must be correctly sited, and placements are best tolerated in older infants. It takes 6–8 weeks to gain maximum advantage.[37]

Hepatobiliary and Gastro-Intestinal Tract

The liver is shared in all thoraco-omphalopagus twins. Ultrasound, CT, and radio nucleotide scanning provide the best overall picture of hepatic conjunction, the biliary drainage system including the gall bladder and configuration of the pancreas. For successful hepatic division, each liver has to have an inferior vena cava to its own heart; absence thereof is incompatible with survival after surgery. Hepatic conjunction is along an oblique plane, and venous connections may consist of a labyrinth of small venous channels, which may bleed excessively during surgery. In our experience, hepatic division has always been possible. Cardiac disconnection must be accomplished before hepatic division, as a large volume of blood can circulate through the liver, creating a false impression that both hearts are able to sustain independent life.

As 25% of thoracopagus twins share a biliary system, the anatomy of the extra hepatic biliary system (EHBS) needs to be evaluated. This is best achieved with dynamic biliary scintigraphy and two gallbladders with independent excretion into separate duodenums are indicative of two EHBS. However, intraoperative cholangiography may also be required.[38,47] Two gallbladders do not always equate with two EHBSs, espe-

cially if there is fusion of the proximal duodenum. This may be demonstrated by upper contrast radiography. Bile drainage is imperative and in the presence of a single EHBS, one twin should be allocated the EHBS, while every attempt should be made to establish bile drainage through a Roux-Y hepaticojejunostomy in the other twin.[5] Anatomically, the pancreas belongs to the duodenum, and is best left with the EHBS if there is a single pancreas.

The upper gastrointestinal tract from the duodenum distally is shared in 50% of thoracopagus conjunction. This junction can extend to the level of Meckel's point where it will divide into two separate distal ilea. High duodenal conjunction is a pointer appointed toward a single or shared EHBS.

Musculoskeletal System

Children with hemivertebrag asymmetrical or diminutive chest cavities, and even those with caudal junction are prone to develop progressive scoliosis of the spine, sometimes in areas remote from the area of conjunction. Long-term follow up is therefore mandatory.

Cardiorespiratory System and Chest Wall

The twins should be anesthetized on their sides. The whole of the twins below the separate cervical areas should be skin prepared and draped to be included in the operative field. If two survivors are possible arrangements for two separate operating tables and teams of surgeons should be made in preparation for the chest and abdominal reconstruction after separation. (It may be that a decision has yet to be made on the necessity to sacrifice one twin, depending on anatomy found.). The skin incision is made circumferentially along the sternum on the upper side. If only one survivor is possible then a curved incision on Twin A's side of the thorax is made from the cervical conjunction and curving across to beyond the nipple and extending caudally down into the abdomen incorporating a substantial part of the chest wall of the other twin. This donated thoracic cage can be used to reconstruct the chest wall after the separation (Fig. 45.1b). The pericardium is opened and the two hearts inspected.

The thoracotomy approach to the heart is very limited in terms of assessing the anatomy. The pericardium and hearts can only be adequately exposed and examined once the incision is taken across into twin B's chest, and the anterior of both hearts can be seen. We found this in both sets we have done with fused left ventricles: very little could be assessed until both chests had been opened quite widely.

The cardiac anatomy will of course have been determined to some extent before surgery, and there would be at least a working supposition of the anatomy, and what needs to be confirmed.

Decisions are made according to the anatomy. If the two hearts are separate and can maintain cardiovascular autonomy, the general surgeons can then open the abdomen and divide the single liver mass into two along an oblique median plane.

If the hearts are completely separate the issue is uncomplicated. If there is any bridge of tissue the most important first determination to be made if they are to be separated is the nature of the coronary supply to each heart, and the coronary sinus drainage. If they are in any way codependent for coronary supply or coronary venous drainage they cannot be separated. Beyond that, atrial connections can generally be divided, and ventricular connections cannot (or never have been with any survivors.) In our two sets with ventricular connections, we elected to leave the fused heart unseparated totally in twin B's chest.

The separation of the thorax is then completed from anterior to posterior. The diaphragms are attached in the normal manner posteriorly and to a large central tendon and inferior floor of the pericardium anteriorly. After separation there is a very large central defect. The pericardium can be replaced with a Gore-Tex patch but primary skin cover is not possible unless tissue expanders have been placed prior to separation. Even with skin expanders and skin cover, the anterior diaphragmatic attachment needs to be stabilized to facilitate normal respiratory ventilatory function. Staged closure with eventual skin graft is another method of achieving wound closure. What is important is that closure under tension is to be avoided as cardiac and respiratory compromise will result.

In a case with a single fused heart, one being rudimentary, the following procedure was carried out. The thoracic cavity was opened via thoracotomy in Twin A's side at the level of the fifth intercostal space. The heart and great vessels were exposed as far as possible with dissection and carefully examined. The cardiac abnormalities were as predicted (Figs. 45.6 and 45.7).

Twin A had a double-outlet univentricular heart of LV morphology, with a vestigial anterior ventricle and large ventricular septal defect, with transposition of the great vessels (Taussig-Bing type), and the major ventricle was fused with Twin B's left ventricle. The preoperative decision was that this twin could not survive with this cardiac anatomy.

Twin B had dextrocardia, probably situs inversus, with ventricular apices towards the right. The left ventricle was fused to Twin A's heart with a communication through the common wall, but there was no VSD or outflow obstruction.

The coronary artery system of twin B was separate from that of twin A. All the great vessels and left pulmonary veins (we could not access the right pulmonary veins) and both venae cavae of twin A were identified. A's ductus arteriosus was divided and oversewn, as was the azygos vein and a small left SVC. Silk ties were placed around the great vessels and the venae cavae, and around the left pulmonary veins. By snaring them a trial occlusion of all of the vessels leading to and from the heart of twin A was attempted. Because there was a concern for this side of the heart lacking coronary supply after occluding the vessels, and causing a general arrhythmia of both hearts, and an attempt was to be made to connect A's ascending aorta to B's with a synthetic shunt. However, it proved impossible to side-clamp the aortas, so trial occlusion was done instead. Although it significantly darkened,

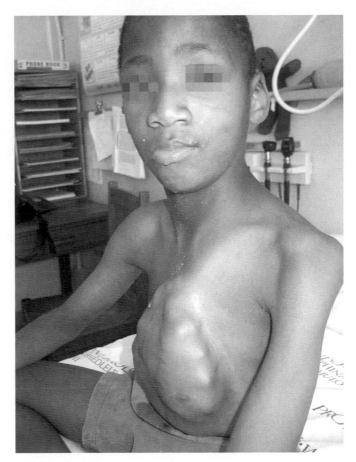

FIG. 45.6. One of a very few survivors (10 years) of a twin from a set of thoracopagus twins with a fused heart. Note gross chest deformity. At the time of initial surgery, the chest wall of the other twin was used to cover the chest wall defect. Any change in position of the heart resulted in arrhythmia. Late reconstruction of the chest wall is planned. [A personal comment: Our survivor of almost 10 years has had a very unhappy course including severe cerebrovascular accidents from thrombus discharged from the "appendage" heart, which has also significantly interfered with his own heart's function. There is a strong opinion amongst the clinicians caring for him that we should never have embarked on the procedure in the first place. I have wondered about it myself, and think I would probably support doing it again, though we have some experience now on which to build. (J.H. author)]

and there was some distension especially of the vestigial right ventricle, A's heart continued to function well, and after about 10 min looked healthy again. No other adverse events occurred during the test occlusion and the arterial and venous structures were individually ligated and divided. Occlusion of the great vessels resulted in the cessation of circulation in twin A. The separation was completed with the division of the thoracic cage well onto Twin A's side about 2 cm outside the nipple line. Twin A's body was removed from the operating table. The heart now protruded anteriorly from the thoracic cavity of Twin B. Any attempt at manipulating the heart to put it within the thoracic cavity resulted in ventricular arrhythmias. The bony defects in the chest wall were thus closed using a

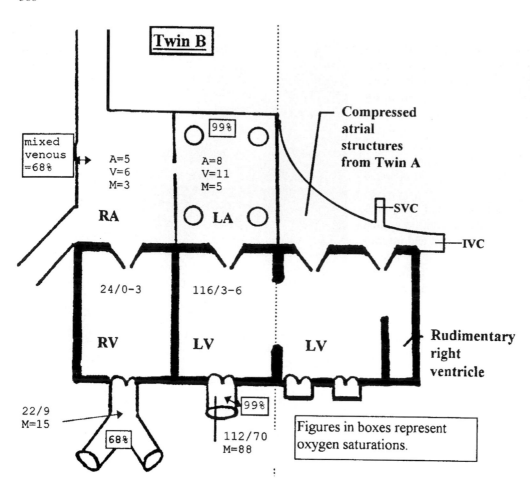

FIG. 45.7. Diagram of the ventricular and atrial arrangement of a set of twins with a single heart after separation to save the life of one

section of the ribcage of twin A. Skin closure was achieved using skin from Twin A.

No twin with ventricular conjunction has ever been successfully separated with both twins surviving. However there is a report of thoracopagus twins with two normal hearts joined by a myocardial bridge who were seperated successfully.[48,49] In a situation where one twin is acardiac or with shared ventricles successful separation is impossible without sacrificing one infant. The chest wall and skin of the sacrificed twin can be used to obtain skin cover and to create a firm structure to protect the protuberant fused single heart as any dislocation of the heart from its natural position is likely to cause disturbance of function. All the main inflow and outflow vessels from one twin have to be disconnected from the heart and the whole cardiac complex assigned to the infant selected to survive. We have had two such infants surviving a sacrifice procedure one survived 30 days and died from aspiration, and the other is a long-term survivor of nearly 9 years (Figs. 45.6 and 45.7). Subsequent reconstruction of the deformed chest is possible at a later stage.[50]

Postoperative Management

Cardiovascular and respiratory failure remain the most frequent causes of death in the immediate postoperative period. Further operations may be required for secondary wound closure or

dehiscence and skin grafting. There is also hidden long-term morbidity and mortality. A number of infants died later from factors such as unresolved aspiration, bronchopneumonia, poor respiratory function, gastro oesophageal reflux, and cerebral anoxia.

Postoperative challenges maybe regarded as early or late, and are determined by all the other predictors of survival after thoracopagus surgery for separation.[27]

Postoperatively, the separated twins should be transported to the Intensive Care Unit and continually monitored for bleeding, hypotension, hypothermia, hypoxia, hypercarbia, acidosis, and electrolyte disturbances. Ongoing volume losses, respiratory impairment, and cardiogenic instability commonly occur in separated twins. Cardiovascular, respiratory failure and sepsis remain the most frequent causes of morbidity and mortality in the immediate postoperative care. Additional postoperative complications include chest wall and sternal insufficiency, diaphragmatic dysfunction, gastro-oesophageal reflux, and the risk of inadequate skin cover.

Further operations may be required for secondary wound closure, wound dehiscence, and vascular access.

Results

Over a period of 43 years (1964–2007), the Red Cross War Memorial Children's Hospital has managed 47 sets of symmetrical and asymmetrical conjoined twins. The relevant information is shown in Table 45.2. There was a tendency toward premature labor and CS for obstructive labor. There were few postnatal maternal complications.

The surgical management of conjoined twins has been divided into three categories (Tables 45.3 and 45.4).

1. *Nonoperative management:* Ten sets were stillborn, 8 of which were thoracopagus, 1 ischiopagus, and 1 triplet. Intrauterine death was either due to elective abortion (13–32 weeks), obstetric error or complex cardiac anomalies incompatible with life, confirmed by postmortem examination. These fetuses were lost during the 26–30th week of gestation. Six sets of thoracopagus twins were born alive but subsequently died from complex cardiac anomalies with cardiac failure at 9 days – 2 months postbirth. One symmetrical ischiopagus twin died as a result of a perforated colon and peritonitis.

2. *Emergency separation:* Emergency operations were performed on three symmetrical sets during the neonatal period. A thoracopagus twin deteriorated on day 15 necessitating emergency separation. Great difficulty was encountered closing the thoraco-abdominal defects primarily, which resulted in irreversible respiratory failure. An omphalopagus twin was born with a ruptured exomphalos with evisceration of liver and loops of bowel and demise of the other. The one parapagus twin was moribund at birth necessitating surgical separation within 17 h once preliminary investigations were performed. Only two of six children survived separation with one dying at 6 weeks from bronchopneumonia.

3. *Elective separation:* Elective separations were performed on 14 sets at ages ranging from 4 days to 11 months, when tissues were still pliable and the infants in the optimal physiological state. Reasons for the wide variation included allowing time for the infants to grow and to bond with their families and also completion of the multitude of investigations required. On occasion it was also necessary to resolve complex moral and ethical issues when there was a threat to the survival of one or both infants. Additional delay was due to the use of tissue expanders in two sets of ischiopagus twins to facilitate wound closure, repeated operative rehearsals, and reordering of selected investigations, where uncertainty existed. Twenty-two of a potential 28 children survived. In one set of thoracopagus twins with a combined complex heart, the decision was made to sacrifice the one child, with the parents' permission to save the life of his brother. This child is the only long-term survivor following a procedure of this kind.

An assessment of the cardiac anomalies encountered in 16 thoracopagus infants during presurgical investigations, during surgery and at postmortem, revealed the following: a shared pericardial sac with separate hearts in 5, conjoined hearts in 8 who manifested varying types of atrial or ventricular fusion, while 3 had a single heart.

Other abnormalities identified included anomalous pulmonary veins, atrio-ventricular septal defects, hypoplastic pulmonary vessels, abnormal vena caval drainage and abnormal origin of major arterial vessels from the aortic arch 9.

TABLE 45.2. Obstetric implications implications of conjoined twins (based on data from 54 sets of twins).[a]

Maternal history		
	Maternal age in years	23 (16–45 range)
	Parity – Nulliparous	38% (17 of 45 sets)
	Family history of twinning	14.3% (8 of 54 sets)
	Stillbirths	39.6% (21 of 54 sets)
	Antenatal diagnosis	41% (32 sets)
Birth		
	Presentation:	
	○ Breech	52% (13 of 25 sets)
	○ Vertex	48% (12 of 25 sets)
	Vaginal delivery	41% (19 of 46 sets)
	Mean gestational age weeks	35.3 (20 sets)
	Combined weight/kg	3.9 (2.7–4.9 in 13 sets)
	Elective Cesarean section	59% (27 of 46 sets)

[a]Obstetrical information extrapolated from available data **5**

TABLE 45.3. Conjoined twins 1964–2006.

	Sets	Operations	Survivors
Symmetrical twins			
Thoracopagus	23	9	10
Omphalopagus	1	1	1
Ischiopagus	5	3	6
Pygopagus	2	2	4
Parapagus	1	1	1
Craniopagus	1	1	0
Cephalopagus	1	0	0
Total	34	17	22
Incomplete or asymmetrical twins			
Ischiopagus	4	3	3
Parasitic	5	5	5
Fetus in fetus	3	3	3
Total	12	11	11
Conjoined triplets			
	1	0	0

TABLE 45.4. Outcome in three major studies on conjoined twins.

			Operated			
Symmetrical twins			Emergency surgery		Elective surgery	
Source	No of sets	Not operated sets	No of sets	No of Survivors (%)	No of sets	No of survivors (%)
Spitz and Kiely[34]	22	6	7	4 (29)	9	15 (83)
O'Neill[37]	18	5	5	1 (10)	8	13 (81)
Red Cross Hospital Series	34	17	3	2 (33)	14	20 (72)

Surgical Outcome

The surgical outcome of our series is depicted in Table 45.3 and compared with two international series in Table 45.4. The overall survival for symmetrical twins was 33.3% but 64.7% for those that were operated upon. Emergency surgery had a dismal outcome with only two infants surviving (33%.). Asymmetrical separation had a 92% survival rate.

Late deaths are reported in those babies who have been separated but have poor respiratory dynamic function and have died from aspiration.[27,4] Sepsis is another significant contributor to morbidity and mortality of these babies.

Conclusions

Prenatal diagnosis allows careful planning for delivery and for preoperative assessment. Emergency surgery may be required, but it is preferable to delay surgery to allow growth and the completion of investigations. Inevitably, the ultimate prognosis will depend on the state of the conjoined organs and the potential for successful separation. Tragically in some, separation will not be possible. Detailed preoperative assessment is essential to determine the best surgical approach, reconstruction methods, and ultimate outcome. Despite successful separation, some children are left crippled and disabled, requiring life-long follow-up and care.

References

1. Spencer R. Anatomic description of conjoined twins: a plea for standardized terminology. J Pediatr Surg 1996: 3; 941–4.
2. Spencer R. Conjoined Triplets and Beyond. In: Conjoined Twins. Developmental Malformations and Clinical Implications. Spencer R. John Hopkins University Press, Baltimore, 2003: 376–391.
3. Magnus KG, et al. Intrahepatic fetus-in-fetu: a case report and review of the literature. J Pediatr Surg 1999: 34; 1861–1864.
4. Cywes S, Millar AJW, Rode H, Brown RA. Conjoined twins–the Cape Town experience. Pediatr Surg Int 1997: 12; 234–248.
5. Hall JG. Twinning. Lancet 2003: 362(9385); 735–43.
6. Viljoen DL, Nelson MM, Beighton P. The epidemiology of conjoined twinning in Southern Africa. Clin Genet 1983: 24; 15–21.
7. Mackenzie TC, Crombleholme TM, Johnson MP, et al. The natural history of prenatally diagnosed conjoined twins. J Pediatr Surg 2002: 37; 303–309.
8. Spencer R. Theoretical and analytical embryology of conjoined twins: part I: embryogenesis. Clin Anat 2000: 13; 36–53.
9. Spencer R. Theoretical and analytical embryology of conjoined twins: part II: adjustments to union. Clin Anat 2000: 13; 97–120.
10. Kaufman MH. The embryology of conjoined twins. Childs Nerv Syst 2004: 20; 508–525.
11. Mayer A. The Monstrous Birth: The Theory of Maternal Impression and Congenital Malformations. Proceedings of the 10th Annual History of Medicine Day 2001: pp. 48–52.
12. Bondeson J. The Biddenden Maids: a curious chapter in the history of conjoined twins. J R Soc Med 1992: 85; 217–221.
13. Rickham PP. The dawn of Paediatric Surgery: Johannes Fatio (1649–1691)- His life, his work and his horrible end. Prog Pediatr Surg 1986: 20; 95–105.
14. Van der Weiden RM. The First Successful Separation of Conjoined (1689). Twin Res 2004: 7; 125–127.
15. Maggio M, Nancy A, Callan MD, et al. The first-trimester ultrasonographic diagnosis of conjoined twins. Am J Obstet Gynecol 1985: 152; 833–5.
16. Gray CM, Nix HG, Wallace AJ. Thoracopagus twins: prenatal diagnosis. Radiology 1950: 54; 398–400.
17. Basgül A, Kavak ZN, Sezen D, Basgul A, Gokaslan H. Thoraco-omphalopagus conjoined twins detected at as early as 9 weeks of gestation: transvaginal two-dimensional ultrasound, color Doppler and fetoplacental Doppler velocity waveform findings. Fetal Diagn Ther 2006: 21; 477–480.
18. Maymon R, Mendelovic S, Schachter M, et al. Diagnosis of conjoined twins before 16 weeks' gestation: the 4-year experience of one medical center. Prenat Diagn 2005: 25; 839–843.
19. Harper RG, Kenigsberg K, Sia CG, et al. Xiphopagus conjoined twins: a 300-year review of the obstetric, morphopathologic, neonatal, and surgical parameters. Am J Obstet Gynecol 1980: 137; 617–629.
20. Rode H, Fieggen AG, Brown RA, et al. Four decades of conjoined twins at Red Cross Children's Hospital--lessons learned. S Afr Med J 2006: 96; 931–940.
21. Kingston CA, McHugh K, Kumaradevan J, et al. Imaging in the preoperative assessment of conjoined twins. Radiographics 2001: 21; 1187–1208.
22. Mann MD, Coutts JP, Kaschula RO, et al. The use of radionuclides in the investigation of conjoined twins. J Nucl Med 1983: 24; 479–84.
23. Pepper C. Ethical and Moral Considerations in the Separation of Conjoined Twins. Birth Defects Original Article Series 1967: 3; 128–134.
24. Spitz L. The conjoined twins. Transcript of the speeches given at the BAFS annual dinner on 28 February 2002. British Academy of Forensic Sciences. Med Sci Law 2002: 42; 284–7
25. Bratton MQ, Chetwynd SB. One into two will not go: conceptualising conjoined twins. J Med Ethics 2004: 30; 279–285.
26. Raffensperger JA. philosophical approach to conjoined twins. Pediatr Surg Int 1997: 12; 249–255.
27. Thomas JM, Lopez JT, Conjoined twins--the anaesthetic management of 15 sets from 1991-2002. Paediatr Anaesth 2004: 14; 117–129.
28. Diaz JH, Furman EB. Perioperative management of conjoined twins. Anesthesiol 1987: 67; 965–973.
29. Hoyle RM. Surgical separation of conjoined twins. Surg Gynecol Obstet 1990: 170; 549–562.
30. Bouchard S, Johnson MP, Flake AW, et al. The EXIT procedure: experience and outcome in 31 cases. J Pediatr Surg 2002: 37; 418–426.
31. Ossowski K, Suskind DL. Airway management in conjoined twins: a rare indication for the EXIT procedure. Arch Otolaryngol Head Neck Surg 2005: 131; 58–60.
32. Shank EN, Manohar N, Schmidt U. Anesthetic management for thoracopagus twins with complex cyanotic heart disease in the magnetic resonance imaging suite. Anesth Analg 2005: 100; 361–364.
33. Szmuk P, Rabb MF, Curry B, et al. Anaesthetic management of thoracopagus twins with complex cyanotic heart disease for cardiac assessment: special considerations related to ventilation and cross-circulation. Br J Anaesth 2006: 96; 341–5.
34. Spitz L, Kiely EM. Conjoined twins. JAMA 2003: 289; 1307–1310.
35. Cywes S, Davies MR, Rode H. Conjoined twins–the Red Cross War Memorial Children's Hospital experience. S Afr J Surg 1982: 20; 105–18.
36. Spitz L, Kiely E. Success rate for surgery of conjoined twins. Lancet 2000: 356(9243); 1765.
37. O'Neill JA. Conjoined Twins. In: Pediatric Surgery, 6th Edition. Grosfeld J, O'Neill JA, Coran AG, Fonkalsrud EW (Editors). Mosby, 2006.

38. Lobe TE, Oldham KT, Richardson CJ. Successful separation of a conjoined biliary tract in a set of omphalopagus twins. J Pediatr Surg 1989: 24; 930–932.
39. Filler RM, Conjoined twins and their separation. Semin Perinatol 1986: 10; 82–91.
40. Spitz L. Surgery for conjoined twins. Ann R Coll Surg Engl 2003: 85; 230–235.
41. Fitzpatrick C. Psychosocial Study of a Surviving Conjoined Twin. Clin Child Psychol Psychiatr 2000: 5; 513–519.
42. Hisano K, Nakamura K, Okada M, Iwai S. Separation of conjoined twins using chest wall prosthesis. J Pediatr Surg 1989: 24; 928–929.
43. Spitz L, Capps AN, Kiely EM. Xiphoomphaloischiopagus tripus conjoined twins: successful separation following abdominal wall expansion. J Pediatr Surg 1991: 26; 26–29.
44. Ricketts R, Zubowicz VN. Use of tissue expansion for separation and primary closure of thoracopagus twins. Pediatr Surg Int 1987: 2; 365–368.
45. Hilfiker ML, Hart M, Holmes R, et al. Expansion and division of conjoined twins. J Pediatr Surg 1998: 33; 768–770.
46. Zubowicz VN, Ricketts R. Use of skin expansion in separation of conjoined twins. Ann Plast Surg 1988: 20; 272–6.
47. Spitz L, Crabbe DC, Kiely EM. Separation of thoraco-omphalopagus conjoined twins with complex hepato-biliary anatomy. J Pediatr Surg 1997: 32; 787–789.
48. Benjamin LC, Nahar J, Sable C, et al. Separation of thoracopagus-cardiopagus twins joined by a myocardial bridge. J Thorac Cardiovasc Surg 2005: 130; 1212–1213.
49. Norwitz ER, Hoyte LP, Jenkins KJ, et al. Separation of conjoined twins with the twin reversed-arterial-perfusion sequence after prenatal planning with three-dimensional modelling. N Engl J Med 2000: 343; 399–402.
50. Fishman SJ, Puder M, Geva T, et al. Cardiac relocation and chest wall reconstruction after separation of thoracopagus conjoined twins with a single heart. J Pediatr Surg 2002: 37; 515–517.

46
Chylothorax

David Lasko and Jacob C. Langer

Introduction

Chylothorax is defined as a collection of lymphatic fluid within the pleural spaces, and is an uncommon but potentially serious condition in infants and children. Asellius and Bartolet first described chylothorax more than 400 years ago, but Quincke reported the first case in 1875. The first case reports of spontaneous chylous pleural effusion in children appeared in 1917 and 1926 by Pisek and Stewart. Blalock provided the earliest understanding of the underlying pathophysiology of the disease in 1936 when he showed experimentally that superior vena cava occlusion produced chylothorax an average of 17 days later. Preemptive ligation of the thoracic duct prevented development of the effusion.[1] This led to the introduction of therapeutic thoracic duct ligation by Lampson in 1948.

Subsequent developments focused on understanding the physiology of chyle production and flow. In recent decades basic and clinical research has led to advances in both medical and surgical therapy for chylothorax. On the medical side understanding the metabolism of medium versus long-chain fatty acids led to the introduction of low fat diets to treat chylothorax. Subsequently, the development of total parenteral nutrition with complete bowel rest has greatly improved outcomes. Modern surgical advances include pleuroperitoneal shunting, which was introduced to pediatric surgery by Azizkahn and colleagues in 1983.[2,3]

Embryology

The lymphatic system begins its initial development in the sixth gestational week. This diffuse system of endothelial-lined channels develops from six different outpouchings of the venous endothelium: two jugular sacs, two femoral sacs, a retroperitoneal sac, and the cisterna chyli. These sacs grow longitudinally and link together by the ninth gestational week, eventually forming a bilateral system of lymphatic trunks connected across the midline by numerous horizontal and diagonal anastomoses. Regression of the superior portion of the right trunk and the inferior portion of the left trunk, with maintenance of a diagonal connection at the level of the fourth to sixth thoracic vertebra, ultimately yields the final thoracic duct.[1,4]

Anatomy

The thoracic duct represents the most important lymphatic channel in the development of chylothorax. It arises from the cisterna chyli near the midline at the level of the second lumbar vertebra, and passes through the aortic hiatus of the diaphragm into the right chest medial to the azygos vein. The duct remains as a single structure in the inferior aspect of the chest, but on its upward passage numerous lymphatic tributaries empty into it from the chest wall. In the majority of patients the thoracic duct crosses as a single structure into the left chest at the fourth or fifth thoracic vertebra and continues into the left neck, where it forms an arch that rises 3–4 cm above the clavicle. It then drains into the left subclavian vein near the junction of the subclavian and left internal jugular veins.

Chyle Physiology

Chyle is a milky fluid consisting of lymph and emulsified fats, which is produced by the mucosal cells of the small intestine during the process of digestion. It is taken up by lacteals, which join with larger lymphatics that are carrying lymph fluid from the rest of the body. Ultimately these converge to form the cisterna chyli, which empties into the thoracic duct. The high lymphocyte content of chyle is important both diagnostically and clinically (see the section "Pathophysiology of Chylothorax") as chylothorax patients can become lymphopenic with up to threefold increased susceptibility to infection after long courses of therapeutic drainage.[5]

Pathophysiology of Chylothorax

Chylothorax in children falls into two main categories: congenital and acquired. Most reports identify congenital etiology in approximately 10% of pediatric chylous effusions,

D.H. Parikh et al. (eds.), *Pediatric Thoracic Surgery*,
DOI: 10.1007/b136543_46, © Springer-Verlag London Limited 2009

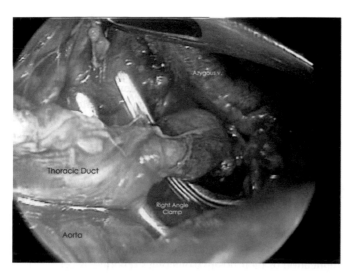

FIG. 46.1. Thoracoscopic thoracic duct ligation

Although widely cited as the most common surgical approach to recalcitrant pediatric chylothorax, thoracic duct ligation has generally yielded equivocal results. In one large series of postcardiac surgery chylothorax, all four of the patients treated with duct ligation failed and three of them died.[21] Other authors have reported success rates between 25 and 100%, but no series includes more than five patients treated with this procedure.[6,22,23] It is likely that the equivocal results are related to selection bias toward sicker patients.[21] As such, some authors have suggested that a more aggressive approach earlier in the course of the chylothorax might improve both surgical and overall outcomes.

Pleuroperitoneal Shunt

While traditional medical and surgical approaches are usually successful, a subset of patients remains refractory to dietary manipulation, medications, thoracic duct ligation, and external drainage. Approximately 25 years ago, Azizkahn introduced the technique of pleuroperitoneal shunting for such patients.[3] Several series since then have demonstrated greater than 75–85% success rates in treating refractory pediatric chylothorax.[2,3,23]

The procedure involves creation of subcutaneous tunnels in both the chest wall (mid-axillary line of the affected side) and abdominal wall. The two cuffed ends of the shunt are passed through the tunnels and into the pleural and peritoneal cavities. The middle of the shunt tube contains a 1.5–2.5-cc pumping chamber that can be positioned either externally[24] or subcutaneously.[3] The chamber includes a one-way valve, and when manually pumped pushes fluid from the chest cavity into the abdomen. The fluid is then absorbed by peritoneal vessels. The chest cavity is emptied several times daily until the pumping sessions can be weaned and ultimately discontinued.[24]

Wolff et al. reported successful clearance of 16 out of 19 refractory chylothoraces in patients aged 1 month to 11 years (median 3 months) who had failed at least 2 weeks (and up to 2 years) of parenteral nutrition and external drainage.[24] The patients required from 12 to 365 days of pleuroperitoneal shunting for their effusions to disappear (median 14 days of therapy). Complications included six shunt malfunctions requiring further surgical intervention and two shunt infections requiring removal.

Treatment Recommendations

Clearly, chylothorax in children represents a difficult management dilemma. New therapies and management strategies have increased the therapeutic armamentarium but no adequately sized trials exist to define the optimal order, dosing, and duration of the various therapeutic approaches. On the basis of available data, we suggest the treatment algorithm detailed in Fig. 46.2, which can be tailored to the availability and experience of the individual physician or institution.

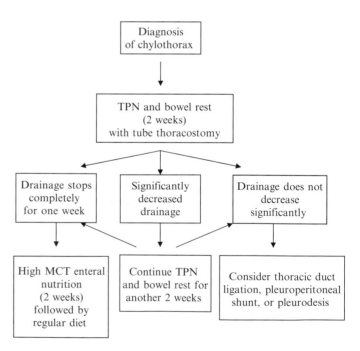

FIG. 46.2. Treatment algorithm for chylothorax

References

1. Le Coultre C. Chylothorax. In: Operative Pediatric Surgery. Ziegler MM, Azizkahn RG, Weber TR (editors). McGraw Hill, New York, 2003.

2. Murphy MC, Newman BM, Rodgers BM. Pleuroperitoneal shunts in the management of persistent chylothorax. Ann Thorac Surg 1989: 48; 195–200.

3. Azizkhan RG, Canfield J, Alford BA, Rodgers BM. Pleuroperitoneal shunts in the management of neonatal chylothorax. J Pediatr Surg 1983: 18; 842–50.

4. Gray SW, Skandalakis JE. The lymphatic system. In: Embryology for Surgeons: The Embryological Basis for the Treatment of Congenital Defects. W.B. Saunders, Philadelphia, PA, 1972.

5. Allen EM, van Heeckeren DW, Spector ML, Blumer JL. Management of nutritional and infectious complications of postoperative chylothorax in children. J Pediatr Surg 1991: 26; 1169–74.

6. Beghetti M, La Scala G, Belli D, et al. Etiology and management of pediatric chylothorax. J Pediatr 2000: 136; 653–8.

7. Antonetti M, Manuck TA, Schramm C, Hight D. Congenital pulmonary lymphangiectasia: a case report of thoracic duct agenesis. Pediatr Pulmonol 2001: 32; 184–6.

8. Guleserian KJ, Gilchrist BF, Luks FI, et al. Child abuse as a cause of traumatic chylothorax. J Pediatr Surg 1996: 31; 1696–7.

9. Winters RW, Stephens HB, Olney MB. Traumatic chylothorax; report of two cases and review of pediatric literature. J Pediatr 1954: 45; 446–56.

10. Cannizzaro VB, Frey B, Bernet-Buettiker V. The role of somatostatin in the treatment of persistent chylothorax in children. Eur J Cardiothorac Surg 2006: 30; 49–53.

11. Aubard Y, Derouineau I, Aubard V, et al. Primary fetal hydrothorax: a literature review and proposed antenatal clinical strategy. Fetal Diagn Ther 1998: 13; 325–33.

12. Longaker MT, Laberge J-M, Dansereau J, et al. Primary fetal hydrothorax: natural history and management. J Pediatr Surg 1989: 24; 573–6.

13. Wasmuth-Pietzuch A, Hansmann M, Bartmann P, Heep A. Congenital chylothorax: lymphopenia and high risk of neonatal infections. Acta Paediatr 2004: 93; 220–4.

14. Cormack BE, Wilson NJ, Finucane K, West TM. Use of monogen for pediatric postoperative chylothorax. Ann Thorac Surg 2004: 77; 301–5.

15. Bond SJ, Guzzetta PC, Snyder ML, Randolph JG. Management of pediatric postoperative chylothorax. Ann Thorac Surg 1993: 56; 469–72; discussion 472–3.

16. Landvoigt MT, Mullett CJ. Octreotide efficacy in the treatment of chylothoraces following cardiac surgery in infants and children. Pediatr Crit Care Med 2006: 7; 245–8.

17. Yildirim SV, Kervancioğlu M, Saritas B, et al. Octreotide infusion for the treatment of chylothorax in pediatric cardiac intensive care unit. Anadolu Kardiyol Derg 2005: 5; 317–18.

18. Rosti L, De Battisti F, Butera G, et al. Octreotide in the management of postoperative chylothorax. Pediatr Cardiol 2005: 26; 440–3.

19. Helin RD, Angeles ST, Bhat R. Octreotide therapy for chylothorax in infants and children: a brief review. Pediatr Crit Care Med 2006: 7; 576–9.

20. Berkenbosch JW, Withington DE. Management of postoperative chylothorax with nitric oxide: a case report. Crit Care Med 1999: 27; 1022–4.

21. Chan EH, Russell JL, Williams WG, et al. Postoperative chylothorax after cardiothoracic surgery in children. Ann Thorac Surg 2005: 80; 1864–70.

22. Liu CS, Tsai HL, Chin TW, Wei CF. Surgical treatment of chylothorax caused by cardiothoracic surgery in children. J Chin Med Assoc 2005: 68; 234–6.

23. Milsom JW, Kron IL, Rheuban KS, Rodgers BM. Chylothorax: an assessment of current surgical management. J Thorac Cardiovasc Surg 1985: 89; 221–7.

24. Wolff AB, Silen ML, Kokoska ER, Rodgers BM. Treatment of refractory chylothorax with externalized pleuroperitoneal shunts in children. Ann Thorac Surg 1999: 68; 1053–7.

the fourth branchial pouches. Lymphoid cells from bone-marrow progenitors migrate into the thymus at a later stage and coalesce to form the lymphoid follicles.

The upper poles of the thymus extend into the neck while the lower poles drape over the pericardium. The right lobe is slightly larger than the left, and the two lobes interconnect by a bridge of loose areolar tissue. The thymus receives blood supply from the internal mammary arteries and the venous drainage enters the brachio-cephalic and internal thoracic veins. The lymphatic drainage of the thymus is along the internal mammary vessels, anterior mediastinal lymph nodes, and hilar lymph nodes.

The thymus progressively decreases in size during late childhood and adult life.

Significant variations in size, shape, and extent of the thymus have been described. These anatomical variations are of clinical importance when complete thymectomy is contemplated for myasthenia.[6] Thymic tissue may be found beyond the anatomical capsule of the gland in up to 72% of individuals.[7,8] The thymus extends into the neck in 32% of individuals and thymic tissue may be found anywhere from the anterior triangle of the neck to the diaphragm. Thymic tissue is commonly found in the mediastinum beyond the confines of the thymus gland in the region of phrenic nerves, behind the innominate vein, in the aorto-pulmonary window, in the aorto-caval groove and in the cardio-phrenic groove (Fig. 47.1). In approximately 4% of cases the left lobe of the thymus lies inferior to left innominate vein.

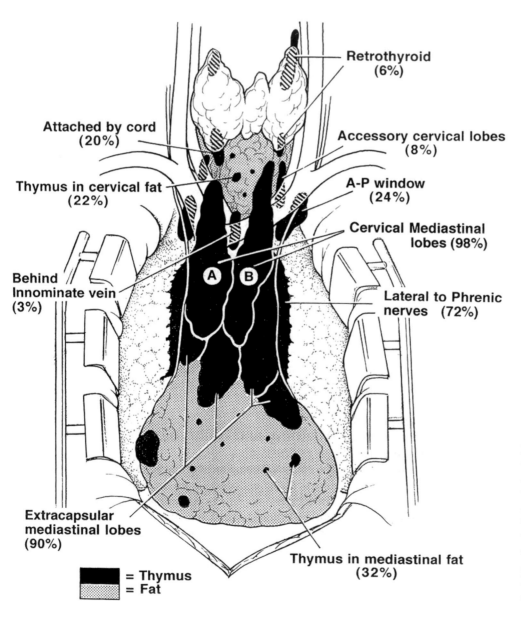

FIG. 47.1. Variations in the surgical anatomy of the thymus and sites of ectopic thymic tissue. Numbers in parentheses are the frequencies with which these variations occur. *Black* = thymus, *grey* = fat which may contain islands of thymus. AP = aorticopulmonary window. From: Neurology 1997; 48(suppl 5): S52–63. With permission

Consequences of Thymectomy

The human thymus is required for establishment of the T cell pool in fetal life. Following thymectomy in infancy there are measurable changes in T lymphocyte subtypes. Numbers of $CD4^+$ T cells (mature helper T cells) are reduced by 30–50%, and some studies report reductions in $CD3^+$ and $CD8^+$ T cells.[9,10] Other studies have shown evidence for extra-thymic maturation of T cell following thymectomy.[11] No studies have shown any clinical consequence of thymectomy in terms of frequency of infections, response to childhood vaccinations, or presence of organ-specific autoantibodies.

Thymic Hyperplasia

True thymic hyperplasia is rare in children. Most instances of thymic "hyperplasia" are physiological. Thymic "rebound" is a relatively common condition in childhood and adolescence. It can be seen following recovery from severe thermal burns, cardiac surgery, tuberculosis, treatment of malignancies (especially lymphoma), and after discontinuation of oral steroids.[12] Most cases of rebound thymic hyperplasia occur within a year and the gland typically returns to normal size.

It is important to differentiate thymic hyperplasia from residual/recurrent lymphoma and other thymic tumors.[13] The thymus should appear symmetrically enlarged on CT/MR scanning with no discrete mass. Early experience with FDG-PET scanning is promising – high concentrations of FDG in the thymus are suggestive of malignancy.[14]

DiGeorge Syndrome

DiGeorge syndrome is a rare congenital malformation caused by a deletion on chromosome 22 at locus 22q11.2.[15] DiGeorge described this condition in 1965. Although the cardinal features of the DiGeorge syndrome relate to hypoplasia of the thymus and parathyroids, the phenotype is very variable (Table 47.1) even among members of the same family.[16,17] Because the signs and symptoms of 22q11.2 deletion syndrome are so

TABLE 47.1. Abnormalities seen in the DiGeorge syndrome.

- Congenital heart disease (75%), typically conotruncal malformations (tetralogy of Fallot, interrupted aortic arch, ventricular septal defect, and persistent truncus arteriosus)
- Palatal abnormalities (70%), particularly velopharyngeal incompetence, submucosal cleft palate, and cleft palate
- Characteristic facies, including hypertelorism, low-set ears, micrognathia
- Developmental delay (70–90%)
- Immune deficiency (80%)
- Hypocalcaemia (50%)
- Renal anomalies (37%)
- Feeding problems (30%)
- Deafness (conductive and sensorineural)
- Schizophrenia

varied, different groupings of features were once described as separate conditions. These included the velo-cardio-facial syndrome, Shprintzen's syndrome, CATCH-22, and the DiGeorge syndrome.

The incidence of DiGeorge syndrome is approximately 1 in 4,000 population with an equal sex incidence and no clear racial or ethnic predilections. About 93% of cases have a de novo deletion of 22q11.2 but about 7% inherit the deletion from a parent in an autosomal dominant manner. Prenatal testing is possible by amniocentesis. Genetic testing may also be offered after antenatal detection of congenital heart disease and/or cleft palate.

DiGeorge syndrome is often first recognized when the affected newborn develops seizures from hypocalcaemia. Hypocalcaemia is managed by oral calcium and vitamin D supplements. Infants may suffer from recurrent viral or fungal infections due to a deficient T cell response. Live vaccines should be avoided. Most children outgrow this problem by the first year, although some continue to have trouble into adulthood. There is an increased incidence of autoimmune disease including juvenile rheumatoid arthritis and Grave's disease. Microdeletions in chromosomal region 22q11 are associated with a 30-fold increased risk of schizophrenia.

Thymoma

Thymoma is rare in children and account for less than 1% of all anterior mediastinal tumors.[18–20] The majority of thymomas arise in the third and fourth decades of life. Less than 2% thymomas arise in children, although the majority of these are malignant.

Diagnosis

Between a third and half of patients with thymic tumors are asymptomatic, and the diagnosis is found on routine examination or investigation.[21–23] Of those with symptoms up to 50% are related to paraneoplastic syndromes, predominantly myasthenia.[24] A further 40% present with symptoms related to intrathoracic mass, for example compression of neighboring structures. The remainder have generalized systemic symptoms such as weight loss or malaise.

Paraneoplastic Conditions

Thymomas are associated with a variety of paraneoplastic conditions.[22] Myasthenia gravis (MG) is the most common and is characterized by the development of autoimmune antibodies to the acetylcholine receptor. Approximately 30% of patients with a thymoma develop myasthenia while only 10–12% of patients with myasthenia have thymomas.[25] Pure red cell aplasia (PRCA) is the second most common paraneoplastic syndrome associated with thymoma.[22] PRCA occurs in 5–10% of patients with a thymoma and is thought to result from immune-mediated suppression of erythropoiesis. Other paraneoplastic conditions associated with thymomas include polymyositis, systemic lupus erythematosus, rheumatoid arthritis, thyroiditis, ulcerative colitis, acute pericarditis, myocarditis, hemolytic anemia, Addison's disease, and Cushing's syndrome.

Pathology

Thymomas vary in size and appearance from a small fibrotic plaque to a large lobulated mass. Degenerative cysts, calcification, and hemorrhage are all common. Encapsulated tumors have a good prognosis following complete resection in contrast with tumors that invade adjacent structures.

Traditionally, thymomas are classified into three histological types based on the predominant cell type: lymphocytic, epithelial, and lymphoepithelial. Histopathological classification of thymomas is, however, difficult because of the wide variation in morphological appearance. A number of systems have been proposed but none is perfect and none bears a particularly close correlation with clinical prognosis.[26] The World Health Organization (WHO) classification[27] is shown in Table 47.2.

Carcinoma of the thymus comprises 1% of thymic malignancies.[28] Paraneoplastic syndromes are uncommon in thymic carcinomas. The usual presentation is with cough, chest pain, phrenic nerve palsy, superior vena cava syndrome or as an incidental finding. Local invasion of contiguous mediastinal structures is present in up to 80% of patients at the time of presentation. Metastatic or lymph node spread is present in 40% of patients at presentation, and the commonest sites for metastatic spread are bones, lung, pleura, and liver.

Diagnosis and Imaging

An anterior mediastinal mass may be identified on a plain chest radiograph.[29] CT and MRI are both good methods for imaging the thymus, identifying nodal involvement and metastatic spread.[30,31] The normal thymus has been extensively studied using both modalities.[32] Positron emission tomography (PET) and integrated FDG-PET/CT are promising techniques for imaging thymic tumors.[33] PET is a nuclear medicine imaging technique, which produces a three-dimensional image of functional processes in the body. PET scanning with the tracer fluorine-18 fluorodeoxyglucose (FDG-PET) is widely used in clinical oncology. This tracer is a glucose analogue that is taken up by glucose-using cells and phosphorylated by hexokinase. High levels of mitochondrial hexokinase are found in most rapidly-growing malignant tumors.

Preresection biopsy of a thymoma is generally not helpful unless there is real doubt about the nature of a malignant anterior mediastinal tumor. Biopsy will, by definition, breach the tumor capsule and this may increase the risk of local recurrence.

Staging

The surgical staging of thymomas is controversial. The Masoka surgical staging is widely used, although many authors have modified it.[34] This system is based on macroscopic and microscopic features of tumor invasion beyond the capsule of the thymus (Table 47.3).

Management

Surgical resection is the mainstay of treatment for thymomas since most tumors are localized (85–90%) at presentation.[23] Complete surgical resection offers the best outcome for thymic tumors. In stage 1 thymomas complete surgical resection should be possible in 100% cases. This success rate falls with higher stage tumors, to an average of 47% (0–89%) for stage 3 and 26% (0–78%) for stage 4 tumors.

Median sternotomy is the easiest incision to remove a thymoma.[23] Trans-cervical thymectomy avoids the sternotomy but this is a technically challenging procedure. Thoracoscopic and robot-assisted thymectomy is growing in popularity, although it remains to be seen how long-term survival rates will compare with open surgery. For malignant tumors sternotomy remains the incision of choice. Neo-adjuvant chemotherapy prior to surgery is accepted practice for advanced thymic carcinomas. The role of adjuvant radiotherapy or chemotherapy for early stage tumors is unclear.[23]

Myasthenia Gravis

Myasthenia gravis is a chronic autoimmune disease characterized by varying degrees of skeletal muscle weakness.[35–37] The muscle weakness characteristically worsens during periods of activity and improves after periods of rest. Bulbar muscles are most frequently affected, although peripheral muscles and the diaphragm may also be affected.

TABLE 47.2. World Health Organization classification of thymic tumors.

Type	Histological description
A	Medullary thymoma
AB	Mixed thymoma
B1	Predominantly cortical thymoma
B2	Cortical thymoma
B3	Well-differentiated thymic carcinoma
C	Thymic carcinoma

TABLE 47.3. Masoka staging system for thymoma and associated survival data.

Masoka stage	Criteria
I	Encapsulated tumor
IIA	Microscopic capsular invasion
IIB	Macroscopic invasion into fatty tissue
III	Invasion into great vessels, pericardium or lung
IV A	Pleural and/or pericardial dissemination
IV B	Lymphatic or hematogenous metastases

The earliest description of myasthenia was probably made by a London physician Thomas Willis in 1672.[38] Myasthenia was recognized as a distinct clinical entity around 1880 by the German neurologists Erb and Jolly. They noticed that the muscle weakness in myasthenia was fatigable. The term myasthenia gravis was first used in 1895. Claude Bernard elucidated the mechanism of neuromuscular contraction in the 1850s and demonstrated that curare could block this. A decade later Fraser found that the calabar bean poison protected against curare and purified physostigmine. In 1934 Walker used physostigmine clinically to treat a patient with myasthenia.[39] Dale and Feldberg discovered that acetylcholine was the mediator of neuromuscular conduction the same year.[40]

Thymic tumors had been recognized in myasthenics in the late nineteenth century but it was not until 1937 that Blalock successfully resected the first thymoma with dramatic clinical improvement.[41] In the 1960s Miller and Good showed that the thymus was responsible for generating T lymphocytes.[38] The realization that myasthenia was an autoimmune disease came during this period. During the following decade assays for antibodies to the acetylcholine receptor were developed, and it became clear that most patients with myasthenia had high levels of these. This led to the use of plasmaphareisis and immunosuppressants as treatments for myasthenia.

Basic Science

Myasthenia gravis is caused by an abnormality in neuromuscular transmission.

Antibodies block the nicotinic acetylcholine receptors at the neuromuscular junction preventing muscle contraction from occurring.

Propagation of an action potential across the neuromuscular junction involves release of acetylcholine from the synaptic vesicles. Acetylcholine diffuses across the synaptic cleft and binds to acetylcholine receptors (AChR) in the motor end-plate. This causes membrane depolarization triggering muscle contraction. Comparatively few acetylcholine receptors need to be occupied on the motor end-plate to produce muscle contraction and normally there is a large excess of receptors so that repetitive stimulation can take place without fatigue. Acetylcholine must be removed from the synaptic space rapidly for repolarization to occur. This is accomplished by hydrolysis of ACh catalysed by acetylcholinesterase, which is present in high concentrations on the motor end-plate cell membrane.

In classical MG autoantibodies accelerate degradation of the AChR and prevent normal neuromuscular conduction.[42] This reduces the number of receptors available for repetitive conduction leading to muscle fatigue and weakness. Antibodies to the AChR can be detected in approximately 80% of patients with myasthenia.[43,44] Approximately 10–20% of patients with typical symptoms of MG do not have AChR antibodies. Previously these patients were considered to have seronegative MG. Muscle specific tyrosine kinase (MuSK) is a cell-surface membrane enzyme that is responsible for aggregating AChR during development of the neuromuscular junction. Its role in mature muscle is not yet clear but recent studies have shown that antibodies to MuSK are present in 40–50% of patients with seronegative MG.[45] Anti-MuSK antibodies have not been found in patients with ocular myasthenia nor in those who have anti-AChR antibodies.

Role of the Thymus in Myasthenia Gravis

The relationship between the thymus gland and myasthenia gravis is not yet fully understood. The thymus has been implicated in the production of AChR antibodies. In adults with MG lymphoid hyperplasia can be seen in the thymus in 50–60% cases. B lymphocytes from these lymphoid follicles secrete AChR-antibodies in vitro. Between 10 and 25% adult myasthenic patients develop thymic tumors.[46] Remission of the symptoms of myasthenia following thymectomy is well documented.

Clinical Features

Myasthenia gravis occurs in all ethnic groups and both genders. Myasthenia most commonly affects adult women in their second or third decades and men over the age of 70.[35-37]

Three subtypes of myasthenia are seen in childhood.[47,48] Neonatal MG is a transient disease resulting from transplacental transfer of antibodies from a myasthenic mother to her baby during pregnancy. Neonatal myasthenia gravis is transient, resolving around 2–3 months after birth. The congenital myasthenic syndrome (CMS) is a term used for a group of uncommon hereditary disorders of the neuromuscular junction. A variety of different structural and functional abnormalities of the neuromuscular junction can be identified with differing patterns of inheritance, clinical symptoms, electrophysiology, and response to therapy. Children with congenital myasthenia tend to have lifelong but relatively stable symptoms of generalized fatigable weakness. These disorders are nonimmune and consequently patients do not respond to immune therapy often used in patients with autoimmune myasthenia gravis, including thymectomy. Juvenile myasthenia gravis (JMG) is indistinguishable from the adult disease. Children account for 10–30% of all patients with immune myasthenia gravis.

Although myasthenia gravis may affect all voluntary muscles, the muscles that control eye and eyelid movement, facial expression, and swallowing are most severely affected. The onset of the disorder may be sudden and often the symptoms are not immediately recognized as myasthenia gravis. In most cases, the first symptom is weakness of the extra-occular muscles with diplopia, ptosis, and blurred vision. Less often dysphagia and dysarthria are the first signs. The degree of muscle weakness varies greatly among patients ranging from a localized form, limited to eye muscles (ocular myasthenia), to a severe generalized form which affect the respiratory muscles.

TABLE 47.4. Osserman and Genkins grading of myasthenia severity.

Grade I	Focal disease (ocular myasthenia)
Grade II	Generalized disease
Grade IIa	Mild
Grade IIb	Moderate
Grade III	Severe generalized disease
Grade IV	Myasthenic crisis with respiratory impairment

Osserman and Genkins[49] described five grades of increasing severity of MG (Table 47.4). Neurological examination reveals specific muscle group weakness worsening as the day progresses and improving with rest. The child gradually develops increasing fatigue and exhaustion.

Clinical Course

The clinical course of juvenile myasthenia is variable, although most children will develop progressive weakness and fatigue without treatment.[50–54] In approximately two thirds of patients maximum weakness develops during the first year after diagnosis. Two thirds of children with occular myasthenia will develop generalized disease within this period.[52] If spontaneous improvement is destined to occur this is most likely early in the course of the disease. A myasthenic crisis occurs when the muscles that control breathing weaken to the point that ventilation is inadequate. Myasthenic crises may be triggered by infection, fever, or an adverse reaction to medication.

Diagnosis

The diagnosis of MG is usually confirmed with a Tensilon® test.[55] Electromyography and serological testing are also valuable, although children with occular myasthenia may be seronegative.[48] Acetylcholine receptor antibodies can be detected in approximately 85% of patients with MG. Antibodies to MuSK can be identified in 40–70% patients who do not have AChR antibodies. A chest X-ray and contrast CT scan of the thorax should be performed once the diagnosis of MG is established to identify thymic pathology.

Edrophonium chloride (Tensilon®) is a short acting acetylcholinesterase inhibitor, which is administered intravenously in a dose of 0.15–0.2 mg/kg (up to 10 mg). If the test is positive an increase in muscle strength should be observed within 30 s of injection. The effects should wane after 10 min. The Tensilon test has 85% sensitivity for ocular and 95% sensitivity for generalized myasthenia gravis.[56]

Electromyography studies can provide support for the diagnosis of MG.[57] Repetitive nerve stimulation will identify a post-synaptic defect with fatigue. Muscle fibres in myasthenia gravis, as well as other neuromuscular disorders, do not respond as well to repeated electrical stimulation compared with normal individuals. Single fiber electromyography (SFEMG) involves stimulating a single muscle fiber to detect impaired nerve-to-muscle transmission, although this is a difficult examination to perform in children. This technique detects jitter or blocking and identifies subclinical cases of myasthenia. The test is abnormal in 90% of patients with mild generalized myasthenia and virtually 100% of cases with moderate to severe cases.

Management

There are no controlled trials to guide the management of myasthenia gravis in children, although the goal of treatment is clear to establish and maintain remission.

Medical Management

Anticholinesterases (Pyridostigmine) provide reasonable symptom relief in early disease.[48] The onset of action is about 30 min after ingestion and the effect lasts for about 4 h. Pyridostigmine is generally well-tolerated, although some children complain of abdominal pain and diarrhoea. Corticosteroids are recommended if the response to pyridostigmine is suboptimal. Steroids are useful for children awaiting thymectomy and those who continue to have symptoms after thymectomy. Steroids are also used for ocular myasthenia. Corticosteroids improve symptoms in 80% of cases. Immunosuppression with cyclosporine or azathioprine has been used to treat myasthenia, although this is controversial. Plasmapharesis may be of value in a myasthenic crisis. It is also useful in severe generalized weakness as a preparation for thymectomy. Four to five plasma exchanges are performed over 10–15 days. Some children respond to intravenous immunoglobulin with a clinical improvement after 1–2 weeks, which may last for several months.

Surgical Management

Although myasthenia associated with a thymoma is an absolute indication for thymectomy, there continues to be a debate about the role of thymectomy in the treatment of non-thymomatous myasthenia gravis. This debate persists primarily because of the lack of controlled prospective studies. There is also debate regarding the best approach for thymectomy. The Quality Standards Sub-committee of the American Academy of Neurology recently carried out a systematic review to analyze the role of thymectomy in adults with myasthenia.[58] Over 310 articles discussing MG and thymectomy were included in the review. Twenty-eight controlled studies were identified but none were randomized. The reviewers concluded that the benefit of thymectomy in non-thymomatous autoimmune myasthenia has not been established. They did, however, offer the rather cautious advice that thymectomy was "an option to increase the probability of remission or improvement."

Given the uncertainty over the role of thymectomy in adults with myasthenia, it is not surprising that there is even greater uncertainty in children. Indications for thymectomy in children with myasthenia include[48]:

- Thymoma
- Early-onset generalized anti-AChR positive myasthenia
- Progressive generalized weakness
- Non-thymoma-related autoimmune myasthenia unresponsive to treatment

Thymectomy is not recommended for seronegative myasthenia, anti-MuSK antibody positive myasthenia, and pure ocular myasthenia.[48] Preoperative assessment of respiratory function is mandatory prior to thymectomy for children with generalized and severe disease. Plasmapharesis may be indicated in children with severe disease to minimize postoperative respiratory morbidity.

Surgical Exposure of the Thymus

There are three basic options for thymectomy: trans-sternal, trans-cervical, and thoracoscopic. Debate has continued for over two decades regarding whether there is a relationship between the extent of resection and remission rate. In turn, this debate colors the choice of thymectomy technique. Jaretzki has long been a proponent of radical thymectomy, citing improved long-term outcome compared with simple thymectomy.[59] The same authors have, more recently, proposed a classification system for the approach to and extent of thymic resection to allow meaningful comparison of data (Table 47.5).[60]

Median Sternotomy

This incision provides excellent exposure for removal of the thymus.[61] Some surgeons add a cervical incision to allow radical extirpation of thymic tissue from the neck to the diaphragm.[59] Sternotomy is the incision of choice for removal of a thymoma. Thymectomy can often be achieved without opening the pleura. The phrenic nerves on either side must be identified and protected during the dissection, particularly in the root of the neck if a radical dissection is performed. The recurrent laryngeal nerves are also vulnerable during a radical thymectomy. The chest is closed over an anterior drain using sternal wires. Simple thymectomy can be performed through a partial sternal split. In this approach the manubrium is divided through an upper midline incision.

TABLE 47.5. Thymectomy classification.

T1 Trans-cervical thymectomy
    (a) Basic
    (b) Extended
T2 Thoracoscopic thymectomy
    (a) Conventional
    (b) Video-assisted extended thymectomy (VATET)
T3 Trans-sternal thymectomy
    (a) Simple
    (b) Extended
T4 Combined trans-cervical and trans-sternal thymectomy
    (Radical thymectomy)

Trans-Cervical Approach

This approach gives good access to upper mediastinum, and a good cosmetic result but trans-cervical thymectomy is technically challenging.[62] Pronounced extension of the neck, a headlight for the surgeon, and specially designed self-retaining Pearson retractors facilitate exposure. A transverse incision is made just above the sternal notch. The upper poles of thymus are identified under the sternomastoid muscles and the blood supply from the inferior thyroid artery divided. Blunt dissection proceeds inferiorly and posteriorly to ligate and divide the venous drainage into the innominate vein. Subsequent retraction allows sternum to be elevated anteriorly allowing dissection of the thymus to continue under direct vision. In a series of 164 myasthenic patients, Shrager et al. reported response rates comparable to trans-sternal thymectomy.[63] Henze et al., however, reported incomplete thymectomy in 27% patients undergoing trans-cervical thymectomy and concluded that the procedure should be abandoned.[64]

VATS Thymectomy

Several groups have now reported small series of patients treated by VATS thoracoscopy.[65–67] More recently reports of robotically-assisted thoracoscopic thymectomy have appeared.[68,69] The thymus can be approached through either hemithorax using a thoracoscope.[70] The right sided approach is more popular for a number of reasons. Dissection of the thymus in a caudal-cranial direction is ergonomically more efficient for a right-handed surgeon through the right chest. The confluence of the innominate veins and the superior vena cava is easier to identify through the right thorax, and therefore, ligation of the thymic vein(s) is safer. The main argument in favor of the left-sided approach is access to the aortopulmonary window for removal of mediastinal fat containing ectopic thymic tissue. Mineo et al. induced a pneumomediastinum to facilitate dissection of the thymus but this has not gained widespread popularity.[71]

Results After Thymectomy

Mortality should be negligible and morbidity minimal in children undergoing thymectomy for myasthenia. Establishing the long-term benefit of thymectomy conclusively is difficult in adults and consequently almost impossible in children.

The natural history of myasthenia is variable.[72] Debate regarding the benefits of radical over simple thymectomy complicates matters. Differing outcome measures makes comparison between studies exceedingly difficult. Although most large studies include some children, studies confined to children and generally small.[73–79]

Summarizing the adult literature leads to the conclusion that the long-term benefit of thymectomy in MG is variable. Most patients begin to improve within one year following a thymectomy, and a variable number eventually enter permanent remission

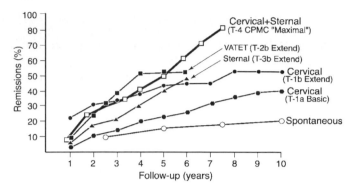

FIG. 47.2. Remission rates (life table analysis) following five thymectomy techniques for non-thymomatous MG
Cervical + Sternal – Combined transcervical and transsternal thymectomy (T-4)[82]
VATET (T-2b Extend) – Video-Assisted Thoracoscopic Extended Thymectomy[83]
Sternal (T-3b Extend) – Extended transsternal thymectomy[83]
Cervical (T-1b Extend) – "Extended" transcervical thymectomy[63]
Cervical (T-1a Basic) – Original "basic" transcervical thymectomy[84]
Spontaneous – Spontaneous remissions in children[72]
From: Jaretzki A. Video-assisted thoracoscopic extended thymectomy and extended transsternal thymectomy in non-thymomatous myasthenia gravis patients. J Neurol Sci 2004; 217: 233–4. With permission

off medication. Whether remission rates vary according to the type of thymectomy performed is hotly debated.[80,81] The proponents of radical thymectomy cite significant long-term benefits over simple thymectomy (Fig. 47.2). The counter-argument over the morbidity of simple vs. radical thymectomy and endoscopic thymectomy is equally important.[85]

Other Thymic Tumors

Thymolipoma

Thymolipoma is a rare benign slow-growing neoplasm of the thymus that usually affects young adults, although it has been reported in children.[86,87] Approximately half of the patients are asymptomatic. Thymolipomas are composed of mature adipose cells and thymic tissue. Radiologically, thymolipomas are large soft anterior mediastinal masses, which changes in shape with changes in patient position. CT and MRI appearances are characteristic with a combination of fat and soft-tissue elements. Surgical excision is curative.

Mediastinal Lymphangioma

Mediastinal lymphangiomas are benign lymphatic malformations that appear in young children.[88,89] Fifty percent are present at birth, and 90% are discovered by 2 years of age. Mediastinal lymphangiomas typically occur in the superior aspect of the anterior mediastinum and are usually contiguous with a cervical or axillary component. Radiologically these are rounded, lobulated, multicystic tumors that can reach massive sizes. Lymphangiomas may infiltrate tissue planes and they may surround or displace mediastinal structures. Because of the infiltrative nature of this condition complete surgical resection is often impossible.

Thymic Cysts

Thymic cysts may be congenital or acquired.[90,91] Congenital thymic cysts derive from remnants of the thymopharyngeal duct. These cysts are generally unilocular and may occur anywhere along the course of the embryonic thymus from the mandible to the manubrium. Acquired thymic cysts are most often multilocular and are induced by thymic inflammation. They may be found within thymomas or thymic germ cell neoplasms. The cyst wall is lined by squamous, transitional, or simple cuboidal or columnar epithelium. Ulceration with underlying fibrosis and chronic inflammation is common as is evidence of previous hemorrhage.

Thymic cysts are indistinguishable from other thymic masses on chest X-ray. CT scans show a well-defined cystic mass demonstrating low attenuation values consistent with fluid, although the appearance may vary if hemorrhage or infection has occurred. Surgical excision is the treatment of choice.

Conclusion and Future Perspective

Although the thymus plays a crucial role in prenatal development of the immune system, postnatal thymectomy has no clinical consequences. Changes in the size and shape of the thymus with age often lead to confusion with anterior mediastinal tumors. The precise role of thymectomy in the management of childhood myasthenia gravis is uncertain because of the lack of randomized trials. It does, however, seem likely that thymectomy increases the prospect of remission for children with myasthenia. The optimum route and technique for thymectomy remain a matter for debate.

References

1. Jacobs MT, Frush DP, Donnelly LF. The right place at the wrong time: historical perspective of the relation of the thymus gland and pediatric radiology. Radiology 1999; 210: 11–16.
2. Moncrieff A. Enlargement of the thymus in infants with special reference to clinical evidence of so-called status thymolymphaticus. Proc R Soc Med 1937; 31: 537–544.
3. Duffy BJ Jr, Fitzgerald PJ. Thyroid cancer in childhood and adolescence: report of 28 cases. Cancer 1950; 3: 1018–1032.
4. Hildreth NG, Shore RE, Dvoretsky PM. The risk of breast cancer after irradiation of the thymus in infancy. N Engl J Med 1989; 321: 1281–1284.

5. Caffey J. The mediastinum. In: Caffey J (Ed). Pediatric x-ray diagnosis. Chicago, Ill: Year Book, 1945; 344–345.

6. Jaretzki A, Wolff M. "Maximal" thymectomy for myasthenia gravis. Surgical anatomy and operative technique. J Thorac Cardiovasc Surg 1988; 96: 711–716.

7. Masaoka A, Nagaoka Y, Kotake Y. Distribution of thymic tissue at the anterior mediastinum. Current procedures in thymectomy. J Thorac Cardiovasc Surg 1975; 70: 747–754.

8. Fukai I, Funato Y, Mizuno T, Hashimoto T, Masaoka A. Distribution of thymic tissue in the mediastinal adipose tissue. J Thorac Cardiovasc Surg 1991; 101: 1099–1102.

9. Brearley S, Gentle TA, Baynham MI, et al. Immunodeficiency following neonatal thymectomy in man. Clin Exp Immunol 1987; 70: 322–327.

10. Wells WJ, Parkman R, Smogorzewska E, Barr M. Neonatal thymectomy: does it affect immune function? J Thorac Cardiovasc Surg 1998; 115: 1041–1046.

11. Torfadottir H, Freysdottir J, Skaftadottir I, et al. Evidence for extrathymic T cell maturation after thymectomy in infancy. Clin Exp Immunol 2006; 145: 407–412.

12. Bogot NR, Quint LE. Imaging of thymic disorders. Cancer Imaging 2005; 5: 139–149.

13. Aribal ME, Canpolat C, Berrak SG, Berik P. Anterior mediastinal mass in children following chemotherapy: thymic hyperplasia v recurrence. Radiog 2003; 9: 139–145.

14. Brink I, Reinhardt MJ, Hoegerle S, et al. Increased metabolic activity in the thymus gland studied with 18 F-FDG PET. Age dependency and frequency after chemotherapy. J Nucl Med 2001; 42: 591–595.

15. http://en.wikipedia.org/wiki/DiGeorge_Syndrome.

16. Robin NH, Shprintzen RJ. Defining the clinical spectrum of deletion 22q11.2. J Pediatr 2005; 147: 90–96.

17. Ryan AK, Goodship JA, Wilson DI, et al. Spectrum of clinical features associated with interstitial chromosome 22q11 deletions: a European collaborative study. J Med Genet 1997; 34: 798–804.

18. Rothstein DH, Voss SD, Isakoff M, Puder M. Thymoma in a child: case report and review of literature. Pediatr Surg Int 2005; 21: 548–551.

19. Welch KJ, Tapper D, Vawter GP. Surgical treatment of thymic cysts and neoplasms in children. J Pediatr Surg 1979; 14: 691–698.

20. Dehner LP, Martin SA, Sumner HW. Thymus related tumors and tumor-like lesions in childhood with rapid clinical progression and death. Hum Pathol 1977; 8: 53–66.

21. Lewis JE, Wick MR, Scheithauer BW, et al. Thymoma. A clinicopathologic review. Cancer 1987; 60: 2727–43.

22. Detterbeck FC, Parsons AM. Thymic tumors. Ann Thorac Surg 2004; 77: 1860–1869.

23. Srirajaskanthan R, Toubanakis C, Dusmet M, Caplin ME. A review of thymic tumours. Lung Cancer 2008; 60: 4–13.

24. López-Cano M, Ponseti-Bosch JM, Espin-Basany E, et al. Clinical and pathologic predictors of outcome in thymoma-associated myasthenia gravis. Ann Thorac Surg 2003; 76: 1643–1649.

25. Drachman DB. Myasthenia gravis. N Engl J Med 1994; 330: 1797–810.

26. Suster S, Moran CA. Thymoma classification: current status and future trends. Am J Clin Pathol 2006; 125: 542–554.

27. Okumura M, Ohta M, Tateyama H, et al. The World Health Organization histologic classification system reflects the oncologic behavior of thymoma: a clinical study of 273 patients. Cancer 2002; 94: 624–632.

28. Eng TY, Fuller CD, Jagirdar J, et al. Thymic carcinoma: state of the art review. Int J Radiat Oncol Biol Phys 2004; 59: 654–664.

29. Williams HJ, Alton HM. Imaging of paediatric mediastinal abnormalities. Paediatr Respir Rev 2003; 4: 55–66.

30. Pediatric Chest Imaging: Chest Imaging in Infants and Children. Lucaya J, Strife JL. Springer-Verlag, New York, Springer-Verlag, 2001.

31. Bogot NR, Quint LE. Imaging thymic disorders. Cancer Imaging 2005: 5: 139–149.

32. Boothroyd AE et al. The magnetic resonance appearances of the normal thymus in children. Clin Radiol 1992; 45: 378–381.

33. Quint LE. PET: other thoracic malignancies. Cancer Imaging 2006; 6: S82–S88.

34. Masaoka A, Monden Y, Nakahara K, Tanioka T. Follow-up study of thymomas with special reference to their clinical stages. Cancer 1981; 48: 2485–2492.

35. Drachman DB. Myasthenia gravis (first of two parts). N Engl J Med 1978; 298: 136–142.

36. Drachman DB. Myasthenia gravis (second of two parts). N Engl J Med 1978; 298: 186–193.

37. Nicolle MW. Myasthenia gravis. Neurologist 2002; 8: 2–21.

38. http://www.mgauk.org/

39. Walker MB. Treatment of Myasthenia Gravis with pyridostigmine Lancet 1934; 1:1200.

40. Dale HH, Feldberg W, Vogt M. Release of acetylcholine at voluntary motor nerve endings. J Physiol 1936; 86: 353–380.

41. Blalock A, Harvey AM, Ford RF, Lilienthal JL Jr. The treatment of myasthenia gravis by removal of the thymus gland. JAMA 1941; 117:1529.

42. Drachman DB, Adams RN, Stanley EF, Pestronk A. Mechanisms of acetylcholine receptor loss in myasthenia gravis. J Neurol Neurosurg Psychiatr 1980; 43: 601–610.

43. Seybold ME. Myasthenia gravis: a clinical and basic science review. JAMA 1983; 250: 2516–2521.

44. Vincent A. Immunology of disorders of neuromuscular transmission. Acta Neurol Scand Suppl 2006; 183: 1–7.

45. Hoch W, McConville J, Helms S, et al. Auto-antibodies to the receptor tyrosine kinase MuSK in patients with myasthenia gravis without acetylcholine receptor antibodies. Nat Med 2001; 7: 365–368.

46. Rivner MH, Swift TR. Thymoma: diagnosis and management. Semin Neurol 1990; 10: 83–88.

47. Ashraf VV, Taly AB, Veerendrakumar M, Rao S. Myasthenia gravis in children: a longitudinal study. Acta Neurol Scand 2006: 114: 119–123.

48. Parr JR, Jayawant S. Childhood myasthenia: clinical subtypes and practical management. Dev Med Child Neurol 2007, 49: 629–635.

49. Osserman KE, Genkins G. Studies in myasthenia gravis: review of twenty year experience in over 1200 patients. Mt Sinai J Med 1971; 38: 497.

50. Evoli A, Batocchi AP, Bartoccioni E, et al. Juvenile myasthenia gravis with prepubertal onset. Neuromuscul Disord 1998; 8: 561–567.

51. Lindner A, Schalke B, Toyka KV. Outcome in juvenile-onset myasthenia gravis: a retrospective study with long-term follow-up of 79 patients. J Neurol 1997; 244: 515–520.

52. Mullaney P, Vajsar J, Smith R, Buncic JR. The natural history and ophthalmic involvement in childhood myasthenia gravis at the hospital for sick children. Ophthalmology 2000; 107: 504–510.

53. Rodriguez M, Gomez MR, Howard FM Jr, Taylor WF. Myasthenia gravis in children: long-term follow-up. Ann Neurol 1983; 13: 504–510.

54. Snead OC 3rd, Benton JW, Dwyer D, Juvenile myasthenia gravis. Neurology. 1980; 30: 732–739.

55. Seybold ME. The office Tensilon test for ocular myasthenia gravis. Arch Neurol 1986; 43: 842–843.

56. Phillips LH, Melnick PA.. Diagnosis of myasthenia gravis in the 1990's. Semin Neurol 1990; 10: 62–69.

57. Massey JM. Electromyography in disorders of neuromuscular transmission Semin Neurol 1990; 10: 6–11.

58. Gronseth GS, Barohn RJ. Practice parameter. Thymectomy for autoimmune myasthenia gravis (an evidence-based review) – Report of the Quality Standards Subcommittee of the American Academy of Neurology. Neurology 2000; 55: 7–15.

59. Jaretzki A, Wolff M. "Maximal" thymectomy for myasthenia gravis. Surgical anatomy and operative technique. J Thorac Cardiovasc Surg 1988; 96: 711–716.

60. Task Force of the Medical Scientific Advisory Board of the Myasthenia Gravis Foundation of America. Myasthenia gravis. Recommendations for clinical research standards. Neurology 2000; 55: 16–23.

61. Jaretzki A, Steinglass KM, Sonett JR. Thymectomy in the management of myasthenia gravis. Semin Neurol 2004; 24: 49–62.

62. Calhoun RF, Ritter JH, Guthrie TJ, Pestronk A, Meyers BF, Patterson GA, Pohl MS, Cooper JD. Results of transcervical thymectomy for myasthenia gravis in 100 consecutive patients. Ann Surg 1999; 230: 555–559.

63. Shrager JB, Nathan D, Brinster CJ, et al. Outcomes after 151 extended transcervical thymectomies for myasthenia gravis. Ann Thorac Surg 2006; 82: 1863–1869.

64. Henze A, Biberfeld P, Christensson B, et al. Failing transcervical thymectomy in myasthenia gravis. An evaluation of transsternal re-exploration. Scand J Thorac Cardiovasc Surg 1984; 18: 235–238.

65. Mack MJ, Landreneau RJ, Yim AP, et al. Results of video-assisted thymectomy in patients with myasthenia gravis. J Thorac Cardiovasc Surg 1996; 112: 1352–1359.

66. Tomulescu V, Ion V, Kosa A, Sgarbura O, Popescu I. Thoracoscopic thymectomy mid-term results. Ann Thorac Surg 2006; 82: 1003–1007.

67. Wright GM, Barnett S, Clarke CP. Video-assisted thoracoscopic thymectomy for myasthenia gravis. Intern Med J 2002; 32: 367–371.

68. Augustin F, Schmid T, Sieb M, Lucciarini P, Bodner J. Video-assisted thoracoscopic surgery versus robotic-assisted thoracoscopic surgery thymectomy. Ann Thorac Surg 2008; 85: S768–S771.

69. Rea F, Marulli G, Bortolotti L, et al. Experience with the "da Vinci" robotic system for thymectomy in patients with myasthenia gravis: report of 33 cases. Ann Thorac Surg 2006; 81: 455–459.

70. Mineo TC, Pompeo E, Ambrogi V. Video-assisted thoracoscopic thymectomy: from the right or from the left? J Thorac Cardiovasc Surg 1997; 114: 516–517.

71. Mineo TC, Pompeo E, Ambrogi V, et al. Adjuvant pneumomediastinum in thoracoscopic thymectomy for myasthenia gravis. Ann Thorac Surg 1996; 62: 1210–1212.

72. Rodriguez M, Gomez MR, Howard FM Jr, Taylor WF. Myasthenia gravis in children: long-term follow-up. Ann Neurol 1983; 13: 504–510.

73. Youssef S. Thymectomy for myasthenia gravis in children. J Pediatr Surg 1983; 18: 537–541.

74. Skelly CL, Jackson CC, Wu Y, et al.Thoracoscopic thymectomy in children with myasthenia gravis. Am Surg 2003; 69: 1087–1089.

75. Essa M, El-Medany Y, Hajjar W, et al. Maximal thymectomy in children with myasthenia gravis. Eur J Cardiothorac Surg 2003; 24: 187–189.

76. Kogut KA, Bufo AJ, Rothenberg SS, Lobe TE. Thoracoscopic thymectomy for myasthenia gravis in children. J Pediatr Surg 2000; 35: 1576–1577.

77. Lakhoo K, Fonseca JD, Rodda J, Davies MR. Thymectomy in black children with juvenile myasthenia gravis. Pediatr Surg Int 1997; 12: 113–115.

78. Adams C, Theodorescu D, Murphy EG, Shandling B. Thymectomy in juvenile myasthenia gravis. J Child Neurol. 1990; 5: 215–218.

79. Ryniewicz B, Badurska B. Follow-up study of myasthenic children after thymectomy. J Neurol 1977; 217: 133–138.

80. Jaretzki A. Video-assisted thoracoscopic extended thymectomy and extended transsternal thymectomy in non-thymomatous myasthenia gravis patients. J Neurol Sci 2004; 217: 233–234; author reply 235–236.

81. First WH, Thirumalai S, Doehring CB, et al. Thymectomy for the myasthenia gravis patient: factors influencing outcome. Ann Thorac Surg 1994; 57: 334–338.

82. Jaretzki A, Penn AS, Younger DS, et al. "Maximal" thymectomy for myasthenia gravis. Results. J Thorac Cardiovasc Surg 1988; 95: 747–757.

83. Mantegazza R, Baggi F, Bernasconi P, et al. Video-assisted thoracoscopic extended thymectomy (VATET) and extended transsternal thymectomy (T-3b) in non-thymomatous myasthenia gravis patients: remission after 6 years of follow-up. J Neurol Sci 2003; 212: 31–36.

84. Papatestas AE, Genkins G, Kornfield P, et al. Effects of thymectomy in myasthenia gravis. Ann Surg 1987; 206: 79–88.

85. Jaretzki A, Sonett JR. Evaluation of results of thymectomy for MG requires accepted standards. Ann Thorac Surg 2007; 84: 360–1; author reply 361.

86. Damadoglu E, Salturk C, Takir HB, et al. Mediastinal thymolipoma: an analysis of 10 cases. Respirology 2007; 12: 924–927.

87. Kitano Y, Yokomori K, Ohkura M, et al. Giant thymolipoma in a child. J Pediatr Surg 1993; 28: 1622–1625.

88. Brown LR, Reiman HM, Rosenow EC, et al. Intrathoracic lymphangioma. Mayo Clin Proc 1986; 61: 882–892.

89. Strollo DC, Rosado de Christenson ML, Jett JR. Primary mediastinal tumors. Part 1: tumors of the anterior mediastinum. Chest 1997; 112: 511–522.

90. Indeglia RA, Shea MA, Grage TB. Congenital cysts of the thymus gland. Arch Surg 1967; 94:149–152.

91. Suster S, Rosai J. Multilocular thymic cyst: an acquired reactive process. Am J Surg Pathol 1991; 15:388–389.

48
Hyperhidrosis and Thoracic Sympathectomy

David C.G. Crabbe and Dakshesh H. Parikh

Introduction

Generalized sweating is a normal physiological response to reduce body temperature. Humans are the smallest mammals that sweat. Smaller mammals, such as dogs, lose heat by panting. Limited sweating of the palms and soles controls the humidity of the stratum corneum of the skin and improves grip.

Hyperhidrosis or excessive sweating of the hands, axillae, and soles of the feet can be a debilitating condition. Children suffering from palmar hyperhidrosis find writing difficult as the page becomes wet and their academic work may suffer. They may find holding a pen or pencil difficult. Sports that involve a strong grip may be impossible as may also playing musical instruments. The child may become withdrawn and find difficulty mixing socially with peers. Occasionally hyperhidrosis affects the whole body but the debilitating areas for which they seek treatment are usually the palms and axillae.

Hyperhidrosis affects 1–3% of the population.[1,2] The condition is more common in hot humid climates, and in certain racial groups especially middle eastern Jews, Japanese, and Taiwanese. Most cases are idiopathic. Secondary hyperhidrosis is exceedingly rare in childhood but lymphoma, hyperthyroidism, phaeochromocytoma, and anxiety disorders should be considered in the differential diagnosis.

Historic Perspective

Galen described the sympathetic trunk but incorrectly he considered the vagus nerve to be part of the sympathetic chain. Claude Bernard recognized the physiological significance of the sympathetic chain in 1852. The first sympathectomy was performed by Alexander 1889. Naively sympathectomy was recommended for various conditions including epilepsy, exophthalmic goiter, idiocy, and glaucoma. Subsequently sympathectomy was offered as a treatment for angina pectoris,

Raynaud's disease, and Sudeck's atrophy, conditions for which the procedure still has limited application.[3]

The first use of the sympathectomy for vascular disorders was reported by Leriche and Fontaine in 1932.[3] Most surgeons including Jaboulay, who was first to recognize that sympathectomy might improve the circulation, used an anterior approach.[4] Adson and Brown described a posterior approach to the sympathetic chain, which involved resecting the second rib.[5] Variations in this approach involving paravertebral, posterolateral incisions, and resection of the third and fourth ribs have been described. More recently the transaxillary approach has become popular, particularly since thoracoscopic sympathectomy has become routine. Kux reported the first large series of patients undergoing thoracoscopic sympathectomy in 1978.[6]

The main indication for sympathectomy today is hyperhidrosis. The technique of sympathectomy has been modified over recent decades with a trend to minimize the extent of surgery from open to endoscopic approaches, from resection of ganglia to thermoablation, transection, and clipping. Despite this compensatory hyperhidrosis remains a significant problem for a number of patients.

Basic Science

The surface of the body is covered with sweat glands of two types.[7,8] Eccrine sweat glands secrete a clear odorless fluid that serves to aid thermoregulation by evaporation. Eccrine glands are widespread but present in higher density on the soles of the feet, forehead, and palms. Apocrine sweat glands are restricted to the axillae and groin. Apocrine glands produce a thick fluid that undergoes bacterial decomposition to produce a strong odor.

The thermoregulatory center in the hypothalamus controls body temperature by regulating blood flow to the skin and eccrine sweat production. The thermoregulatory center

D.H. Parikh et al. (eds.), *Pediatric Thoracic Surgery*,
DOI: 10.1007/b136543_48, © Springer-Verlag London Limited 2009

Systemic medication can be used for the treatment of generalized or focal hyperhidrosis but side effects are common and limit widespread use.[16] Anticholinergics block the sympathetic stimulation of eccrine glands. Anticholinergics used for hyperhidrosis include propantheline, glycopyrronium bromide, oxybutynin, and benztropine.

Botulinum toxin blocks the release of acetylecholine from cholinergic nerves supplying the sweat glands. Multiple intradermal injections are required and repeated injection is really only feasible in the axilla. A large double blind randomized control trial involving 230 patients between botulinum and placebo reported by Naumann showed that after four week significantly improved response and patient satisfaction (94% with botulinum toxin vs. 36% with placebo).[17] Compensatory sweating does not seem to occur with this treatment.

Ionotophorosis

Ionotophorosis involves the use of an electrical current to draw ionized molecules through intact skin.[18] In the 1940s, Takata and Shelley discovered independently that iontophoresis with tap water could stop sweating.[19,20] How iontophoresis reduces sweating is not well-understood, although it probably involves occlusion of the sweat ducts by reversibly altering the outer layer of the skin. Commercially available iontophoreisis equipment for home use is relatively expensive, and although there is plenty of anecdotal evidence for the effectiveness of this treatment, controlled trials are lacking.

During an iontophoresis session, the patient sits with hands or feet, or both, immersed in shallow trays of water for 20–40 min. Electrodes are placed in each tray and the electrical circuit is completed through the patient. The current is increased to around 10–20 mA. The anode has a better inhibitory effect on sweating than cathode, so electrode polarity is reversed half way through the treatment. Intensive treatment is necessary until sweating ceases followed by weekly maintenance treatment. If iontophoresis with tap water is not effective glyocpyrrolate can be added to the water. Side effects seen during tap water iontophoresis are usually mild. Most patients notice a mild tingling from the electricity, although cuts and abrasions can be very painful during iontophoreisis.

Surgical Management

Surgical options for the treatment of hyperhidrosis include sympathectomy, which is applicable to palmar and axillary hyperhidrosis, and local excision, which is applicable only to the axillary sweat glands.

Excision or curetting the sweat glands from the undersurface of the axillary skin is an effective and permanent treatment for hyperhidrosis.[21–23] The area to be treated must be mapped by drying the skin then applying iodine and starch. Sweat results in a blue discoloration as the iodine and starch react. Complications rates can be high, particularly infection and wound dehiscence.

Thoracic Sympathectomy

Sympathectomy has been used to treat axillary and palmar hyperhidrosis for several decades. The earliest operations involved removal of the stellate ganglion but this was soon abandoned because of the accompanying Horner's syndrome.

The sympathetic chain can be approached through posterior, supraclavicular, and transaxillary incisions.[24–28] Although endoscopic sympathectomy was first described in detail by Kux in 1951, the technique remained obscure.[29] With improvements in endoscopic imaging and lighting over the last decade, the thoracoscopic approach has become the procedure of choice for upper limb sympathectomy. The only contraindication to thoracoscopic sympathectomy is impenetrable adhesions around the apex of the lung, and this would also make sympathectomy through an open incision very difficult.

The extent and technique for interruption of the sympathetic nerve supply to the upper limb remains a subject for debate. In part this is because of concern about the incidence of compensatory sweating in other parts of the body following sympathectomy. However, it is also recognized that complete sympathetic denervation of the palm may be undesirable because the hand becomes so dry that grip becomes affected. Terminology is confusing and in many publications it is difficult to determine exactly how the sympathetic innervation to the arm has been interrupted (Table 48.3). The original description by Kux suggested a number of options: "… by means of a thoracoscope, a long needle is then introduced, through which the sympathetic chain can be injected or divided by cautery by direct vision at any given point above the diaphragm. With a suitable instrument, the sympathetic chain, including the nerves from below the diaphragm, can then be avulsed."[29]

The majority of the sympathetic innervation of the upper limb arises from T2 and T3 levels. Consequently division of the sympathetic chain above and below the T2 ganglion (Fig. 48.2) is probably the technique used most widely for palmar hyperhidrosis. Most authors also ensure accessory rami from T2 joining the T1 root are divided – the nerve of Kuntz. This will result in complete cessation of palmar sweating in almost 100% patients. Division of the sympathetic chain above and below the T3 ganglion seems to be equally effective and may reduce the incidence of compensatory hyperhidrosis. Neumayer et al. reported satisfactory results clamping the sympathetic chain above and below the T4 ganglion with 65% palms being completely dry and substantial reduction in sweating in 36%.[45] Division of the sympathetic chain above and below the T5 ganglion is not effective for palmar hyperhidrosis.[46]

Several different techniques can be used to interrupt the sympathetic chain. Division of the chain and excision of one or more ganglia (Fig. 48.3) guarantees a sympathectomy and allows histological confirmation, although, of course, this does not confirm the level of the sympathectomy.[47] Wittmoser described selective division of rami communicates with a thoracoscope without interruption of the sympathetic chain (Fig. 48.4).[48] This technique is relatively complicated and may

TABLE 48.3. Data from published series of sympathectomy for hyperhidrosis.

Authors	No of patients	No of operations	Operative details	Outcome	Recurrence	Compensatory sweating (%)	Over dry hands (%)	Horner's syndrome (%)	Open conversion (%)	Chest drain (%)
Kopelman[30]	53		T2 and T3 ganglia removed. Accessory rami divided	100% success		67		17	0	0
Montessi[31]	521	162	T2 ablation	94% v good, 3% good		67		0.4		1.8
		65	T3 ablation	89% v good, 6% good		67				
		294	T4 ablation	80% v good, 12% good		62				
Jeganathan[32]	163		Sympathetic chain divided between T2 and T3	98.5% success, 1.5% failed	5%	77		0	1	4
			Sympathetic chain divided T2–4 ± T5	98% success, 2% failed	9%					
Moya[33]	458	918	Palmar: sympathicolysis T2–3 ganglia	97% no sweating, 2.4% reduced sweating, 0.2% failed		86	0.4	0.3	1	0.5
			Axillary: sympathicolysis T2–4 ganglia							
Kwong[34]	202	397	Palmar: sympathetic chain divided T2 + T3 levels	92% improved quality of life		40		0.5	0	0.5
			Axillary: sympathetic chain divided T3 + T4 levels							
Gossot[35]	398		Sympathetic chain divided and removed T2–T4 (T5 if axilla involved)	100% success		51	33	0.4	0.3	100
	69		Wittmoser – rami communicantes divided T2–T4 (T5 if axilla involved)	11 sides relapsed, remainder successful	8%			0		
Herbst[36]	270	480	Interganglionic fibres and postganglionic rami divided D1/2 to D4. Accessory rami divided	98.1% success, 19.% failed	1.5%	67.4		2.5	0	2.5
Chou[37]	25		Sympathetic chain divided above and below T4 ganglion	0% regretted surgery	0%	0		0	0	0
	324		Sympathetic chain clipped above and below T4 ganglion. Accessory rami divided.	0% regretted surgery	0%	0		0	0	0
Lin[38]	326		Sympathetic chain clipped above and below T2 ganglion, accessory rami divided	Satisfactory except for 3 patients						
Lin[39]	1520 palmar		Sympathetic chain divided above and below T2. Accessory rami divided		1.3% after 5 years	86		0		0.5
	480 axillary		Sympathetic chain divided above and below T3 and T4 ganglia. Accessory rami divided	16.7% after 5 years						
Dewey[40]	222		Palmar: excision of T3 ganglion. Axillary: excision T3 and T4 ganglia. Accessory rami divided	Would you undergo repeat surgery ? 6% palmar no, 15% axillary no		85		0.5	0.5	0
Rex[41]	785 palmar		Sympathetic chain divided above and below T2	99% effective reoperation 4.3%		60		0.4	0	1.3
	93 axillary		Sympathetic chain divided above and below T4 ganglion.	94% effective reoperation 2.2%						
Cohen[42]	223	402	Sympathetic chain divided at T2 and T3 (+ T4 if axilla involved)	98% satisfied			0.5		0	
Duarte[43]	31 palmar		Sympathetic chain divided T2–5. Accessory rami divided	100% cured		3		0	0	0
	50 axillary			98% cured		4		2	0	2
Chang[44]	234	86	Sympathetic chain divided above and below T2 ganglion	All operations effective	26%	92	36	0		4
		78	Sympathetic chain divided above and below T3 ganglion		8%	92	40	0		
		70	Sympathetic chain divided above and below T4 ganglion		23%	80	9	0		
Neumayer[45]	91	176	Sympathetic chain divided over 2nd, 3rd, 4th ribs. Accessory rami divided	88% no sweating, 10% reduced sweating		56		1	0	1
	53	106	Sympathetic chain clipped above and below T4	65% no sweating, 36% reducued sweating		9		0	0	1

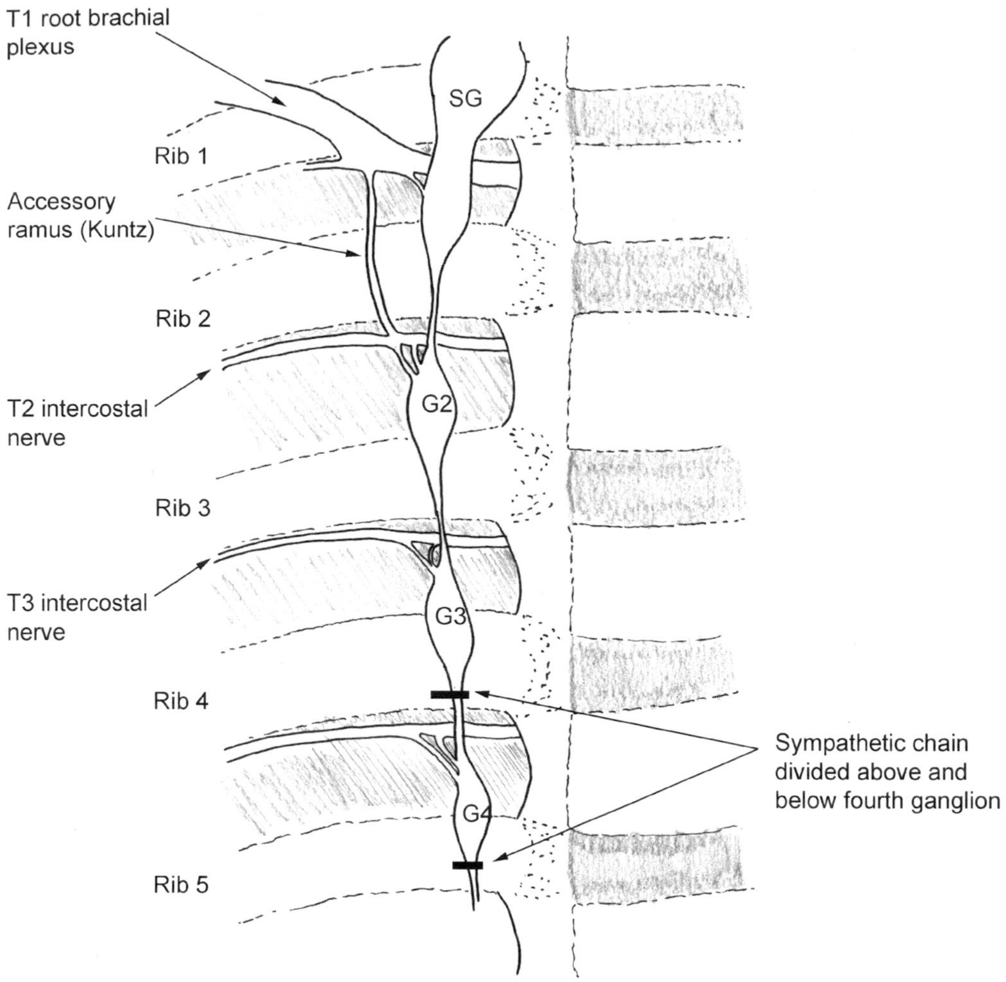

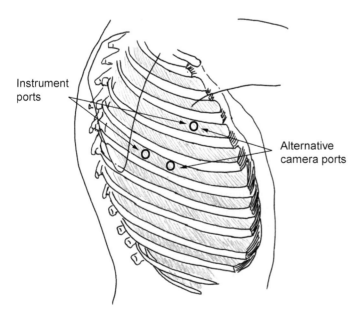

FIG. 48.5. T4 sympathectomy by cautery or clipping without ganglion excision

Labels (Fig. 48.5): T1 root brachial plexus; SG; Rib 1; Accessory ramus (Kuntz); Rib 2; T2 intercostal nerve; G2; Rib 3; T3 intercostal nerve; G3; Rib 4; G4; Rib 5; Sympathetic chain divided above and below fourth ganglion

Labels (Fig. 48.6): Instrument ports; Alternative camera ports

FIG. 48.6. Port placement for thoracoscopic sympathectomy

interrupted at the chosen level(s) using one of the techniques described previously.[50] If a segment of the sympathetic chain is to be resected, the chain is divided at the upper and lower levels and collateral branches transected as the dissection proceeds from each end.

Accessory communicating rami can be divided reliably by dissection and coagulation along the second rib 3–4 cm lateral to the sympathetic chain. Frequently, there is a small vein overlying the sympathetic chain between the second and third ganglia. This should be coagulated and divided if the sympathetic chain is to be interrupted at this level to avoid troublesome bleeding. Care must be taken to avoid damage to the stellate ganglion because a Horner's syndrome will result.

Sympathectomy is accompanied by an almost immediate vasodilatation in the ipsilateral hand. Characteristic changes in pulse oximetry waveforms have been reported.[51] The lung is then inflated under direct vision, the trocar(s) removed and the wound(s) closed maintaining a high level of positive end expiratory airway pressure. This step eliminates the need for a chest drain. The procedure can then be repeated on the opposite side.

Postoperative Management

A chest X-ray should be performed in the recovery room after surgery to confirm complete lung expansion. Bilateral sympathectomy may be performed as a day case procedure provided postoperative discomfort is minor.

Results

Upper limb sympathectomy is a highly effective long-term treatment for palmar hyperhidrosis (Table 48.3). The results for isolated axillary hyperhidrosis are less good and also more variable. Gossot reported a high initial success rate but a 65% relapse rate leading him to the conclusion that local therapy should be the treatment of choice for axillary hyperhidrosis.[52] De Campos et al. found better results with 100% initial success and only a 2.5% recurrence rate.[53] The authors attributed these impressive results to resection of the T4 ganglion.

Side Effects of Sympathectomy

Sympathectomy was used as a treatment for angina pectoris in the past, and has been likened to long-term beta blockade. Sympathectomy results in a decrease in maximal heart rate of around 10%, although no functional consequences can be identified using objective methods.[54–56] Modest reduction in the rise of blood pressure in response to exercise have been noted. Some authors have noted minor reductions in resting heart rate, although others have failed to observe any change, which may be because resting heart rate is regulated by vagal rather than sympathetic tone. Sympathectomy produces slight bronchial constriction suggesting that in patients with essential hyperhidrosis bronchial motor tone is influenced by the sympathetic nervous system. Again, this is not associated with any measurable reduction in exercise tolerance. Noppen looked specifically for alterations in lung function in children following sympathectomy and concluded that the changes were statistically insignificant and of no functional consequences.[57]

Compensatory sweating (CS) is the single most important side effect of sympathectomy. CS may occur on the back, chest, abdomen, legs, face, and buttocks as a side effect of sympathectomy. This side effect is grave because it can be equally or even more extreme than the original hyperhidrosis. The reported incidence of CS is highly variable with some authors suggesting zero[37] and others close to 100%.[58] Steiner et al. studied the time course of CS after sympathectomy in 265 patients.[59] CS developed immediately in 50% of affected patients, in 80% after 3 months, and in 90% after 3 more months. The severity of CS remained static in 70% during the first two postoperative years, and it increased in severity in 10% and decreased in severity in 20%.

The cause of CS is unclear and it is undoubtedly more complex than compensatory thermoregulation. Chou et al. outline an attractive hypothesis based on loss of negative feedback following sympathectomy and coin the term "reflex sweating" instead of "compensatory hyperhidrosis."[37] They suggest that changes in sweating patterns are not compensatory but a reflex response originating in the hypothalamus. Sympathetic afferent fibers convey negative feedback information from target organs (i.e., sweat glands) to the hypothalamus from where the efferent positive feedback signals originate (Fig. 48.7). They found the incidence of compensatory hyperhidrosis to be highest after T2 sympathectomy, less severe after T3 sympathectomy, and least after T4 sympathectomy. They postulated that T2 sympathectomy caused most interruption to the afferent sympathetic negative feedback to the hypothalamus (Fig. 48.8). Consequently an exaggerated efferent signal is released inducing severe compensatory sweating. The same mechanism can be applied to T3, T4 sympathectomy. In contrast to the T2 block, sympathectomy at T3 or T4 level preserves some negative feedback and, as a result, the efferent signals are less intensive than after T2 sympathectomy with less compensatory sweating (Fig. 48.9).

Several studies comparing the incidence of CS with sympathectomy at various levels support this theory (Table 48.3). However, other authors report no difference in the incidence of CS with sympathectomy at different levels.[60]

Gustatory sweating is facial sweating, which occurs when eating typically spicy or acidic foods. Gustatory sweating may occur as a complication of sympathectomy, although the physiological basis for this is unknown. The reported incidence varies considerably.[45,61] Licht et al. studied gustatory sweating after sympathectomy by questionnaire and discovered that it affected one third of patients.[61] Options for treatment include oral anticholinergics, topical aluminium chloride, and botulinum toxin injection.

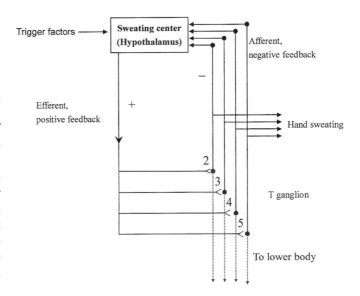

FIG. 48.7. Negative feedback regulation of normal sweating (with kind permission from Springer[37])

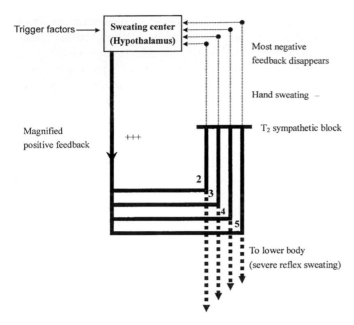

FIG. 48.8. Interuption of negative feedback following T2 sympathectomy (with kind permission from Springer[37])

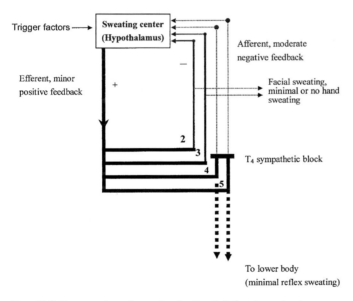

FIG. 48.9. Preservation of negative feedback following selective sympathectomy with kind permission from Springer[37])

Horner's syndrome (HS) is an uncommon complication of sympathectomy, although it is reported in almost all series. Horner's syndrome can be total or partial (without miosis), and it may be temporary or permanent. It is caused by damage to the T1 ganglion either by excessive traction on the sympathetic chain during dissection or by conduction of stray diathermy current. The reported incidence of postoperative Horner's syndrome ranges from 0% to 17%.[30,39] Most authors agree that the endoscopic approach reduces the rate of HS because of better visualization.

Other rare complications of endoscopic sympathectomy include bleeding, pneumothorax, chylothorax, and hypoxic cerebral injury.[62,63] Routine use of a chest drain following thoracoscopic sympathectomy is unnecessary, particularly if reexpansion of the lung is monitored thoracoscopically as the pneumothorax is released. Open conversion rates following endoscopic sympathectomy are less than 1% in experienced hands.

Conclusions and Future Perspective

Endoscopic sympathectomy is a safe and effective treatment for severe palmar hyperhidrosis. There is a significant incidence of compensatory sweating after sympathectomy and this is sufficiently troublesome in some patients for them to regret surgery. The best level for sympathectomy and the technique used to interrupt the sympathetic chain remain the subject of debate. There is growing evidence that limited sympathectomy (T3 or T4 level) is effective for palmar hyperhidrosis with a lower incidence of compensatory sweating than conventional T2 sympathectomy. The results of sympathectomy for isolated axillary hyperhidrosis are frequently unsatisfactory.

Predictably there is comparatively little published specifically on the management of hyperhidrosis in children.[64–68] These series are small in comparison to the large adult series but it is clear that the results and complications are directly comparable.

References

1. Collin J. Treating hyperhidrosis: Surgery and botulinum toxin are treatment for severe cases. Brit Med J 2000; 320:1221–1222.
2. Strutton DR, Kowalski JW, Glaser DA, et al. US prevalence of hyperhidrosis and impact on individuals with axillary hyperhidrosis: results from a national survey. J Am Acad Dermatol 2004; 51: 241–248.
3. Hashmonai M, Kopelman D. History of sympathetic surgery. Clin Auton Res 2003; 13 (Suppl 1): I6–9.
4. Jaboulay M. Le traitment de quelques troubles trophiques de le pied et de la jambe par la denudation de l'artere et la distension des nerfs vasculaires. J Med Lyon 1899; 91:467.
5. Adson AW, Brown GE. The treatment of Raynaud's disease by resection of the upper thoracic and lumber sympathetic ganglia and trunks. Surg Gynecol Obstet 1929; 48:577.
6. Kux M Throacoscopic endoscopic sympathectomy in palmer and axillary hyperhidrosis Arch Surg 1978; 113:264
7. Sato K, Kang WH, Saga K, Sato KT. Biology of sweat glands and their disorders. I. Normal sweat gland function. J Am Acad Dermatol 1989; 20:537–563.
8. Hölzle E. Pathophysiology of sweating. Curr Probl Dermatol 2002; 30:10–22.
9. Kuntz A. Distribution of the sympathetic rami to the brachial plexus: its relationto sympathectomy affecting the upper extremity. Arch. Surg 1927; I5:871–877.
10. Cho HM, Lee DY, Sung SW. Anatomical variations of rami communicantes in the upper thoracic sympathetic trunk. Eur J Cardiothorac Surg 2005; 27:320–324.

11. Sato K, Kang WH, Saga K, Sato KT. Biology of sweat glands and their disorders. II. Disorders of sweat gland function. J Am Acad Dermatol 1989; 20:713–726.

12. Heckmann M. Hyperhidrosis of the axilla. Curr Probl Dermatol 2002; 30:149–155.

13. Ro KM, Cantor RM, Lange KL, Ahn SS. Palmar hyperhidrosis: evidence of genetic transmission. J Vasc Surg 2002; 35:382–386.

14. Hund M, Kinkelin I, Naumann M, Hamm H. Definition of axillary hyperhidrosis by gravimetric assessment. Arch Dermatol. 2002; 138:539–541.

15. http://www.sweathelp.org/English/HCP_Treatment_Topical.asp

16. Hölzle E. Topical pharmacological treatment. Curr Probl Dermatol. 2002; 30:30–43.

17. Naumann M, Lowe NJ. Botulinum toxin type A in treatment of bilateral primary axillary hyperhidrosis: randomised, parallel group, double blind, placebo controlled trial. Brit Med J 2001; 323:596–599.

18. Anliker MD, Kreyden OP. Tap water iontophoresis. Curr Probl Dermatol 2002; 30:48–56.

19. Shelley WB, Horvath PN, Weidman FD, Pillsbury DM. Experimental miliaria in man. I. Production of sweat retention anhidrosis and vesicles by means of Iontophoresis. J Invest Dermatol 1948; 11:275.

20. Shrivastava SN, Singh G. Tap water iontophoresis in palmoplantar hyperhidrosis. Brit J Dermatol 1977; 96:189–195.

21. Hafner J, Beer GM. Axillary sweat gland excision. Curr Probl Dermatol 2002; 30:57–63.

22. Swinehart JM. Treatment of axillary hyperhidrosis: combination of the starch-iodine test with the tumescent liposuction technique. Dermatol Surg 2000; 26:392–396.

23. Naumann M, Hamm H.Treatment of axillary hyperhidrosis. Br J Surg 2002; 89:259–261.

24. Atkins HJB. Sympathectomy by the axillary approach. Lancet 1954; I:538

25. Nanson EM. The anterior approach to upper dorsal sympathectomy. Surg Gynecol Obstet 1957; 104:118–120.

26. Palumbo LT. Upper dorsal sympathectomy without Horner's syndrome. AMA Arch Surg 1955; 71:743–751.

27. Mackay HJ. Improved approach for posterior upper thoracic sympathectomy. J Am Med Assoc 1955; 159:1261–1263.

28. Ray BS. Sympathectomy of the upper extremity; evaluation of surgical methods. J Neurosurg 1953; 10:624–633.

29. Kux E. The endoscopic approach to the vegetative nervous system and its therapeutic possibilities; especially in duodenal ulcer, angin-a pectoris, hypertension and diabetes. Dis Chest 1951; 20:139–147.

30. Kopelman D, Hashmonai M, Ehrenreich M, et al. Upper dorsal thoracoscopic sympathectomy for palmar hyperhidrosis: improved intermediate-term results. J Vasc Surg 1996; 24:194–199.

31. Montessi J, Almeida EP, Vieira JP, et al. Video-assisted thoracic sympathectomy in the treatment of primary hyperhidrosis: a retrospective study of 521 cases comparing different levels of ablation. J Bras Pneumol 2007; 33:248–254.

32. Jeganathan R, Jordan S, Jones M, et al. Bilateral thoracoscopic sympathectomy: results and long-term follow-up. Interact Cardiovasc Thorac Surg 2008; 7:67–70.

33. Moya J, Ramos R, Morera R, et al. Thoracic sympathicolysis for primary hyperhidrosis: a review of 918 procedures. Surg Endosc 2006; 20:598–602.

34. Kwong KF, Cooper LB, Bennett LA, et al. Clinical experience in 397 consecutive thoracoscopic sympathectomies. Ann Thorac Surg 2005; 80:1063–1066.

35. Gossot D, Toledo L, Fritsch S, Célérier M. Thoracoscopic sympathectomy for upper limb hyperhidrosis: looking for the right operation. Ann Thorac Surg 1997; 64:975–978.

36. Herbst F, Plas EG, Függer R, Fritsch A. Endoscopic thoracic sympathectomy for primary hyperhidrosis of the upper limbs. A critical analysis and long-term results of 480 operations. Ann Surg 1994; 220:86–90.

37. Chou SH, Kao EL, Lin CC, et al. The importance of classification in sympathetic surgery and a proposed mechanism for compensatory hyperhidrosis: experience with 464 cases. Surg Endosc 2006; 20:1749–1753.

38. Lin CC, Mo LR, Lee LS, Ng SM, Hwang MH. Thoracoscopic T2-sympathetic block by clipping – a better and reversible operation for treatment of hyperhidrosis palmaris: experience with 326 cases. Eur J Surg Suppl 1998; 580:13–6.

39. Lin TS, Kuo SJ, Chou MC. Uniportal endoscopic thoracic sympathectomy for treatment of palmar and axillary hyperhidrosis: analysis of 2000 cases. Neurosurgery 2002; 51(5 Suppl):S84–S87.

40. Dewey TM, Herbert MA, Hill SL, et al. One-year follow-up after thoracoscopic sympathectomy for hyperhidrosis: outcomes and consequences. Ann Thorac Surg 2006; 81:1227–1232.

41. Rex LO, Drott C, Claes G, et al. The Borås experience of endoscopic thoracic sympathicotomy for palmar, axillary, facial hyperhidrosis and facial blushing. Eur J Surg Suppl 1998; 580:23–26.

42. Cohen Z, Levi I, Pinsk I, Mares AJ. Thoracoscopic upper thoracic sympathectomy for primary palmar hyperhidrosis–the combined paediatric, adolescents and adult experience. Eur J Surg Suppl 1998; 580:5–8.

43. Duarte JB, Kux P. Improvements in video-endoscopic sympathicotomy for the treatment of palmar, axillary, facial, and palmarplantar hyperhidrosis. Eur J Surg Suppl 1998; 580:9–11.

44. Chang YT, Li HP, Lee JY, et al. Treatment of palmar hyperhidrosis: T(4) level compared with T(3) and T(2). Ann Surg 2007; 246:330–336.

45. Neumayer C, Zacherl J, Holak G, et al. Limited endoscopic thoracic sympathetic block for hyperhidrosis of the upper limb: reduction of compensatory sweating by clipping T4. Surg Endosc 2004; 18:152–156.

46. Reisfeld R. The importance of classification in sympathetic surgery and a proposed mechanism for compensatory hyperhidrosis: experience with 464 cases. Surg Endosc 2007; 21:1249–1250.

47. Ribas Milanez de Campos J, Kauffman P, Wolosker N, et al. Axillary hyperhidrosis: T3/T4 versus T4 thoracic sympathectomy in a series of 276 cases. J Laparoendosc Adv Surg Tech A 2006; 16:598–603.

48. Wittmoser R. Thoracoscopic sympathectomy and vagotomy. In: Operative manual of endoscopic surgery. Cuschieri A, Buess G, Perissat J (Editors). Springer, New York. 1992.

49. Moya J, Ramos R, Morera R, et al. Results of high bilateral endoscopic thoracic sympathectomy and sympatholysis in the treatment of primary hyperhidrosis: a study of 1016 procedures. Arch Bronconeumol 2006; 42:230–234.

50. http://www.youtube.com/watch?v=Qf_Pvh6yJsM

51. Klodell CT, Lobato EB, Willert JL, Gravenstein N. Oximetry-derived perfusion index for intraoperative identification of

successful thoracic sympathectomy. Ann Thorac Surg 2005; 80:467–470.

52. Gossot D, Galetta D, Pascal A, et al. Long-term results of endoscopic thoracic sympathectomy for upper limb hyperhidrosis. Ann Thorac Surg 2003; 75:1075–1079.

53. de Campos JR, Kauffman P, Werebe Ede C, et al. Quality of life, before and after thoracic sympathectomy: report on 378 operated patients. Ann Thorac Surg 2003; 76:886–891.

54. Hashmonai M, Kopelman D. The pathophysiology of cervical and upper thoracic sympathetic surgery. Clin Auton Res 2003; 13 Suppl 1: 140–144.

55. Vigil L, Calaf N, Codina E, et al. Video-assisted sympathectomy for essential hyperhidrosis: effects on cardiopulmonary function. Chest 2005; 128:2702–2705.

56. Noppen M, Vincken W. Thoracoscopic sympathicolysis for essential hyperhidrosis: effects on pulmonary function. Eur Respir J 1996; 9:1660–1664.

57. Noppen M, Dab I, D'Haese J, et al. Thoracoscopic T2-T3 sympathicolysis for essential hyperhidrosis in childhood: effects on pulmonary function. Pediatr Pulmonol 1998; 26:262–264.

58. Chiou TS, Chen SC. Intermediate-term results of endoscopic transaxillary T2 sympathectomy for primary palmar hyperhidrosis. Br J Surg 1999; 86:45–47.

59. Steiner Z, Kleiner O, Hershkovitz Y, et al. Compensatory sweating after thoracoscopic sympathectomy: an acceptable trade-off. J Pediatr Surg 2007; 42:1238–1242.

60. Lesèche G, Castier Y, Thabut G, et al. Endoscopic transthoracic sympathectomy for upper limb hyperhidrosis: limited sympathectomy does not reduce postoperative compensatory sweating. J Vasc Surg 2003; 37:124–128.

61. Licht PB, Pilegaard HK. Gustatory side effects after thoracoscopic sympathectomy. Ann Thorac Surg 2006; 81:1043–1047.

62. Ojimba TA, Cameron AE. Drawbacks of endoscopic thoracic sympathectomy. Br J Surg 2004; 91:264–269.

63. Gossot D, Kabiri H, Caliandro R, et al. Early complications of thoracic endoscopic sympathectomy: a prospective study of 940 procedures. Ann Thorac Surg 2001; 71:1116–1119.

64. Imhof M, Zacherl J, Plas EG, et al. Long-term results of 45 thoracoscopic sympathicotomies for primary hyperhidrosis in children. J Pediatr Surg 1999; 34:1839–1842.

65. Hehir DJ, Brady MP. Long-term results of limited thoracic sympathectomy for palmar hyperhidrosis. J Pediatr Surg 1993; 28:909–911.

66. Kao MC, Lee WY, Yip KM, et al. Palmar hyperhidrosis in children: treatment with video endoscopic laser sympathectomy. J Pediatr Surg 1994; 29:387–391.

67. Lin TS, Huang LC, Wang NP, Chang CC. Endoscopic thoracic sympathetic block by clipping for palmar and axillary hyperhidrosis in children and adolescents. Pediatr Surg Int 2001; 17:535–537.

68. Steiner Z, Cohen Z, Kleiner O, et al. Do children tolerate thoracoscopic sympathectomy better than adults? Pediatr Surg Int 2008; 24:343–347.

Index

Rhabdomyosarcoma, 269–270
Rigid bronchoscopy, 65–66, 368
Rigid endoscopy technique, 359

S
Saccular bronchiectasis, 171
Sandifer syndrome, 344
Schatzki's rings, 314
Scimitar syndrome, 53, 404
Scintigraphic ventilation, 36
Scoliosis, 272–273
Seldinger technique, 117
Serology, 100
Serratus anterior muscle, 6
Serratus anterior myoplastic flap technique, 122
Sibson's fascia, 6
Single-lung ventilation (SLV)
   management
      double-lumen endobronchial tube (DLT), 62–63
      univent bronchial-blocker tube, 63–64
   physiology, 59–60
Sinusitis, 439
Sniff nasal inspiratory pressure (SNIP), 34, 35
Sonic hedgehog gene, 283–284
Spontaneous pneumothorax (SP). *See* Pneumothorax
Sternal tumor
   clinical features, 273–274
   diagnosis and management, 274
   enchondroma and osteoblastoma, 273
Sternum, 3
Stomach
   gastric pull-up, 322–323
   gastric tubes, 322
Stortz ventilating bronchoscopes, 369
Streptococcus pneumoniae, 95, 112
Strictures, 330
Subglottic stenosis, 67
Superior vena cava (SVC), 181
   azygos vein, 14
   phrenic nerve, 9
   right pulmonary hilum, 10
   superior mediastinum, 8
Supreme intercostal artery, 5
Surfactant, 412
Surfactant protein disorders, 461
Surgical management, bronchiectasis, 176–177
Sweat test, 428–429
Syndrome of inappropriate antidiuretic hormone (SIADH)
   fluid management, 102
   hyponatremia, 103
Systemic lupus erythematosus (SLE), 447

T
Tensilon®, 584
Thoracic anesthesia
   anterior mediastinal mass, 68–69
   bronchoscopy, 61
   chest roentgenogram, 60
   computed tomography (CT), 60–61

echocardiography and angiography, 61
history, 57–58
infection, 67–68
magnetic resonance imaging (MRI), 61
management
   monitoring, 62
   postoperative analgesia, 64–65
neonates
   anatomical and physiological consideration, 58–59
   infants, 66–67
Nuss procedure, 71
procedures, 65–66
pulmonary function tests (PFTs), 61–62
single-lung ventilation (SLV)
   management, 62–64
   physiology, 59–60
sonography and bronchography, 61
thymectomy, 70
trauma, 69–70
Thoracic duct, 13–14
Thoracic incisions
   axillary thoracotomy, 84
   chest drain, 85–87
   consideration, 81–82
   history, 81, 82
   intraoperative complication, 91–92
   limited thoracotomy, 83–84
   lobectomy, 88–91
   median sternotomy, 84–85
   pneumonectomy, 91
   posterolateral thoracotomy, 82–83
   postoperative complication, 92
   pulmonary resection, 87–88
   segmental resection, 91
   thoracoabdominal incision, 85
Thoracic outlet compression syndrome (TOCS).
      See Thoracic outlet syndrome
Thoracic outlet syndrome
   anatomical considerations, 547–548
   arterial TOCS, 549
   causation and pathological anatomy, 548
   conservative management, 552
   neurogenic TOCS, 548–549
   outcomes, 554
   surgical techniques for
      supraclavicular approach, 552–553
      transaxillary approach, 553–554
   venous TOCS
      deep venous thrombosis (DVT), 549
      effort thrombosis, 550
      venography, 551–552
Thoracic skeleton and soft tissues
   CT and ultrasound examination, 55
   dysphagia and respiratory distress, 53, 54
   generalized abnormality, 53
   mediastinal/intrathoracic extension, 54, 55
Thoracic trauma
   assosiated injuries, 196
   emergency department, 196–197